ATLAS OF

Procedures in Respiratory Medicine

A Companion to Murray and Nadel's Textbook of Respiratory Medicine

•

Warren M. Gold, M.D.
Professor of Medicine
University of California, San Francisco
Attending Physician
Moffitt-Long Hospitals
Associate Staff and Director
Adult Pulmonary Laboratories, Clinical Physiological Services
Cardiovascular Research Institute
University of California, San Francisco
San Francisco, California

John F. Murray, M.D., D.Sc. (HON), FRCP
Professor Emeritus of Medicine
University of California, San Francisco
Senior Staff, Pulmonary and Critical Care Division
San Francisco General Hospital
Senior Staff, Cardiovascular Research Institute
San Francisco, California

Jay A. Nadel, M.D., D.Sc. (HON)
Professor of Medicine
Physiology and Radiology
University of California, San Francisco
Senior Staff, Cardiovascular Research Institute
San Francisco, California

W.B. SAUNDERS COMPANY
A Harcourt Health Sciences Company
Philadelphia London New York St. Louis Sydney Toronto

W.B. SAUNDERS COMPANY
A Harcourt Health Sciences Company

The Curtis Center
Independence Square West
Philadelphia, Pennsylvania 19106

Library of Congress Cataloging-in-Publication Data

Atlas of procedures in respiratory medicine: companion to accompany Textbook of respiratory medicine / [edited by] Warren M. Gold, John F. Murray, Jay A. Nadel.—1st ed.
p. ; cm.
ISBN 0–7216–4086–9
1. Respiratory therapy–Atlases. 2. Respiratory organs–Diseases–Atlases. I. Gold, Warren M. II. Murray, John F. (John Frederic), III. Nadel, Jay A., IV. Textbook of respiratory medicine.
[DNLM: 1. Respiratory Tract Diseases–Atlases. WF 17 A8809 2002]
RC735.I5 A874 2002
616.2'0046--dc21 2001049543

Editor-in-Chief: Richard Zorab
Acquisitions Editor: Catherine Carroll
Project Manager: Tina Rebane
Production Manager: Guy Barber
Illustration Specialist: Peg Shaw
Book Designer: Lynn Foulk

ATLAS OF PROCEDURES IN RESPIRATORY MEDICINE:
Companion to Murray and Nadel's Textbook of Respiratory Medicine ISBN 0–7216–4086–9

Printed in the United States of America.

Last digit is the print number: 9 8 7 6 5 4 3 2 1

To my father,

Herman Gold, M.D.

(1908–2001)

CONTRIBUTORS

Sergio Cavaliere, M.D.
Assistant Professor, University Medical School
Director, Center for Respiratory Endoscopy
and Laser Therapy
Spedali Civili, Brescia, Italy
BRONCHOSCOPY

Walter E. Finkbeiner, M.D., Ph.D.
Professor and Director, Anatomic Pathology
Department of Pathology
University of California, Davis, and
University of California Medical Center
Sacramento, California
MORPHOLOGICAL PROCEDURES IN RESPIRATORY ANATOMY AND PATHOLOGY; ANATOMY OF THE RESPIRATORY SYSTEM; RESPIRATORY PATHOLOGY

Warren M. Gold, M.D.
Professor of Medicine
University of California, San Francisco
Attending Physician
Moffitt-Long Hospitals
Associate Staff and Director
Adult Pulmonary Laboratories
Clinical Physiological Services
Cardiovascular Research Institute
University of California, San Francisco
San Francisco, California
PULMONARY FUNCTION TESTING

W. Keith Hadley, M.D., Ph.D.
Professor Emeritus of Clinical Laboratory Medicine
University of California, San Francisco
Formerly Chief, Microbiology Division
Clinical Laboratories
San Francisco General Hospital
San Francisco, California
MICROBIOLOGY

David L. Levin, M.D., Ph.D.
Assistant Professor of Radiology
University of California, San Diego, School of Medicine
La Jolla; and
University of California Medical Center
San Diego, California
RADIOGRAPHY AND IMAGING

Udaya B. S. Prakash, M.D.
Edward W. Scripps Professor of Medicine
Mayo Medical School and
Mayo Graduate School of Medicine
Consultant, Pulmonary, Critical Care
and Internal Medicine
Director of Bronchoscopy
Mayo Clinic and Mayo Medical Center
Rochester, Minnesota
BRONCHOSCOPY

David C. Price, M.D.
Professor of Radiology and Medicine and
Section Chief, Pulmonary Nuclear Medicine
University of California, San Francisco
San Francisco, California
NUCLEAR MEDICINE TECHNIQUES AND APPLICATIONS

W. Richard Webb, M.D.
Professor of Radiology and
Chief, Thoracic Imaging
University of California, San Francisco
San Francisco, California
RADIOGRAPHY AND IMAGING

Jennifer M. Wu, M.D.
Clinical Fellow in Obstetrics, Gynecology
and Reproductive Biology
Brigham and Women's Hospital
Boston, Massachusetts
ANATOMY OF THE RESPIRATORY SYSTEM

FOREWORD

About three decades ago, the specialty of respiratory medicine began to blossom, with support from the National Institutes of Health and the entrance of talented young investigators into the field. New diagnostic tools were developed, including tests of pulmonary function, fiberoptic bronchoscopy, and refined radiographic and nuclear technologies. Improved diagnostic tools such as measurement of blood gases and equipment for efficient assisted ventilation led to the development of critical care facilities. Sophisticated methods for visualizing pathologic conditions also evolved. Textbooks have attempted to incorporate this vast new array of information concerning the diagnosis and treatment of respiratory diseases, with varying success.

The *Textbook of Respiratory Medicine* aimed to integrate the rapidly expanding knowledge of respiratory disease in an authoritative and carefully documented manner.

This atlas takes a different approach: It emphasizes the extensive use of diagrams, illustrations, and various visual pictures to clarify methods that have been developed in respiratory medicine. This "visual approach" goes back to lessons learned years ago by Dr. Warren Gold, the editor of *Atlas of Procedures in Respiratory Medicine,* from his teacher, Dr. Julius Comroe. Dr. Comroe was director of the Cardiovascular Research Institute in San Francisco, a visionary, and teacher of a multitude of famous pulmonologists. In a classic textbook on pulmonary function tests, Dr. Comroe used simple diagrams to describe methods and procedures. These illustrations show the effectiveness of visual images in explaining technical procedures. Dr. Comroe also invented a "fantasy" instrument, which he called the "retrospectroscope," a device that enables the viewer to look backward in many directions to find the seeds and roots of modern miracles. He showed that discovery takes many different paths!

The present text describes many of the instruments examined by Comroe's retrospectroscope and describes how these tools are used effectively in the diagnosis and treatment of respiratory diseases. Dr. Gold has assembled experts in various procedures used in respiratory medicine. The text emphasizes the use of visual methods such as illustrations, diagrams, and photographs to explain the pathways, mechanisms, and methods used in pulmonary medicine and their application. Just as Dr. Comroe used his retrospectroscope to determine how discoveries are made, Dr. Gold and his colleagues have used visual pictures to assist in the understanding of pulmonary diseases. The authors have worked long and hard. I hope the readers find the text interesting and useful.

Jay A. Nadel, M.D.
Professor of Medicine and Physiology
University of California, San Francisco

PREFACE

The third edition of the *Textbook of Respiratory Medicine* by John F. Murray and Jay A. Nadel was recently published. This single work covers almost all of the many new and important scientific discoveries and their clinical applications in respiratory medicine. It continues to focus on integrating basic science with the practice of respiratory medicine supported by an exhaustive list of references. In my view, however, the emphasis of this book is on words. The *Atlas of Procedures in Respiratory Medicine,* on the other hand, is designed to supplement and complement the *Textbook of Respiratory Medicine* with illustrations. The *Atlas* aims to present the often complex and esoteric procedures with pictures and diagrams of the highest quality. The goal is to provide the readers, whether practicing chest physicians or internists, graduate physicians-in-training, medical students, or others who want to know, with a picture book that illustrates how things are done in respiratory medicine. It will also illustrate how the methods were used to accumulate information about specific diseases.

The job of creating the *Atlas* was made easier by the expert authors who skillfully completed their assignments. At W.B. Saunders Company in Philadelphia, Judith Fletcher had the foresight to help us initiate the project, Dolores Meloni provided excellent editorial help, and Catherine Carroll gave superb production assistance, enthusiasm, and devotion to excellence. Lynn Foulk and Tina Rebane provided ingenious solutions to difficult production problems, particularly with the tables and text. I hope the outcome of this enterprise, especially when used in conjunction with the *Textbook of Respiratory Medicine,* will enrich the education of my readers and improve the care of patients with respiratory diseases.

Warren M. Gold, M.D.

NOTICE

CONTENTS

Morphologic Procedures in Respiratory Anatomy and Pathology

Walter E. Finkbeiner, M.D., Ph.D.

INTRODUCTION

The study of anatomy relies on observations made with the naked eye or with vision enhanced by special tissue preparations and microscopic methods. The gross and microscopic identification of changes in normal anatomy induced by disease (morbid anatomy) is a significant component of both the scientific and clinical practice of pathology. Analysis of the anatomic and pathologic features of the respiratory system in all its complexity requires a myriad of morphologic techniques, each with its own advantages and disadvantages. The method chosen will depend on the question or hypothesis being asked or tested and the degree of resolution required to arrive at an accurate answer. In TABLE 1–1 the limit of resolution of gross examination is compared with the resolution achieved with the two most commonly used microscopic methods—light and electron microscopy.

TABLE 1–1

Limit of Resolution by Gross and Microscopic Evaluation

Technique	Limit of Resolution	Effective Limit of Magnification	Structures Detectable
Naked eye	0.2 mm		Organs; larger anatomic structures; anatomic relationships
Light-based microscopy	0.2–0.25 μm	1000–1200	Animal cells; bacteria; some cell organelles
Electron microscopy	0.10–0.20 nm	500,000	Animal cells; cell organelles; macromolecules; small molecules; elements

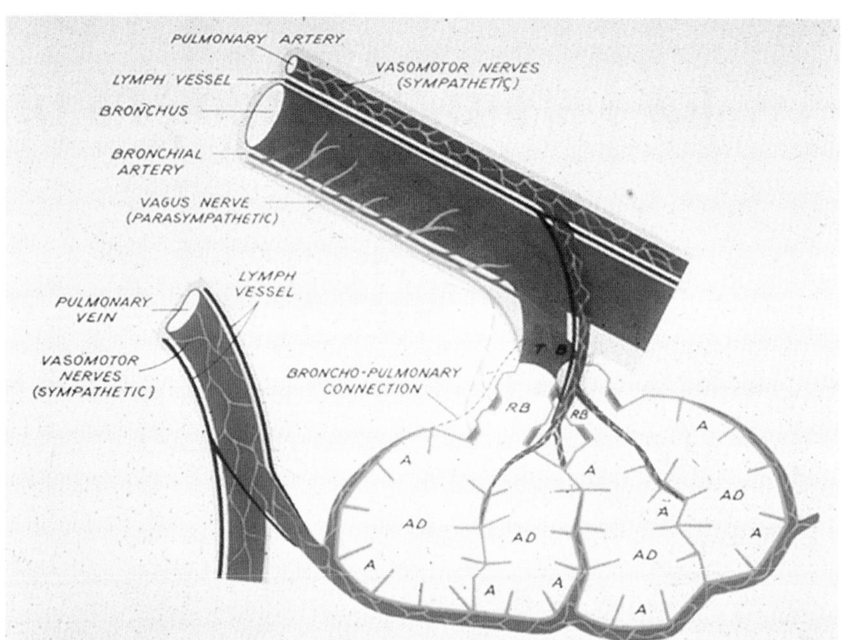

This model illustrates the proper anatomic and physiologic relationships of the major anatomic structures of the lung, which will be described in detail in this and subsequent chapters. Each bronchus with its accompanying pulmonary artery (plus bronchial artery, lymphatics, and vagus and sympathetic nerves) is surrounded by a loose binding connective tissue. There is a potential space within this bronchovascular bundle that is in direct communication with the pleural space. The alveoli (A) and alveolar ducts (AD) branch from the respiratory bronchiole (RB) to form the terminal respiratory unit. This terminal respiratory unit forms an ovoid structure in three dimensions and is the true "alveolus" of gas exchange. Within this structure, O_2 and CO_2 concentrations are uniform and the poorly oxygenated venous blood entering from the pulmonary artery (blue) is distributed within the fine capillary network so that oxygen and carbon dioxide can be exchanged in less than 1 second, yielding arterialized blood (red), which enters the pulmonary veins. The alveolar wall parenchyma connects directly with the loose-binding connective tissue of the bronchovascular bundle. (Modified from Staub NC. Edema. New York: Raven Press, 1984, p. 721.)

GROSS EXAMINATION OF THE RESPIRATORY SYSTEM

Supplementary techniques used in conjunction with anatomic dissection and gross examination enhance the ability to visualize anatomic or pathologic features of the respiratory system. These techniques often identify specific structures to best advantage, or they provide an intermediate step prior to sampling tissue for microscopic examination. Several techniques and their primary uses, advantages, and disadvantages are listed in TABLE 1–2.

TABLE 1–2

Supplementary Examination Techniques

Technique	Primary Uses	Advantages	Disadvantages
Fresh, unfixed	Study of anatomic relationships; pathologic diagnosis	Simple; continuous view of dissected large airways and vessels	Parenchymal anatomy and disease visualized poorly; subsequent microscopy poor due to alveolar collapse; no long-term storage
Perfusion (inflation) fixation and serial sectioning	Initial step for optimal microscopic examination; gross pathologic diagnosis	Simple; versatile method for evaluating most lung diseases; additional techniques can be applied to cut sections; optimal technique for selecting tissue for subsequent microscopic examination	Disruption of material within perfused airspace or vessel; sites of lung infection are fixed prior to visualization precluding microbiologic studies; degradation with long-term storage (years)
Barium sulfate impregnation	Quantifying airspace disease	Makes lung tissue opaque for better visualization and photography	Degradation with long-term storage; significant preparation time
Air drying	Pathologic diagnosis	Simple; particularly good for evaluation of emphysema; tissue can be fixed before drying to delay degradation	Limited to study of diseases that do not produce solid lesions; may interfere with microscopic examination; delay before lung can be sectioned
Paper-mounted thin (Gough-Wentworth) sections	Quantifying airspace disease	Excellent correlation with modern in vivo imaging studies; long-term storage of sections without degradation (decades)	Moderately laborious
Injection of acid-resistant substances followed by tissue digestion	Anatomic studies	Excellent for examination of vascular and airway anatomic relationships	Digestion destroys tissue prohibiting microscopic examination
Injection of radiopaque substances	Anatomic and pathologic studies	Excellent for examination of vascular and airway structure; does not preclude subsequent gross and microscopic analysis	Requires x-ray analysis

GROSS EXAMINATION OF THE RESPIRATORY SYSTEM

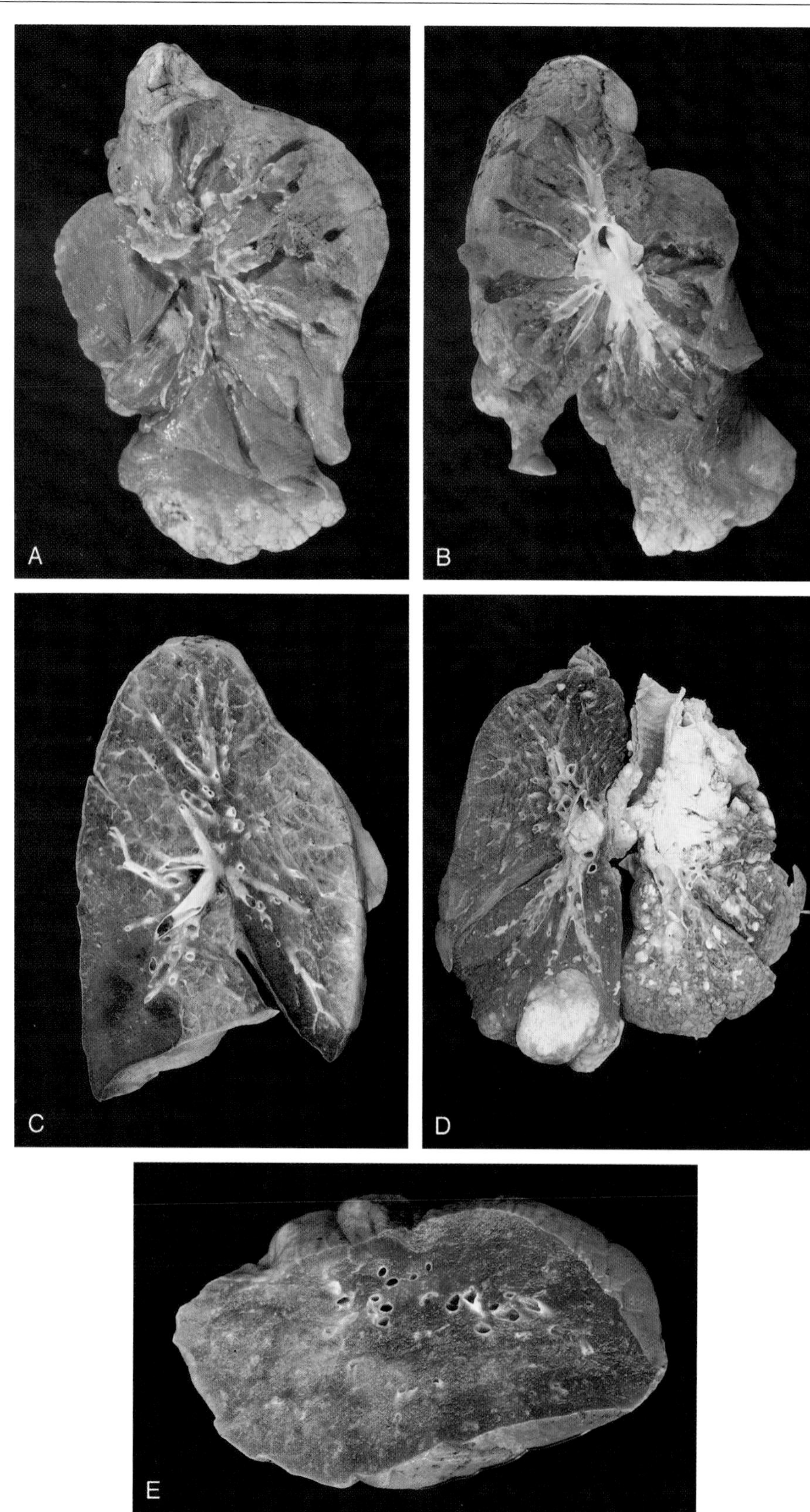

FIGURE 1-1

Gross examination of lungs, comparing fresh, unfixed lungs with lungs prepared by inflation fixation. **A,** Postmortem left lung, hilar aspect, cut while fresh. The bronchi have been opened longitudinally into the periphery. Although this technique provides a continuous view of the conducting airways, parenchymal diseases are not seen to advantage. **B,** Same lung, antihilar aspect, cut while fresh. The pulmonary arteries and their branches have been opened longitudinally into the periphery. **C,** Postmortem right lung, same patient as in *A* and *B*. This lung was inflated with fixative (10% neutral buffered formalin) via the mainstem bronchus at a pressure of approximately 30 cm H_2O until the pleura was evenly distended. Next, it was sliced at intervals of 1.0 to 2.0 cm along the sagittal plane, preserving the hilar structures (not shown). This technique affords a better gross examination of the parenchyma. In this specimen two thromboemboli lodged in pulmonary artery branches are readily identified, as are the acute pulmonary infarcts in the inferior upper and lower lobe parenchyma corresponding to the regions supplied by the vessels. Also note that emphysema in the upper lobe (not readily detected in *A* or *B*) is recognized by the inward collapse of the visceral pleura. Minor disadvantages of inflating the lung prior to sectioning are that airway perfusion obscures edema fluid and may transport material in the airway (mucus, pus) distally.[1] **D,** A midcoronal slice (posterior view) through the trachea and mainstem bronchi of a lung that has been inflated through the trachea demonstrates to best advantage the central airways and destruction and obstruction of the right mainstem bronchus by a squamous cell carcinoma. **E,** Horizontal sections of inflated lung allow comparison to clinical computed tomographic scans.

GROSS EXAMINATION OF THE RESPIRATORY SYSTEM

FIGURE 1-2

Simple apparatuses for achieving uniform inflation of whole lungs or lobectomy specimens are easily constructed.[2] In this example, an immersed electrical pump (P) protected by a filter (F) refills an upper reservoir (B). Lung specimens immersed in container A inflate by overflow through pipe D, which is adjusted to a height of 25 to 30 cm between the levels of fixative in each tank. A manifold allowing multiple specimens is supplied by tube E. Tap C controls the flow of fixative into the upper reservoir. Alternatively, an immersed pump under control of a variable transformer can be used to regulate flow. Manometer M serves to check that no unused taps on the manifold are inadvertently left open. (From Heard BE: Pathology of pulmonary emphysema: Methods of study. Am Rev Respir Dis 82:792–799, 1960.)

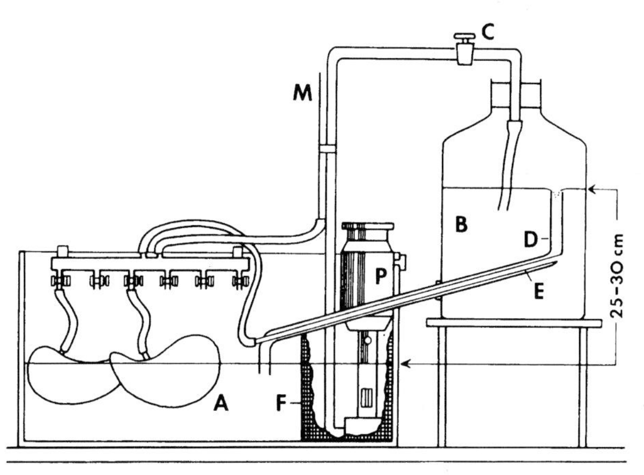

FIGURE 1-3

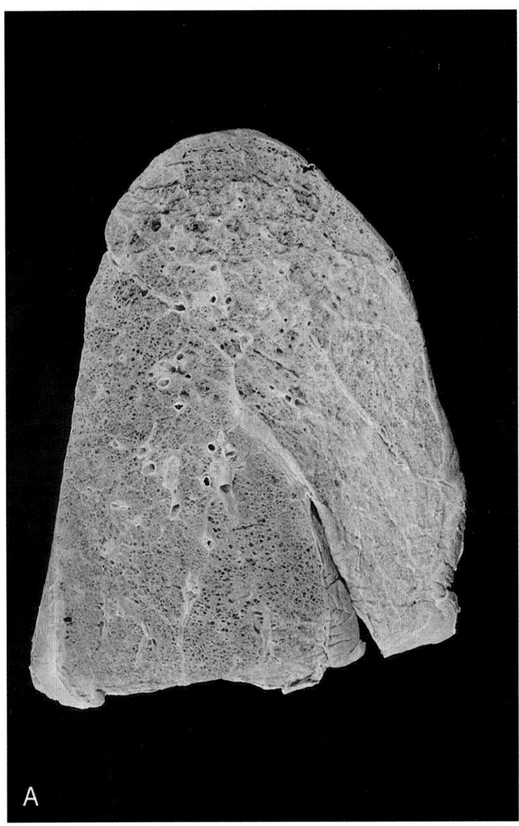

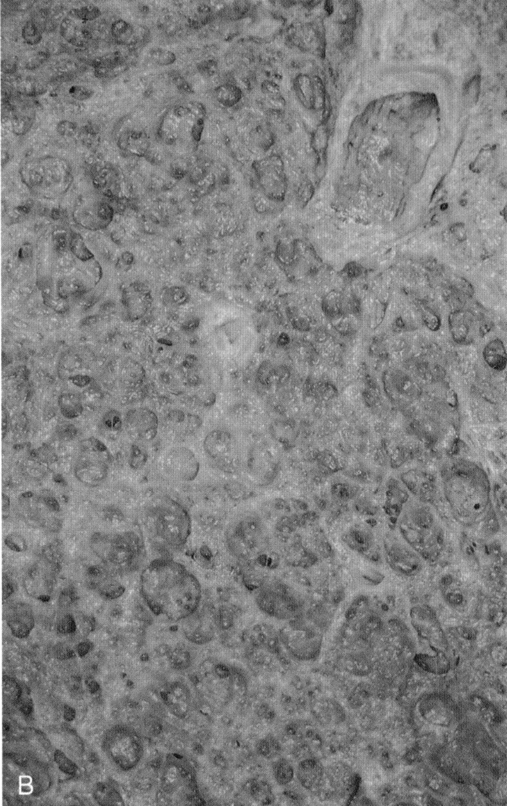

Barium sulfate impregnation of lung slices reduces the translucency of airspace walls.[2] A section of lung is submerged in a flat container containing aqueous barium nitrate (75 g/L). Gentle compression of the lung encourages penetration of the barium nitrate. After approximately 1 minute, the lung is squeezed gently and transferred, face down, to a container containing aqueous sodium sulfate (100 g/L). After 1 minute or so, the lung tissue becomes impregnated by a fine white precipitate of barium sulfate. Repetition of the process completes the deposition of precipitate. **A,** A barium sulfate–impregnated lung affected by centriacinar emphysema is examined underwater. **B,** A dissecting microscope improves resolution and demonstrates the marked parenchymal loss and dilation of the airspaces.

GROSS EXAMINATION OF THE RESPIRATORY SYSTEM

FIGURE 1–4

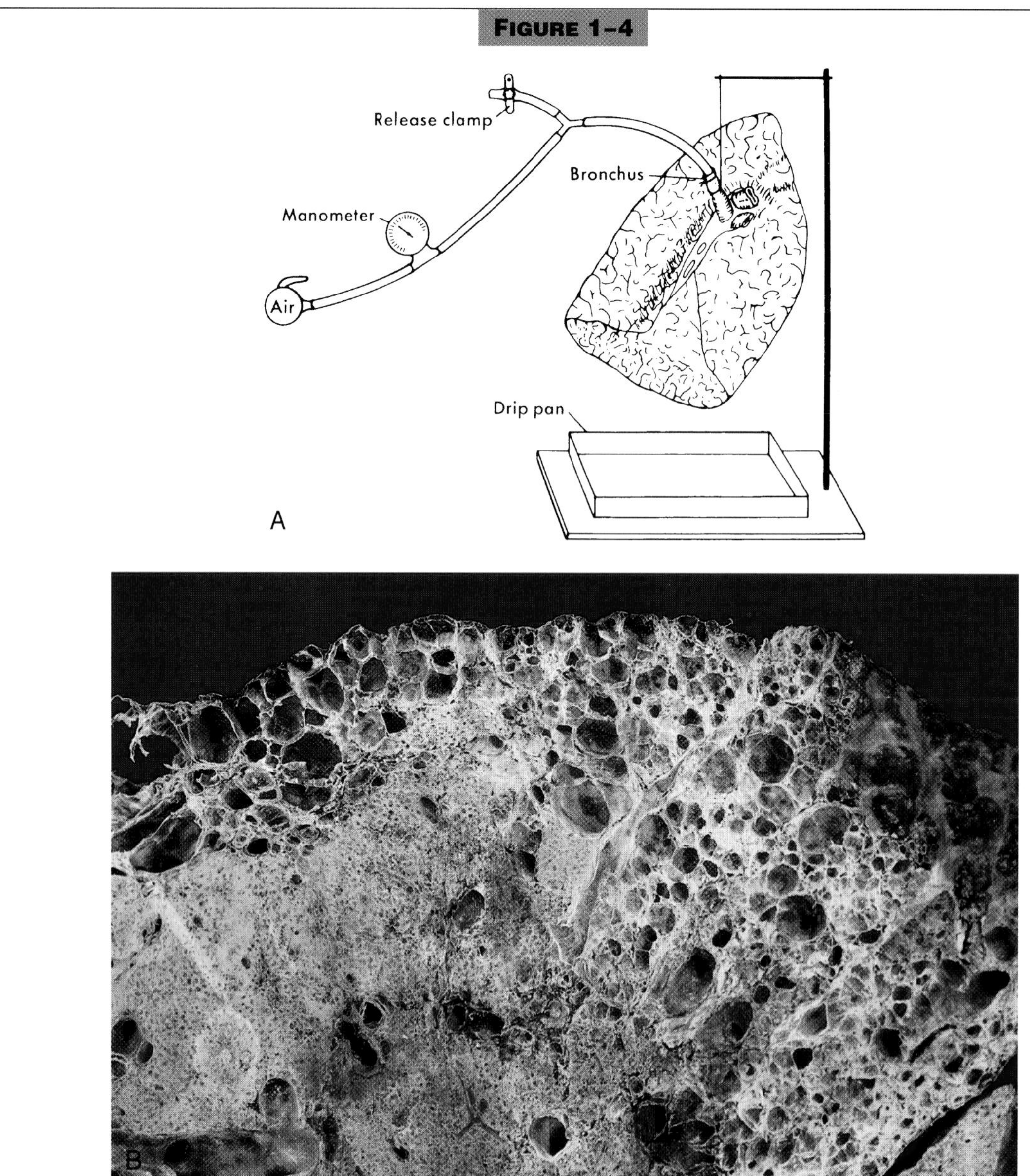

Following intrabronchial fixation, the lung can be air-dried and sectioned producing an excellent specimen for gross examination, photography, and correlation with imaging studies.[3, 4] **A,** Apparatus for preparing air-dried specimen. The mainstem bronchus is cannulated and the lung is suspended on a ring stand from a string around the cannula. The cannula is connected to plastic tubing containing a Y connector that has a C-clamp attached to one end. The other end is connected to an air supply with a manometer interposed. A constant stream of air is forced through the system at a pressure of 25 to 30 mmHg by adjusting the release clamp until the lung is absolutely dry (at least 1 week). (From Heitzman ER: The Lung: Radiologic-Pathologic Correlations, 2nd ed. St. Louis, CV Mosby, 1984.) **B,** Air-dried and then sagittally sectioned lung from a patient with idiopathic pulmonary fibrosis. Note the extensive subpleural honeycomb cysts.

GROSS EXAMINATION OF THE RESPIRATORY SYSTEM

FIGURE 1-5

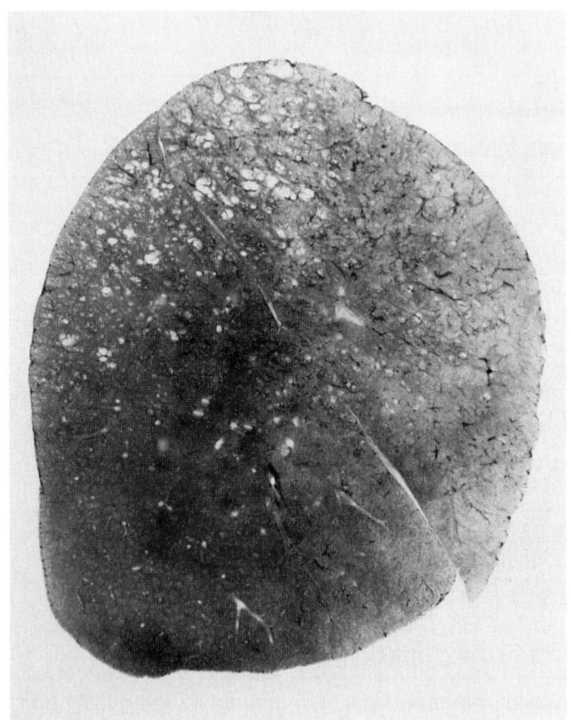

The Gough and Wentworth technique[5] of preparing thin sections of lung mounted on paper as modified by others[6-8] provides very thin, whole lung slices that are especially useful for studying emphysema, pneumoconiosis, and other diseases that affect the lung parenchyma, particularly at early stages of disease when subtle changes may go unnoticed in thicker sections of lung. In this example, centriacinar emphysema is evident in the upper lobe.

FIGURE 1-6

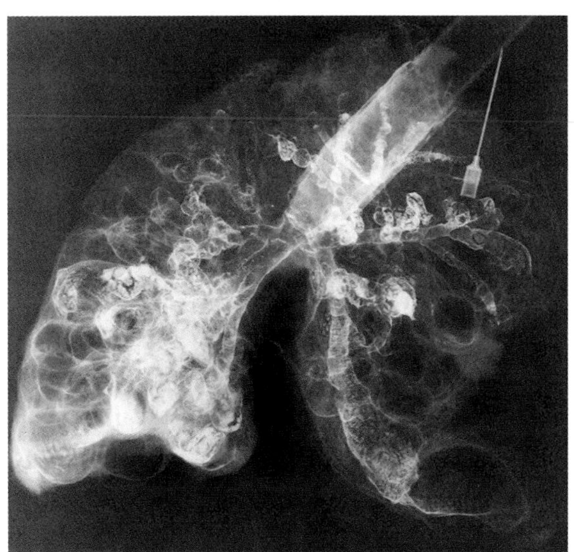

Radiopaque substances such as barium are injected easily into pulmonary arteries, pulmonary veins, or the bronchial tree. A mixture containing some gelatin will prevent leakage into the alveoli, will harden with fixation, and will remain visible in microscopic sections.[9] Nadel et al.[10] used powdered tantalum, a superb radiopaque marker that outlines airways from the trachea to those less than 1 mm in diameter, for in vivo and ex vivo bronchography. In this postmortem tantalum bronchogram of a lung from a patient with emphysema, the fine details of large and small airways are evident. (Courtesy of J. A. Nadel, M.D., University of California, San Francisco.)

FIGURE 1-7

Simple apparatus for performing injections under a constant pressure. A pulmonary vessel or a bronchus is cannulated, and plastic tubing connects the cannula to a flask. The flask contains the injection mass which is perfused into the lung at a controlled pressure, typically 50 to 150 mm Hg for vascular injections and somewhat less for bronchial injections. Injections of latex or plastic used for making corrosion casts may require even higher pressures. (From Heitzman ER: The Lung: Radiologic-Pathologic Correlations, 2nd ed. St. Louis, CV Mosby, 1984.)

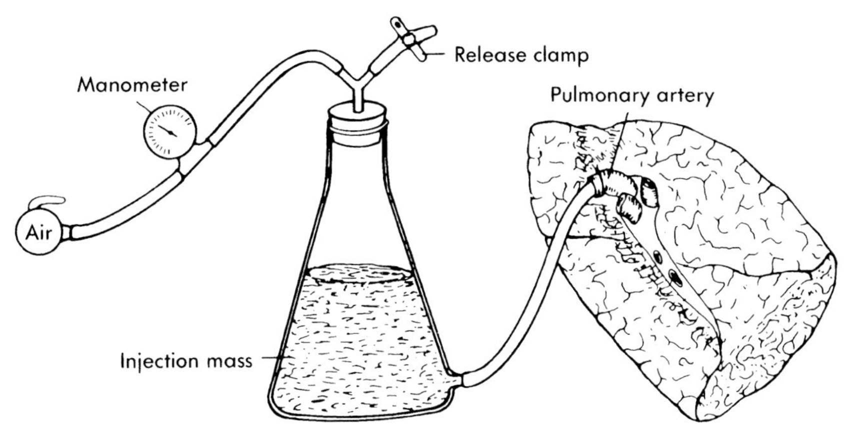

MICROSCOPIC EXAMINATION OF THE RESPIRATORY SYSTEM

Among the various types of microscopy, light and electron microscopy are the primary methods used to study the biology and pathobiology of cells. The different types of light and electron microscopy and their main uses are listed in TABLE 1–3.

TABLE 1–3

Uses of Light and Electron Microscopy

Types of Microscopy	Main Uses
LIGHT-BASED MICROSCOPY	
Bright-field microscopy	Examination of tissues and cells following histochemical staining
Phase-contrast microscopy	Examination of unstained tissues and cells (suitable for living cells)
Dark-field microscopy	Examination of unstained tissues and cells; examination of silver grains from in situ hybridization or autoradiography; examination of edges and boundaries
Differential interference contrast (Nomarski) microscopy	Examination of unstained living tissues and cells; identification of the mass of cellular components
Fluorescence microscopy	Examination of cells and subcellular structures stained with fluorescent markers; spectroscopy at cellular level; identification of autofluorescent biologic substances
Ultraviolet microscopy	Examination of nucleic acids
Polarizing microscopy	Identification of materials that are birefringent or anisotropic
Confocal microscopy	Improved examination of fluorescent markers allowing improved image quality and three-dimensional reconstruction
ELECTRON MICROSCOPY (EM)	
Transmission EM	Resolution of cell organelles
Scanning EM	Three-dimensional view of surfaces
Analytical EM	Analysis of elemental composition of material within tissues
High voltage EM	Three-dimensional analysis of intracellular structure

MICROSCOPIC EXAMINATION OF THE RESPIRATORY SYSTEM

FIGURE 1–8

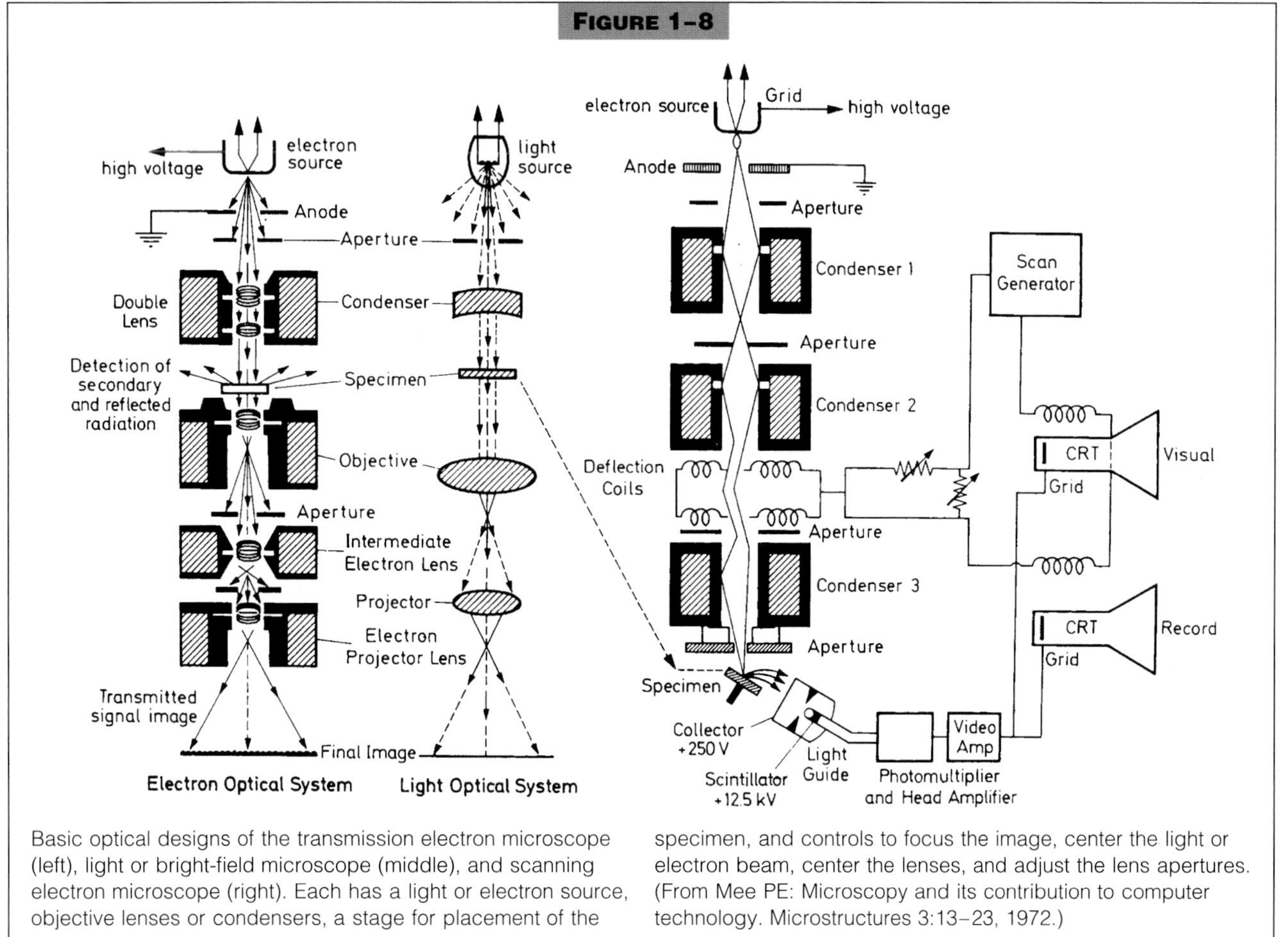

Basic optical designs of the transmission electron microscope (left), light or bright-field microscope (middle), and scanning electron microscope (right). Each has a light or electron source, objective lenses or condensers, a stage for placement of the specimen, and controls to focus the image, center the light or electron beam, center the lenses, and adjust the lens apertures. (From Mee PE: Microscopy and its contribution to computer technology. Microstructures 3:13–23, 1972.)

MICROSCOPIC EXAMINATION OF THE RESPIRATORY SYSTEM

The first step in the preparation of tissues for microscopic examination is generally fixation. The aims of tissue fixation (halting autolysis, limiting diffusion of cellular constituents, preventing postmortem changes, preventing alteration of microanatomic structures during subsequent tissue processing and facilitating subsequent staining reactions) are met to a variable degree by the large number of the fixatives used today. Ten percent neutral buffered formalin is the fixative of choice for most routine light microscopic studies. The use of combination fixatives (e.g., alcoholic formalin, B-5, zinc formalin, Carnoy's) seeks to maximize advantages and minimize deleterious effects or reduce toxicity. For example, fixative B-5 is often used for fixing specimens that are suspected to contain hematologic malignancies because it gives excellent results with special histochemical and immunocytochemical stains with sections prepared from paraffin-embedded tissues. Acetic acid is added to alcohol to counteract tissue shrinkage. Two and one-half percent glutaraldehyde is a popular fixative for electron microscopy as is modified Karnovsky's fixative (5% paraformaldehyde, 2.5% glutaraldehyde). The advantages and disadvantages of several categories of tissue fixatives are listed in TABLE 1–4.

TABLE 1–4

Types of Tissue Fixatives

Fixative	Advantages	Disadvantages
Aldehyde-based (10% neutral buffered formalin, 4% paraformaldehyde, 2.5% glutaraldehyde)	• Fairly rapid tissue penetration • Good preservation of cell organelles • Limited tissue shrinkage • Minimal tissue hardening • Good lipid preservation • Suitable for immunohistochemical studies • Suitable for many molecular studies • Suitable for electron microscopy	• Toxicity • Environmental protection • Cost of disposal
Alcohol-based (ethanol, methanol, Carnoy's)	• Lower toxicity • Rapid penetration • Ethanol or methanol useful for fixation of smears	• Tissue shrinkage • Tissue brittleness
Mercuric chloride–containing (B-5, Zenker's, Helly's, Susa)	• Enhances many histochemical and immunocytochemical stains	• Toxicity • Poor penetration
Zinc sulfate/chloride–containing	• Superior nuclear detail • Better paraffin infiltration • Preservation of antigens	• Zinc precipitation
Picric acid–containing (Bouin's, Gendre's, Rossman's)	• Preserves glycogen	• Tissue shrinkage
Acetic acid	• Noncoagulant • Swells tissue	• Swells tissue
Potassium dichromate	• Enhances tissue affinity for eosin	• Tissue shrinkage • Toxicity
Osmium tetroxide	• Preserves lipids	• Toxicity
Microwave energy	• Fixes rapidly • Good antigen preservation • Antigen retrieval	• Underheating affects sectioning • Overheating produces vacuoles, pyknotic nuclei and over-stained cytoplasm

MICROSCOPIC EXAMINATION OF THE RESPIRATORY SYSTEM

FIGURE 1–9

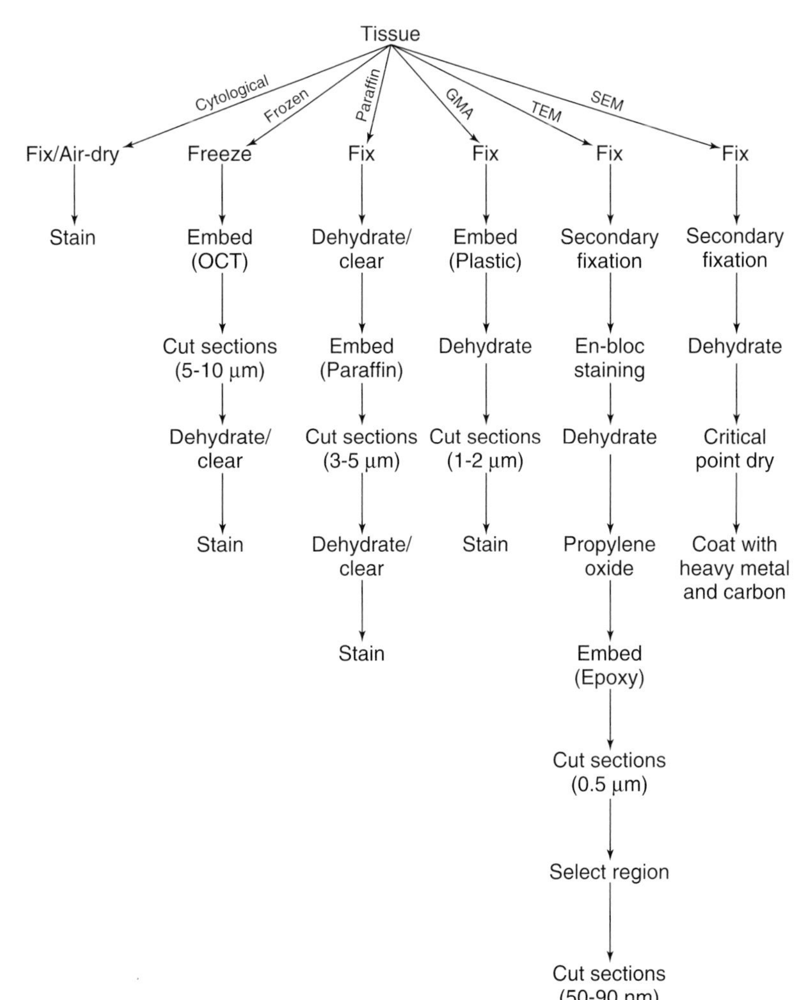

The various types of microscopy require different processes to ready tissue samples for actual viewing. Cytologic preparations placed on glass microscopic slides require the least preparation. They are prepared from tissue imprints (touch preps), tissue aspirates, or smears of bodily fluids previously concentrated by centrifugation and are air-dried or immediately fixed (usually in methanol). Frozen tissue sections are prepared by freezing selected samples rapidly within a viscous embedding solution. Fixation prior to freezing is not required, but it does improve the final appearance of the microscopic section. If tissue has been fixed prior to freezing, infiltration with 30% sucrose acts as a cryoprotectant and reduces freezing artifacts. The embedded frozen tissue is ready for immediate sectioning with a cryostat. Typical frozen sections are 6 to 7 μm thick. For paraffin sections, tissue is dehydrated (stepwise, usually in graded alcohol), cleared (usually in xylene), infiltrated with paraffin wax, and finally embedded in the wax. Sections, typically 5 μm thick, but occasionally as thin as 3 μm or as thick as 100 μm, are cut using a rotary microtome. The sections are floated on warm water to remove wrinkles and then are picked up on glass microscopic slides. Because histochemical reagents are prepared as aqueous solutions, the paraffin slides are returned to water by equilibrating them first in the clearing agent and then back through the dehydrating agent into water before staining. Glycol methacrylate (GMA) is an acrylic resin miscible with water and is excellent for preparing light microscopic sections of hard tissue, such as bone, and for preparing very thin sections demonstrating fine cellular detail. Other advantages of GMA include good preservation of antigens and enzymes. Processing of fixed tissue is initiated with dehydration in graded acetone or alcohol and then followed by infiltration and embedding. Sections are typically cut at 1 to 2 μm with glass knives placed in a water bath before transfer to either glass coverslips or microscopic slides. Preparation of specimens for transmission electron microscopy (TEM) typically begins with perfusion fixation by or immersion of very small pieces of tissue into buffered aldehyde fixative. Next, secondary fixation in osmium tetroxide to better preserve membrane lipids precedes optional en bloc staining with uranyl acetate. Dehydration, typically in graded alcohol, follows. Then, the tissue receives transitional treatments, first with propylene oxide and then with a propylene oxide–epoxy resin mixture prior to infiltration and embedding with pure epoxy resin. For immunoelectron microscopy, London Resin (LR) white, a hydrophilic acrylic monomer, may be used in place of epoxy resins, although slightly different processing steps are required. For TEM, initial semithin (so-called "thick") 0.5-μm sections are cut with glass knives, placed on glass microscope slides, and stained with toluidine blue. The desired area of the section is selected using a light microscope. The unwanted areas of tissue are trimmed from the block, thin (50 to 90 nm) sections are cut with a diamond knife, and the sections are placed on special circular copper grids. Once placed on the grids, the thin sections are stained first with uranyl acetate (if this was not done en bloc) and then with lead citrate before examination in the transmission electron microscope. Tissue samples prepared for scanning electron microscopy (SEM) receive primary aldehyde and secondary osmium tetroxide fixation before alcoholic dehydration. Then, specimens are dried by the critical point method using CO_2 to eliminate potential surface tension forces that might affect the morphology. After drying, the tissue is attached to a specimen holder and coated with heavy metal (gold or palladium) and carbon to prevent electrical charge buildup during examination in the scanning electron microscope. OCT = Optimal Cutting Temperature (Sakura Finetek, U.S.A., Inc., Torrance, CA)

MICROSCOPIC EXAMINATION OF THE RESPIRATORY SYSTEM

TABLE 1–5

Respiratory Cell Samples, Collection Methods and Their Preparation for Cytologic Examination

Sample	Collection Method	Cytologic Preparation
Sputum	Early morning, deep cough, collected over several days Induction with nebulized water or saline	• Tissue fragments and blood removed from fresh sputum and smears prepared from these, fixed in 95% ethanol • Modified Saccomanno method—expectoration into 70% ethanol, specimen homogenized in blender and then concentrated by centrifugation; smears made for concentrated material • Embed prefixed sputum in paraffin and prepare microscopic "cell block" sections
Bronchial washings	Instillation and aspiration of 3–10 mL saline via bronchoscope	• Concentrated by centrifugation, smeared or embedded as cell block
Bronchoalveolar lavage	Bronchoscope wedged distally, distal airways flushed with several aliquots of saline. First aliquot most representative of cellular material from larger airways; subsequent aliquots reflect alveolar compartment	• Concentrated by centrifugation, smeared or embedded as cell block
Bronchial brushings	Under direct visualization, airway is brushed and cells are entrapped in the brush	• Smear, fixed and unfixed
Transbronchial fine-needle aspiration	Aspirated via retractable needle attached to flexible catheter	• Smear, fixed and unfixed
Transthoracic fine-needle aspiration	Aspirated via computed tomography, fluoroscopy, or ultrasound guidance	• Smear, fixed and unfixed
Pleural fluid	Thoracentesis	• Concentrated by centrifugation, smeared or embedded as cell block

MICROSCOPIC EXAMINATION OF THE RESPIRATORY SYSTEM

SUPPLEMENTARY TECHNIQUES

Histochemistry and Enzyme Histochemistry

FIGURE 1-10

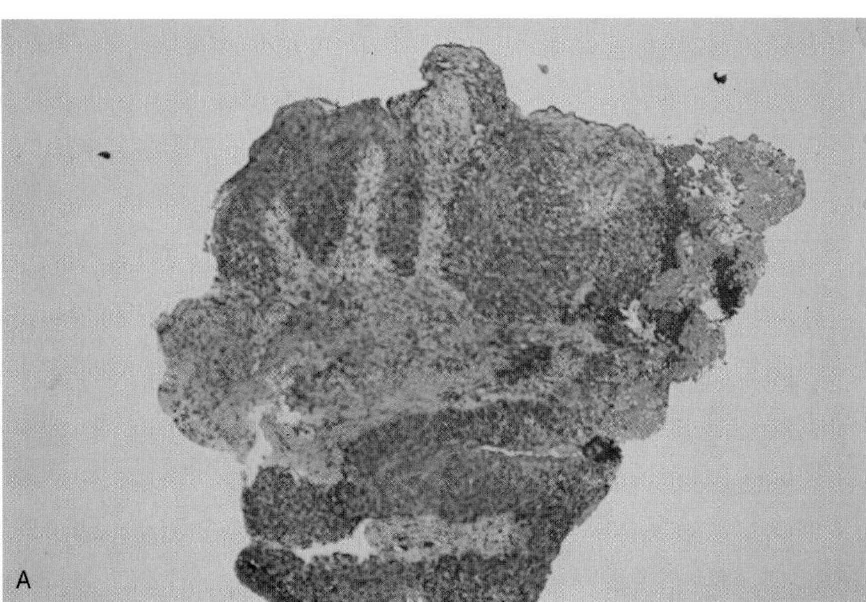

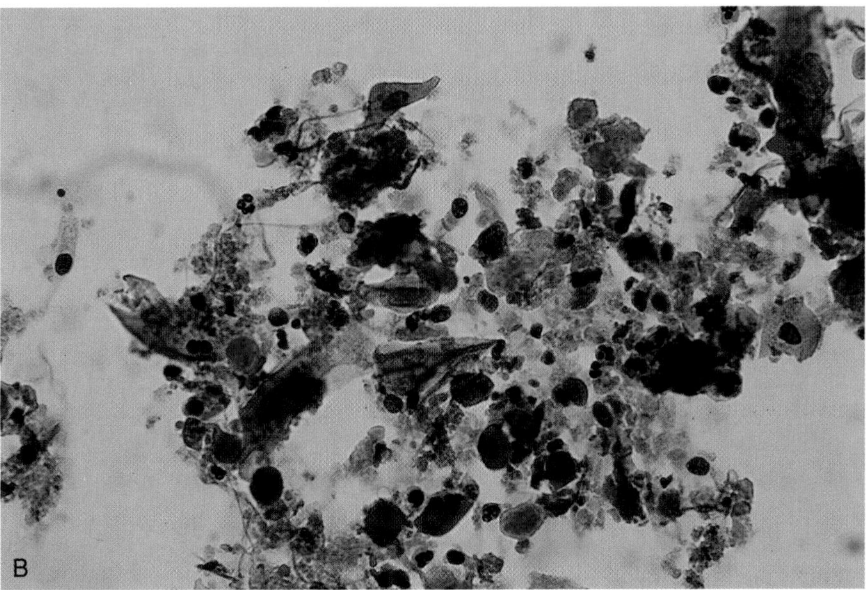

Used primarily for preparing cells and tissues for bright-field microscopy, histochemical staining techniques have evolved over the last 175 years and are described in detail in a number of reference works.[11-14] Three types of chemical reactions are used most frequently in histochemistry: (1) simple ionic interactions; (2) reactions of aldehydes with Schiff's reagent or silver compounds; and (3) coupling of aromatic diazonium salts with aromatic residues on proteins.[15] The mainstay of most light microscopic diagnostic pathologic examinations are the hematoxylin-eosin stain for tissue sections and the Papanicolaou stain for cytologic preparations. Both are performed quickly, easily, and inexpensively. Each demonstrate nuclei, cytoplasm, and other cellular components to great advantage. In this example, a microscopic section of paraffin-embedded airway tissue obtained by endobronchial biopsy is compared to a bronchial brushing sample stained with the Papanicolaou stain. **A,** In the hematoxylin-eosin stained microscopic section from an endobronchial biopsy a well-differentiated squamous cell carcinoma arising from the epithelium invades into the submucosa. Tumor cell, leukocyte, and connective tissue cell nuclei stain blue, cytoplasm stains varying shades of pink, and erythrocytes stain red. **B,** In the Papanicolaou-stained specimen, nuclei stain blue-black and cytoplasm stains variably blue to green in nonkeratinizing cells and pink-orange as the amount of cytoplasmic keratin increases in the keratinizing carcinoma cells.

MICROSCOPIC EXAMINATION OF THE RESPIRATORY SYSTEM

SUPPLEMENTARY TECHNIQUES

Histochemistry and Enzyme Histochemistry

A wide variety of histochemical stains that identify specific tissues, cells, secretions, metabolic products, minerals or microorganisms are useful for histologic studies and pathologic diagnosis of diseases of the respiratory tract. A list of some the most useful histochemical procedures for studying the lung is provided in TABLE 1–6.

TABLE 1–6

Histochemical Stains and Their Uses

Application	Histochemical Stain
SPECIFIC CELLS, TISSUES, AND TISSUE COMPONENTS	
Blood cells	Wright, Romanowsky-Giemsa, hematoxylin-eosin
- Basophils	Toluidine blue
- Plasma cells	Methyl green–pyronine
Mast cells	Toluidine blue
Basement membrane	Periodic acid–Schiff (PAS); PAS-Jones' hexamine silver
Collagen	Masson's trichrome
Elastin	Weigert's elastic van Giesen
Fat	Sudan black B, oil red O (frozen tissue)
Minerals (endogenous)	
- Calcium	Von Kossa
- Iron (hemosiderin)	Perls' Prussian blue
Minerals (exogenous)	
- Aluminum	Chromoxane pure black B
- Asbestos	Perls' Prussian blue detects iron, and alizarin reaction detects calcium deposited on asbestos bodies
- Beryllium	Naphthachrome B
- Nickel	Dimethylglycoxine method
- Zirconium	Morin method
Carbohydrates	
- Glycogen	PAS with diastase
- Hyaluronic acid	Alcian blue pH 2.5 with and without hyaluronidase

Application	Histochemical Stain
SPECIFIC CELLS, TISSUES, AND TISSUE COMPONENTS	
- Mucins	Mayer's mucicarmine, Alcian blue pH 2.5, PAS
Neutral mucins	PAS
Acid mucins	Alcian blue pH 2.5
PIGMENTS, OTHER METABOLIC PRODUCTS	
Alveolar proteinosis	PAS
Amyloid	Congo red
Cholesterol	Perchloric acid–naphthoquinone, digitonin reaction
Fibrin	Mallory's PTAH; Lendrum's Martius yellow-brilliant crystal scarlet-soluble blue (MSB)
Lipofuscin	Long Ziehl-Neelsen
Melanin	Masson-Fontana
MICROORGANISMS	
Gram-positive and gram-negative bacteria	Brown-Brenn Gram stain or other tissue Gram stain
Mycobacterium species	Fite
Legionella species	Dieterle's
Spirochetes and *Rochalimaea* species	Warthin-Starry
Fungi including *Pneumocystis carinii*	Grocott methenamine silver (some also stain with PAS with diastase)
Protozoan	May-Grunwals-Giemsa

MICROSCOPIC EXAMINATION OF THE RESPIRATORY SYSTEM

SUPPLEMENTARY TECHNIQUES

Histochemistry and Enzyme Histochemistry

Enzyme histochemistry depends on the conversion of the primary reaction product of an enzyme acting on a substrate to form a colored precipitate. The techniques of enzyme histochemistry are used most frequently in the diagnosis of hematologic proliferations and neoplasms. However, many enzymes are now detected with greater ease using immunocytochemical methods. In the respiratory system, the identification of specific enzymes may be useful for identification of some specific cell types.

TABLE 1-7

Enzyme Histochemistry

Enzyme	Cells Identified
Chymase	Mast cells
Cytochrome oxidase	Nonciliated bronchiolar (Clara) cells
Naphthol AS-D chloracetate esterase	Myeloblasts, neutrophils, mast cells
Myeloperoxidase	Myeloblasts, neutrophils
Tryptase	Mast cells

Immunocyto(histo)chemistry

FIGURE 1-11

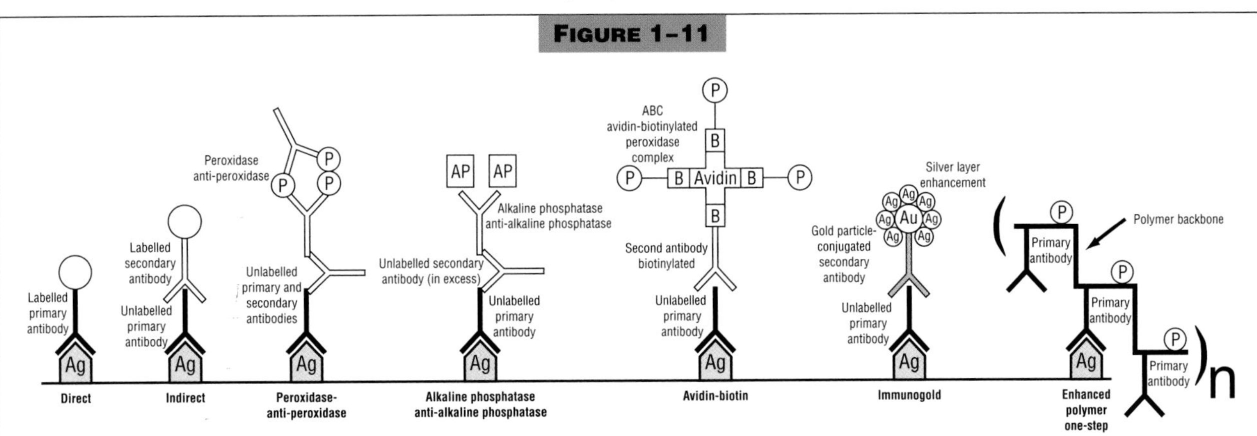

Immunocyto(histo)chemical staining, a technique for localizing substances in cells and tissues using antigen-antibody reactions has revolutionized both experimental histologic and pathologic examinations. Improved immunohistochemical technology and an increasingly diverse array of commercially available antibodies that react with formalin-fixed, paraffin-embedded antigens have greatly expanded the role of immunohistochemistry in diagnostic pathology.[16, 17] Adaptation of these techniques to the electron microscope continues to yield greater information regarding the structure and function at cellular and subcellular levels. Immunostains rely on the specificity of the antibody for a specific epitope in the tissue and a secondary labeling reaction that allows detection of the antibody-antigen complex with a light microscope. In the direct method, antibodies are conjugated with an indicator such as fluorescein. Fluorescence is observed using a microscope equipped with an ultraviolet light source and specialized filters. The more sensitive indirect method uses a secondary heterologous antisera for recognition of the primary antibody. Again, one can use a fluorescein-conjugated antibody. However, the use of enzymes such as peroxidase is favored. Following incubation of the tissue section in the appropriate substrate, enzyme reactions evident as a precipitated color change are observed using a standard light microscope. Recognition of antibody binding with the peroxidase-antiperoxidase or alkaline phosphatase methods or the avidin-biotin complex method have found great utility in paraffin embedded tissues.[18–20] These methods increase sensitivity of the indirect method about tenfold. The immunogold technique uses antibodies labeled with colloidal gold particles. The immunogold reagent may be difficult to see in light microscopic sections; however, antigen recognition sites can be enhanced using silver intensification. Immunogold reagents are readily detected using an electron microscope, and this technique is most often used for immunoelectron microscopy. Enhanced polymer one-step staining provides similar sensitivity to the avidin-biotin technology but requires fewer procedural steps.

MICROSCOPIC EXAMINATION OF THE RESPIRATORY SYSTEM

SUPPLEMENTARY TECHNIQUES

Immunocyto(histo)chemistry

Plant and other lectins having strong and selective affinity for specific saccharides can be used to detect these structures in tissue sections. Saccharide structures are robust and very resistant to fixation and tissue embedding and can be used readily on paraffin sections. For morphologic use, lectins are typically conjugated with a secondary marker such horseradish peroxidase and then visualized using diaminobenzidine and hydrogen peroxide. They may also be conjugated with fluorescent dyes. TABLE 1–8 lists a number of more frequently used lectins and their saccharide specificity.

TABLE 1–8

Saccharide Specificity of Lectins

Common Abbreviation	Source	Nominal Saccharide Specificity
GLUCOSE/MANNOSE GROUPS		
Con A	Jack bean (*Canavalia ensiformis*)	αMan > αGlc ≥ GlcNAc
LCA*	Lentil (*Lens culinaris*)	αMan > αGlc > GlcNAc
PSA	Pea (*Pisum sativum*)	αMan > αGlc = GlcNAc
N-ACETYLGLUCOSAMINE GROUP		
BSA II	*Bandeirea simplicifolia* seed	β and αGlcNAc
GSA-II	Griffonia seed (*Griffonia simplicifolia*)	α and βGlcNAc
DSA	Jimson weed (*Datura stramonium*)	GlcNAc (β1,4GlcNAc)$_{1-3}$ = Galβ1, 4GlcNAc
PWM	Pokeweed (*Phytolacca americana*)	GlcNAc (β1,4GlcNAc)$_{1-5}$ = Galβ1, 4GlcNAc$_{2-5}$
STA	Potato (*Solanum tuberosum*)	GlcNAc (β1,4GlcNAc)$_{1-4}$
UEA-II	Gorse seed (*Ulex europaeus* II)	L-Fucα1,1,2Galβ1,4GlcNAc > GlcNAc (β1,4GlcNAc)$_{1-3}$
WGA	Wheat germ (*Triticum vulgans*)	GlcNAc(β1,4-GlcNAc)$_{1-2}$ > GlcNAc > Neu5-Ac
N-ACETYLGALACTOSAMINE/GALACTOSE GROUP		
BPA	*Bauhinia purpurea* seed	α and βGalNAc > α and βGal
BSA I-B_4	*Bandeirea simplicifolia* seed	αGal > αGalNAc
DBA	Horse gram (*Dolichos biflorus*)	αGalNAc ≫ αGal
GSA-I	Griffonia seed (*Griffonia simplicifolia*)	α GalNAc > αGalI-A_4
HPA	Edible snail (*Heltx pomatia*)	GalNAcα 1,3GalNAc > α GalNAc
LBA	Lima bean (Phaseolus lunatus limensis)	GalNAcα 1,3[L-Fucα1,2] Galβ > GalNAc
MPA	Osage orange seed (*Maclura pomifera*)	αGalNAc > αGal
PNA	Peanut (*Arachis hypogaea*)	Galβ 1,3GalNAc > α and βGal
RCA I	Castor bean (*Ricinus communis*)	βGal > αGal ≫ GalNAc

MICROSCOPIC EXAMINATION OF THE RESPIRATORY SYSTEM

SUPPLEMENTARY TECHNIQUES

Immunocyto(histo)chemistry

TABLE 1-8

Saccharide Specificity of Lectins *continued*

Common Abbreviation	Source	Nominal Saccharide Specificity
N-ACETYLGALACTOSAMINE/GALACTOSE GROUP *CONTINUED*		
SBA	Soybean (*Glycine max*)	α and βGalNAc > α and βGal
SJA	Japanese pagoda tree (*Sophora japonica*)	α and βGalNAc > α and βGal
VVA	Hairy vetch (*Vicia villosa*)	GalNA α1,3Gal = αGalNAc αGalNAc
WFA	Wisteria seed (*Wisteria floribunda*)	GalNAc α1,6Gal > αGalNAc > βGalNAc
L-FUCOSE GROUP		
AAA	Orange peel fungus (*Aleuria aurantia*)	αL-Fuc
LTA	Asparagus pea (*Lotus tetragonolobus*)	αL-Fuc > L-Fucα 1,2 Galβ 1,4GlcNAc $\gg$ L-Fuc α1,2Gal β 1,3GlcNAc
UEA-I	Gorse seed (*Ulex europaeus*)	αL-Fuc
SIALIC ACID GROUP		
LFA	Slug (Limax flavus)	αNeu5Ac > αNeu5Gc
LPA	Horseshoe crab (*Limulus polyphemus*)	Neu5Ac (or Gc)α2,6-GalNAc > Neu5Ac

* Not to be confused with leukocyte common antigen.

Key: Man = mannose, Glc = glucose, Ac = acetyl, GlcNAc = *N*-acetylglucosamine, Gal = galactose, GalNAc = *N*-acetylgalactosamine, Neu = sialic acid (neuraminic acid), Fuc = fucose, Gc = glucuronic acid.

Source: Modified from Damjanov I: Biology of disease. Lectin cytochemistry and histochemistry. Lab Invest 57:5–20, 1987 and Stoward PJ: Histochemical methods available for pathologic diagnosis. *In* Spicer SS (ed): Histochemistry in Pathologic Diagnosis. New York, Marcel Dekker, 1987.

MICROSCOPIC EXAMINATION OF THE RESPIRATORY SYSTEM

SUPPLEMENTARY TECHNIQUES

In Situ Hybridization

The powerful technique of in situ hybridization allows the cellular localization of specific DNA and RNA sequences in tissue processed for microscopy. Among the uses of in situ hybridization techniques are (1) localization of specific mRNA species; (2) identification of specific nucleic acid sequences within a chromosome; (3) diagnosis of chromosomal disorders; and (4) recognition of viruses within cells. DNA is generally more stable than mRNA but the sensitivity of in situ hybridization techniques allows detection of as few as 10 DNA or RNA copies per cell.[21] Numerous factors contribute to the degeneration of the nucleic acids within tissue samples. Therefore, tissue fixation should be performed as soon as possible. Standard 10% buffered formalin appears to be an excellent fixative for purposes of in situ hybridization. In situ hybridization techniques are more refined for detection with the light or fluorescence microscope (fluorescence in situ hybridization or FISH) than the electron microscope. However, some labeling methods that work at the level of the light microscope adapt to the ultrastructural level. Advances in nonradioactive labeling and detection have improved the sensitivity of in situ hybridization and reduced, somewhat, its technical difficulty. TABLE 1–9 lists different reporter molecules used for in situ hybridization and their characteristics.

TABLE 1–9

Molecules Used for In Situ Hybridization

Label	Shelf Life	Time Required for Completion of ISH Testing	Background	Other
Biotin	>5 years	1 day	Low to high	• Liver and kidney have high levels of endogenous biotin
Digoxigenin	>5 years	1 day	Low	• Not present in tissues
^{35}S	90 days	3–14 days	Low to high	• Background highly variable • Requires expensive emulsion
^{3}H	12 years	30–60 days	Very low	• Requires expensive emulsion

Source: Modified from Nuovo, GJ: PCR *in situ* Hybridization: Protocols and Applications (3rd ed). Philadelphia, Lippincott-Raven, 1977.

MICROSCOPIC EXAMINATION OF THE RESPIRATORY SYSTEM

SUPPLEMENTARY TECHNIQUES

In Situ Hybridization

FIGURE 1–12

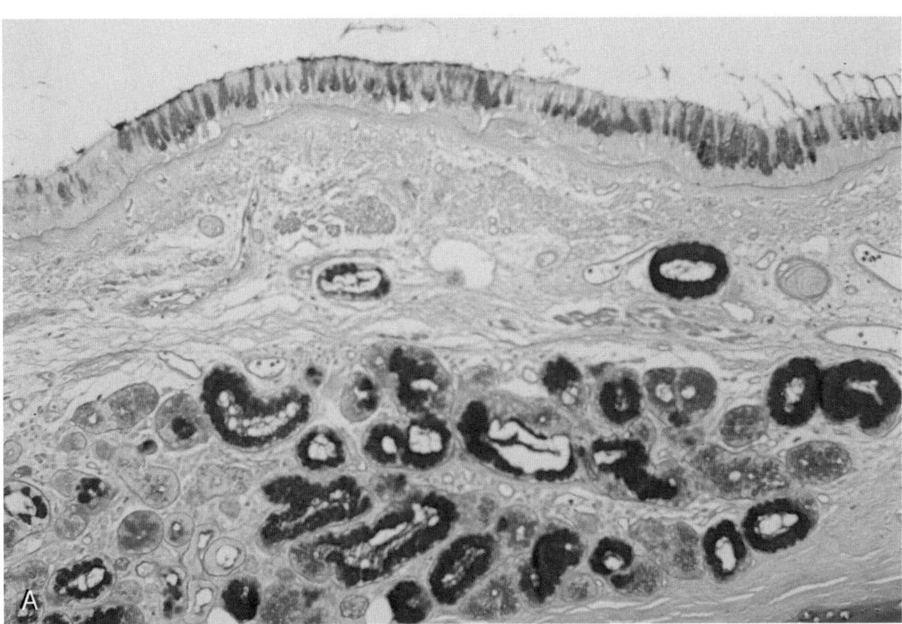

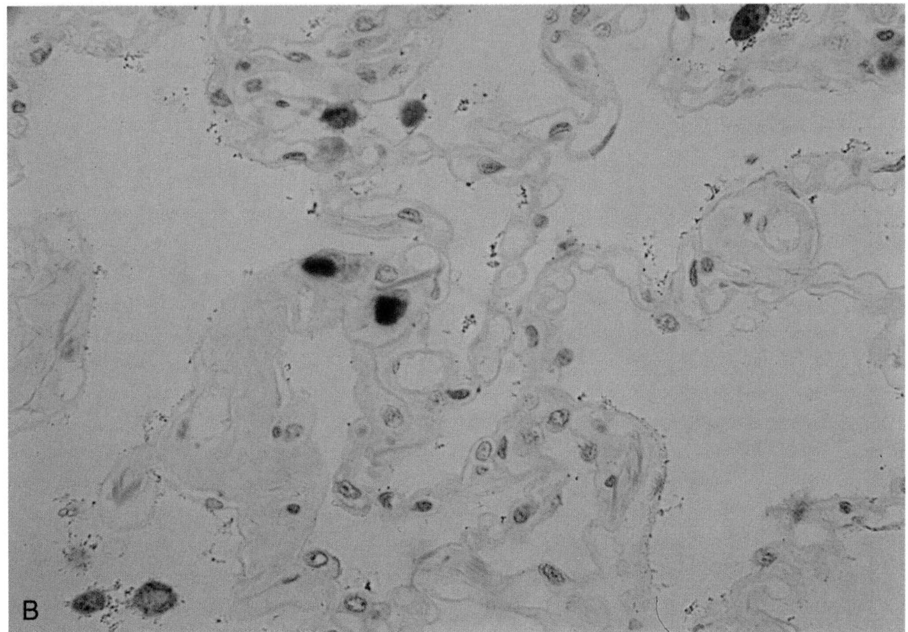

The use of supplementary morphologic techniques. **A,** In formalin-fixed, paraffin-embedded tissue, Alcian blue (pH 2.5)-PAS histochemical staining identifies cells containing both acidic (blue) and neutral (magenta) mucins. **B,** Enzyme histochemistry detects chymase-containing mast cells (blue) in alveolar septa and spaces (glycomethacrylate-embedded tissue).

Illustration continued on following page.

MICROSCOPIC EXAMINATION OF THE RESPIRATORY SYSTEM

SUPPLEMENTARY TECHNIQUES

In Situ Hybridization

FIGURE 1–12

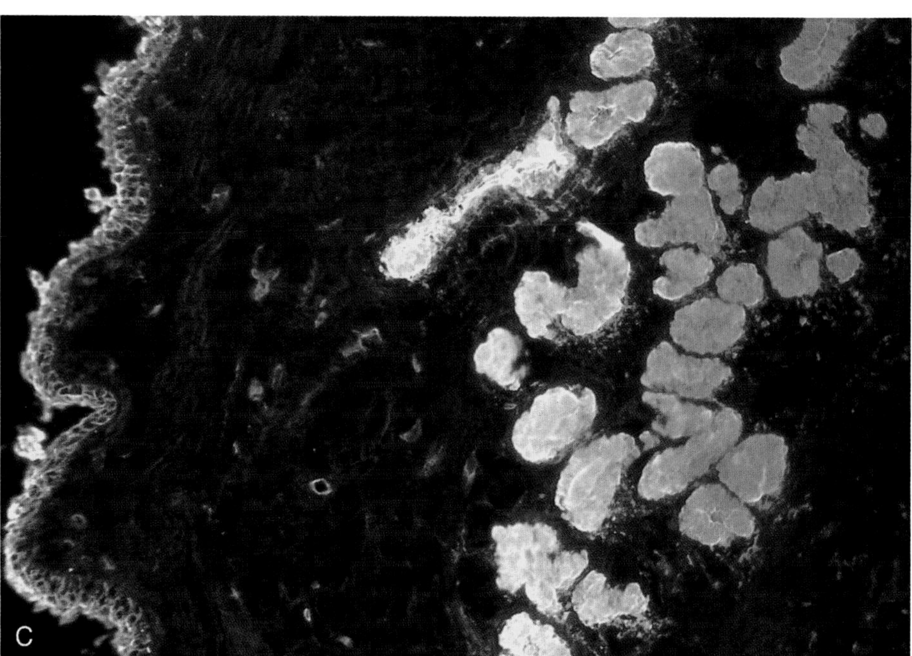

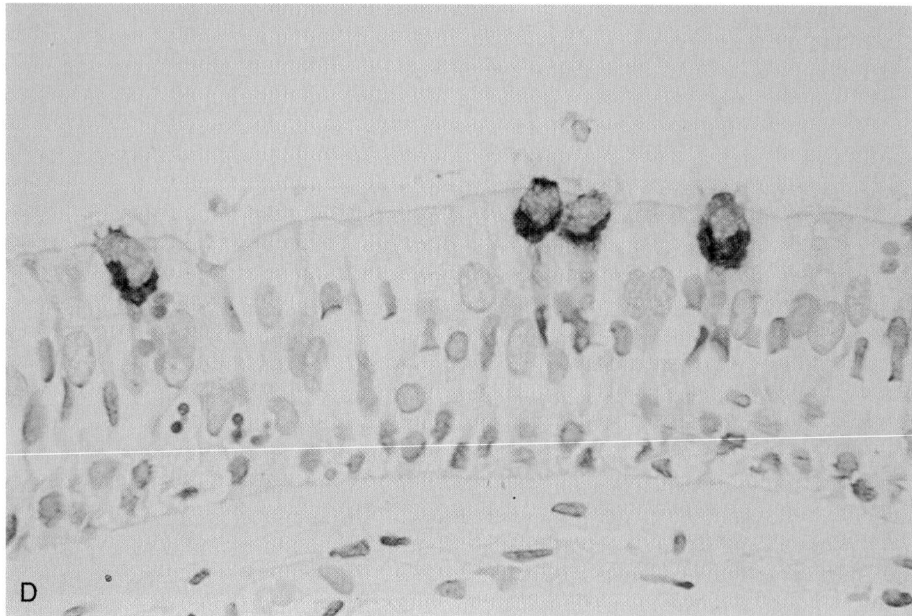

The use of supplementary morphologic techniques *(continued)* **C,** Immunofluorescence microscopy performed on a fixed, frozen section with a mouse hybridoma antibody (B3E8) raised against human mucus.[22] The sites of antibody binding to the luminal surface and tracheobronchial glands are detected using goat anti-mouse IgG-fluorescein isothiocyanate. **D,** Light microscopic immunohistochemistry using avidin-biotin with peroxidase in glycol methacrylate-embedded tissue. In this example, a monoclonal antibody (B8E10) raised against human airway mucus identifies specific human tracheobronchial surface epithelial goblet cells.[22]

MICROSCOPIC EXAMINATION OF THE RESPIRATORY SYSTEM

SUPPLEMENTARY TECHNIQUES

In Situ Hybridization

FIGURE 1–12

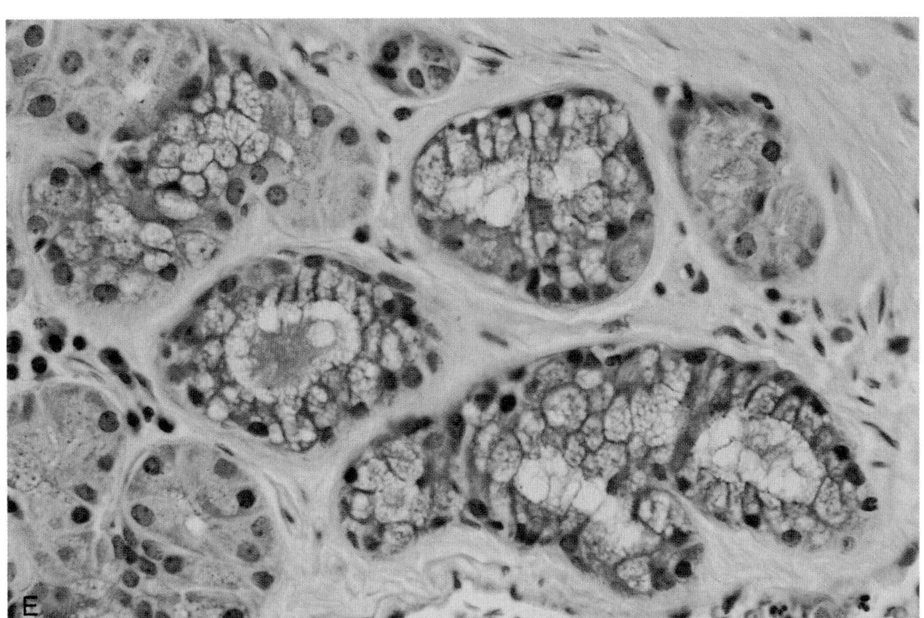

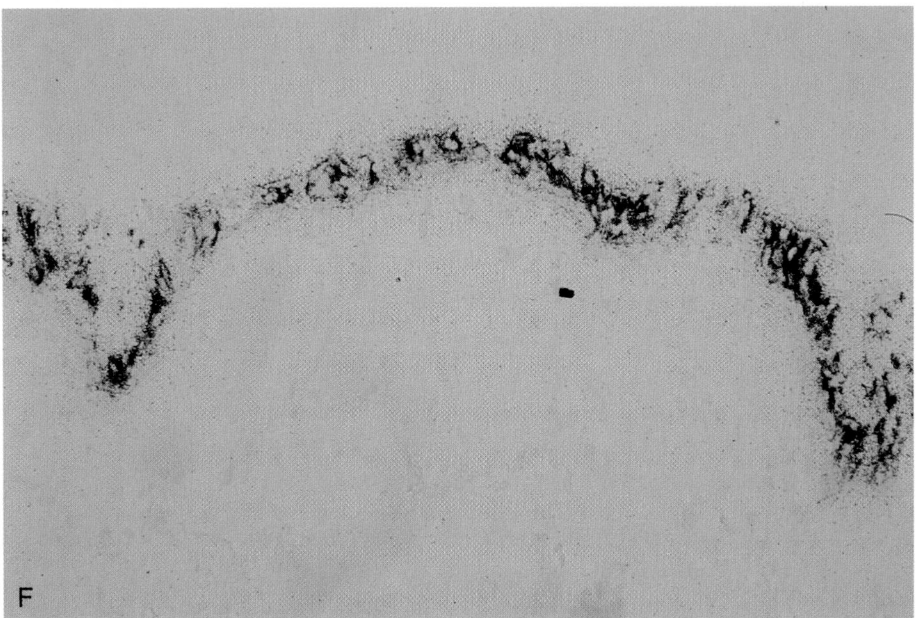

The use of supplementary morphologic techniques *(continued)* **E,** The lectin DBA (*Dolichos biflorus*) recognizes a saccharide structure present in secretions of mucous gland cells. In this example of bronchus embedded in paraffin, alkaline phosphatase conjugated to the lectin is evident as red staining within the mucous gland cell secretory granules and secretory ducts. **F,** In situ hybridization in paraffin-embedded bronchus using ^{35}S as a label to detect upregulated MUC2 RNA in surface epithelial goblet cells of a patient with cystic fibrosis.

Illustration continued on following page.

MICROSCOPIC EXAMINATION OF THE RESPIRATORY SYSTEM

SUPPLEMENTARY TECHNIQUES

In Situ Hybridization

FIGURE 1-12

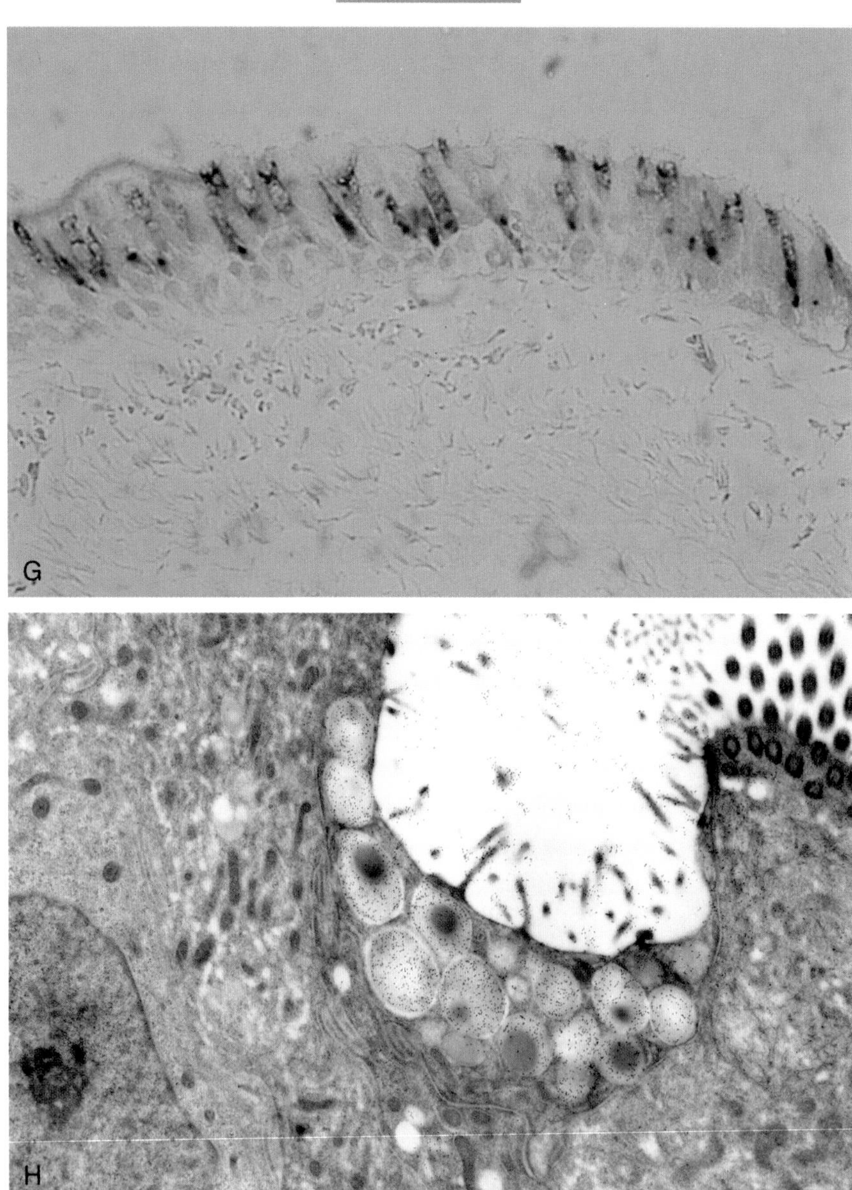

The use of supplementary morphologic techniques *(continued)* **G,** In situ hybridization using digoxigenin as a label to detect MUC5AC in the bronchial goblet cells of a patient with chronic bronchitis. **H,** Immunoelectron microscopy using colloidal gold to localize antibody B5D5 in goblet cell secretory granules.[23]

MICROSCOPIC EXAMINATION OF THE RESPIRATORY SYSTEM

SUPPLEMENTARY TECHNIQUES

In Situ Hybridization

FIGURE 1-12

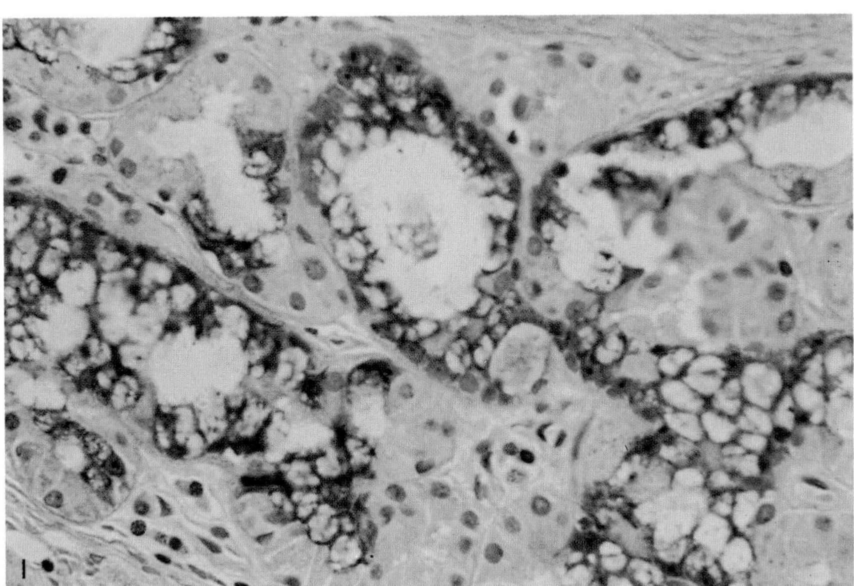

The use of supplementary morphologic techniques *(continued)* **I,** Immunohistochemistry and in situ hybridization on the same paraffin-embedded tissue section using two different colored labels. The red alkaline phosphatase product identifies the lectin DBA in mucous gland cells. The dark grains of silver-enhanced immunogold identify MUC5B in the same cells.

MICROSCOPIC EXAMINATION OF THE RESPIRATORY SYSTEM

SUPPLEMENTARY TECHNIQUES

Microscopic Autoradiography

FIGURE 1–13

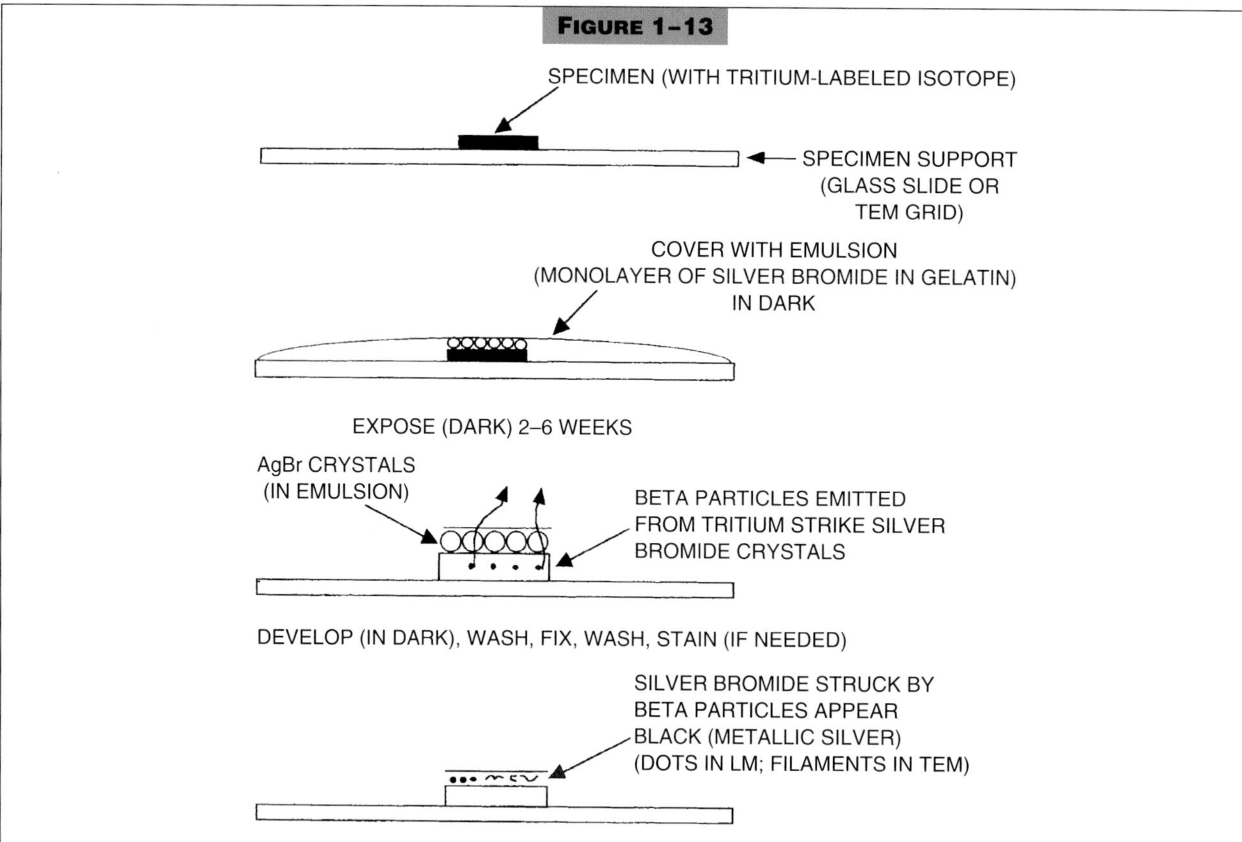

Important steps in the preparation of an autoradiograph for light or transmission electron microscopy. The radiolabel is administered to small experimental animals such as mice or rats orally or by injection. Alternatively, in vitro labeling can be achieved in organ or cell cultures by introducing radiolabeled precursor molecules or tracers into the nutrient media. After appropriate intervals, specimens are prepared for light or electron microscopy. In a darkroom, a thin layer of photographic emulsion (silver halide crystals in gelatin) is layered over the tissue section. At sites of radioactive decay, β particles pass through the emulsion producing a latent image by converting a portion of a silver halide crystal to metallic silver. After an appropriate exposure, the coated tissue section is developed chemically to convert the entire silver halide crystal hit by radiation into metallic silver. The removal of unexposed crystals as silver thiosulfate complexes with a photographic fixer leaves a pattern of metallic silver grains as the true image. The silver grains overlie sites on the tissue section. Standard staining techniques can be applied to the tissue to provide a morphologic backdrop on which the radiolabeled molecule is localized. Histoautoradiography has a resolution of 0.1 μm, adequate for light microscopy. For precise localization at the levels that can be achieved with the electron microscope, statistical analysis is required.[24] (From Kessel RG: Basic Medical Histology. New York, Oxford University Press, 1998, p. 8.)

MICROSCOPIC EXAMINATION OF THE RESPIRATORY SYSTEM

SUPPLEMENTARY TECHNIQUES

Microscopic Autoradiography

The procedure of microscopic autoradiography allows the localization of sites of radioactivity within tissue sections. Because it is a good emitter of β particles, tritium (^3H) is the most commonly used isotope in microscopic autoradiography. Radiolabel can be incorporated into macromolecules or small molecular weight compounds or target tracers. TABLE 1–10 lists some experimental uses of microscopic autoradiography.

FIGURE 1–14

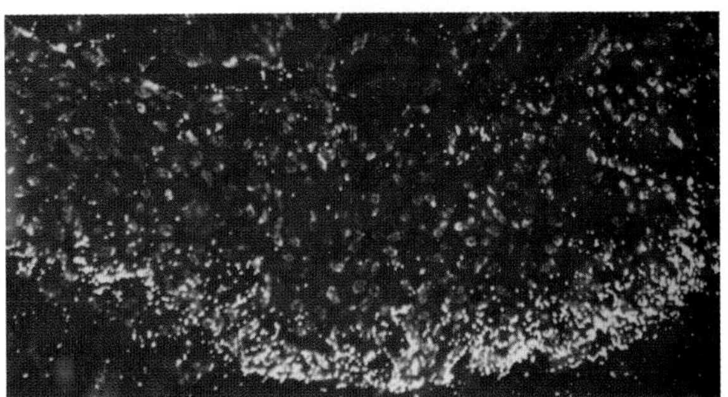

Darkfield micrograph showing distribution of muscarinic receptors in tracheal smooth muscle as detected by microscopic autoradiography using a radiolabeled muscarinic antagonist, [^{3}H]propylbenzylcholine. Autoradiographic silver grains indicating binding sites are clustered at the adventitial surface. (From Basbaum CB, Grillo MA, Widdicombe JH: Muscarinic receptors: Evidence for a nonuniform distribution in tracheal smooth muscle and exocrine glands. J Neurosci 4:508–520, 1984.)

TABLE 1–10

Experimental Uses of Microscopic Autoradiology

Research Purpose	Radiolabeled Compounds
NUCLEIC ACIDS	
DNA synthesis/ cell proliferation	[^{3}H]-thymidine
RNA synthesis	[^{3}H]-uridine
OTHER MACROMOLECULES	
Proteins	
- Secretory granules	[^{3}H]-glycine; [^{3}H]-leucine, etc
- Collagen	[^{3}H]-proline; [^{3}H]-hydroxyproline
Carbohydrates	
- Simple polysaccharides	[^{3}H]-glucose; [^{3}H]-glucosamine
- Complex glycoconjugates	[$^{35}SO_4$]
Lipids	[^{3}H]-glycerol; [^{3}H]-fatty acids, etc
TRACERS AND SMALL MOLECULES	
Hormones	[^{3}H]-steroids; [^{3}H]-insulin, etc
Neurotransmitters	[^{3}H]-GABA; [^{3}H]-dopamine, etc
Receptors (density/distribution)	[^{3}H]-receptor antagonist
Vitamins	[^{3}H]-vitamin
Inorganic substances	[^{22}Na]Cl; [^{45}Ca]Cl_2; [^{203}Hg]Cl_2; etc
Drugs	[^{3}H]-antibiotics, [^{14}C]-aspirin; etc
Toxins	[^{3}H]-ouabain; [^{3}H]-strychnine; etc

Source: Modified from Nagata T: Techniques and application of microscopic radioautography, Histo Histopatho 12: 1091–1124, 1997.

MICROSCOPIC EXAMINATION OF THE RESPIRATORY SYSTEM

SUPPLEMENTARY TECHNIQUES

Laser Capture Microdissection

FIGURE 1–15

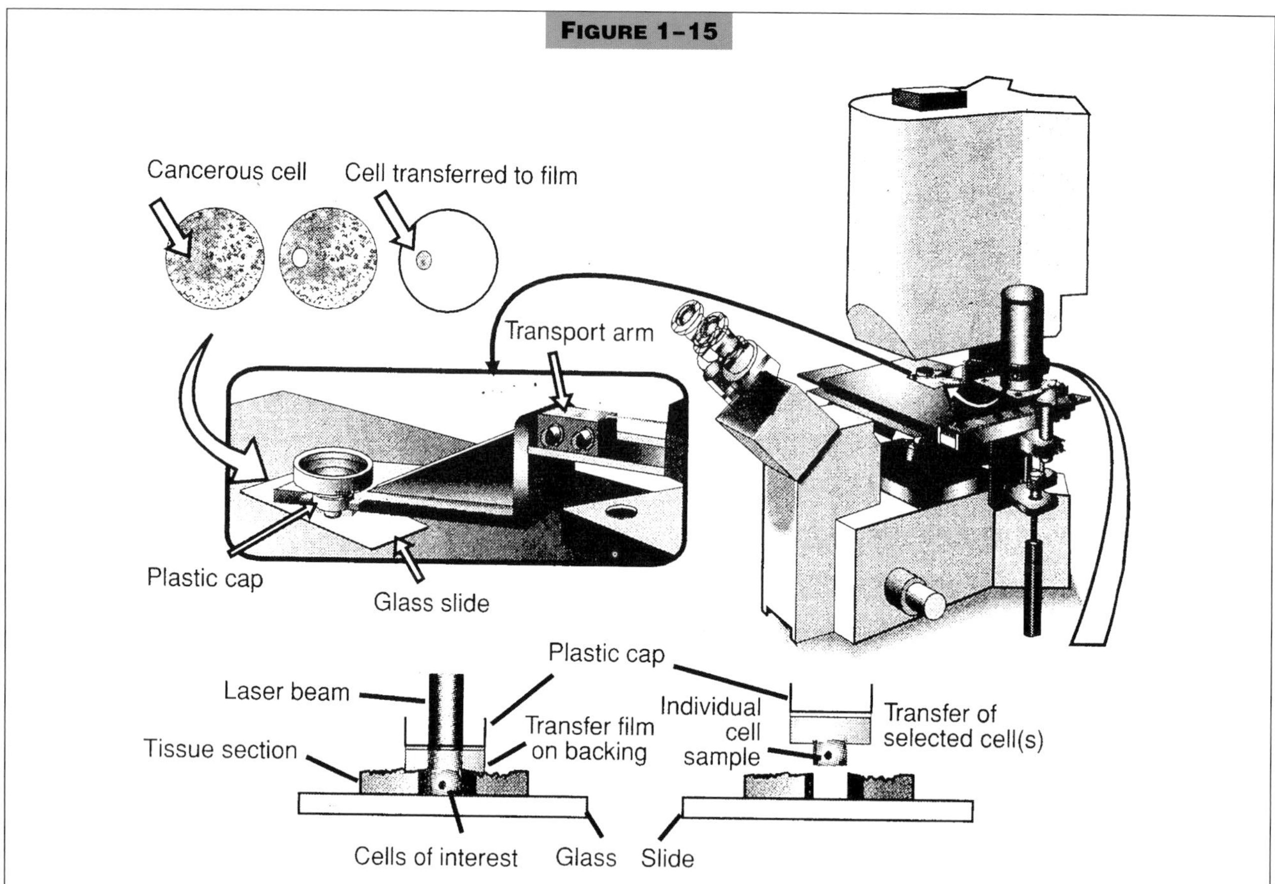

Laser capture microdissection system. Laser capture microdissection provides a method for obtaining specific cells from tissue sections.[25, 26] Once an area of interest is identified with the specialized microscope, a pulsed laser beam activates a thermal polymer transfer film that fuses to the target area. The transfer film with the bonded region is lifted off the tissue section, leaving unwanted tissue on the glass slide. The targeted cells are held in a transparent vial cap, and the cap is placed onto a processing vial where isolation of DNA, RNA, or protein can be initiated. The starting tissue may be embedded in paraffin or frozen and stained to facilitate cell selection. Targeting precision of 1 μm with targeted spots as small as 3 to 5 μm have been achieved. (From Bonner RF: Laser capture microdissection: Molecular analysis of tissue. Science 278:1481–1483, 1997.)

MICROSCOPIC EXAMINATION OF THE RESPIRATORY SYSTEM

SPECIALIZED TECHNIQUES FOR ELECTRON MICROSCOPY

Specialized techniques for electron microscopy and their use. Transmission electron microscopy of thin sections provides excellent resolution of two-dimensional cell structure; however, in the absence of laborious reconstruction from serial sections, do not depict three-dimensional relationships. The scanning electron microscope provides 300 to 500 times the depth of field of the light microscope allowing three-dimensional study of surfaces but not of internal structures. The high-voltage electron microscope can be used to examine thicker sections than the standard transmission microscope. Thus, these instruments can reveal spatial information about internal cell structure. Unfortunately, high voltage electron microscopes are extremely expensive and available to very few investigators. Fortunately, the techniques listed in TABLE 1–11 provide the transmission electron microscopist with several ways to obtain high resolution images that convey three-dimensional information of subcellular structure.

TABLE 1–11

Specialized Techniques Used in Electron Microscopy

Technique	Use and/or Advantage
Metal shadowing	High resolution study of surfaces with three-dimensional effect
Freeze-fracture	Visualizing interior of cell membranes
Freeze-etch	Determining three-dimensional organization of the exterior and interior cell structures
Negative staining	Viewing large macromolecules, e.g., subunit structure of proteins
Cryoelectron microscopy	Viewing without fixation, staining, or dehydrating providing high resolution of small structures without tissue processing artifacts

FIGURE 1–16

(a) Cell or tissue is frozen in nitrogen
(b) Fracture ruptures the cell
(c) Etching: surface ic
is removed by sublimation
Exposed nuclear membrane with membrane proteins and particles
Carbon
(d) Carbon is added to form a continuous surface
Platinum
(e) Surface is shadowed with a thin layer of platinum
(f) Tissue is dissolved with acid; carbon-metal replica can be viewed under the electron microscope

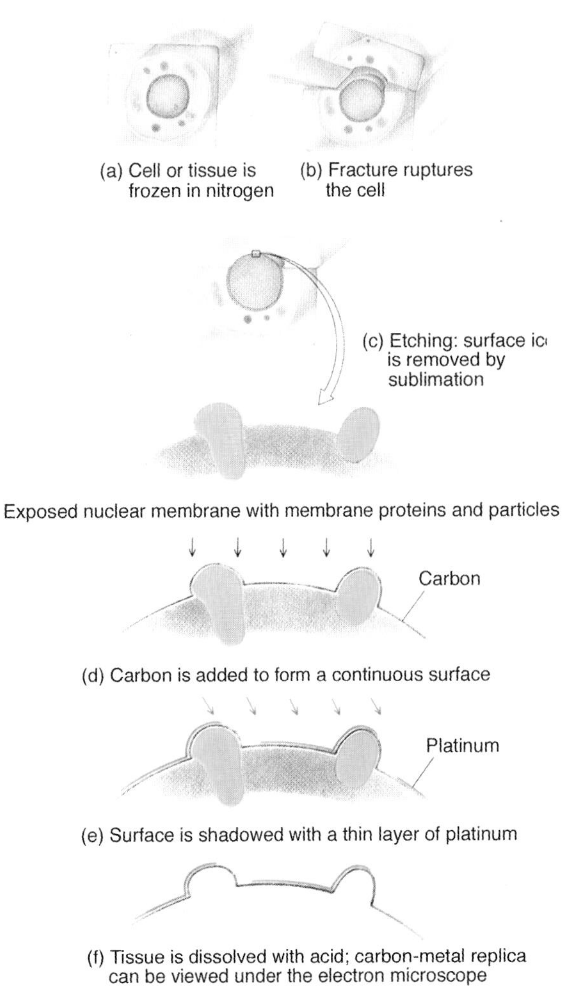

Preparation of freeze-fracture, deep-etched image of a cell: (a) the sample is quickly frozen in liquid nitrogen at −196°C, which instantly immobilizes cell structures. (b) A cold knife is used to fracture the sample. (c) In a vacuum, the surface ice is removed from the sample by sublimation (deep-etching). (d) A thin layer of carbon is evaporated onto the sample surface producing a carbon replica. (e) The specimen is shadowed with platinum. (f) The organic material is dissolved with acid leaving a carbon-metal replica of the tissue that can be examined using an electron microscope. (From Lodish H, Baltimore D, Berk A, et al: Molecular Cell Biology, 3rd ed. New York, Scientific American Books, 1995.)

MICROSCOPIC EXAMINATION OF THE RESPIRATORY SYSTEM

SPECIALIZED TECHNIQUES FOR ELECTRON MICROSCOPY

FIGURE 1–17

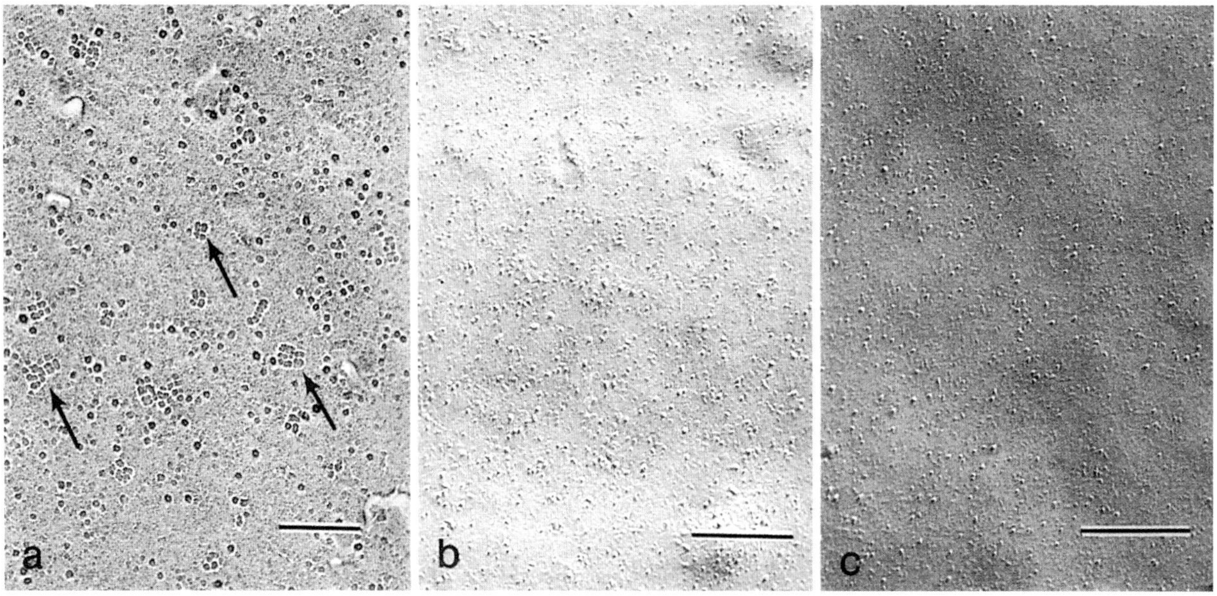

Freeze-fracture, rotary shadowed images of the lateral (a), basal (b), and apical (c) plasma membranes of tracheal ciliated epithelial cells. The lateral portion of the plasma membrane contains specific water channels that are seen as square arrays (*arrows*) while the basal and apical epithelium do not. Scale bars = 200 nm. (From Widdicombe JH, Coleman DL, Finkbeiner WE, Friend DS: Primary cultures of the dog's tracheal epithelium: Fine structure, fluid, and electrolyte transport. Cell Tissue Res 247: 95–103, 1987.)

MICROSCOPIC EXAMINATION OF THE RESPIRATORY SYSTEM

SPECIALIZED TECHNIQUES FOR ELECTRON MICROSCOPY

Analytical electron microscopes allow identification of a wide range of inorganic fibers and particulates, and therefore are of great value in the analysis of mineral dusts, e.g., within lung tissue in suspected cases of pneumoconiosis.[27] TABLE 1–12 lists a number of analytical methods and applications.

TABLE 1–12

Analytical Methods Used in Electron Microscopy

Method	Applications and Limitations	Examples of Actual or Potential Uses
Bulk (macroanalytic) techniques	Localization of particle not usually possible; sample generally destroyed	Identification of quartz polymorphs; sometimes specific identification of silicates
X-ray diffraction	Qualitative, quantitative; overlapping silicate peaks are a problem; can be used with as little as 100 ng of sample; can identify elements, minerals, and polymorphs of minerals	—
X-ray fluorescence	Qualitative, quantitative	Chemical composition of fly ash
Atomic absorption spectroscopy*	Very sensitive for trace elements (down to 0.003 ppm); not all elements identifiable	Analysis of beryllium content
Neutron activation analysis	Relatively high sensitivity (to about 10 ppm) for trace elements; not all elements identifiable; requires on-site nuclear reactor	Largely used for tracers in experimental animal work
Proton-induced x-ray emission spectroscopy	Element detection down to 1 to 10 ppm	—
Microanalytic techniques	Identification of specific particle at least theoretically possible; tissue section or digested specimen can be used	—
Energy-dispersive x-ray spectroscopy*	Equipment available in many labs; very high resolution (depending on electron microscope) and provides simultaneous analysis of all elements; most systems do not detect elements lighter than sodium	Widely used for analysis of asbestos fibers; also good for identification of other silicates
Wavelength-dispersive x-ray spectroscopy	Good resolution (depending on instrument); can detect all elements; slow	Able to identify light elements such as beryllium
Electron energy loss spectroscopy	Deflects light elements in thin sections	Potentially useful for identification of beryllium and other light elements in EM sections
Laser Raman spectroscopy	Detects down to picogram amounts of individual elements; resolution limited to particles several microns and up	Has been used to detect quartz, calcite, and rutile in tissue sections
Auger electron spectroscopy	Detects light elements; also good for analysis of materials on particle surfaces	—
Secondary ion or laser microprobe mass spectroscopy	Sensitivity for trace elements in ppm range. Resolution 0.5–1 μm	Has been used for in situ beryllium analysis and element mapping
Electron diffraction	Identification of individual crystals of any size; time-consuming and often difficult to interpret	Confirmation of particle identification when chemical composition alone is not sufficient

* Commonly available techniques. EM = electron microscope.

Source: Modified from Churg A, Green FHY: Analytic methods for identifying and quantifying mineral particles in lung tissue. *In* Churg A, Green FHY (eds): Pathology of Occupational Lung Disease (2nd ed). Baltimore, Williams & Wilkins, 1998.

FLOW CYTOMETRY, IMAGE ANALYSIS, AND STEREOLOGY

Similar to a flow cytometer, the laser scanning cytometer measures laser excited fluorescence at multiple wavelengths and light scatter from cells. However, the laser scanning cytometer can obtain these measurements from cells on microscopic slides. Thus it provides both a visual and spectral analysis at higher resolution than the flow cytometer. TABLE 1–13 lists some uses of the laser scanning cytometer.

TABLE 1–13

Uses of the Laser Scanning Cytometer

- DNA ploidy analysis
- DNA analysis of complex aneuploid specimens (when combined with FISH)
- Immunophenotyping
- Analysis of cell proliferation
- Analysis of apoptosis
- Cytotoxic drug targeting assays

FIGURE 1–18

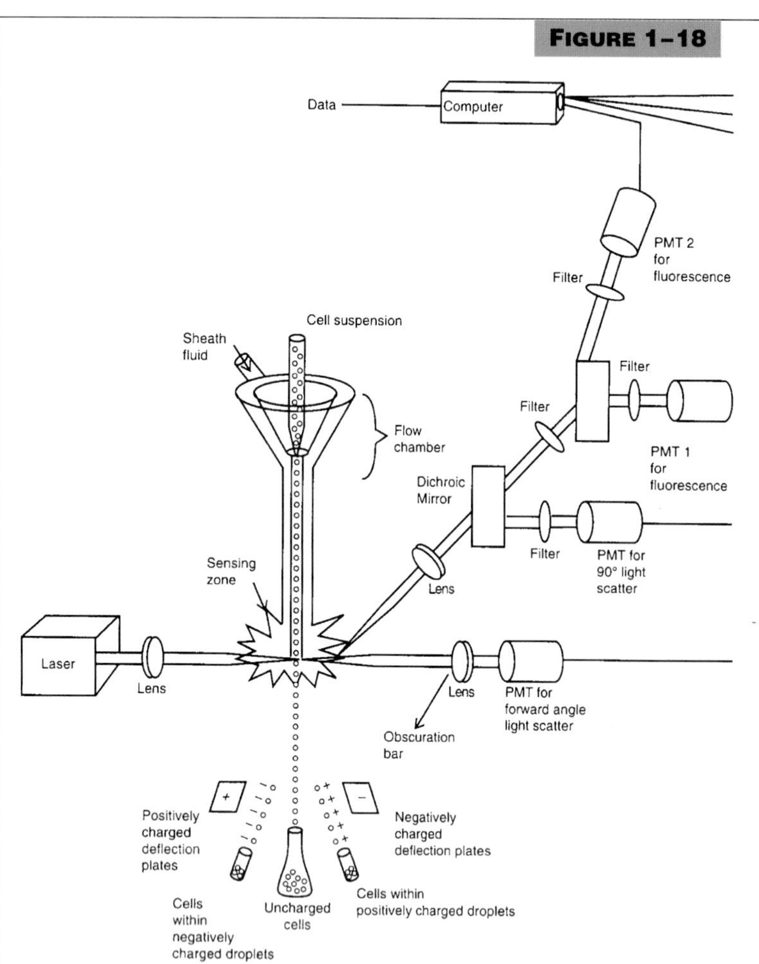

Components of a flow cytometer and cell sorter. The analysis of how cells flowing in single file interact with a focused beam of light is the basis for flow cytometry. The light is an approximately 650 μm-in-diameter beam generated from a laser (argon or krypton) or high-pressure vapor lamp (mercury, xenon). The analytical instrumentation measures electrical resistance, light scatter, and fluorescence. Data collected as analog signals is converted to digital signals, amplified and stored either as histograms or preferably as a list (listmode) that allows additional data analysis. Electrical resistance measurements provide a determination of cell volume. Light scatter, both forward angle scatter and scatter at right angles (side scatter), provides data on sample particle size and granularity, respectively, and can be used to distinguish some cell types. Cytochemically bound fluorescent dyes (fluorochromes) of different wavelengths conjugated with specific monoclonal antibodies or used alone provide additional information for cell phenotyping or measurement of RNA content, DNA content (ploidy), cell proliferation, and cell death (apoptosis).

Flow cytometers may also be used to sort cells based on technology that allows the formation of single cell-containing droplets and electrostatic deflection of droplets based on discrimination of measurable cell parameters. Fluorescently stained cells are passed through a focused laser beam, and the generated light scatters. Fluorescence emission signals are sensed, digitized, and displayed as frequency distributions. After the sensing area, the fluid stream breaks up into uniform droplets generated by a piezoelectric transducer. Sorting is accomplished by selectively charging the fluid stream (positively or negatively for the two defined sorting windows) with an electrode, exactly at the moment that the cell of interest is about to pinch off into a droplet. Charged droplets are consequently deflected in an electric field downstream and collected. The example shown allows detection of forward-angle light scatter and one fluorescence parameter. Extensions may include the counter sensor or additional photomultipliers for measurements of multicolor fluorescence or for perpendicular light scatter. (PMT = photomultiplier tube) (From Ward KM, Lehmann CA, Leiken AM: Clinical Laboratory Instrumentation and Automation; Principles, Applications, and Selection. Philadelphia, WB Saunders, 1994, p. 75.)

FLOW CYTOMETRY, IMAGE ANALYSIS, AND STEREOLOGY

FIGURE 1-19

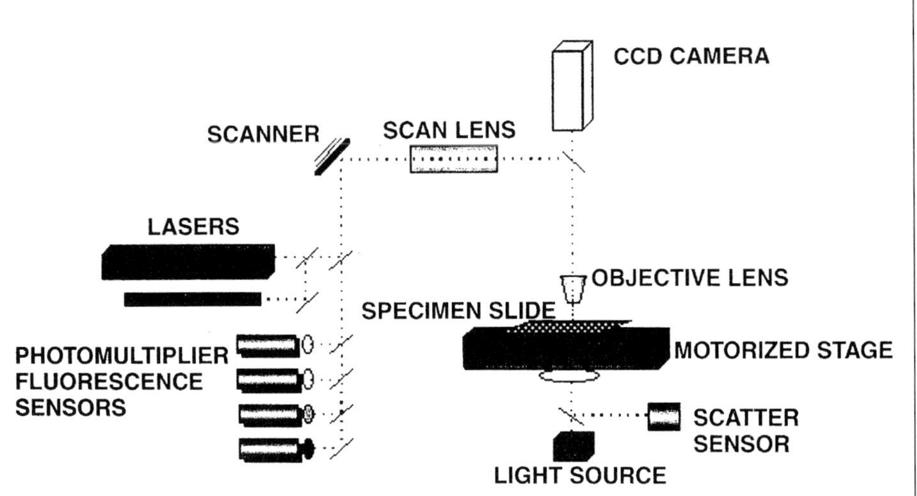

Diagram of the optical arrangement of the laser scanning cytometer. In this example, the laser scanning cytometer accommodates two lasers and four photomultiplier tubes. The image from the CCD camera is linked to a computer. (CCD = closed circuit device.) (From Kamentsky LA, et al: Slide-based laser scanning cytometry. Acta Cytol 41:123–143, 1997.)

FIGURE 1-20

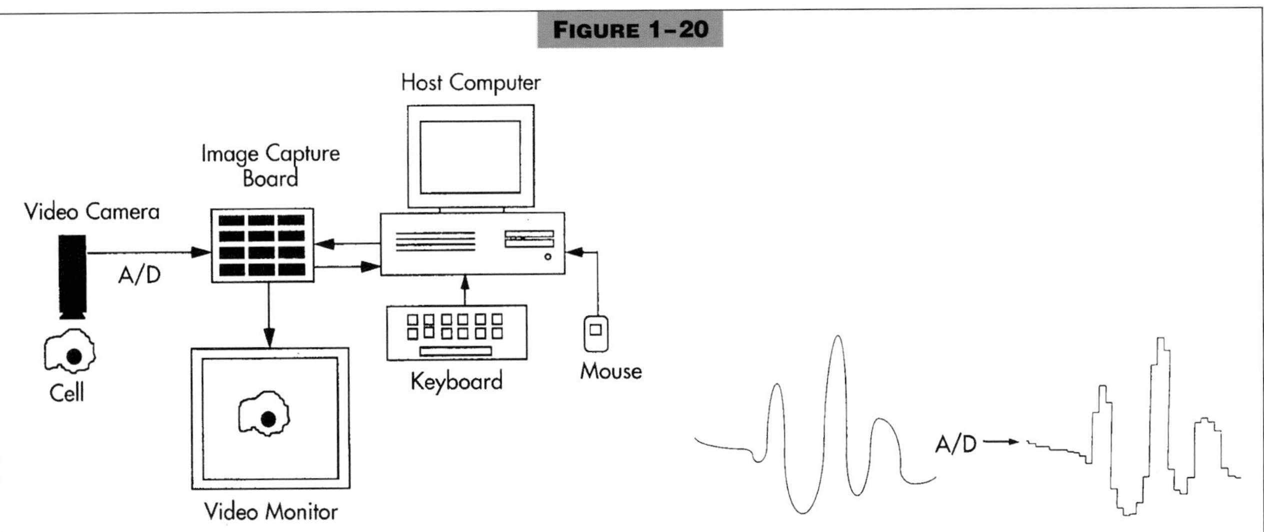

Components of an image analysis system. Image analysis, or image cytometry, refers to the quantitative measurement of morphologic features of cells or tissues on microscopic slides, and as such, complements flow cytometry and laser scanning cytometry. A variety of different parameters such as laser-induced fluorescence, stoichiometric binding of dyes, enzymatic reduction of chromogens may be quantified and thus, compared among clinical or experimental samples.[28] The typical image analysis system is based on capture of an image with a camera and conversion of the analog image to a digital image. The digital image can be analyzed using specifically designed computer software.

FLOW CYTOMETRY, IMAGE ANALYSIS, AND STEREOLOGY

Stereologic techniques provide methods to determine geometric characteristics including length, surface area, volume, number, and connectivity of three-dimensional objects. Classical stereologic methods for estimating particle number and size have relied on biased assumptions about particle shape, size, and orientation.[29] However, the so-called "new stereology" techniques introduced beginning in 1984 provide efficient and unbiased design-based methods through the use of the disector and optical sectioning techniques.[34–36] These methods may be applied to the respiratory system from the level of gross anatomy down to subcellular structure.

TABLE 1–14

Useful Cellular Parameters Measured by Image Analysis

Morphometry
- Nuclear diameter, circumference, area
- Cytoplasmic diameter, circumference, area
- Nuclear shape (roundness, contour index)
- Ratio nucleus to cytoplasm area
- Distance (thickness, vessel caliber)
- Fractal dimension (architectural complexity)
- Texture (chromatin)
- Percentage positivity (immunohistochemistry, in situ hybridization)

Counting
- Number of cells or nuclei
- Grains (autoradiography, in situ hybridization)

Optical Density
- Sum optical density (for DNA by Feulgen stain)
- Average optical density
- Standard deviation (texture)

Source: Modified from Weinberg DS, Carey JL: Flow and imaging cytology. *In* Damjanov I, Linder J (eds): Anderson's Pathology. St. Louis, Mosby, 1996.

TABLE 1–15

Stereologic Techniques

Technique	Measure Estimate or Use	Reference
IUR plane sample*	Length	30
Vertical sections	Surface area	31
Cavalieri's direct estimator	Volume	30
Star volume	Volume of complex structures	32
Point sample intercept	Volume weighted average volume	32
Orientator	Making isotropic sections	33
Disector	Uniform sampling	34
Optical disector	Uniform sampling in one microscopic section	35
Selector	Mean particle volume in a disector of unknown thickness	36
Nucleator	Mean particle volume; spatial distribution	37
Fractionator	Counting	38

* IUR = isotropic, uniformly and randomly distributed.

REFERENCES

1. Thurlbeck WM: Examination of the lung: Autopsy. *In* Thurlbeck WM, Churg AM (eds): Pathology of the Lung (2nd ed). New York, Thieme Medical Publishers, 1995, pp 129–136.

2. Heard BE: Pathology of pulmonary emphysema: Methods of study. Am Rev Respir Dis 82:792–799, 1960.

3. Sills B: A multidisciplinary method for study of lung structure and function. Am Rev Respir Dis 86:238–245, 1962.

4. Markarian B: A simple method of inflation-fixation and air drying of lungs. Am J Clin Pathol 63:20–24, 1975.

5. Gough J, Wentworth JE: The use of thin sections of entire organs in morbid anatomical studies. J Roy Micros Soc 69:231–235, 1949.

6. Whimster WF: Rapid giant paper sections of the lungs. Thorax 24:737–741, 1969.

7. Gevenois PA, Koob M-C, Jacobovitz D, et al: Whole lung sections for computed tomographic-pathologic correlation. Invest Radiol 28:242–246, 1993.

8. Gevenois PA, Zanen J, De Maertelaer V, et al: Macroscopic assessment of lung emphysema by image analysis. J Clin Pathol 48:318–322, 1995.

9. Whimster WF: Techniques for the examination of excised lungs. Hum Pathol 1:305–314, 1970.

10. Nadel JA, Wolfe WG, Graf PD: Powdered tantalum as a medium for bronchography in canine and human lungs. Invest Radiol 3:229–238, 1968.

11. Pearse AGE: Histochemistry, Theoretical and Applied (4th ed). Edinburgh, Churchill Livingstone, 1980.

12. Filipe MI, Lake BD: Histochemistry in Pathology. Edinburgh, Churchill Livingstone, 1983.

13. Spicer SS: Histochemistry in Pathologic Diagnosis. New York, Marcel Dekker, 1987.

14. Bancroft JD, Stevens A: Theory and Practice of Histological Techniques (4th ed). New York, Churchill Livingstone, 1996.

15. Beckstead JH: Histochemistry. *In* Damjanov I, Linder J (eds): Anderson's Pathology (10th ed). St. Louis, CV Mosby, 1996, pp 176–189.

16. Taylor CR, Cote RJ: Immunomicroscopy: A Diagnostic Tool for the Surgical Pathologist (2nd ed). Philadelphia, WB Saunders, 1994.

17. Cote RJ, Taylor CR: Immunohistochemistry and related marking techniques. *In* Damjanov I, Linder J (eds): Anderson's Pathology (10th ed). St. Louis, CV Mosby, 1996, pp 136–175.

18. Sternberger LA, Hardy PH, Cuculis JJ, et al: The unlabeled antibody-enzyme method of immunohistochemistry: Preparation and properties of soluble antigen-antibody complex (horseradish peroxidase-anti-horseradish peroxidase) and its use in identification of spirochetes. J Histochem Cytochem 18:315–333, 1970.

19. Guesdon JL, Ternynck T, Aurameas S: The use of avidin-biotin interaction in immunoenzyme techniques. J Histochem Cytochem 27:1131–1139, 1978.

20. Hsu SM, Raine L: Protein A, avidin and biotin in immunohistochemistry. J Histochem Cytochem 11:1349–1353, 1981.

21. Nuovo GJ: PCR in situ Hybridization: Protocols and Applications (3rd ed). Philadelphia, Lippincott-Raven, 1997.

22. Finkbeiner WE, Basbaum CB: Monoclonal antibodies directed against human airway secretions: Localization and characterization of antigens. Am J Pathol 131:290–297, 1988.

23. Yamaya M, Finkbeiner WE, Chun SY, et al: Differentiated structure and function of cultures from human tracheal epithelium. Am J Physiol 262 (Lung Cell Mol Physiol 6):L713–L724, 1992.

24. Padykula HA: Histochemistry and cytochemistry. *In* Weiss L (ed): Cell and Tissue Biology (6th ed). Baltimore, Urban & Schwarzenberg, 1988.

25. Bonner RF, Emmert-Buck M, Cole K, et al: Laser capture microdissection: Molecular analysis of tissue. Science 278:1481–1483, 1997.

26. Simone NL, Bonner RF, Gillespie JW, et al: Laser-capture microdissection: Opening the microscopic frontier to molecular analysis. Trends Genet 14:272–276, 1998.

27. Churg A, Green FHY: Analytic methods for identifying and quantifying mineral particles in lung tissue. *In* Churg A, Green FHY (eds): Pathology of Occupational Lung Disease (2nd ed). Baltimore, Williams & Wilkins, 1998, pp 45–55.

28. Frierson HF Jr, Linder J: Flow and image cytometry. *In* Silverberg SG (ed): Principles and Practice of Surgical Pathology and Cytopathology. New York, Churchill Livingstone, 1997, pp 95–111.

29. Mayhew TM, Gundersen HJG: 'If you assume, you can make an ass out of u and me': A decade of the disector for stereological counting of particles in 3D space. J Anat 188:1–15, 1996.

30. Gundersen HJG, Bendtsen TF, Korbo L, et al: Some new, simple and efficient sterological methods and their use in pathological research and diagnosis. APMIS 96:379–394, 1988.

31. Baddeley AJ, Gundersen HJG, Cruz-Orive LM: Estimation of surface area from vertical sections. J Microsc 142:259–276, 1986.

32. Gundersen HJG, Jensen EB: Stereological estimation of the volume-weighted mean volume of arbitrary particles observed on random sections. J Microsc 138:127–142, 1985.

33. Mattfeldt T, Mall G, Von Herbay A, et al: Stereological investigation of anisotropic structures with the orientator. Acta Stereol 8:671–676, 1989.

REFERENCES

34. Sterio DC: The unbiased estimation of number and sizes of arbitrary particles using the disector. J Microsc 134:127–136, 1984.

35. Gundersen HJG: Stereology of arbitrary particles. A review of unbiased number and size estimators and the presentation of some new ones, in memory of William R. Thompson. J Microsc 143:3–45, 1986.

36. Cruz-Orive L-M: Particle number can be estimated using a disector of unknown thickness: The selector. J Microsc 145:121–142, 1986.

37. Gundersen HJG, Bagger P, Bendtsen TF, et al: The new stereological tools: Disector, fractionator, nucleator and point sample intercepts and their use in pathological research and diagnosis. APMIS 96:857–881, 1988.

38. Braendgaard H, Gundersen HJG: The impact of recent stereological advances on quantitative studies of the nervous system. J Neurosci Meth 18:39–78, 1986.

Anatomy of the Respiratory System

Jennifer M. Wu, M.D.

and

Walter E. Finkbeiner, M.D., Ph.D.

GROSS ANATOMY

FIGURE 2–1

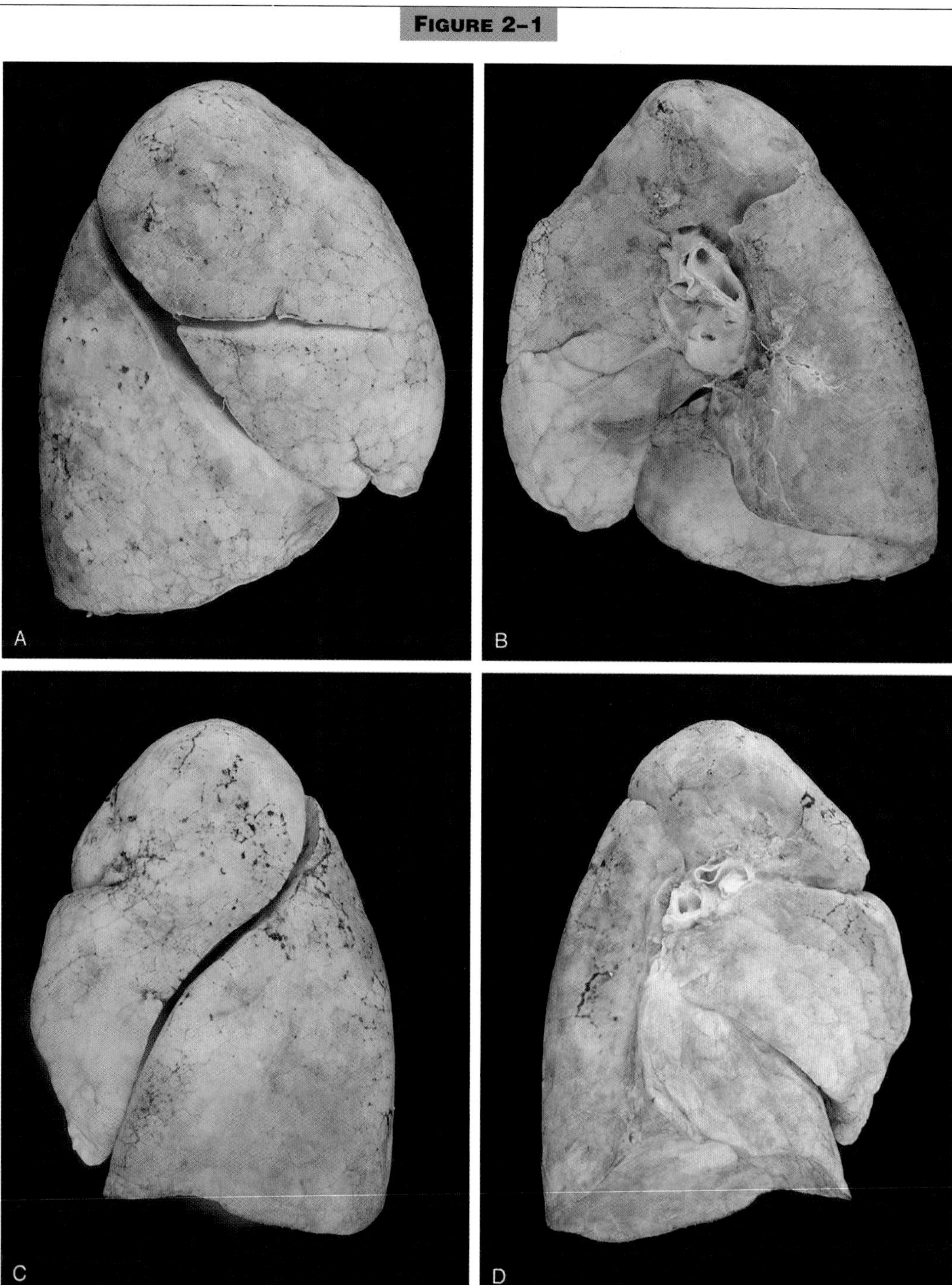

External appearance of inflated human lungs. **A,** Right lung, lateral side. **B,** Right lung, medial side. **C,** Left lung, lateral side. **D,** Left lung, medial side. The lungs are paired organs of respiration, with the right lung weighing 360 to 570 g and the left lung weighing 325 to 480 g. They consist of soft, spongy tissue with a smooth, shiny, pink-to-black mottled surface, depending on the amount of carbon particle deposition. The lungs move freely within the thoracic cavity and are attached at the hila, where the major vessels, nerves, and lymphatics enter the lung. The orientation of the hilar structures varies from right to left, as the pulmonary artery lies anterior to the bronchus on the right and superior to the bronchus on the left.

Each lung is covered by visceral pleura, and this serous membrane reflects over the mediastinum, diaphragm, and chest wall as the parietal pleura. These two layers are in contact with each other around and below the hila and are lubricated by a thin film of pleural fluid within the pleural cavity. In addition, the visceral pleura dips into fissures of the lung that subdivide the right lung into upper, middle, and lower lobes and the left lung into upper and lower lobes.

GROSS ANATOMY

FIGURE 2-2

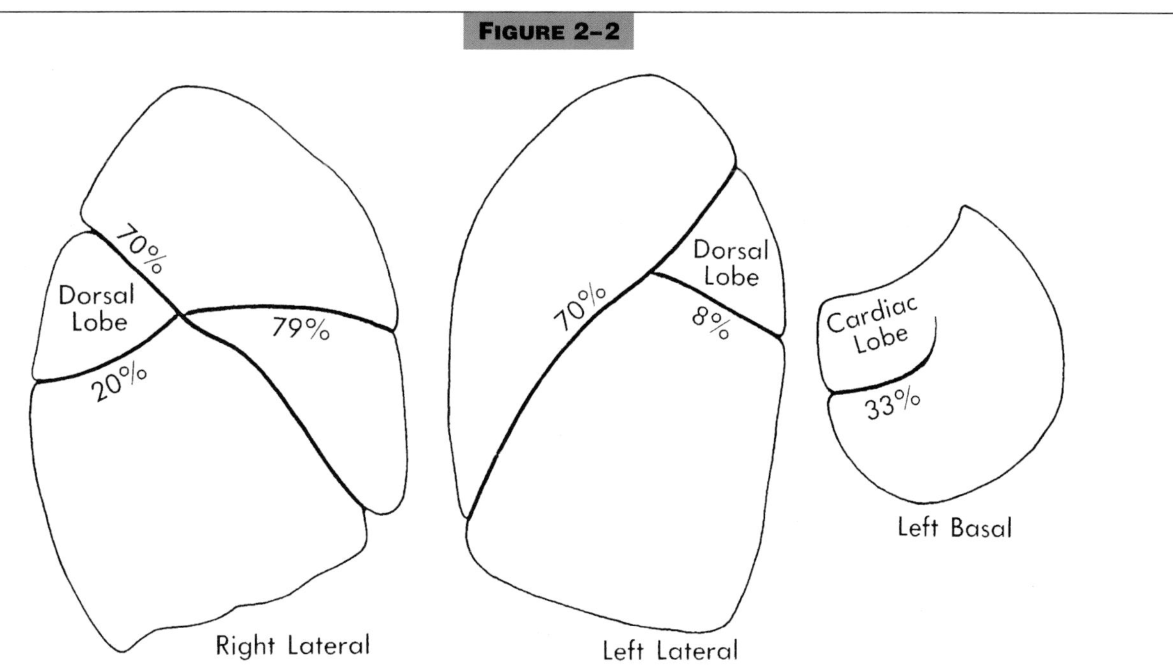

Anomalies of the pulmonary fissures or lobation and the frequency of their occurrences. The pattern and completeness of the pulmonary fissures is variable and generally of no clinical consequence. Variations may be classified into three groups: (1) variations without alteration of the underlying bronchial pattern (supernumerary fissures or lobes); (2) superficial septation produced by an extrinsic blood vessel (azygous lobe); and (3) variations of the bronchial pattern with or without external evidence (left parterial bronchus or tracheal lobes). (From Gray SW, Skandalakis JL: Embryology for Surgeons: The Embryological Basis for the Treatment of Congenital Defects. Philadelphia, WB Saunders, 1972, p. 307.)

FIGURE 2-3

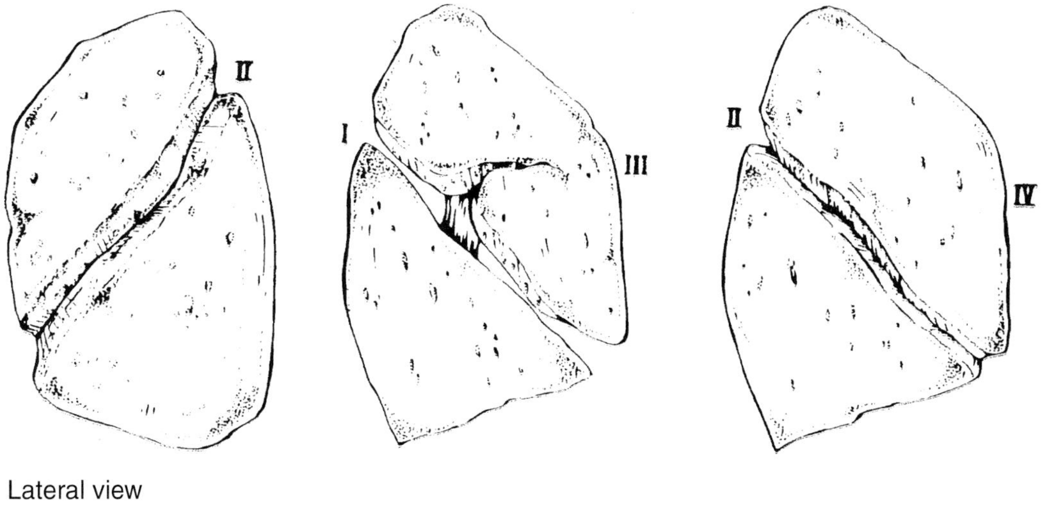

II I III II IV

Lateral view

Grading of the completeness of pulmonary fissures and balance of the oblique fissures. One method of assessing the anatomic variability of the lung fissures is by describing their completeness and balance. Completeness of fissures may be divided into four grades: grade I, fissure complete; grade II, lobes partially fused at fissure but visceral cleft complete; grade III, lobes partially fused at fissure and visceral cleft incomplete; grade IV, lobes completely fused without evidence of a fusion line. Fissural balance refers to the relationship of the pulmonary artery to the oblique fissure: the pulmonary artery may be central to the oblique fissure (fissures balanced), anterior to the midpoint of the oblique fissure (anterior imbalance), or posterior to the midpoint of the oblique fissure (posterior imbalance). (From Craig SR, Walker WS: A proposed anatomical classification of the pulmonary fissures. J R Coll Surg Edinb 42:233–234, 1997.)

GROSS ANATOMY

FIGURE 2–4

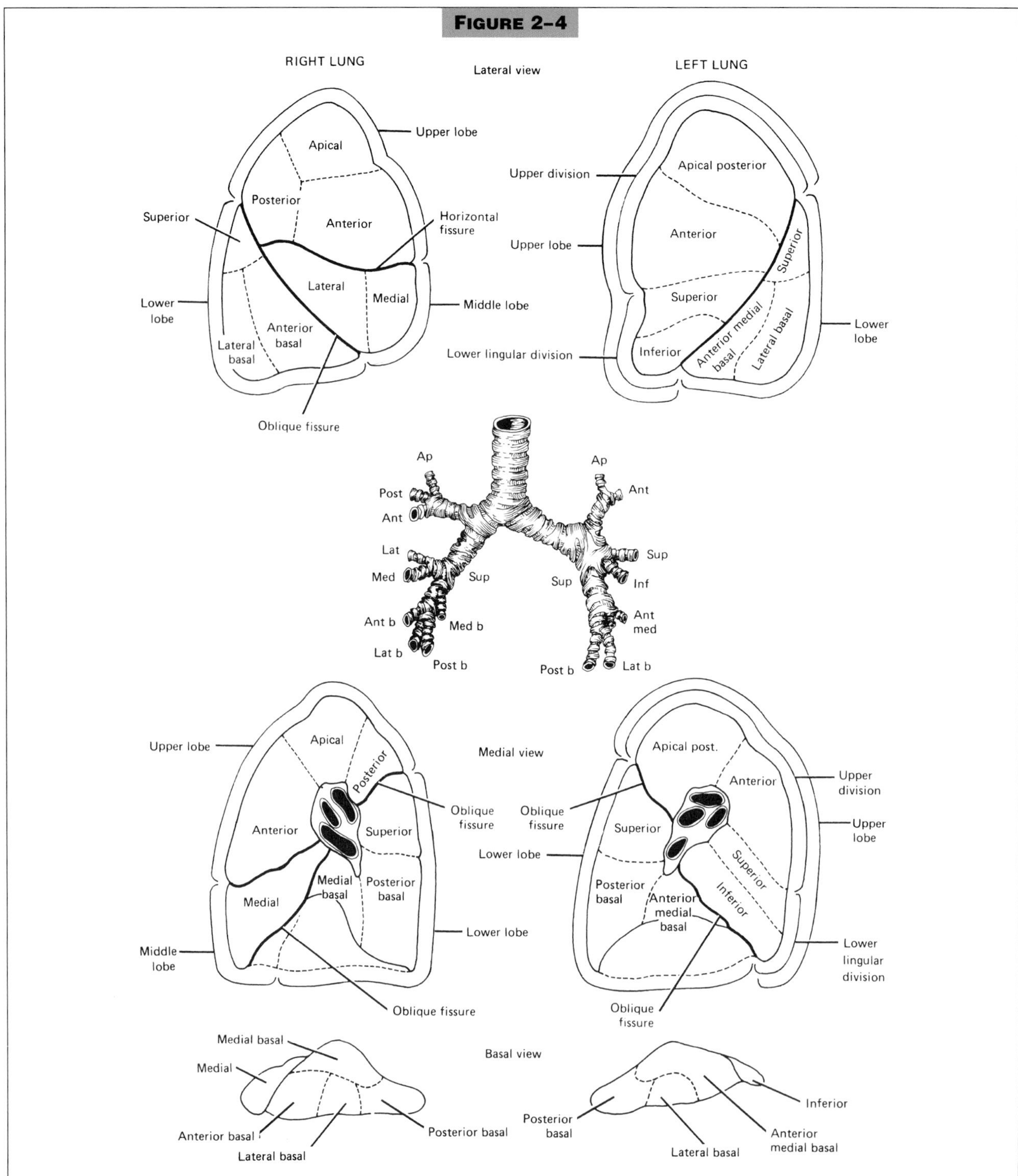

Bronchopulmonary segments and segmental bronchi of the right and left lungs. The conducting airways, which deliver air to the gas-exchanging regions of the lung, begin with the trachea. The trachea divides asymmetrically into the right and left main bronchi at the level of T4–T5, with the right being wider, shorter, and more vertically oriented than the left. Arising from the main bronchi are the lobar bronchi, which branch into the segmental bronchi and subsequently, the subsegmental bronchi. Each segmental bronchus and its accompanying pulmonary artery supplies a region of a lobe known as a bronchopulmonary segment. Bronchopulmonary segments and their associated bronchi are named according to their positions in the lobes. The segments are roughly pyramidal in shape and are separated from one another by connective tissue septa. These subunits can be defined radiologically and can be removed surgically without significant hemorrhage or air leakage. (From Lindner HH: Clinical Anatomy. Norwalk, CT, Appleton & Lange, 1989, p. 261.)

GROSS ANATOMY

FIGURE 2-5

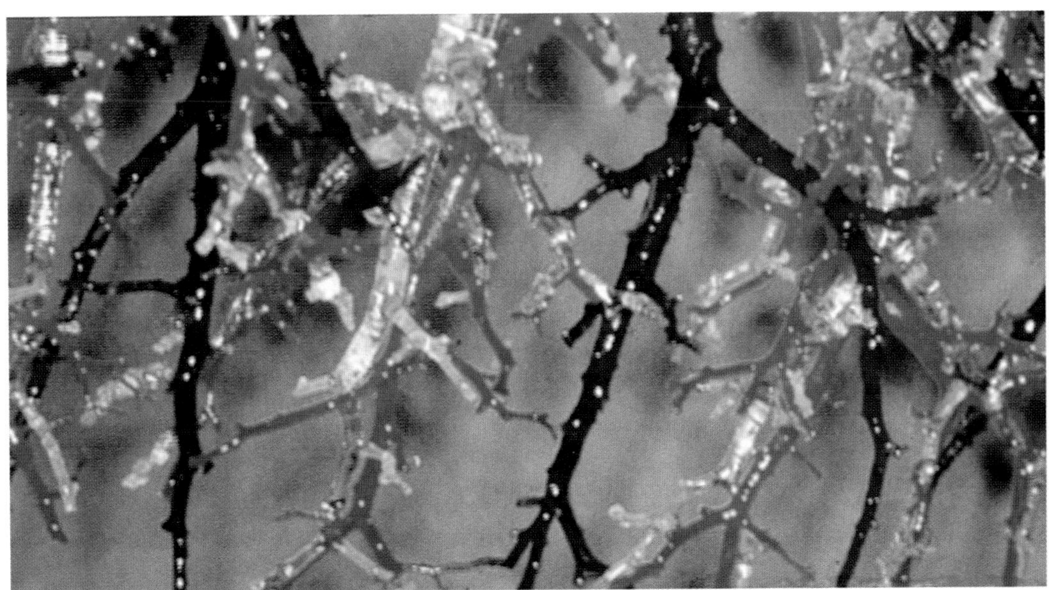

This corrosion cast of the human airways (clear), pulmonary arteries (red) and pulmonary veins (blue) illustrates the complex branching pattern of these structures and the intimate relationship of airways and pulmonary arteries.

CONDUCTING AIRWAYS AND ACINI

FIGURE 2-6

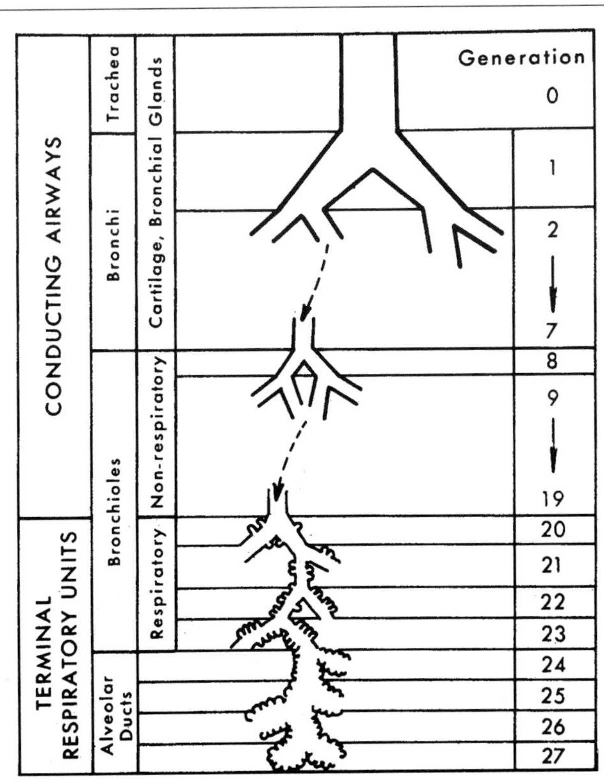

Diagram of the conducting airways and acini. The trachea, bronchi, and nonrespiratory bronchioles are the conducting airways, which distribute air to the gas-exchanging sites. When the cartilage and submucosal glands disappear from the bronchi, the airways are defined as bronchioles. Bronchioles lead into the alveolar ducts and then alveolar sacs. An acinus, or terminal respiratory unit, is the functional gas-exchanging unit of the lung. It is composed of all the structures distal to the terminal bronchiole, which includes the respiratory bronchioles, alveolar ducts, alveolar sacs, and alveoli. Another structural subunit of the lung is the lobule, which consists of three to five terminal bronchioles and their associated acini. Adjacent lobules are separated by connective tissue septa and are visible grossly. (From Weibel ER: Morphometry of the Human Lung. Berlin, Springer Verlag, 1968, p. 111.)

CONDUCTING AIRWAYS AND ACINI

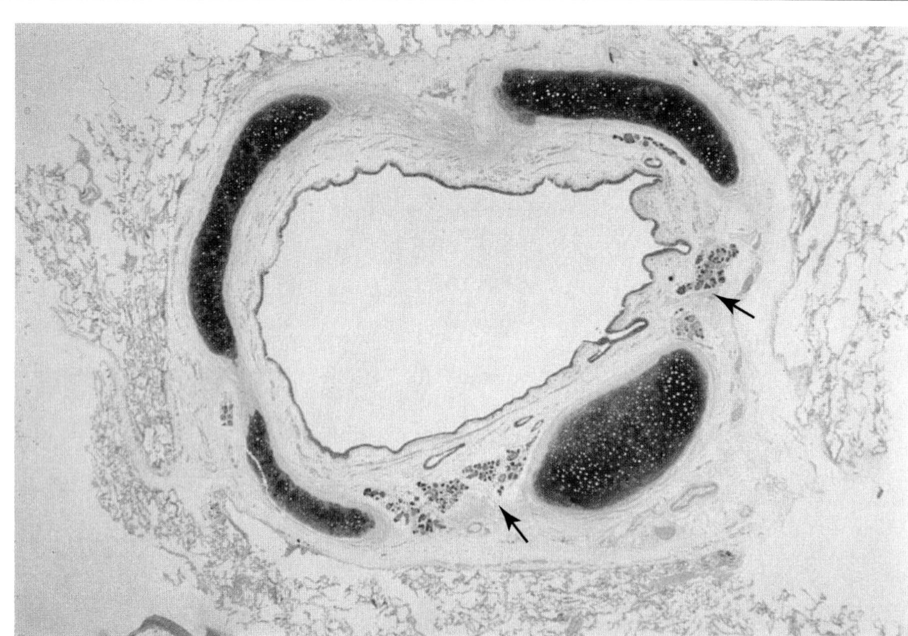

FIGURE 2-7

Bronchus (light microscopy, hematoxylin-eosin stain). The bronchi are lined by pseudostratified columnar epithelium containing ciliated, goblet, and basal cells. Beneath the epithelium, longitudinal elastic fibers run through the lamina propria, and a layer of smooth muscle circumferentially surrounds the airways. Submucosal glands are located between the smooth muscle and the outermost layer of cartilage (*arrows*).

FIGURE 2-8

Bronchiole (light microscopy, hematoxylin-eosin stain). The simple columnar epithelium (*arrows*) of the bronchioles consists of ciliated cells and Clara cells. The secretory Clara cells replace goblet cells in the bronchioles. The bronchiolar wall lacks cartilage and is supported by elastic fibers and smooth muscle.

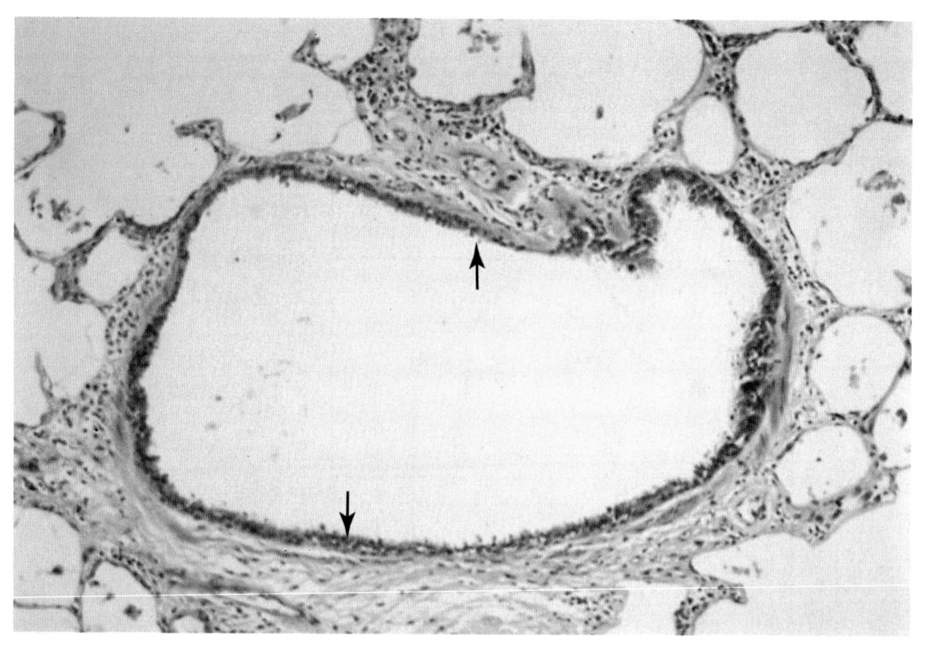

CONDUCTING AIRWAYS AND ACINI

FIGURE 2-9

Acinus—terminal bronchiole (TB), respiratory bronchioles (RB), alveolar ducts (AD), alveolar sacs (AS) (light microscopy, hematoxylin-eosin stain). In the respiratory bronchiole, there is a transition from respiratory epithelium to alveolar epithelium. When the airspace is lined entirely by alveolar epithelium, it is called an alveolar duct. Eventually, the alveolar duct terminates in blind-ended alveolar sacs that are also lined by alveolar epithelium.

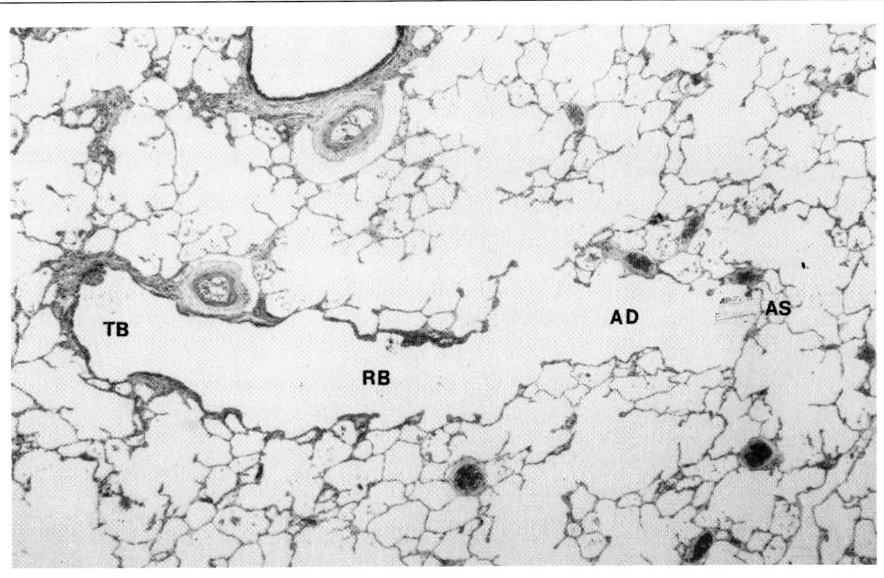

TABLE 2-1

Structural Characteristics of the Airways

Structure	Number	Average Diameter (mm)	Area Supplied	Cartilage	Muscle	Epithelium	Blood Supply
Trachea	1	18	Both lungs	U-shaped	Trachealis muscle—links together open end of cartilage	Ciliated, columnar	• Upper trachea: from inferior thyroid arteries • Lower trachea: from bronchial arteries
Main bronchi	2	13	Right or left lung				
Lobar bronchi	4	7	Lobes	Irregularly shaped and helical plates	Helical bands		From the bronchial circulation
	8	5					
Segmental bronchi	16	4	Broncho–pulmonary segments				
Small bronchi	32	3	Lobules				
	2,000	1					
Terminal bronchioles	4,000	1	—	Absent	Strong helical muscle bands	Cuboidal	
	65,000	0.5					
Respiratory bronchioles	130,000 500,000	0.5	Acini		Muscle bands between alveoli	Cuboidal to flat between alveoli	From the pulmonary circulation
Alveolar ducts	1,000,000 4,000,000	0.3	Alveoli		Thin bands in alveolar septa	Alveolar epithelium	
Alveolar sacs	8,000,000	0.3					

Source: Modified from Nunn JF: Functional anatomy of the respiratory tract. *In* Nunn JF (ed): Applied Respiratory Physiology (3rd ed). London, Butterworth & Co., 1987, p. 7.

LUNG DEVELOPMENT

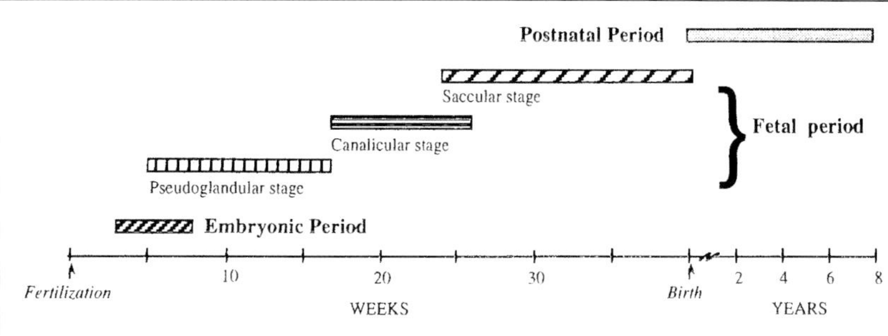

FIGURE 2-10

Human lung development can be divided into three stages—the embryonic, fetal, and postnatal periods. The embryonic period is characterized by the formation of the basic structure of the upper and lower respiratory tracts. The fetal period is subdivided into the pseudoglandular, canalicular, and saccular stages, each of which corresponds to the morphologic changes seen in the airways and airspaces. During the postnatal period, or alveolar period, the number and size of the alveoli increases, until the lung reaches maturity at approximately 8 years of age. (Adapted from Burri P: Fetal and postnatal development of the lung. Ann Rev Physiol 46:618, 1984.)

LUNG DEVELOPMENT

EMBRYONIC PERIOD (GESTATIONAL AGE: 3 TO 8 WEEKS)

FIGURE 2-11

Diagrams showing the growth of the developing lung during the embryonic period. A to C corresponds to 4 weeks; D and E to 5 weeks; F to 6 weeks; and G to 8 weeks. (From Moore KL: The respiratory system. *In* The Developing Human, 5th ed. Philadelphia, WB Saunders, 1993, p. 230.)

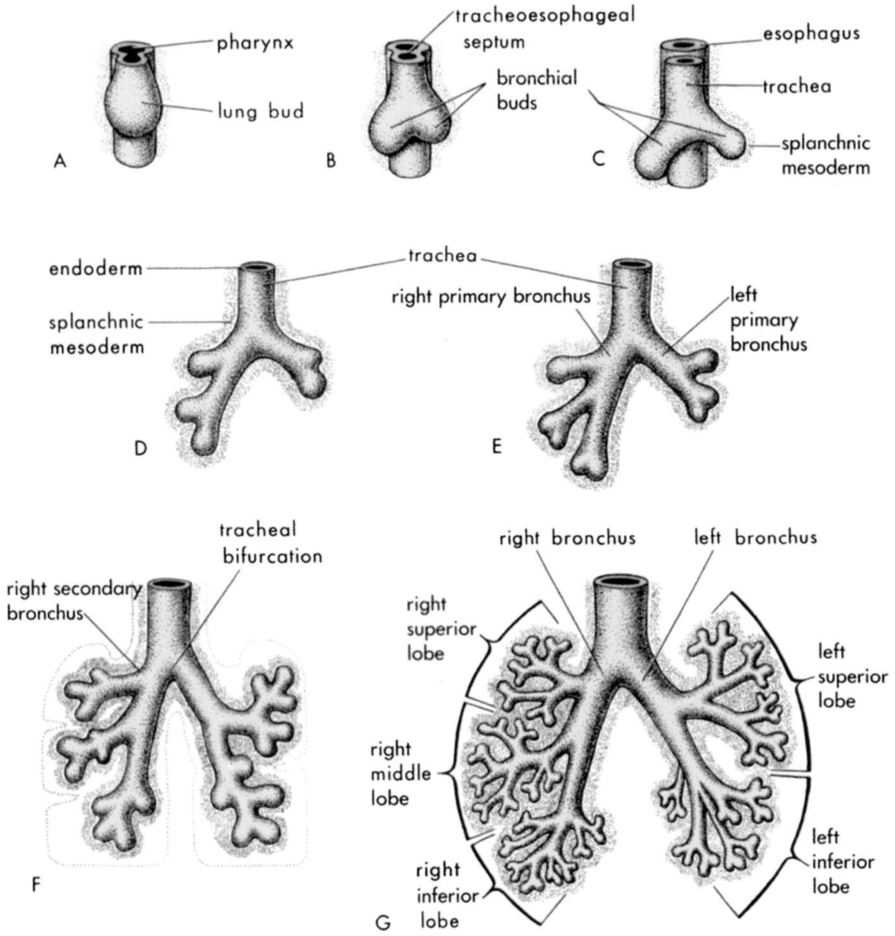

TABLE 2-2

Characteristics of the Successive Phases During the Embryonic Period of Lung Development

Gestational Age	Developmental Features
3 weeks	• Respiratory bud appears as a ventral diverticulum off the foregut endoderm. • Respiratory epithelium and alveoli develop from the endoderm. • Splanchnic mesoderm, surrounding the endoderm, differentiates into cartilage, muscle, connective tissue, blood vessels, and lymphatics.
4 weeks	• Respiratory bud divides into right and left lung buds, which represent the main-stem bronchi. • A primitive pulmonary artery develops from right and left aortic arches. • The common pulmonary vein develops from dorsal atrial wall of the heart. • Arterial and venous channels develop in the mesenchymal tissue and connect to the main pulmonary arteries and veins.
5 weeks	• Lung buds elongate into right and left lung sacs. • Lung sacs branch into three lobar buds on the right and two on the left. • Tall pseudostratified columnar epithelium lines these ducts.
6 weeks	• Segmental buds arise off the lobar buds. • Bronchopulmonary segments develop from the segmental buds and the surrounding tissue.
7–8 weeks	• Subsegmental buds develop.

LUNG DEVELOPMENT

FETAL PERIOD (GESTATIONAL AGE: 5 WEEKS TO BIRTH)

FIGURE 2-12

Features of the three stages of the fetal lung development[2,3] and corresponding light photomicrographs.

Stage and Age	Features	Histology (Hematoxylin–Eosin Stain)
Pseudoglandular stage 5–17 weeks	• Formation of the conducting airways by successive branching to form the terminal bronchioles. • Branching epithelial tubes resemble glands, thus the name pseudoglandular stage. • The columnar epithelium is surrounded by abundant mesenchyme. • 7 weeks: Smooth muscle differentiates. • 9 weeks: Bronchial arteries and lymphatics appear. • 10 weeks: Cartilage forms in the main bronchi. • 12 weeks: Ciliated cells are present in the bronchi. • 13 weeks: Goblet cells and submucosal glands appear.	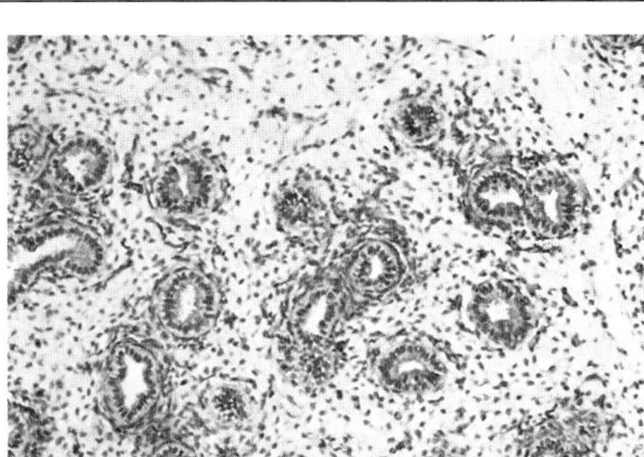
Canalicular stage 17–26 weeks	• Distal airways widen with a concomitant decrease in amount of mesenchymal tissue. • Airways, lined by cuboidal epithelium, resemble canaliculi. • By 24 weeks, each terminal bronchiole has developed 2 or more respiratory bronchioles. • The number of capillaries increases, and they move closer to airways.	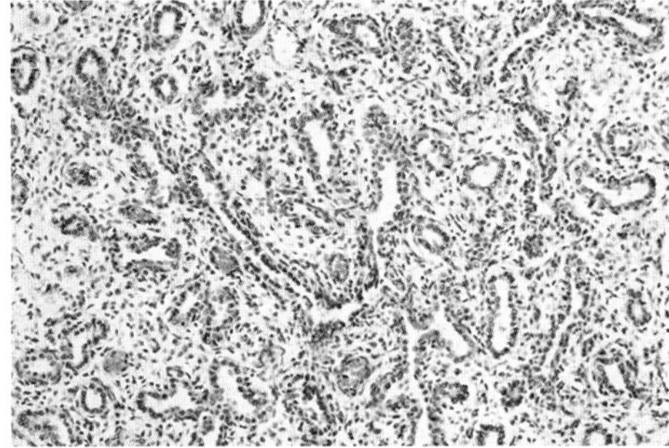
Saccular stage 24–40 weeks	• Airways end in groups of terminal sacs, which are lined by the flat type I epithelial cells. • Type II epithelial cells differentiate at around 23 weeks and begin to secrete surfactant. • Capillaries proliferate with a continued decrease in amount of connective tissue. • By 25–28 weeks, adequate alveolar surface area, vascularity and surfactant production are present for the survival of a premature infant.	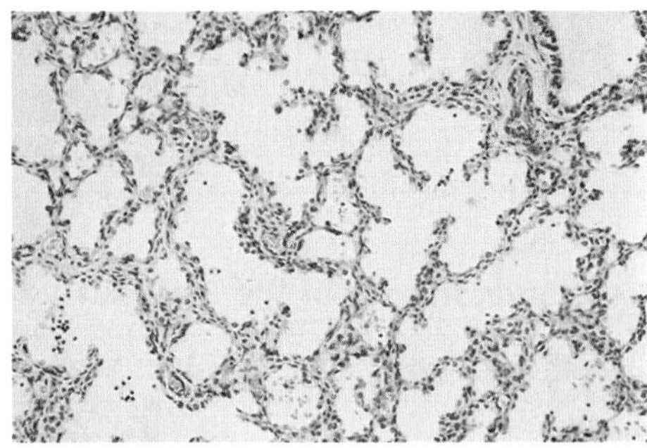

LUNG DEVELOPMENT

POSTNATAL PERIOD (BIRTH TO 8 YEARS)

TABLE 2-3

Features of the Postnatal Period, or Alveolar Period, of Lung Development

- At birth, the airway number and branching pattern are established.
- However, the number and size of the alveoli, and thus alveolar surface area, continue to increase until approximately 8 years of age.
- Initially, there are 24×10^6 alveoli with an alveolar-capillary surface area of 2.8 m^2, and the adult has 300×10^6 alveoli with a surface area of 150 m^2 (see Fig. 2–11).
- Through successive septations, the thick alveolar wall of the newborn is remodeled to form the thin alveolar-capillary membrane of the adult.
- Postnatally, the pulmonary arteries become thinner with a decrease in the medial smooth muscle thickness and an increase in the number of branches.

FIGURE 2-13

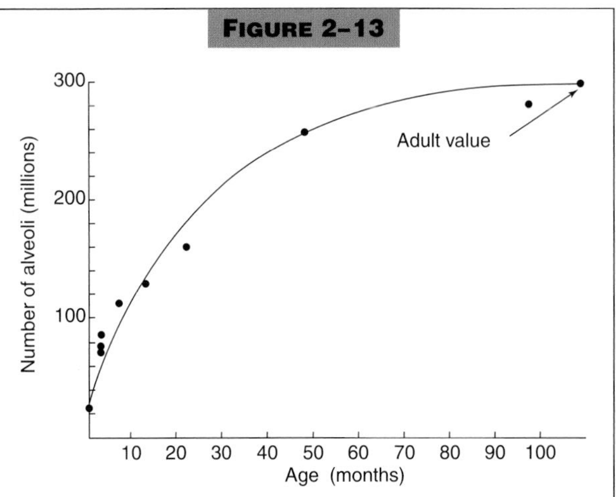

Graph illustrating the change in the number of alveoli with age. (From Dunnill MS: Postnatal growth of the lung. Thorax 17:329–333, 1962.)

AIRWAY EPITHELIUM

FIGURE 2-14

Eight epithelial cell types of the airways. The predominant cell of the respiratory epithelium is the ciliated cell, which covers the majority of the luminal surface of the conducting airways and respiratory bronchioles. Interspersed between the ciliated cells are the mucous (goblet) and serous epithelial cells, the latter of which are found in many species but are rare in humans, except during development. The intermediate cells, which may undergo differentiation into secretory or ciliated cells, form a poorly defined layer above the basal cells. The columnar brush cells have numerous apical microvilli and thus may have a role in liquid absorption. In the bronchioles, nonciliated columnar epithelial (Clara) cells are the predominant secretory cells. Scattered along the airways are the neuroendocrine or Kulchitsky cells of the lung.[6] (Modified from Reid LM, Jones R: Mucous membrane of respiratory epithelium. Environ Health Perspect 35:114 1980.)

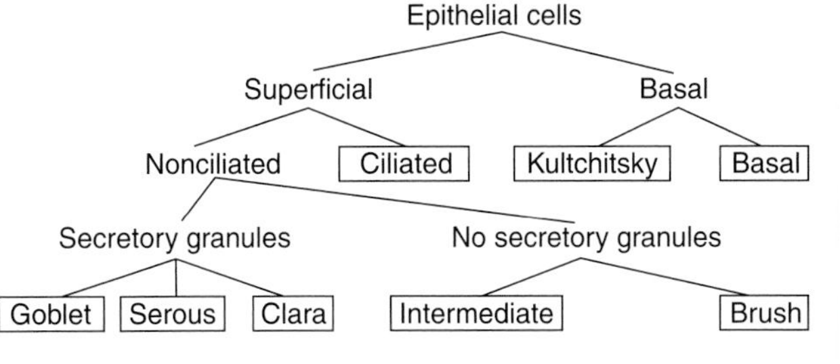

AIRWAY EPITHELIUM

BRONCHIAL EPITHELIUM

FIGURE 2-15

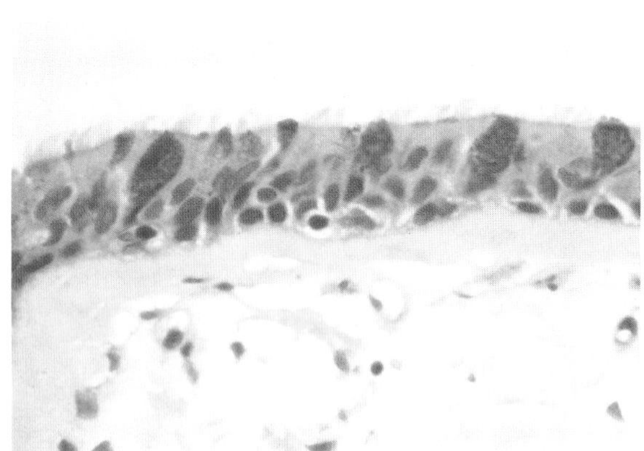

Bronchial mucociliary epithelium (light microscopy, hematoxylin-eosin stain). Located along the basement membrane, basal cells are pluripotential stem cells with the ability to differentiate into both ciliated and goblet cells. They are triangular with large nuclei, few organelles, and hemidesmosomes anchoring them to the basement membrane. In contrast to the other epithelial cells, basal cells usually withstand mucosal injury, and their survival allows them to reconstitute the epithelium. However, chronic irritation may lead to basal cell hyperplasia, squamous metaplasia, dysplasia, or neoplasia.

FIGURE 2-16

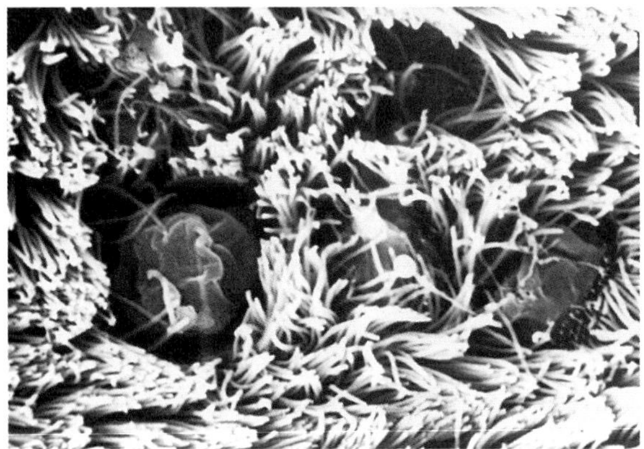

Bronchial mucociliary epithelium (scanning electron microscopy). Dispersed among the ciliated cells are several goblet cells undergoing exocytosis. When quiescent, the apical surfaces of the goblet cells are finely granular. These fine granules represent individual secretory granules. In a healthy lung, the ciliated cells occur four times more frequently than goblet cells.

FIGURE 2-17

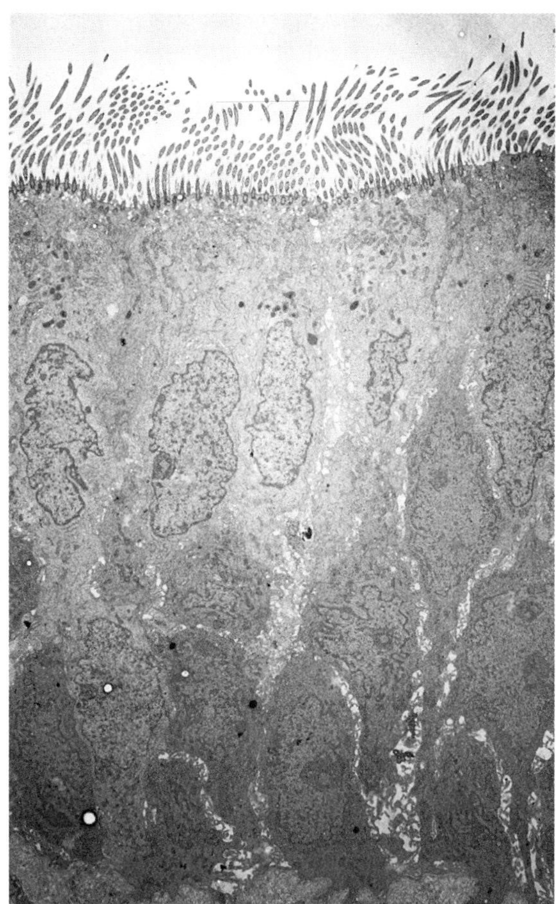

Ciliated cells (transmission electron microscopy). Ciliated cells have a columnar shape with basally located nuclei. They have loosely packed cytoplasm, numerous apical mitochondria that provide adenosine triphosphate to the cilia, and relatively large Golgi apparatuses for nonsecretory cells. The main function of the bronchial epithelium is protective. The goblet cells and submucosal glands secrete mucus that traps or neutralizes particulates, infectious agents, and other foreign material. Cilia beat in a sequential, rhythmic pattern, resulting in waves of movement that constantly propel mucus toward the oropharynx, where it is removed by cough or swallowing. The number of ciliated cells and the length and beat frequency of the cilia decrease as the diameter of the bronchi decreases. These changes result in a slower mucus propulsion velocity in the smaller airways.

AIRWAY EPITHELIUM

CILIA

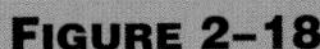
Figure 2-18

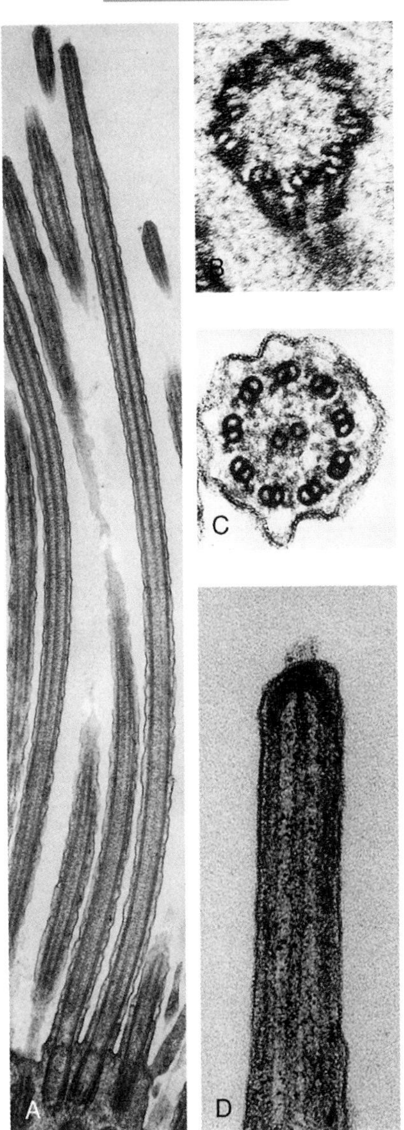

Cilia (transmission electron microscopy). **A,** Longitudinal section of cilia. There are approximately 40 to 200 cilia per ciliated cell, each of which measures 5 to 8 μm in length and 0.3 μm in diameter. In addition, branched microvilli, measuring 1 to 2 μm in length, cover the surface between cilia. Modified centrioles, the intracytoplasmic basal bodies, are arranged perpendicular to the cell membrane and serve as microtubule-organizing centers during ciliogenesis. The main body of the cilium, or axoneme, arises from a basal body and is attached to the cell at the ciliary neck or necklace. **B,** Cross section of a cilia above the basal body but below the central pair microtubules showing the centriolar portion of the axoneme. **C,** Cross section of cilia showing the 9 + 2 arrangement of the microtubules and radial spokes (see Fig. 2–19). **D,** Longitudinal section at the tip of the cilia shows the terminal hooklets that are thought to help propel the overlying mucus.

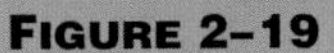
Figure 2-19

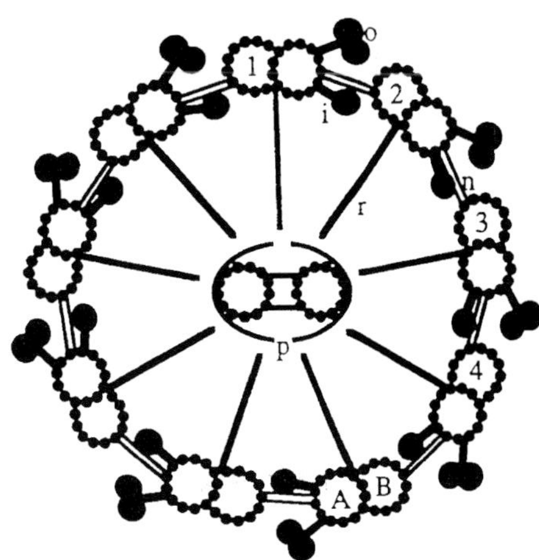

Cilia in cross section and a diagram of cilia structure. The structure of respiratory cilia is similar to that of most eukaryotic organisms. The axoneme, which is surrounded by an extension of the cell membrane, is composed of two central, single microtubules and nine peripheral doublet microtubules (9 + 2 arrangement). The doublets consist of an A and B subunit, with two angulated dynein arms (outer, o; inner, i) attached to each A subunit. These dynein arms are the sites of the majority of ATPase activity. Adjacent doublets are connected by nexin links (n) and the peripheral doublets are attached to the central microtubules by radial spokes. The radial spokes connect the outer doublet microtubules with projections (p) associated with the inner pair microtubules. When oriented with the dynein arms pointing clockwise and the central microtubules positioned horizontally, the doublets are numbered according to the scheme illustrated. (From Wanner A, Salathe M, O'Riordan R: Mucociliary clearance in the airways. Am J Resp Crit Care Med 154:1868–1902, 1996.)

AIRWAY EPITHELIUM

GOBLET CELLS

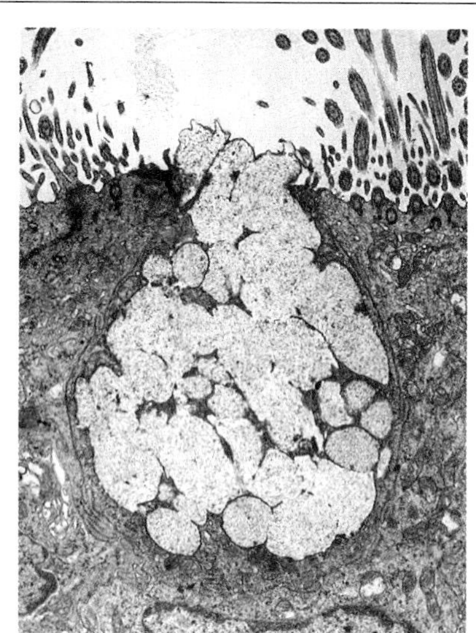

FIGURE 2-20

Goblet cell (transmission electron microscopy). Goblet cells, or mucous epithelial cells, are found distributed individually among ciliated cells of the trachea and bronchi and have a characteristic goblet shape from secretory granules that fill the apical cytoplasm. These cells have basally placed nuclei, electron-dense cytoplasm, a significant rough endoplasmic reticulum, Golgi apparatus, and apical microvilli, which are features of active secretory cells. Although the main function of goblet cells is mucus secretion, the submucosal glands secrete the majority of the mucus in healthy individuals. However, upon bronchial irritation, goblet cells undergo hyperplasia and increase their secretions. In addition, recent studies show that the type of mucin produced is altered in disease.[7]

SUBMUCOSAL GLANDS

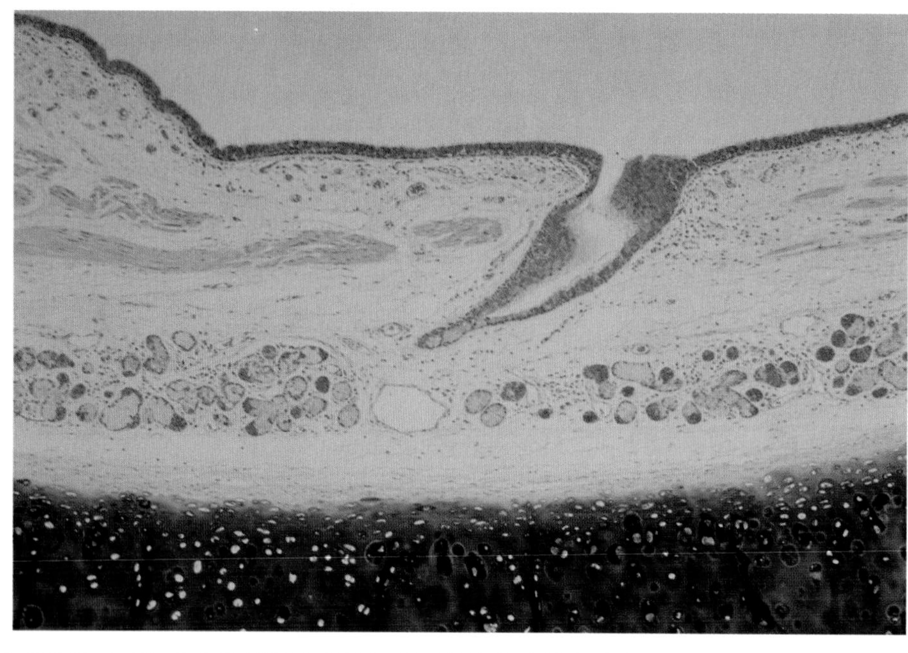

FIGURE 2-21

Submucosal gland (light microscopy, hematoxylin-eosin stain). Submucosal glands are compound tubular glands located in the submucosa between the epithelium and cartilage of the trachea and bronchi. Airway gland secretions empty into the airway lumen via collecting ducts whose proximal ends are in continuity with the overlying airway epithelium.

SUBMUCOSAL GLANDS

FIGURE 2–22

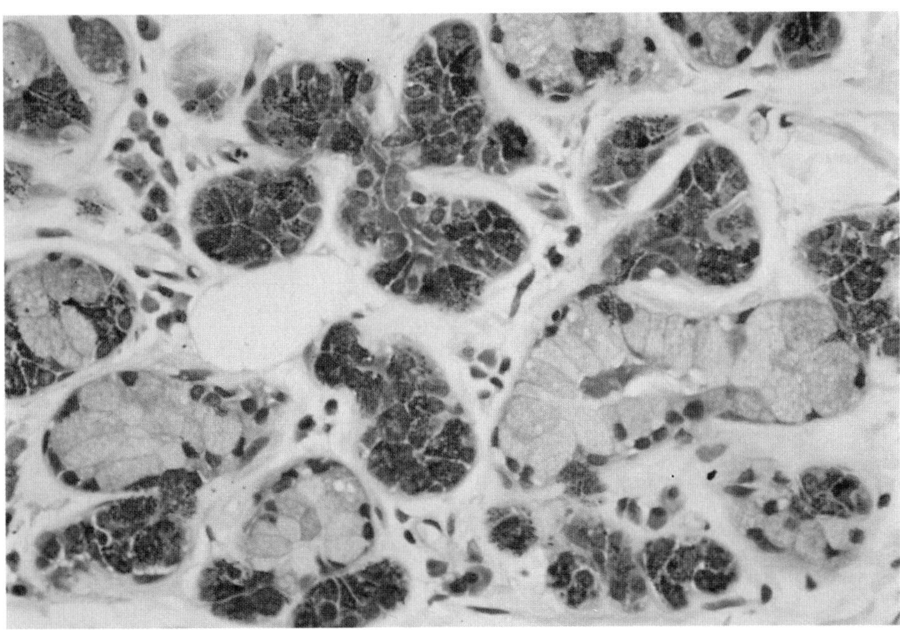

Submucosal gland (light microscopy, hematoxylin-eosin stain). The glands are composed of three major cell types: mucous, serous, and myoepithelial cells though a number of studies suggest heterogeneity among mucous and serous cells.[8, 9] The mucous (pale-staining) and the serous (dark-staining) cells are the secretory cells. The myoepithelial cells are modified smooth muscle cells that are located in the peripheral basal lamina of the gland. Their function may be to aid in the movement of secretions toward the lumen.

FIGURE 2–23

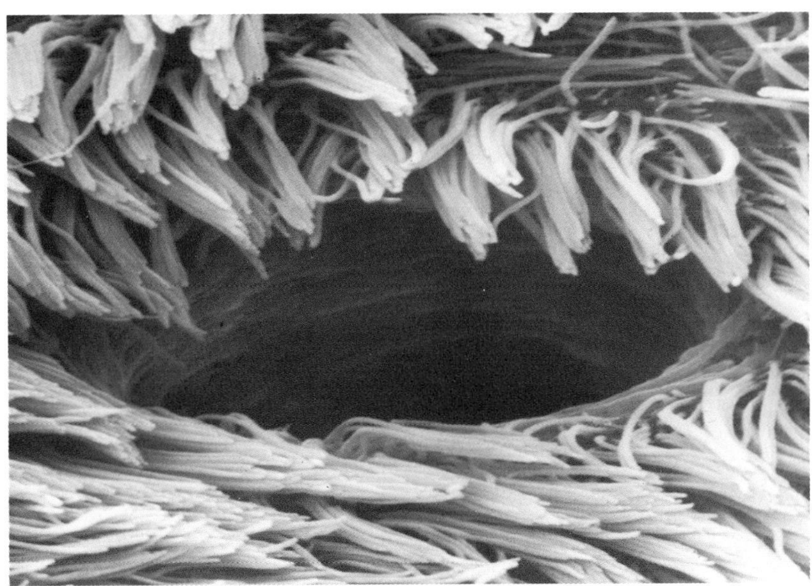

Submucosal gland duct (scanning electron microscopy). The secretions from the mucous and the serous cells empty into secretory tubules, which drain into collecting ducts. The contents of the collecting ducts flow into the ciliated ducts and then into the bronchial lumen. These glands are found approximately every square millimeter and decrease in frequency distally, disappearing with cartilage at approximately the 10th generation.

SUBMUCOSAL GLANDS

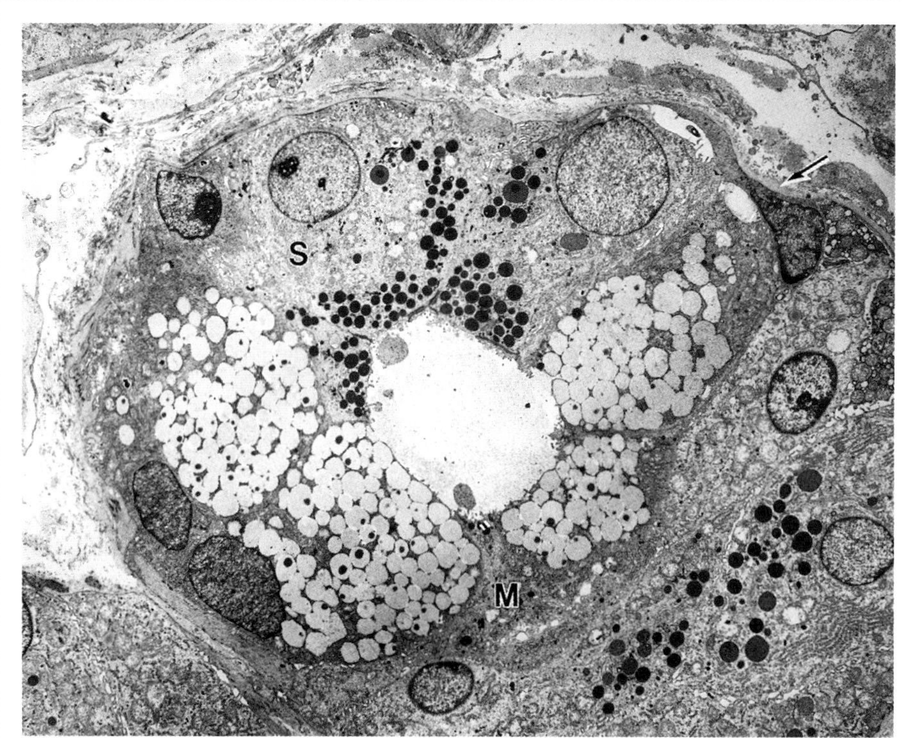

FIGURE 2-24

Submucosal gland acinus (transmission electron microscopy). The mixed acinus contains mucous (M) and serous (S) cells. An arrow indicates a myoepithelial cell. Mucous cells have electron-lucent granules that range in diameter from 300 nm near the Golgi apparatus 1800 nm near the apical membrane. Serous cells are generally located at the end of mucous tubules. These cells have electron-dense secretory granules that range in size between 100 and 1000 nm in diameter, although the majority are from 300 to 1000 nm.

TABLE 2-4

A Comparison between Mucous and Serous Cells of Submucosal Glands

Feature	Mucous Cell	Serous Cell
Location in gland	• Central areas of secretory tubule	• Distal end of secretory tubules
Cell characteristics	• Columnar cell with flattened basal nucleus • Apical microvilli	• Pyramidal cell with round basal nucleus • 50–80 nm long and 50–70 nm in diameter
Granules	• Filled with secretory granules of various sizes • Electron-lucent and may be fused • 300 nm–1800 nm	Apical granules of uniform size • Electron-dense and discrete • 100 nm–1000 nm
Cell products	• Predominantly mucin glycoprotein	• Predominantly antimicrobial compounds

AIRWAY LINING FLUID

FIGURE 2-25

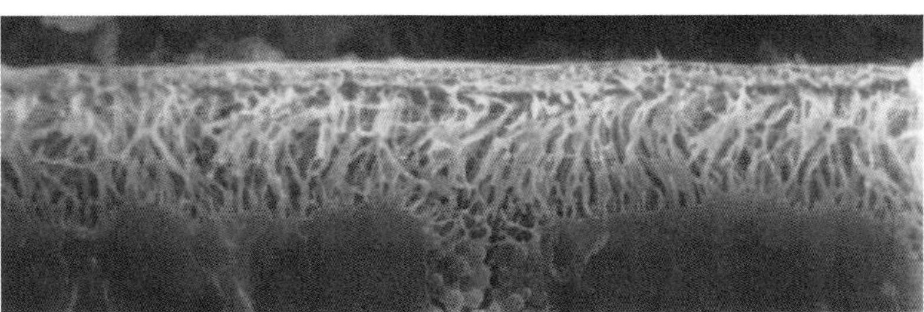

Airway lining fluid (low temperature scanning electron microscopy). The airway lining fluid consists of two layers—the sol (S) and the gel (G) phases. The low viscosity, 5-μm sol layer surrounds the cilia and contains serum glycoproteins. Above the sol is the high viscosity, 2-μm gel layer that contains the mucin glycoproteins. Mucins are very large, heavily glycosylated molecules that impart viscosity and cohesiveness to mucus. The carbohydrate side chains of mucins are extremely variable. The functional significance of this heterogeneity is also unknown, although the mucin carbohydrates may serve as ligands for bacteria and viruses, thus preventing them from reaching the airway epithelial lining cells.[10] The arrow indicates a goblet cell and its secretory granules. (From Wu DXY et al: Regulation of the depth of surface liquid in bovine trachea. Am J Physiol 274 (Lung Cell Mol Physiol 18):L388–395, 1998.)

FIGURE 2-26

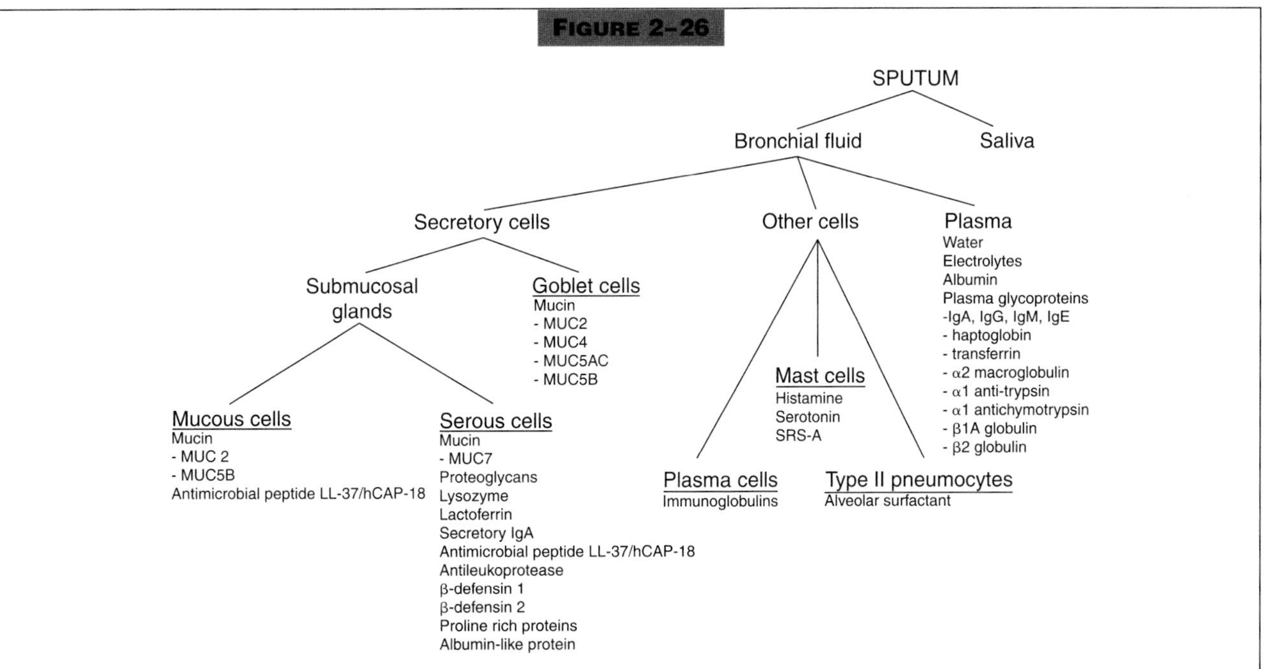

Some constituents of sputum and their major cellular site of origin (underlined). The combination of saliva and airway fluid produces sputum, which is 95% water, 2 to 3% glycoproteins, 0.1 to 0.5% proteins, and 0.3 to 0.5% fat.[11, 12] In the normal adult, the daily bronchial secretion is approximately 100 mL.

AIRWAY EPITHELIUM

BRONCHIOLAR EPITHELIUM

FIGURE 2-27

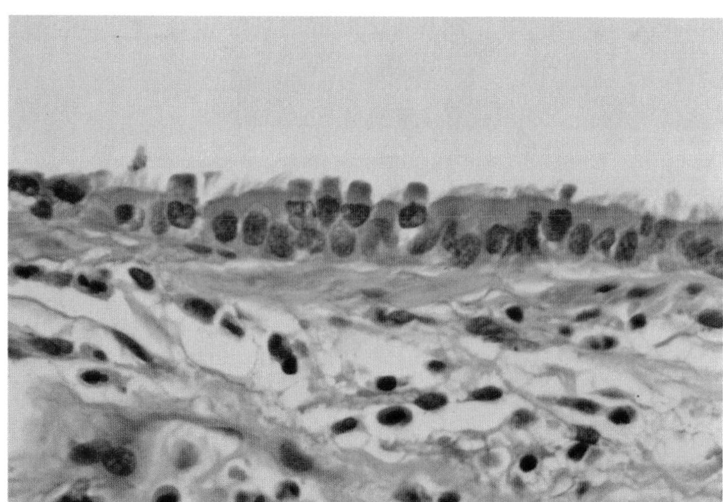

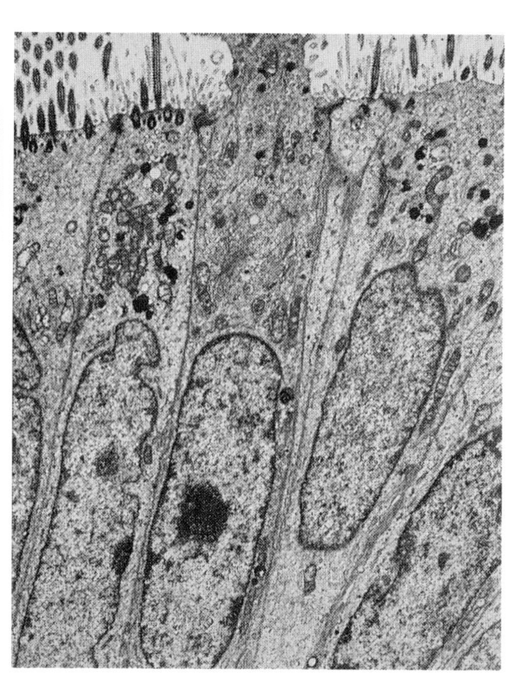

Bronchiolar epithelium (**left,** light microscopy, hematoxylin-eosin stain; **right,** transmission electron microscopy). In the bronchiole, the simple columnar epithelium consists of ciliated cells, similar to those of the bronchi, and the nonciliated columnar epithelial (Clara) cells. The Clara cells are seen scattered among the ciliated cells and are characterized by bulging apical cytoplasm that protrudes into the lumen. These cells contain a basal nucleus, well-developed rough endoplasmic reticulum and Golgi apparatus, numerous mitochondria, and apical secretory granules. Their secretions, which appear to consist primarily of lipid and protein but not of mucin, contribute to the bronchiolar lining fluid. The Clara cell also has a progenitor or reparative role similar to that of basal cells. These cells are rich in smooth endoplasmic reticulum and play an important role in the detoxification of exogenous agents via a cytochrome P-450 pathway.[13] (Courtesy of Dr. Charles Plopper, Department of Anatomy and Cell Biology, School of Veterinary Medicine, University of California, Davis.)

FIGURE 2-28

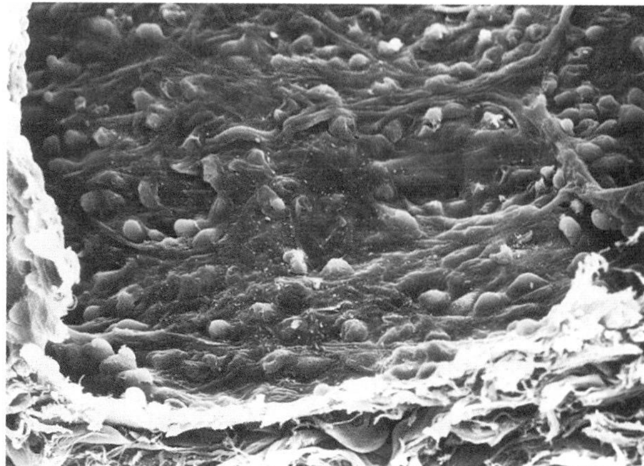

Distal bronchiole (scanning electron microscopy). Clara cells line much of the lumen, and their apical cytoplasm bulges into the lumen.

AIRWAY EPITHELIUM

NEUROENDOCRINE CELL

FIGURE 2–29

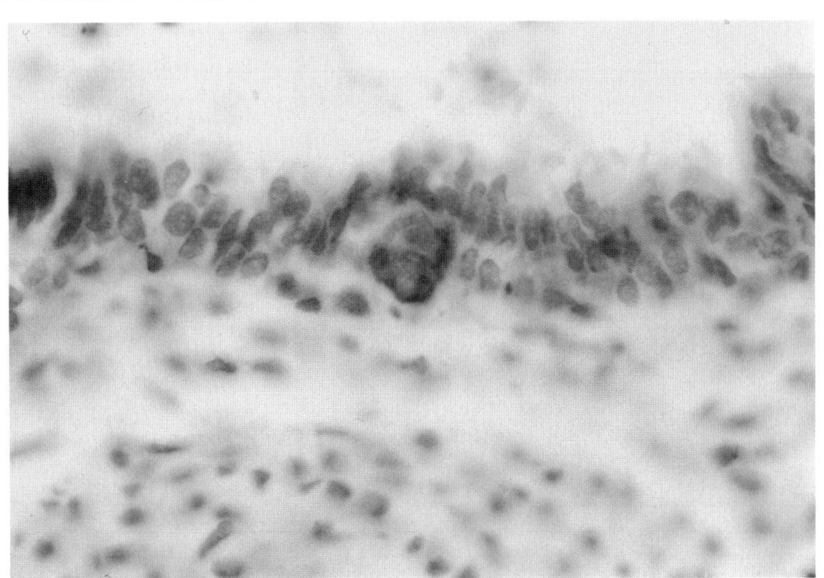

Neuroendocrine cells (light microscopy, chromagranin immunohistochemistry stain). Brown peroxidase reaction product identifies chromagranin within a bronchial neuroendocrine cell. Neuroendocrine cells are characterized by amine and amine-precursor uptake and decarboxylation (APUD cells), and contain numerous basally oriented secretory granules. They are also known as Feyrter cells, Kulchitsky or K cells, and "small granule" cells. They are more numerous in the subsegmental bronchi and bronchioles and more common in fetal than adult lungs. Neuroendocrine cells exist as solitary cells or in groups, and these cells contain a number of granules. The granules contain a variety of amines and peptides, such as serotonin, bombesin, calcitonin, and leu-enkephalin, among others (see TABLE 2–5).[14] Because the secretions are released basally rather than into the airway lumen, they affect structures near the basement membrane, such as nerve fibers, adjacent epithelium, smooth muscles, and capillaries. Although the role of these secretory products is not entirely understood, they presumably have vasoactive and bronchoactive functions.[13] The neuroepithelial bodies are located at bifurcations of airways and are innervated by both afferent and efferent nerves. They may act as chemoreceptors that respond to changes in the composition of air and subsequently alter vascular perfusion and airflow.

TABLE 2–5

Secretory Products of Neuroendocrine Cells

- Serotonin
- Bombesin
- Calcitonin
- Leu-enkephalin
- Neuron-specific enolase
- Chromagranin
- Synaptophysin
- Protein gene product 9.5

FIGURE 2–30

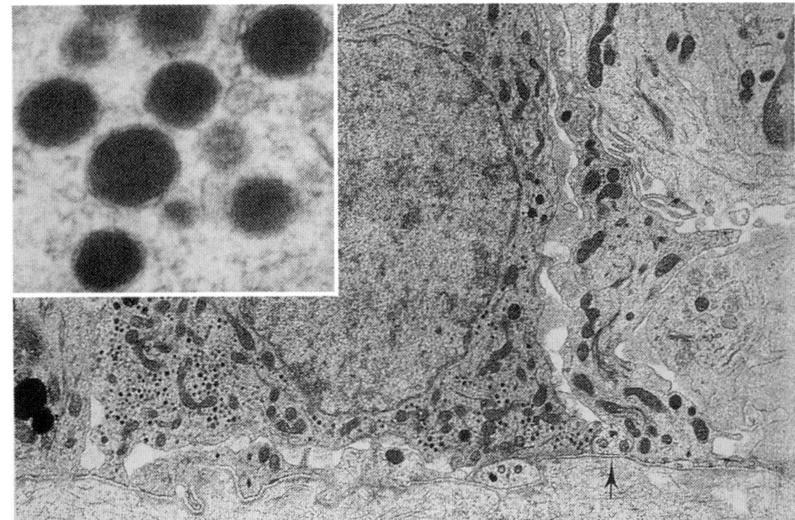

Neuroendocrine cell with dense core granules (transmission electron microscopy). These characteristic granules have electron-dense centers surrounded by a clear zone or halo and a peripheral membrane (see insert). The neuroendocrine cells are typically flasked-shaped cells and lie on the basement membrane with a thin apical extension to the lumen. Their nuclei are round to oval, and their cytoplasm contains abundant endoplasmic reticulum and Golgi apparatus. Intraepithelial nerve fibers (*arrow*) may be found in contact with the cell. (From Jeffrey PK: Microscopic structure of normal lung. *In* Brewis RAL, Corrin B, Geddes DM, Gibson GJ (eds): Respiratory Medicine. London, WB Saunders Co, Ltd, 1995, p. 60.)

ACINUS

GENERAL ORGANIZATION

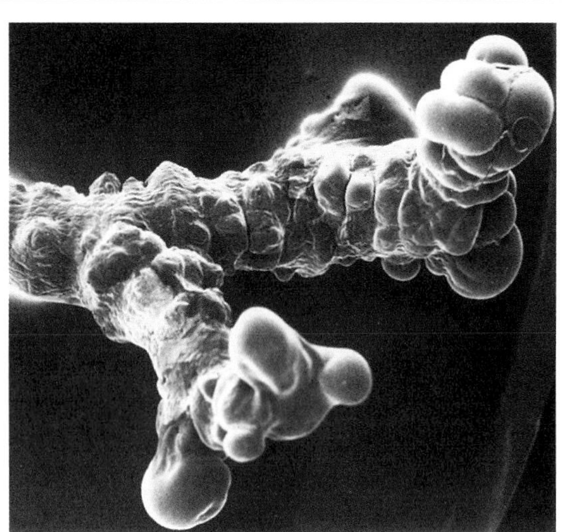

FIGURE 2–31

Silicon corrosion cast of acinus. The acinus is the functional gas-exchanging unit of the lung. Its components, the respiratory bronchiole, alveolar ducts and alveolar sacs, all have alveoli. In the respiratory bronchioles, there is a transition between cuboidal epithelium of Clara cells and ciliated cells to alveolar epithelium. When the epithelial cells are completely replaced by alveoli, the airway is called an alveolar duct. The alveolar duct is lined by smooth muscle and collagen and elastic fibers arranged in a spiral pattern. During inspiration, the duct elongates and dilates, the latter by the uncoiling of the spiral. The alveolar duct eventually terminates in blind-ended alveolar sacs.

This cast illustrates acinar structural variability and complexity. Within one acinus, the respiratory bronchioles and alveolar ducts vary in length, branching pattern, and number of alveoli. In an acinus, there are approximately three generations of respiratory bronchioles, followed by two to six generations of alveolar ducts, each of which may lead to as many as six alveolar sacs.

FIGURE 2–32

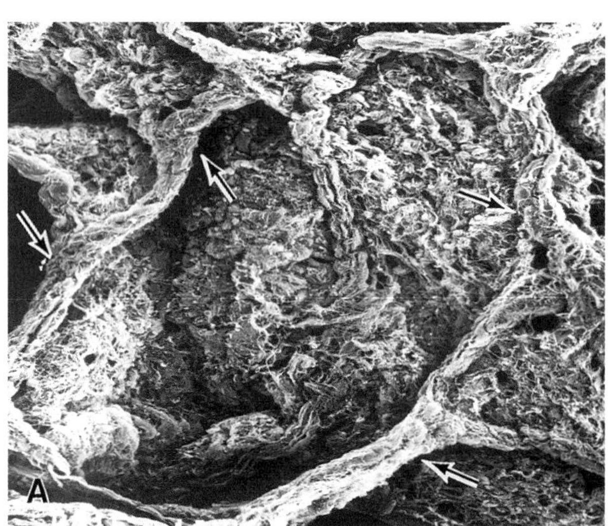

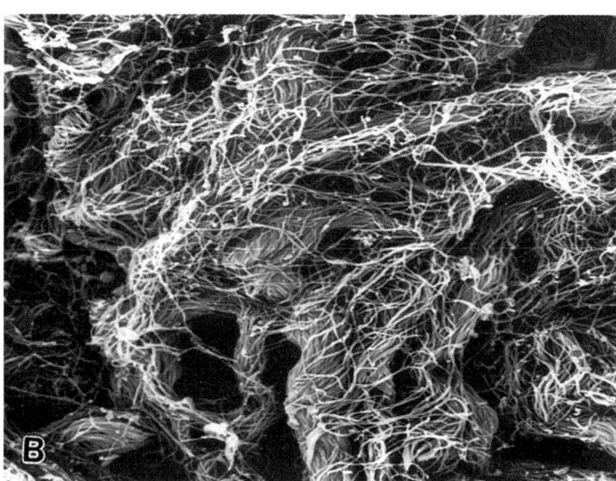

Collagen ultrastructure of the alveolar wall after digestion with 2.5 M NaOH solution (scanning electron microscopy). **A,** The walls of an alveolus are indicated by arrows. The alveoli evaginate from the alveolar ducts and sacs, with their orifices lined by the collagen and elastic fiber bundles that are continuous with the bronchiolar connective tissue framework. **B,** Finer collagen and elastic fibers branch from the orifice bundle to form a mesh of connective tissue. This network supports the alveoli and is essential in the uniform expansion and retraction of the lung during respiration.

ALVEOLUS

FIGURE 2–33

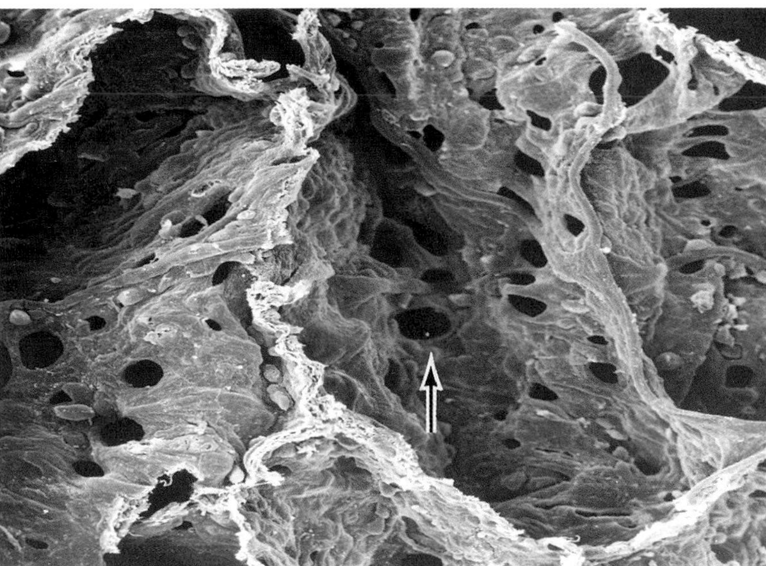

Alveoli (scanning electron microscopy). The alveolus is the smallest unit of the lung, and this cup-shaped structure averages 250 μm in diameter. There are approximately 300 million alveoli in the adult, and this corresponds to a gas-exchanging surface area of approximately 143 m^2. The alveolar walls contain channels, the pores of Kohn (*arrow*). These round to oval openings range in size from 2.5 nm to 15 nm and are usually filled with surfactant-containing liquid film. Theoretically, they provide a means for collateral ventilation and, in disease states, a passageway for infectious agents and excess fluid. Alveolar macrophages, inflammatory cells, or tumor cells could also pass through these pores.

ALVEOLUS

FIGURE 2–34

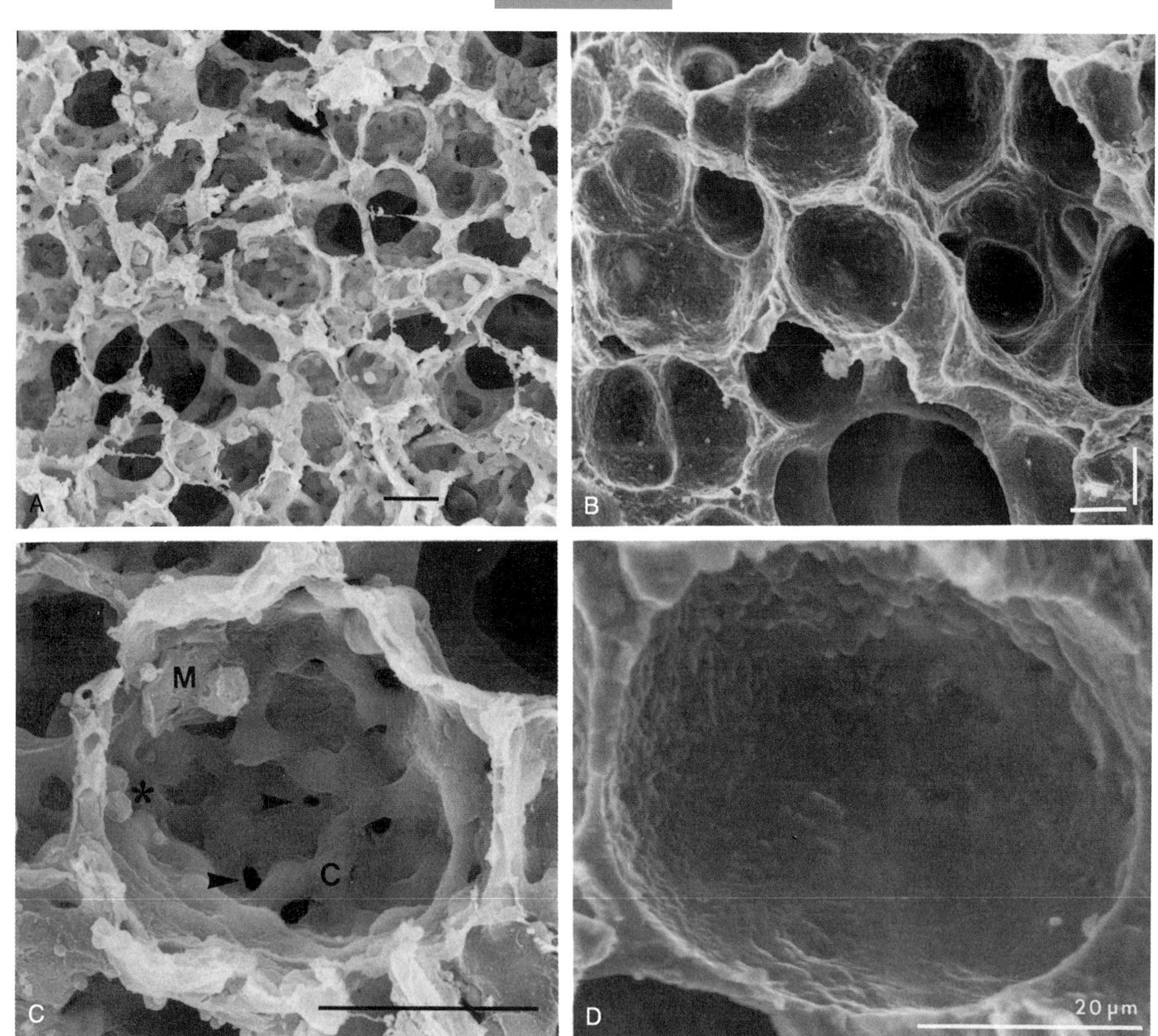

Low-temperature scanning electron microscopy, a technique that preserves the alveolar fluid, shows that the pores of Kohn may allow the components of the aqueous subphase of alveolar lining fluid to spread through the lung.[15] Pores of Kohn, visible in conventionally prepared instillation-fixed dried mouse lung with scanning electron microscope (**A** and **C**), are not evident in another air-inflated frozen hydrated mouse lung held at − 196°C in a low-temperature scanning electron microscope (**B** and **D**). When lung water and air-liquid interface are preserved in a frozen state, the surface contour of the lung is smoother and simplified. **C** and **D,** higher magnification of alveoli in center of **A** and **B.** Note irregular contour of instillation-fixed critical point-dried alveolus (**C**), where surface lining layer has been washed away with liquid fixative and solvents. (M, macrophage on surface; *arrowheads,* patent pores of Kohn; c, prominent capillaries) Capillaries do not protrude in alveoli preserved in a frozen state, although ice-crystal texture is evident. (*Bars,* 20 μm.) (From Bastacky J, Goerke J: Pores of Kohn are filled in normal lungs: Low-temperature scanning electron microscopy. J Appl Physiol 73:88–95, 1992.)

ALVEOLUS

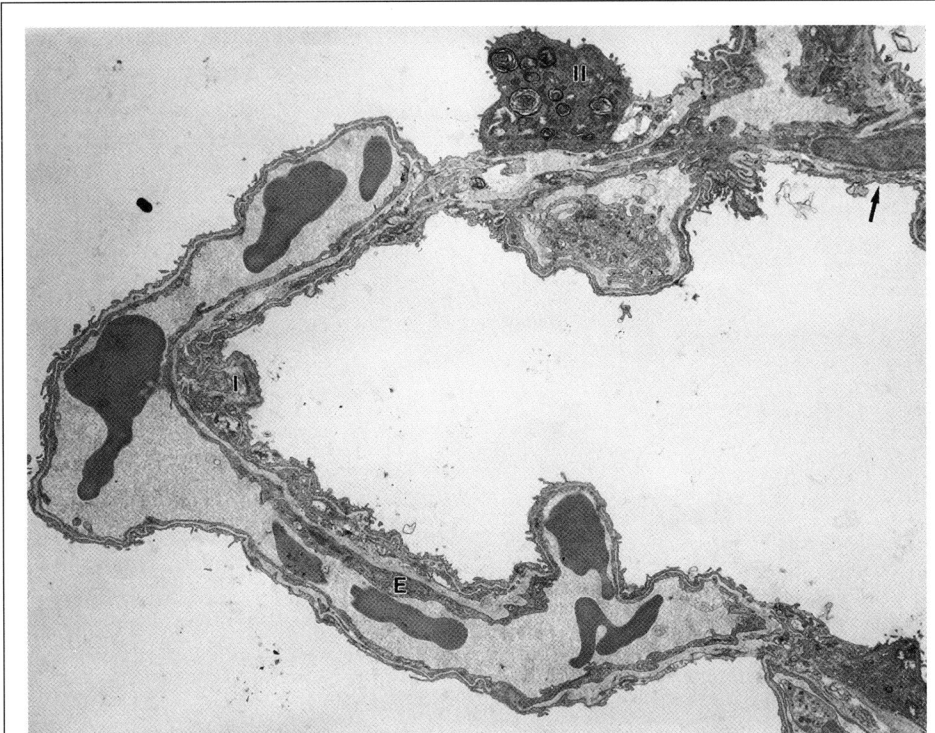

FIGURE 2–35

Alveolus (transmission electron microscopy). The main cells that compose the interalveolar septa are the alveolar epithelial (I and II), interstitial (INT) and endothelial (E) cells. The number of different alveolar cells and their percentages are listed in TABLE 2–6.[16] There are two types of alveolar epithelial cells: type I and type II cells. The type I cell, or membranous pneumocyte, is a flat cell with numerous cytoplasmic extensions, which cover the majority of the alveolar surface. The arrow indicates the thin cytoplasmic extension of the type I cell. The type II cell, or granular pneumocyte, is a cuboidal cell with microvilli that secretes surfactant. Within many alveoli, though none are shown here, there are also macrophages, which phagocytize inhaled bacteria and particulate matter.

TABLE 2–6

Cells of the Alveolar Region

	Cells	Percentage of Total
Alveolar type I cell	19×10^6	8.3
Alveolar type II cell	37×10^6	15.9
Endothelial cell	68×10^6	30.2
Interstitial cell	84×10^6	36.1
Macrophage	23×10^6	9.4

ALVEOLUS

ALVEOLAR TYPE I CELL

FIGURE 2-36

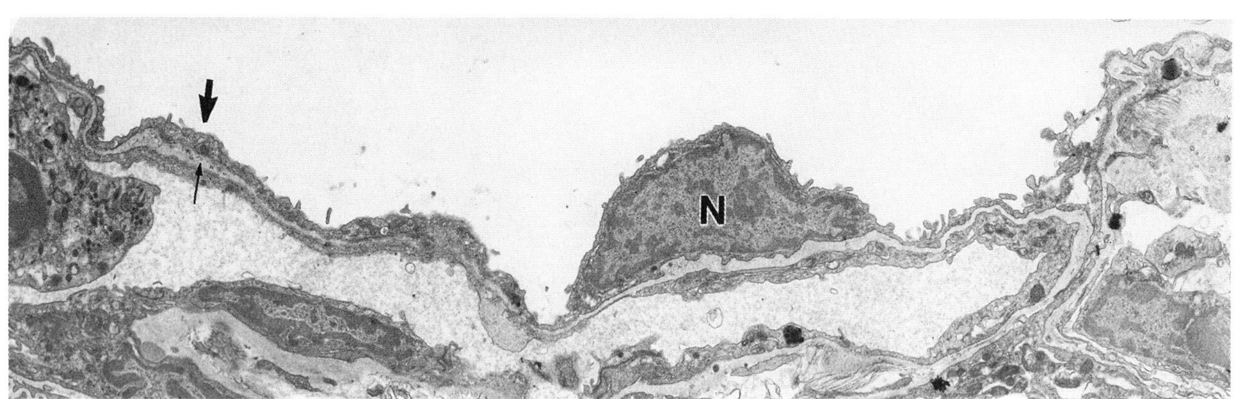

Alveolar type I epithelial cell (transmission electron microscopy). Although these cells make up only 8.3% of total lung cells, their thin cytoplasmic extensions (*large arrow*), which measure approximately 50 μm in diameter and 0.1 μm thick, enable them to cover 90% of the approximately 150 m^2 surface area of the lung. These cells are flat with slightly raised central nuclei (N). In addition, they contain some perinuclear mitochondria and endoplasmic reticulum and few organelles in the cytoplasmic extensions. With such extensive coverage of the alveolar surface, type I cells play an important role in forming the air-blood barrier. This barrier is extremely thin in order to allow for the most efficient exchange of oxygen and carbon dioxide. The thinnest portion of the barrier measures approximately 0.6 μm and is composed of the endothelial and alveolar type I cytoplasm and their fused basal laminas (*small arrow*). This distance may be increased by changes in the constituents of the interstitium (e.g., increased collagen), interstitial cells (e.g., increased numbers of fibroblasts or infiltrates of inflammatory or neoplastic cells), or plasma (e.g., edema fluid).

ALVEOLAR TYPE II CELL

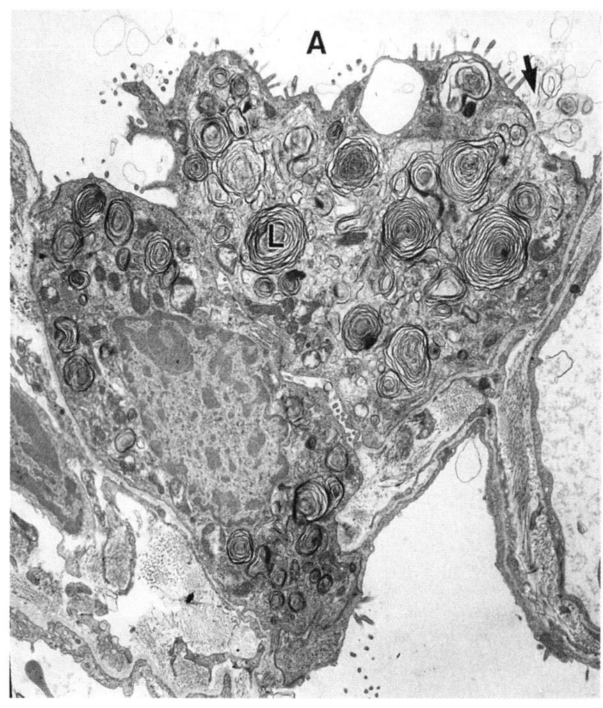

FIGURE 2-37

Alveolar type II epithelial cell (transmission electron microscopy). Type II cuboidal cells are twice as common as type I cells, but cover only approximately 7% of the alveolar surface area. They have a basal nucleus and a prominent Golgi apparatus and endoplasmic reticulum, features of active secretory cells. Their distinctive feature is the presence of 100 to 150 lamellar inclusion bodies (L) per cell, which represents the intracellular form of surfactant. Type II cells synthesize the phospholipid and protein components of surfactant and store them in these lamellar bodies until they are released *(arrow)* into the alveolar space (A).

In addition to their secretory function, type II cells also have a reparative role. In response to alveolar damage, type II cells act as reserve cells with the capacity to divide and differentiate into type I cells, which are very susceptible to injury. Studies also suggest that type II cells may have a role in the metabolism of foreign compounds, the transport of fluid and electrolytes and the defense against oxidant damage to the lungs.[13]

ALVEOLUS

SURFACTANT

FIGURE 2-38

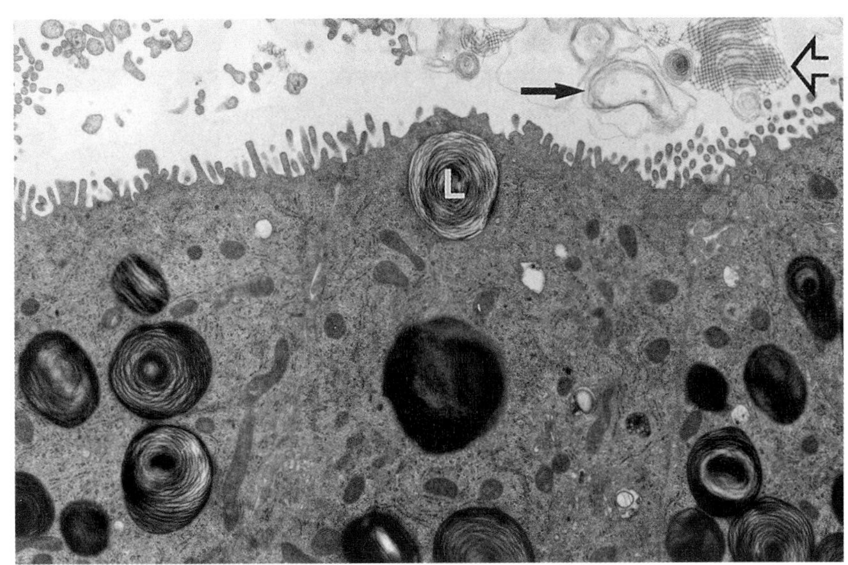

Apical surface of a type II pneumocyte showing surfactant as intracellular lamellar bodies (L), secreted lamellar myelin (*closed arrow*), and the lattice structure of tubular myelin (*open arrow;* transmission electron microscopy.) After secretion and hydration, the contents of the lamellar bodies expand into tubular myelin. The phospholipids from tubular myelin form the surface monolayer of surfactant. This insoluble monolayer on alveolar lining fluid allows surfactant to modify alveolar surface tension depending on the surface area. It promotes lung expansion on inspiration and prevents lung collapse on expiration. (From Finkbeiner WE: Respiratory cell culture. *In* Crystal RG, West JB, Weibel ER, Barnes PJ (eds): The Lung. Philadelphia, Lippincott-Raven, 1997 p. 423, courtesy of L. Dobbs and L. Allen.)

FIGURE 2-39

Components of Surfactant

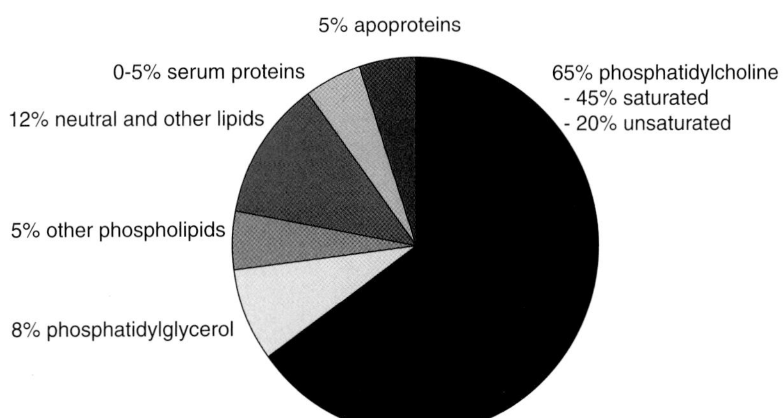

Components of surfactant.[17] Surfactant is a heterogeneous substance made predominantly of lipids (~90%) and proteins (10%). The lipid component consists of mainly phospholipids, in particular, phosphatidylcholine. At an air-fluid interface, phospholipids will form a surface film with their hydrophilic polar head groups contacting water and their hydrophobic nonpolar tails extending into the air, a process called adsorption. The phospholipid intermolecular forces oppose the normal attracting forces between the surface water molecules, which reduces the surface tension of water from 70 mN/m to approximately 25 mN/m. This reduction in surface tension increases lung compliance and thus reduces the work of expanding the lung. In addition, surfactant increases the stability of the alveoli and prevents fluid transudation and thus lung edema.

The protein component of surfactant consists of serum proteins, such as albumin and immunoglobulins, and surfactant-specific proteins, termed SP-A, SP-B, SP-C, and SP-D. These apoproteins are synthesized by both type II epithelial cells and Clara cells and appear to have a role in the formation of tubular myelin and regulating surfactant turnover and metabolism.

ALVEOLUS

SURFACTANT

FIGURE 2-40

The life cycle of surfactant. *Key:* 1, glucose, amino acids and fatty acids, surfactant precursors; 2, endoplasmic reticulum; 3, Golgi apparatus; 4, lamellar bodies; 5, tubular myelin; 6, surface monolayer with adsorbed phospholipids; 7, vesicular forms of surfactant for reuptake into type II cells; 8 and 9, endocytic forms of surfactant, such as multivesicular bodies, which subsequently become lamellar bodies; 10, clearance by macrophages. After synthesizing and storing surfactant in lamellar bodies, type II cells will secrete surfactant in response to a number of different signals, including beta-adrenergic agonists, lung inflation, and hyperventilation. After secretion, the interaction between lamellar bodies, apoproteins, and calcium forms tubular myelin, and ultimately the surface monolayer. During 1 hour, type II cells secrete 10 to 40% of their total intracellular surfactant, and in order to balance this continuous secretion, there must be equally active clearance mechanisms. There are three main routes of clearance. The principal route is reuptake of surfactant by type II cells, which removes up to 90% of the total. The second pathway is phagocytosis by macrophages, and the smallest amount is cleared by the airways.[18] (From Hawgood S, Clements JA: Pulmonary surfactant and its apoproteins. J Clin Invest 86: 1–6, 1990.)

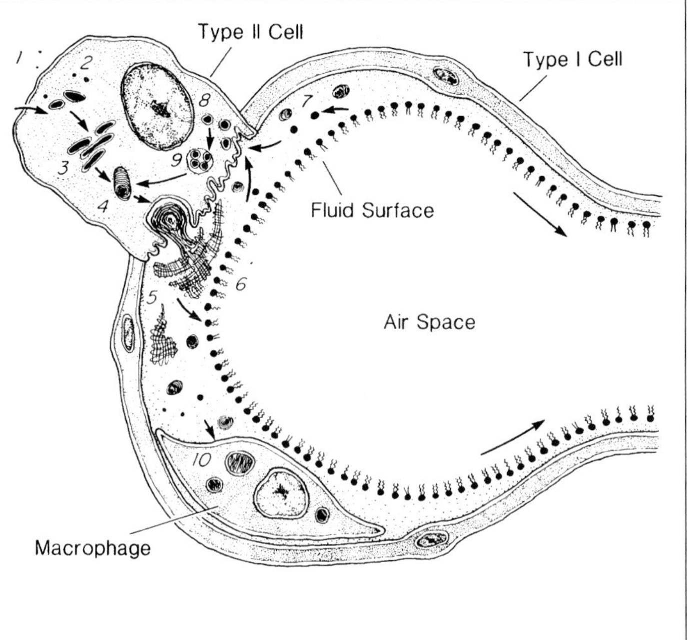

INTERSTITIAL CELLS

FIGURE 2-41

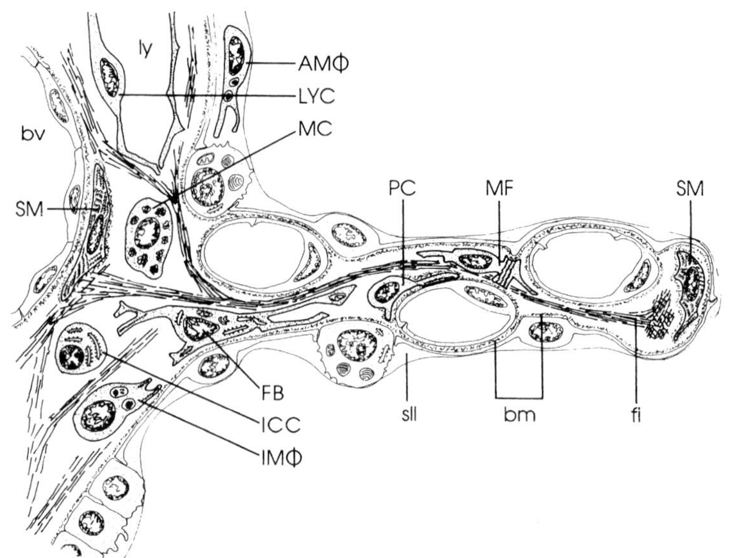

Interstitium and interstitial cells of the alveolar septum. The interstitium is the space between the airway epithelium, vascular endothelium, and pleural mesothelium. Thus, it is continuous from the hilum to the visceral pleura. It consists of connective tissue, a number of different cells, and lymph-like extracellular fluid. The connective tissue system provides mechanical stability to the lung and serves as a framework for alveoli and capillaries. The interstitium also plays an important role in draining interstitial fluid from the alveolar capillaries to the juxta-alveolar lymphatics, as there are no lymphatic vessels in the interalveolar septa.

The principal cells of the interstitium are the mesenchymal cells, which include fibroblasts, myofibroblasts, and pericytes. The fibroblasts synthesize connective tissue fibers, and the myofibroblasts and pericytes have contractile features. There are also a number of inflammatory cells and lymphatic endothelial cells. These different cells are surrounded by an interstitial matrix of collagen and elastic fibers.

Key: alveolar macrophage (AM), basement membrane (bm), blood vessel (bv), fibroblasts (fb), fiber strands (fi), various immune competent cells (ICC), interstitial macrophages (IM), lymphatic endothelial cells (LYC), myofibroblasts (MF), mast cells (MC), pericytes (PC), alveolar surface lining layer (sll), smooth muscle cells (SM). (From Weibel R, Crystal RG: Structural organization of the pulmonary interstitium. *In* Crystal RG, West JB, Weibel ER, Barnes PJ (eds): The Lung. Philadelphia, Lippincott-Raven, 1997, p. 686.)

ALVEOLUS

MACROPHAGES

FIGURE 2–42

Alveolar macrophage (transmission electron microscopy). Although present throughout the respiratory tract, macrophages are dominant in the alveolar spaces, with approximately 50 to 100 per alveolus. Macrophages are derived from blood monocytes and are characterized by eccentrically placed oval nuclei, pseudopods, or elongated cytoplasmic processes, and large lysosomal granules. They migrate around the alveoli and bronchial surfaces to scavenge for and phagocytize debris and bacteria. They also act as antigen-presenting cells, have the ability to recruit and activate other inflammatory cells, and secrete a number of different products, which are listed in TABLE 2–7. (From Kuhn C III: Normal anatomy and histology. *In* Thurlbeck WM, Churg AM (eds): Pathology of the Lung. New York, Thieme Medical Publishers, 1995, p. 23.)

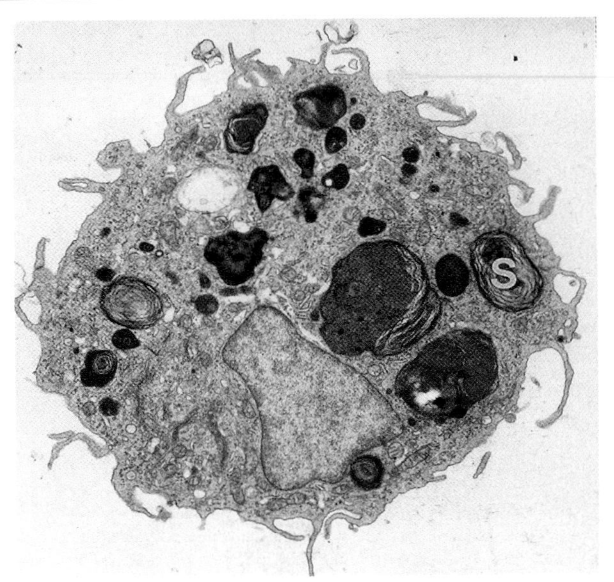

TABLE 2–7

Secretory Products of Macrophages

Enzymes
- Lysosomal enzymes
- Lysozyme
- Urokinase plasminogen activator
- Collagenase
- Other matrix metalloproteinases

Inhibitors
- $Alpha_1$-protease inhibitor
- $Alpha_1$-antichymotrypsin
- $Alpha_2$-macroglobulin
- Tissue inhibitor of metalloproteinases
- Plasminogen activator inhibitors

Modulators of cell activity
- Chemotactic factors
- Growth factors
- Interleukins
- Colony-stimulating factors
- Prostaglandins
- Leukotrienes
- Interferons

Other
- Oxidants (H_2O_2, O_2^-, HO)
- Fibronectin
- Complement proteins

CIRCULATORY SYSTEM

PULMONARY ARTERIES AND ARTERIOLES

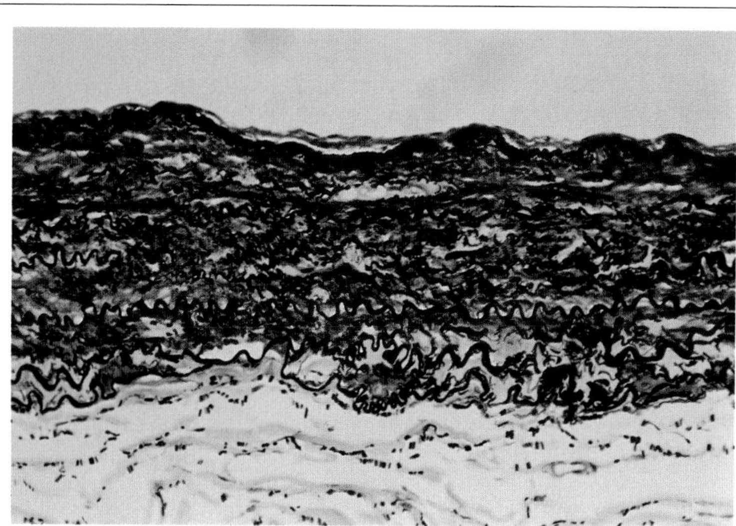

FIGURE 2-43

Elastic pulmonary artery (light microscopy, elastic van Gieson stain). The pulmonary trunk and the main branches of the pulmonary arteries that are larger than 500 μm are elastic arteries. They are characterized by a media of concentric elastic laminas, which are widely separated by smooth muscle. As the diameter of the arteries decrease, the number of elastic laminas diminish and become closer together.

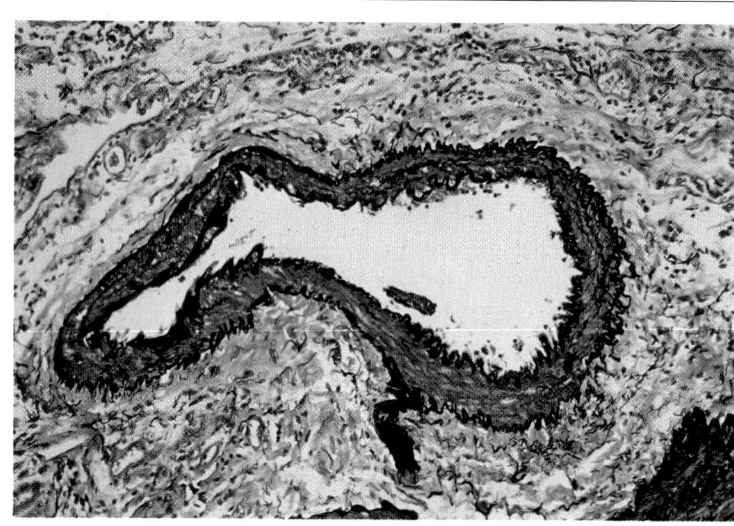

FIGURE 2-44

Muscular pulmonary artery, oblique section (light microscopy, elastic van Gieson stain). The muscular pulmonary arteries accompany small bronchi and respiratory bronchioles and range in size from 70 to 500 μm. They have a thin circumferential layer of smooth muscle bordered by an internal and external elastic lamina. These arteries branch approximately simultaneously with the airways.

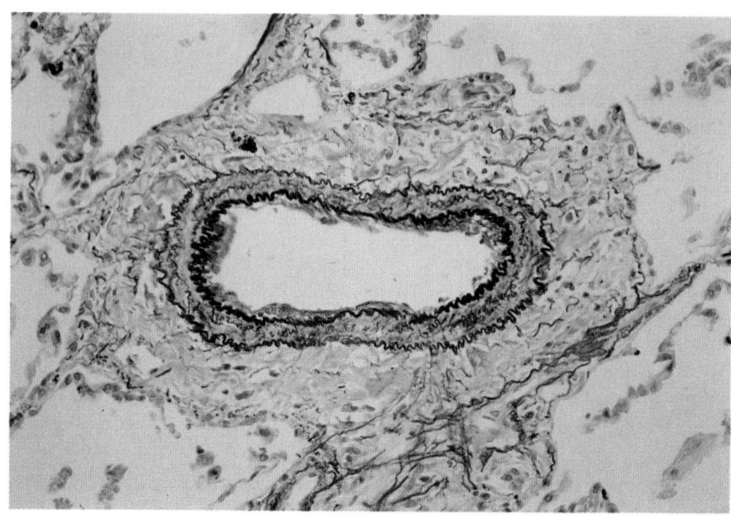

FIGURE 2-45

Arterioles (light microscopy, Weigert elastic van Gieson stain). The pulmonary arterioles, which are less than 70 μm in diameter, supply the alveolar ducts and alveoli. They contain a partial muscular layer that eventually disappears so that the wall consists only of endothelium and an elastic lamina.

CIRCULATORY SYSTEM

PULMONARY VEINS AND VENULES

FIGURE 2-46

Pulmonary venule, longitudinal section (light microscopy, elastic van Gieson stain). The pulmonary venules collect blood from the capillaries in the lobular septi. The smallest venules are histologically indistinguishable from arterioles and are identified by tracing their origin and drainage. They have a single elastic membrane and occasionally smooth muscle cells may be present. As venules become veins, they develop a muscular media.

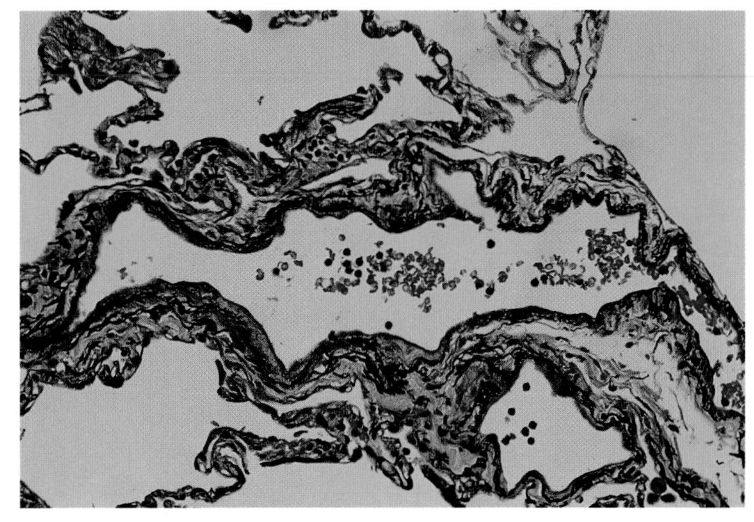

FIGURE 2-47

Pulmonary vein (light microscopy, elastic van Gieson stain). The intima of the pulmonary veins is composed of endothelium overlying an internal elastic lamina. There is no distinct boundary between the media and adventitia, which are composed of smooth muscle fibers, collagen, and elastic fibers. In addition, pulmonary veins do not have valves.

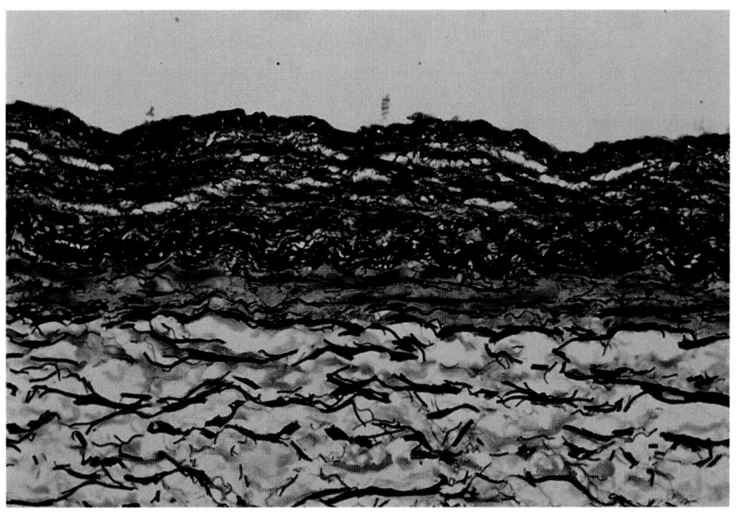

CIRCULATORY SYSTEM

CAPILLARIES

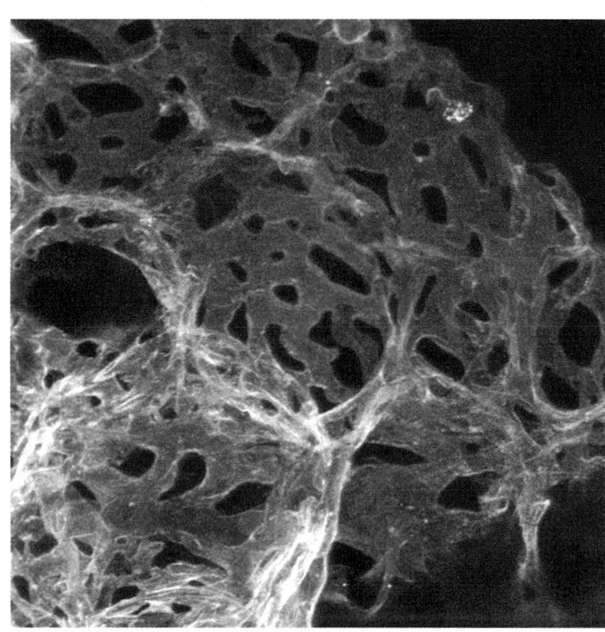

FIGURE 2-48

Confocal fluorescence micrograph of mouse alveolar capillaries stained by vascular perfusion of fluorescein *L. esculentum* lectin. The pulmonary capillary bed is large and extensive, covering 85 to 95% of the alveolar surface, or approximately 126 m^2. These capillaries form hexagonal meshes around the alveolar walls, and each capillary perfuses more than one alveolus as it passes from arteriole to venule.[19] The capillary walls consist of endothelium lying on a thin basement membrane, which sometimes fuses with that of the alveolar epithelium. (Courtesy of Dr. Gavin Thurston, Cardiovascular Research Institute, University of California, San Francisco.)

ENDOTHELIAL CELLS

Endothelial cells play an essential role in forming the air-blood barrier and in the exchange of oxygen and carbon dioxide, water, and solutes. They also have a number of metabolic functions, which include clearing serotonin and norepinephrine from the blood stream, converting angiotensin I to angiotensin II, and metabolizing adenine nucleotides.[13]

FIGURE 2-49

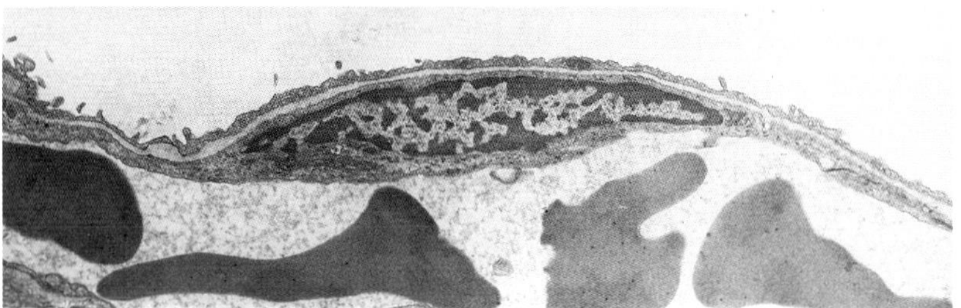

Endothelial cell (transmission electron microscopy). The ultrastructure of endothelial cells varies according to the site. Cells of the pulmonary arteries feature microvilli, complex tight junctions, gap junctions, and Weibel-Palade granules, which are electron-dense granules containing von Willebrand's factor. The endothelium of pulmonary veins is similar to that of the arteries, except that there are fewer microvilli and gap junctions. In contrast, the flat endothelial cells of capillaries (shown here) have few tight junctions, gap junctions, and no Weibel-Palade granules.[20]

TABLE 2-8

Metabolic Functions of Pulmonary Endothelial Cells

Uptake or clearance from the blood stream
- Serotonin
- Norepinephrine
- Prostaglandins E and F
- Adenine nucleotides
- Angiotensin I
- Bradykinin
- Adenosine
- Hormones and drugs

Release into the blood stream
- Adenosine
- Angiotensin I
- Prostaglandins E and F
- Previously accumulated drugs and metabolites
- Lipids

Unaffected by endothelium
- Epinephrine
- Angiotensin II
- Prostaglandins A and I2

Source: Gail DB, Lenfant CJM: Cells of the lung: biology and clinical implications. Am Rev Respir Dis 127: 366–387, 1983.

BRONCHIAL CIRCULATION

FIGURE 2-50

Origin of the bronchial arteries. The lung has a dual blood supply, receiving blood from the pulmonary arteries and bronchial arteries. The bronchial arteries originate directly from the aorta or intercostal arteries. In 80% of cases a right bronchial artery is related to the first right intercostobronchial artery, and in the majority of cases the left bronchial arteries arise form the anterior wall of the descending aorta.[21] An internal elastic lamina, a media of circularly oriented smooth muscle, and the absence of an external elastic lamina characterize the bronchial artery. (From Charan NB, Carvalho PG: Anatomy of the normal bronchial circulatory system in humans and animals. *In* Butler J (ed): The Bronchial Circulation. New York, Marcel Dekker, 1992, p. 49.)

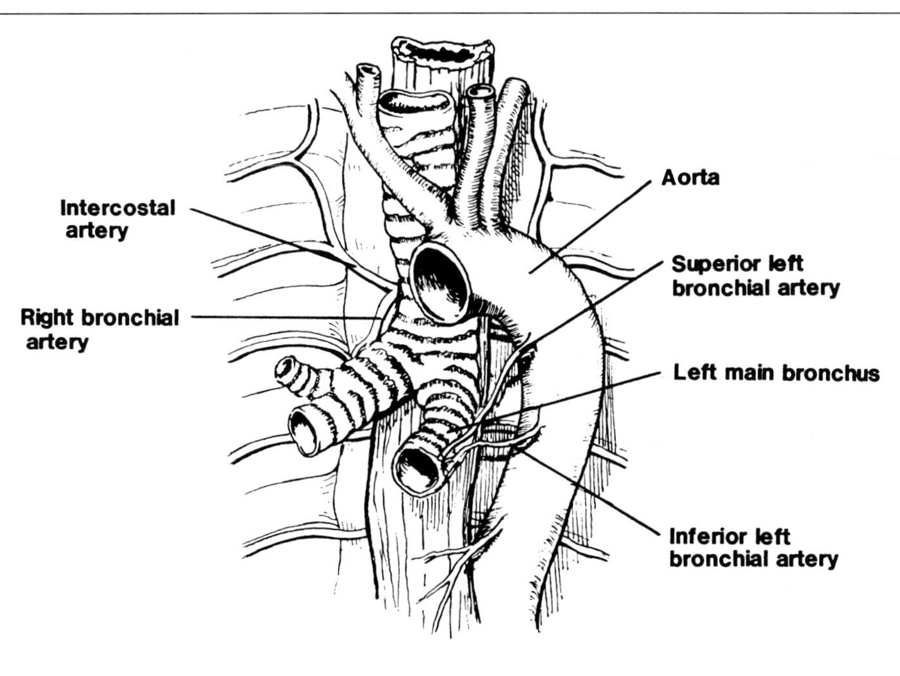

TABLE 2-9

Numbers of Left and Right Bronchial Arteries and Their Combinations in 30 Human Autopsy Cases

Number of Cases	Number of Bronchial Arteries*	
	RIGHT	LEFT
1	1	0
4	1	1
9	1	2
4	1	3
1	1	4
1	1	5
1	2	1
6	2	2
1	2	3
1	2	4
1	3	2
30	41	65

* Right: mean = 1.3. Left: mean = 2.2.
Source: Modified from Schreinemakers H, Cooper JD: The human bronchial circulation: anatomy and lung transplantation. *In* Butler J (ed): The Bronchial Circulation. New York, Marcel Dekker, 1992, p. 730.

BRONCHIAL CIRCULATION

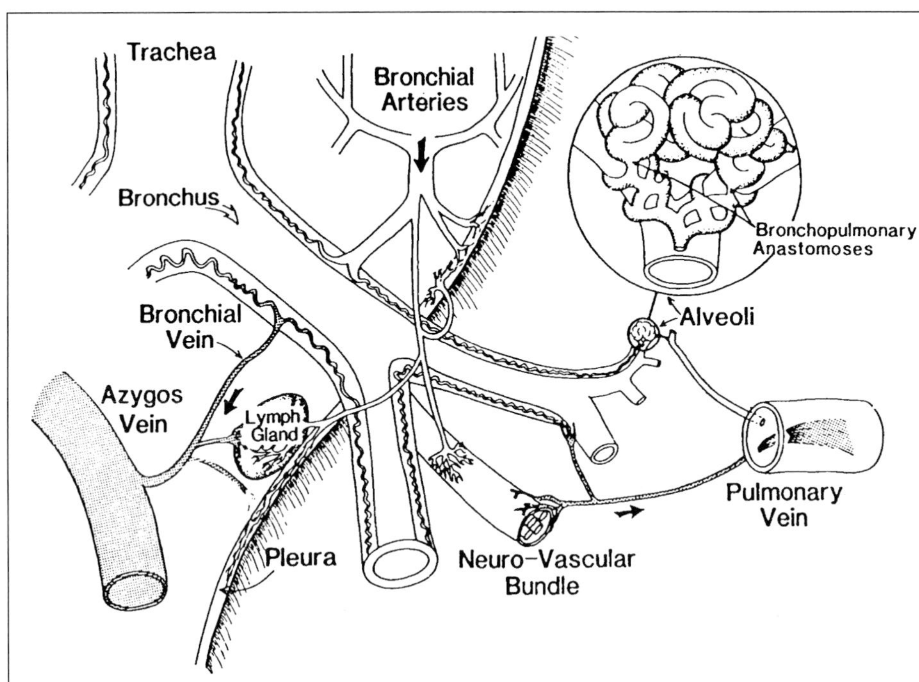

FIGURE 2-51

The systemic blood circulation to the lungs. The bronchial arteries follow the bronchial tree as far as the terminal bronchioles, anastomosing freely and forming a vascular plexus in the peribronchial space.[22] Small branches penetrate the muscular layer to reach the bronchial mucosa to form a submucosal plexus. The bronchial microvascular plexus anastomoses with the pulmonary vasculature both along the airway and distal to the terminal bronchioles. Branches of the bronchial arteries also supply the visceral pleura. Ultimately, the bronchial circulation drains into the azygos or hemiazygous veins. (From Deffebach ME, et al: Am Rev Respir Dis 135:463–481 1987.)

FIGURE 2-52

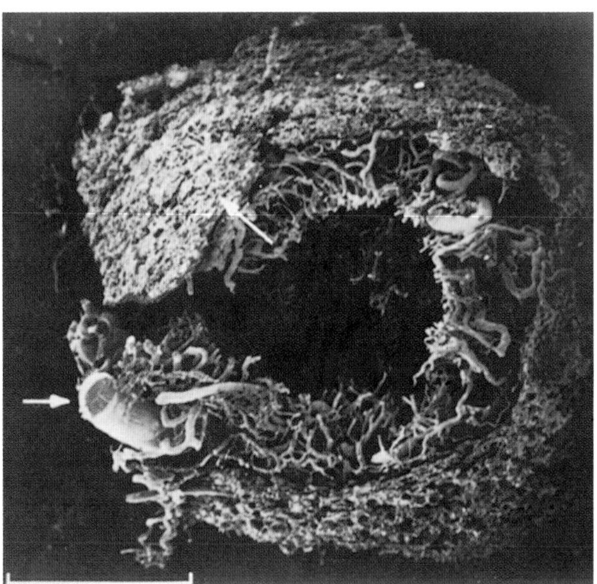

Bronchial microvasculature filled with Batson's solution in the sheep (scanning electron microscopy). Bronchial capillaries are a dense plexus of thin vessels, which originate from a bronchial artery (*lower arrow*). The upper arrow indicates a network of alveolar capillaries. (From Charan NB, et al: Gross and subgross anatomy of the bronchial circulation in sheep. J Appl Physiol 57:658–664, 1984.)

LYMPHATIC SYSTEM

FIGURE 2–53

The distribution of lymphatic vessels. Lung lymphatics, like lymphatic vessels elsewhere in the body, play important roles in fluid homeostasis, the recovery of interstitial fluid and proteins, the response to infection, and the spread of disease. The lymphatics of the lung are organized in two main plexuses—the superficial, or pleural network, and the deep, or the peribronchovascular network. The lymphatics are situated in the connective tissue of the pleura, interlobular septa, and peribronchovascular sheaths. The subpleural vessels, the vessels in the interlobular septa, and those associated with the pulmonary veins compose the superficial network. The lymphatic fluid in this network flows either over the surface of the lung or through the lung to reach the hila. The deep lymphatics begin with the respiratory bronchioles, as there are no lymphatics in the alveolar septa, and they follow the bronchovascular bundles toward the hila. Although the two systems anastomose at the interlobular septa and at the pleura, their drainage remains predominantly separate. (From Okada Y: Lymphatic System of the Human Lung. Kyoto, Japan, Kinopodo, 1989.)

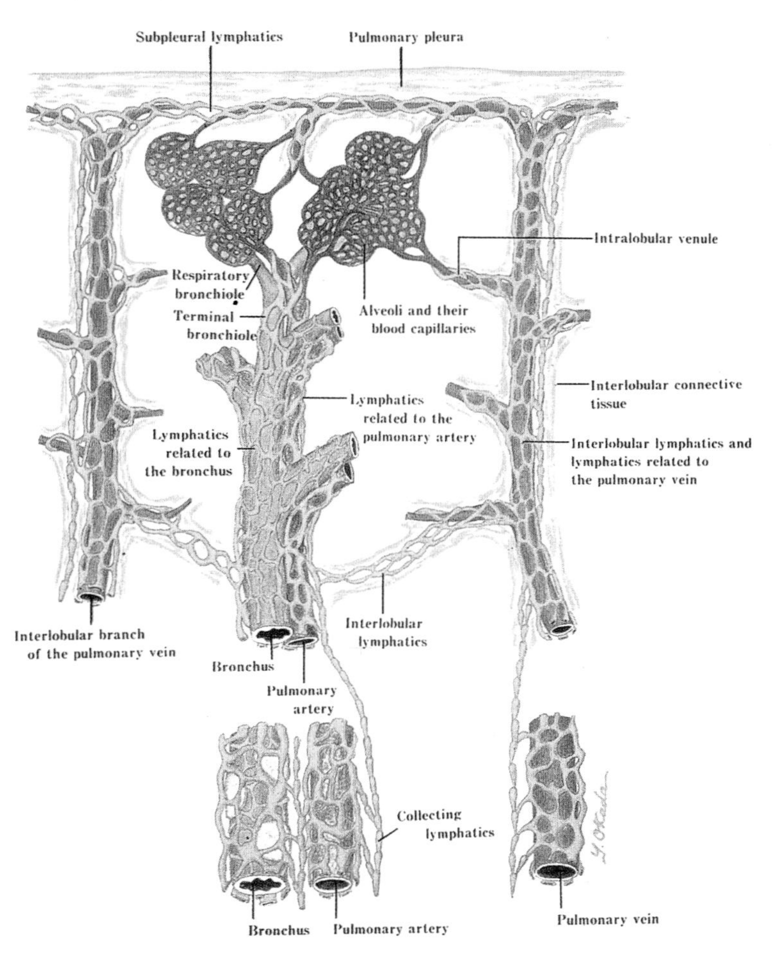

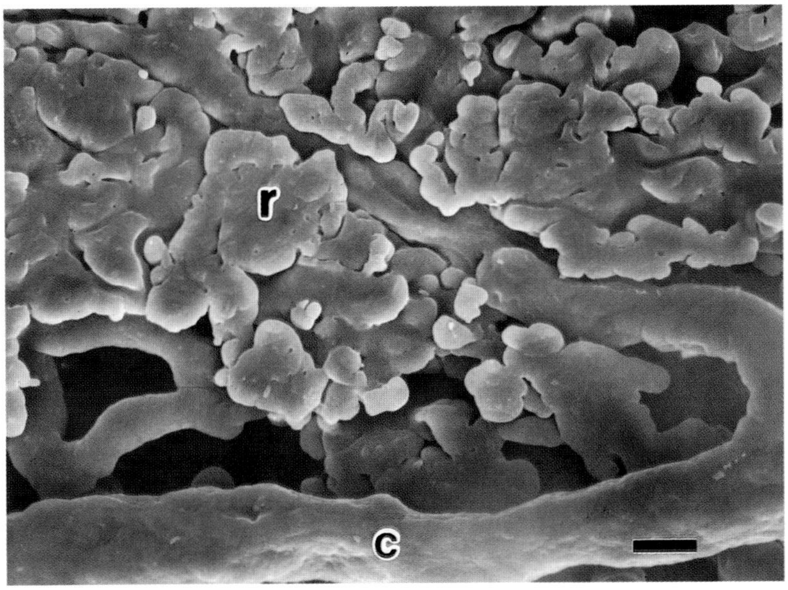

FIGURE 2–54

Lung lymphatic cast (scanning electron microscopy). The lymphatics of the lung have a number of different forms. Prelymphatics are the interstitial spaces that form tissue planes around bronchovascular bundles and beneath the pleura. These drain into reservoir (r), conducting (c), or tubulosaccular lymphatics. Reservoir lymphatics have a flat, ribbon-like structure with blind-ended outpouchings. They are located beneath the visceral pleura and drain into cylindrical conducting lymphatics that are distributed on the pleura, along bronchovascular bundles, and in the interlobular septa. (From Schraufnagel DE: Forms of lung lymphatics: A scanning electron microscopic study of casts. Anat Rec 233:547–554, 1992.)

LYMPHATIC SYSTEM

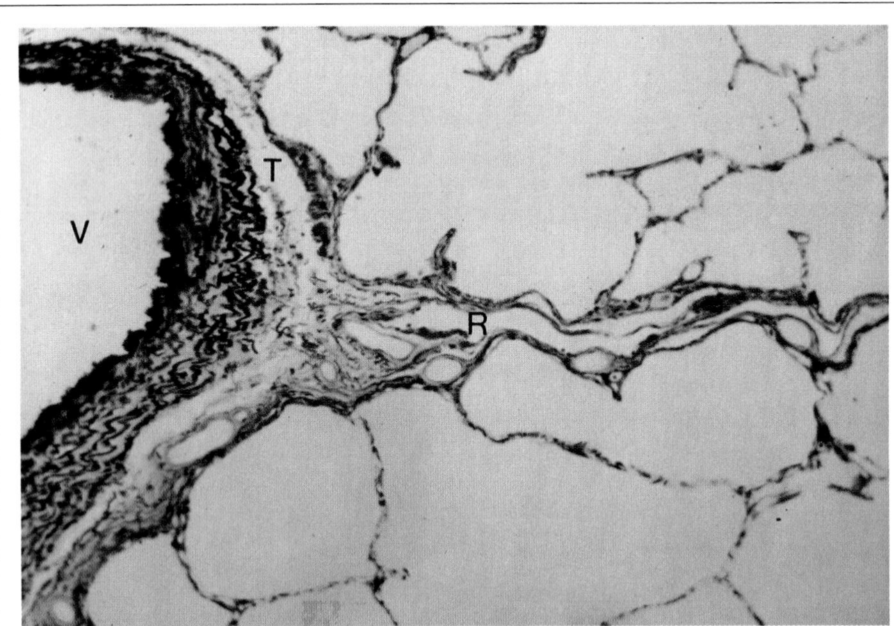

FIGURE 2–55

Lymphatic vessels (light microscopy, elastic van Gieson stain). A tubulosaccular lymphatic (T) lies adjacent to a pulmonary vein (V). The receiving reservoir lymphatic (R) is in the interlobular septa. The basement membrane in the smallest lymphatics is discontinuous, and larger lymphatics develop a muscular media and an adventitia of mainly collagen and fibroblasts. The endothelial cells are connected to the interstitium by anchoring filaments on their basal surface, and adjacent cells may overlap considerably. Within the collecting lymphatics are funnel-shaped valves, which promote the one-way transport of lymph toward the hila of the lungs.

FIGURE 2–56

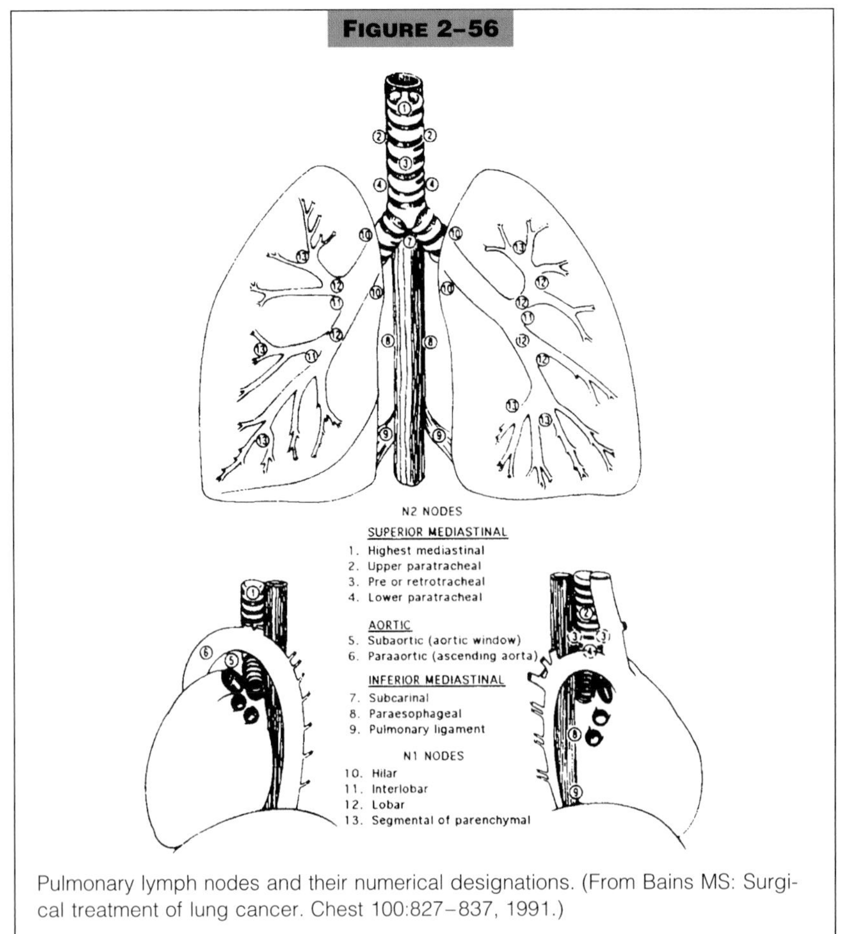

Pulmonary lymph nodes and their numerical designations. (From Bains MS: Surgical treatment of lung cancer. Chest 100:827–837, 1991.)

LYMPHATIC SYSTEM

FIGURE 2–57

Pulmonary lymph nodes and the direction of lymph flow. (From Barkley HT: Lung. *In* Fletcher GH (ed): Textbook of Radiotherapy. Philadelphia, Lea & Febiger, 1980, p. 669.)

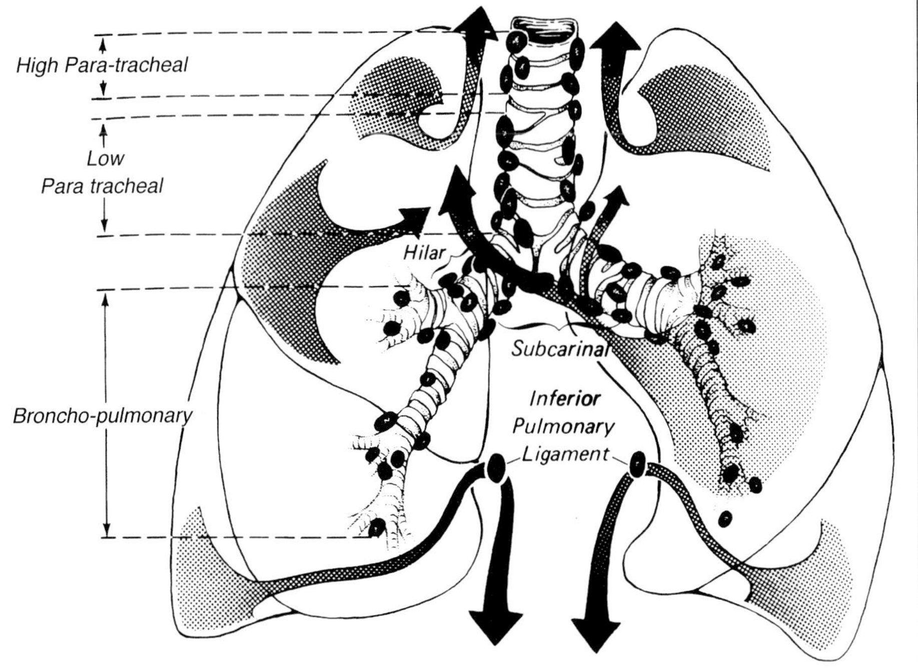

FIGURE 2–58

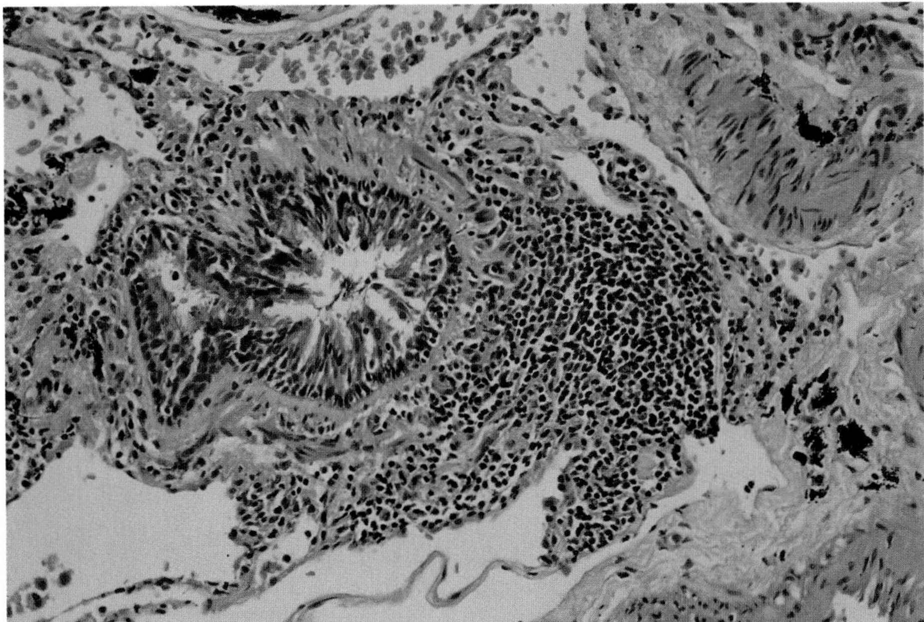

Bronchial-associated lymphoid tissue (light microscopy, hematoxylin-eosin stain). Lymphoid tissue plays an integral role in the defense of the lung. The pulmonary lymphoid tissue can be divided into three main groups—lymphoid nodules, lymphoid aggregates and infiltrates, and lymph nodes. Lymphoid nodules are unencapsulated follicles of lymphocytes present below specialized, nonciliated, flattened epithelium of the bronchus and small bronchioles and usually at airway bifurcations. The lymphoid tissue associated with the tracheobronchial tree is known as the bronchus-associated lymphoid tissue (BALT). Presumably, BALT is involved in the immune response, as a site for environmental antigen sampling and processing. Lymphoid aggregates and infiltrates (shown here) are less organized groups of lymphocytes in peripheral airways, such as terminal bronchioles. These forms of bronchopulmonary lymphoid tissue are relatively rare at birth and increase thereafter. This trend may represent an adaptive response to antigenic stimulation through an individual's life.[6]

NERVOUS SYSTEM

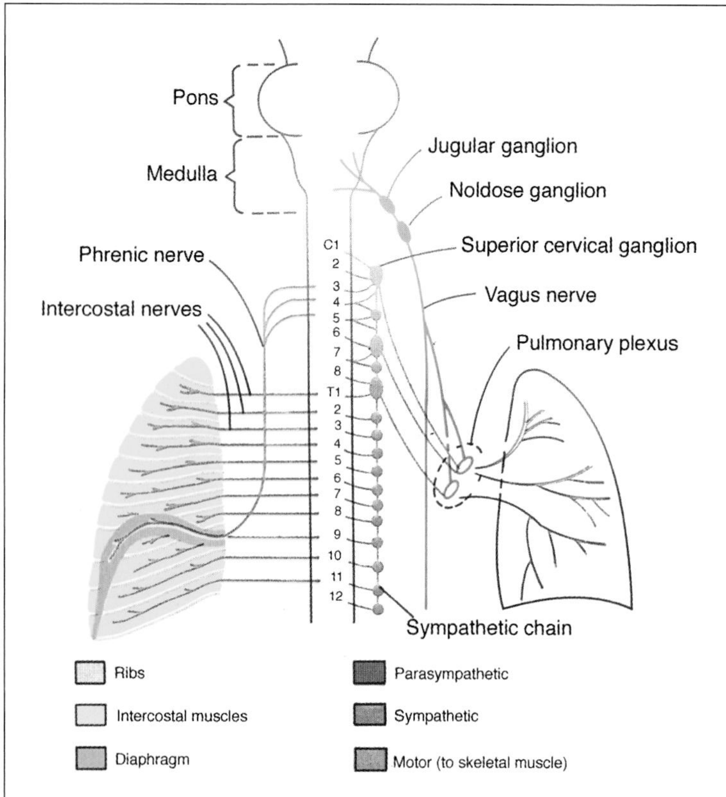

FIGURE 2-59

Diagram of the autonomic innervation of the lung and somatic innervation of the intercostal muscles and diaphragm. The lungs have a dual innervation that results in excitatory and inhibitory neurophysiologic responses. The vagus nerves and the upper four or five thoracic sympathetic ganglion nerves make up the peribronchial plexus and periarterial plexus located at the hila of the lungs, as illustrated here. The peribronchial plexus is further subdivided as the extrachondrial plexus, found between the cartilage and adventitial tissue and the subchondrial plexus, located between the cartilage and the airway epithelium. The periarterial plexus begins as bundles of large nerves, which decrease in size to single fibers that innervate the arterioles and capillaries. (From Murray JF: The Normal Lung (2nd ed). Philadelphia, WB Saunders, 1986, p. 70.)

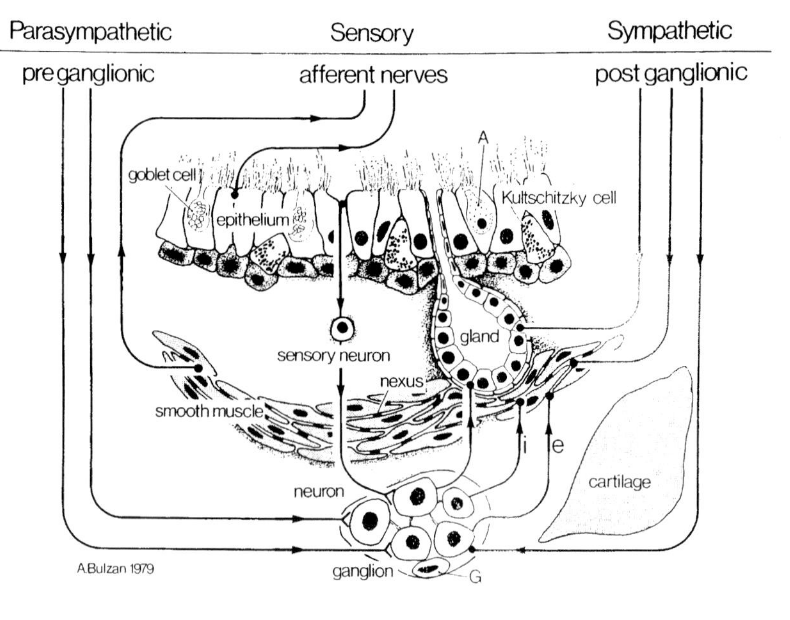

FIGURE 2-60

Schematic diagram of the innervation of the airways (G = glial cells, e = excitatory fibers, i = inhibitory fibers, A = granular cell). In the efferent system, the preganglionic parasympathetic fibers and the postganglionic sympathetic fibers terminate in the ganglia, which are scattered along the perichondrial plexus to the level of the small bronchi. These ganglia contain excitatory neurons that are cholinergic and inhibitory neurons that are nonadrenergic. The postganglionic excitatory or inhibitory fibers innervate smooth muscle, and the excitatory fibers also terminate in the glands. In the afferent system, sensory nerve endings begin in the epithelium and the smooth muscle, and the neurons of the afferent system are found in the vagus or vagal nuclei. (From Richardson JB: Nerve supply to the lungs. Am Rev Resp Dis 119:785–802, 1979.)

NERVOUS SYSTEM

There are three main groups of vagal sensory receptors—the bronchopulmonary stretch receptors, the irritant receptors, and the C-fiber receptors. The stretch receptors function in controlling breathing pattern, and the irritant and C-fiber receptors have a role in regulating airway tone, certain protective reflexes (e.g., cough) as well as in lung disease or abnormal conditions. Some evidence also suggests the existence of a fourth group of receptors, the chemoreceptors, which may respond to changes in air or blood-gas concentrations (Table 2–11).

TABLE 2–10

Neuropeptides Released in the Respiratory Tract*

Peptide	Localization
• Vasoactive intestinal peptide • Peptide histidine isoleucine/methionine • Peptide histidine valine-42 • Helodermin • Pituitary adenylate cyclase-activating peptide • Galanin	Parasympathetic
• Substance P • Neurokinin A • Neuropeptide K • Calcitonin gene-related peptide • Gastrin-releasing peptide	Afferent
• Neuropeptide Y	Sympathetic
• Somatostatin • Enkephalin • Cholecystokinin octapeptide	Afferent/uncertain

* Numerous neuropeptides are relesed from the parasympathetic, sympathetic, and afferent neurons to produce a wide range of effects on airway function.
Source: Barnes PB, Baraniuk MG: Neuropeptides in the respiratory tract. Am Rev Respir Dis 144:1187–1198, 1991.

TABLE 2–11

Characteristics of the Three Pulmonary Vagal Sensory Receptors

Receptor	Location	Fiber Type	Stimulus	Response
Pulmonary stretch, slowly adapting	Associated with smooth muscle of intrapulmonary airways	Myelinated	1. Lung inflation 2. Increased trans-pulmonary pressure	1. Hering-Breuer inflation reflex 2. Bronchodilation 3. Increased heart rate 4. Decreased peripheral vascular resistance
Irritant, rapidly adapting	Epithelium of (mainly) extrapulmonary airways	Myelinated	1. Irritants 2. Mechanical stimulation 3. Anaphylaxis 4. Lung inflation or deflation 5. Hyperpnea 6. Pulmonary congestion	1. Bronchoconstriction 2. Hyperpnea 3. Expiratory constriction of larynx 4. Cough 5. Mucous secretion
C-fibers – Pulmonary (type J) – Bronchial	 Alveolar wall Airways and blood vessels	Nonmyelinated	1. Increased interstitial volume (congestion) 2. Chemical injury 3. Microembolism	1. Rapid shallow breathing 2. Laryngeal and tracheobronchial constriction 3. Bradycardia 4. Spinal reflex inhibition 5. Mucous secretion

Source: Modified from Murray JF: The Normal Lung (2nd ed). Philadelphia, WB Saunders, 1986, p. 73.

PLEURA

FIGURE 2-61

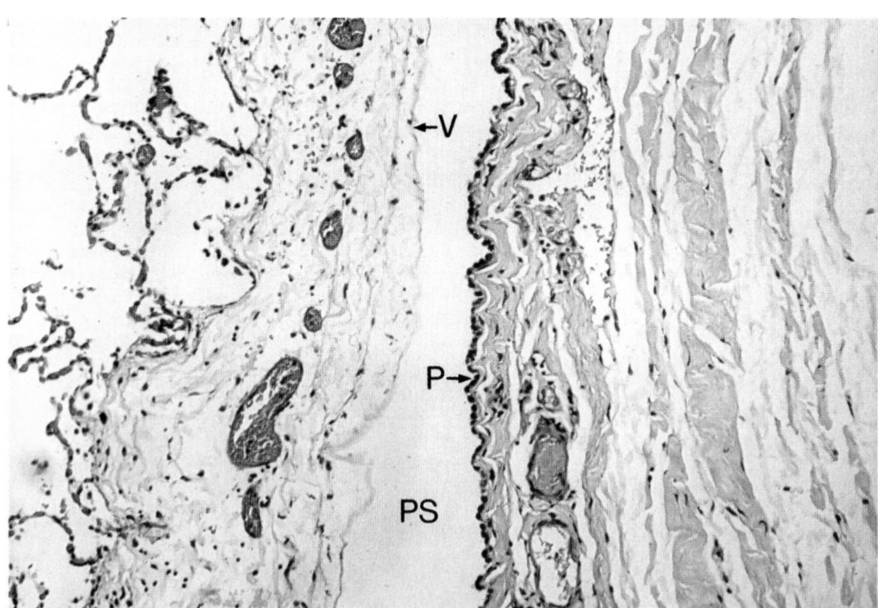

Visceral and parietal pleura (light microscopy, hematoxylin-eosin stain). The visceral pleura (V) is the serous membrane that intimately covers the surfaces of the lungs, including any recesses produced by the fissures. The parietal pleura (P) lines the internal wall of the thoracic cavity and has four parts. The costal pleura lines the ribs, costal cartilages, and sternum. The mediastinal pleura covers the mediastinal structures, and at the lung hilum becomes continuous with the visceral pleura. The diaphragmatic pleura tightly attaches to the diaphragm, especially at its central tendon. The cervical pleura, or capula, covers the apex of the lung above the first rib. The visceral and parietal pleurae are separated by the pleural space or cavity (PS), which is usually filled with a small amount of clear, serous fluid. Mesothelial cells lying on basement membranes form a simple, single cell epithelium that lines both pleural surfaces. Beneath the basement membranes are layers of collagen and elastic tissue layers containing lymphatics, blood vessels, and nerves.[23]

FIGURE 2-62

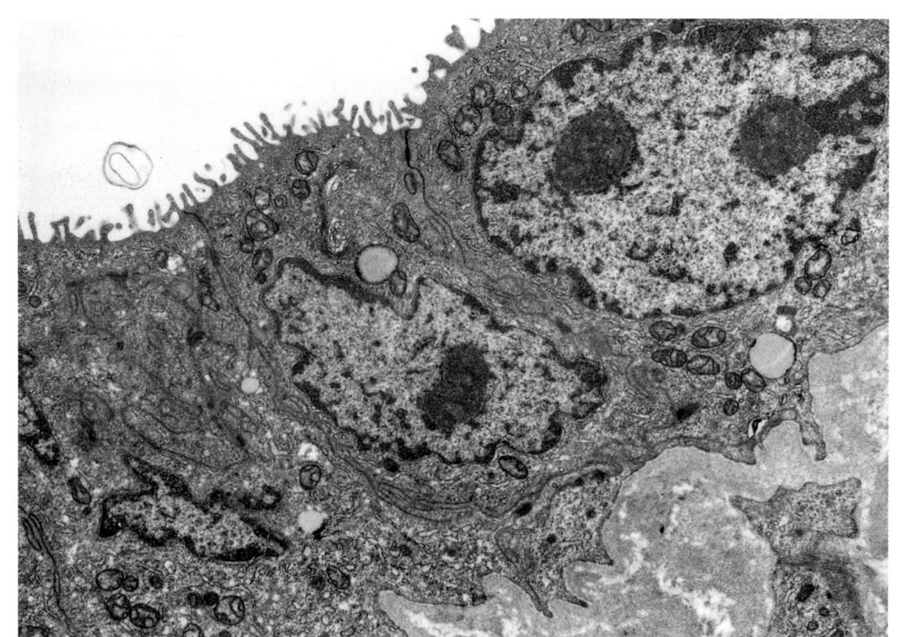

Mesothelial cell (transmission electron microscopy). Mesothelial cells range from 6 to 12 μm in diameter and are characterized by a centrally placed nucleus surrounded by mitochondria, well-developed Golgi apparatus and endoplasmic reticulum, and 200 to 300 microvilli, their most conspicuous feature. Covered with hyaluronic acid glycoprotein, the microvilli are thought to provide a lubricating effect between the two pleural surfaces, as well as aid in cellular transport activities.[23]

Neighboring mesothelial cells are attached by tight intercellular junctions and desmosomes. These cells are quite active producing collagen, elastin, fibronectin, laminin, growth factor β1, fibroblast growth factor, and tissue factor that binds coagulation factor.[24] (Courtesy of Robert Munn, Department of Medical Pathology, University of California, Davis.)

PLEURA

FIGURE 2-63

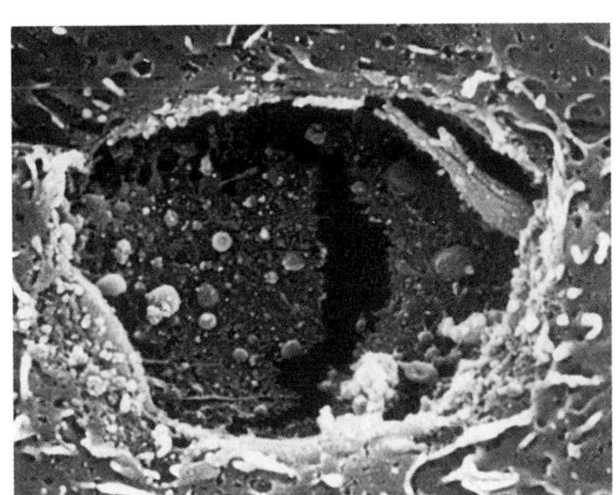

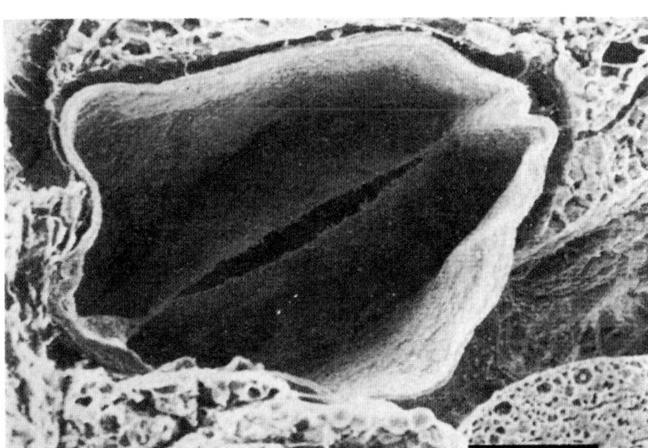

Stoma and valves of the parietal pleura. The lymphatic system of the pleura is quite extensive. The lymphatic vessels of the visceral pleura correspond to the superficial lymphatic network. Thus, the lymph from the visceral pleura flows to the hilum either over the lung surface or through the lung. These lymphatics do not contain any pleural fluid, as they are separated from the pleural space by a connective tissue layer; however, the pleural cavity does communicate directly with the lymphatics of the parietal pleura through 2 to 6-nm pores or stomas (*left*). These stomas, which are more common on the mediastinal and infracostal regions of the parietal pleura and are absent on the visceral pleura, connect the pleural cavity to lacunas, or dilated lymphatic spaces. Fluid and particulate matter is thus removed from the pleural cavity and transported into lymphatic vessels. Movement of the lymphatic fluid is promoted by muscle contractions during respiration, and retrograde movement is prevented by one-way valves in the lacunas (*right*). Eventually, the lymphatic fluid drains into the internal mammary, para-aortic, and diaphragmatic lymph nodes. (From Leak LV: Lymphatic removal of fluids and particles in the mammalian lung. Environ Health Persp 35:55–76, 1980.)

TABLE 2-12

Comparison Between Visceral and Parietal Pleurae

	Visceral Pleura	Parietal Pleura
Vascular supply	Bronchial arteries	Systemic vessels - Costal pleura-intercostal arteries - Diaphragmatic pleura-superior phrenic and musculophrenic arteries - Mediastinal pleura-pericardiacophrenic artery
Lymphatic system	Superficial lymphatic system of the lung	Follow systemic vessels to regional lymph nodes
Nervous supply	Few corpuscular endings (insensitive to pain)	Intercostal, phrenic, and vagus nerves Sympathetic trunk branches (sensitive to pain)

REFERENCES

1. O'Rahilly R: The early prenatal development of the human respiratory system. *In* Nelson GH (ed): Pulmonary Development. New York, Marcel Dekker, 1985, pp. 3–18.

2. Crelin ES: Development of the lower respiratory system. Clin Symposia 27:3–28, 1975.

3. Hislop A, Reid L: Growth and development of the respiratory system: anatomical development. *In* Davis JA, Dobbing J (eds): Scientific Foundations of Paediatrics (2nd ed). Baltimore, University Park Press, 1981, pp. 390–432.

4. Dunnill MS: Postnatal growth of the lung. Thorax 17: 329–333, 1962.

5. Gehr P, Bachofen M, Weibel ER: The normal human lung: Ultrastructure and morphometric estimation of diffusion capacity. Resp Physiol 32:121–140, 1978.

6. Breeze RG, Wheeldon EB: The cells of the pulmonary airways. Am Rev Respir Dis 116:705–777, 1977.

7. Li JD, Dohrman AF, Gallup M, et al: Transcriptional activation of mucin by *Pseudomonas aeruginosa* lipopolysaccharide in the pathogenesis of cystic fibrosis lung disease. Proc Natl Acad Sci (USA) 94:967–972, 1997.

8. Spicer SS, Schulte BA, Chakrin LW: Ultrastructural and histochemical observations of respiratory epithelium and gland. Exp Lung Res 4:137–156, 1983.

9. Mariassy AT, St. George J, Nishio SJ, et al: Tracheobronchial epithelium of the sheep: III. Carbohydrate histochemical and cytochemical characterization of secretory epithelial cells. Anat Rec 221:540–549, 1988.

10. Lamblin G, Aubert JP, Perini JM, et al: Human respiratory mucins. Eur Respir J 5:247–256, 1992.

11. Lopez-Vidriero MT, Reid L: Bronchial mucus in health and disease. Br Med Bull 34:63–74, 1978.

12. Basbaum CB, Jany B, Finkbeiner WE: The serous cell. Ann Rev Physiol 52:97–113, 1990.

13. Gail DB, Lenfant CJM: Cells of the lung: Biology and clinical implications. Am Rev Respir Dis 127:366–387, 1983.

14. Johnson DE, Georgieff MK: Pulmonary neuroendocrine cells. Am Rev Respir Dis 140:1807–1812, 1989.

15. Bastacky J, Goerke J: Pores of Kohn are filled in normal lungs: Low-temperature scanning electron microscopy. J Appl Physiol 73:88–95, 1992.

16. Jones WD, Good RC, Thompson NJ, et al: Bacteriophage types of *Mycobacterium tuberculosis* in the United States. Am Rev Respir Dis 125:640–643, 1982.

17. Hawgood S: Surfactant: Composition, structure, and metabolism. *In* Crystal RG, West JB, Barnes PJ, et al (eds): The Lung, Scientific Foundations (2nd ed). Philadelphia, Lippincott-Raven, 1997, pp. 557–571.

18. Pison U, Neueundank MA, Weibbach S, et al: Host defence capacities of pulmonary surfactant: Evidence for 'non-surfactant' functions of the surfactant system. Eur J Clin Invest 24:586–599, 1994.

19. Staub N, Schultz EL: Pulmonary capillary length in dog, cat and rabbit. Resp Physiol 5:371–378, 1968.

20. Kuhn CI: Normal anatomy and histology. *In* Thurlbeck WM, Churg AM (eds): Pathology of the Lung (2nd ed). New York, Thieme Medical Publishers, 1995, pp. 1–36.

21. Schreinemakers H, Cooper JD: The human bronchial circulation: anatomy and lung transplantation. *In* Butler J (ed): The Bronchial Circulation. New York, Marcel Dekker, 1992, pp. 725–748.

22. Charan NB, Carvalho PG: Anatomy of the normal bronchial circulatory system in humans and animals. *In* Butler J (ed): The Bronchial Circulation. New York, Marcel Dekker, 1992, pp. 45–77.

23. Lee KF, Olak J: Anatomy and physiology of the pleural space. Chest Surg Clin North Am 4:391–403, 1994.

24. Antony VB, Sahn SA, Mossman B, et al: Pleural cell biology in health and disease. Am Rev Respir Dis 145: 1236–1239, 1992.

CHAPTER

3

Respiratory Pathology

Walter E. Finkbeiner, M.D., Ph.D.

INTRODUCTION

All pathologic processes at the cellular level are based on host reaction to injury. Therefore, lung diseases can be grouped according to the underlying type of injury. However, in practice, lung diseases are usually grouped in categories based on a combination of etiology, pathophysiology, or pathology (morbid anatomy) (TABLE 3–1). It must be kept in mind that similar gross and even microscopic pathologic features may be shared among categories and that there may be distinct differences in the pattern of lung damage among diseases of similar etiology (TABLE 3–2). (See Chapter 7, Laboratory Diagnosis of Respiratory Tract Infections.)

TABLE 3–1

Classification of Lung Pathology

Classification Based on Type of Cell Injury	Classification Based on Etiology, Pathophysiology, and Pathologic Features
Hypoxia/anoxia	Lung disease caused by infectious agents
Immunologic reactions	Chronic obstructive pulmonary disease
Biologic agents	Diffuse infiltrative (restrictive) lung disease
Physical agents	Disease of pulmonary vessels
Chemical agents	Neoplastic lung disease
Genetic abnormalities	Congenital lung disease
Nutritional imbalances	Developmental lung disease

INTRODUCTION

TABLE 3-2

Definitions of Important Morphologic and Pathologic Processes

Process	Definition
Necrosis	Cell death
Coagulation necrosis	Necrosis characterized by temporary preservation of basic cell appearance and typically caused by anoxia or severe hypoxia
Liquefaction necrosis	Necrosis characterized by digestion of dead cells and loss of cell and tissue architecture and typically caused by bacterial and occasionally fungal infections
Caseous necrosis	Particular type of mixed coagulation and liquefaction necrosis that develops from infections with *Mycobacterium tuberculosis* complex and some fungal organisms
Apoptosis	Programmed or regulated death of single cells in an asynchronous fashion
Atrophy	Cell shrinkage
Hypertrophy	Cell enlargement and subsequent tissue or organ enlargement
Hyperplasia	Increase in the number of cells in an organ or tissue often contributing to its enlargement
Metaplasia	Reversible replacement of one type of mature cell type by another
Inflammation	Extravascular accumulation of fluid and plasma proteins (edema) along with leukocytes
Acute inflammation	Early phase of inflammation characterized by edema and primarily neutrophils
Chronic inflammation	Later phase of inflammation characterized by presence of lymphocytes, macrophages, angiogenesis, and fibrosis
Fibrinous inflammation	Acute inflammation rich in fibrin developing with severe injury, particularly in body cavities
Granulomatous inflammation	Particular type of chronic inflammation dominated by the presence of epithelioid (activated) macrophages and usually surrounded by lymphocytes and occasionally plasma cells; often epithelioid macrophages fuse to form giant cells
Granulation tissue	Specialized tissue of healing rich in new blood vessels and fibroblasts
Organization	May refer to conversion of a fibrinous inflammation to scar tissue or to fibrosis or scarring
Fibrosis	Repair and remodeling of injured tissue via replacement by extracellular matrix rich in collagen (scarring)
Pneumonia	Inflammation of the lung; pneumonitis
Pneumonitis	Inflammation of the lung; pneumonia
Neoplasia	New and uncoordinated growth of abnormal and autonomous tissue
Dysplasia	Disordered growth, typically of epithelial cells, characterized by loss of cell uniformity and partial loss of polarity
Anaplasia	Loss of cellular differentiation and severe disturbances of architectural orientation

LUNG DISEASE CAUSED BY INFECTIOUS AGENTS

Etiologic classification of lung disease is the most useful because treatments are directed against specific infectious agents.

TABLE 3–3

Classifications of Infectious Pneumonia

Classification	Types of Pneumonia
Chronicity	• Acute pneumonia • Chronic pneumonia
Epidemiology	• Community-acquired pneumonia • Hospital-acquired pneumonia
Host risk factors	• Primary (previously healthy individual) pneumonia • Secondary (underlying disease predisposing to lung infection) pneumonia
Anatomy	• Lobar pneumonia • Bronchopneumonia • Interstitial pneumonia
Etiology	• Infectious organism

VIRAL INFECTIONS

In the 1930s and 1940s the term "primary atypical pneumonia" was coined to refer to a pneumonia syndrome distinct from lobar pneumonia in which no bacteria could be cultured or seen on Gram stain of the sputum. Subsequently, the organisms that caused this syndrome were identified as *Mycoplasma pneumoniae, Chlamydia* species, *Rickettsia* species, and the viruses. The common viral pathogens of the respiratory tract and their major pathologic reactions are listed in TABLE 3–4.

TABLE 3–4

Common Viral Pathogens of the Respiratory Tract

Viral Agent	Major Pathologic Effects	Inclusions	Multinucleation
RNA VIRUSES			
Orthomyxoviridae			
– Influenza A, B, C	Necrotizing bronchitis/bronchiolitis; DAD; BOOP; bacterial superinfection	None	No
Paramyxoviridae			
– Measles	Bronchitis/bronchiolitis; DAD; interstitial pneumonia with multinucleate epithelial giant cells	Intranuclear; intracytoplasmic	Yes
– Parainfluenza 1–4	Laryngotracheobronchitis; occasional bronchiolitis; interstitial pneumonia; DAD	Intracytoplasmic	Occasional
– Respiratory syncytial	Necrotizing bronchiolitis; interstitial pneumonia	Intracytoplasmic	Yes
Picornaviridae			
– Rhinovirus	URI; rarely tracheobronchitis/bronchiolitis or pneumonia in ICH	None	No
– Enterovirus	URI; rarely tracheobronchitis/bronchiolitis or pneumonia in ICH	None	No
– Coxsackie B	URI; rarely tracheobronchitis/bronchiolitis or pneumonia in ICH	None	No
– Echovirus	URI; rarely tracheobronchitis/bronchiolitis or pneumonia in ICH	None	No
Coronaviridae			
– Coronavirus	URI; rarely tracheobronchitis/bronchiolitis or pneumonia in ICH	None	No

LUNG DISEASE CAUSED BY INFECTIOUS AGENTS

VIRAL INFECTIONS

TABLE 3-4

Common Viral Pathogens of the Respiratory Tract *continued*

Viral Agent	Major Pathologic Effects	Inclusions	Multinucleation
DNA VIRUSES			
Adenoviridae			
- Adenovirus	Necrotizing bronchitis/bronchiolitis; DAD	Intranuclear; "smudge" cells	No
Herpetoviridae			
- Herpes simplex 1 and 2	Ulcerative tracheobronchitis/bronchiolitis; hemorrhagic miliary nodules	Intranuclear	Rare
- Varicella-zoster	Hemorrhagic miliary nodules		Rare
- Cytomegalovirus	Hemorrhagic nodular pneumonia; DAD	Intranuclear; intracytoplasmic	No
Bunyaviridae			
- Hantavirus	Massive edema and congestion; DAD; alveolar interstitial infiltrates of T cell–derived immunoblasts	None	No

Key: DAD = diffuse alveolar damage; BOOP = bronchiolitis obliterans organizing pneumonia; URI = upper respiratory tract infection; ICH = immunocompromised host.

FIGURE 3-1

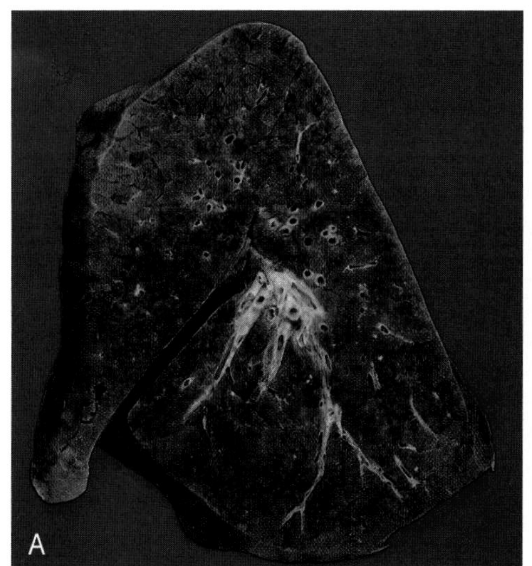

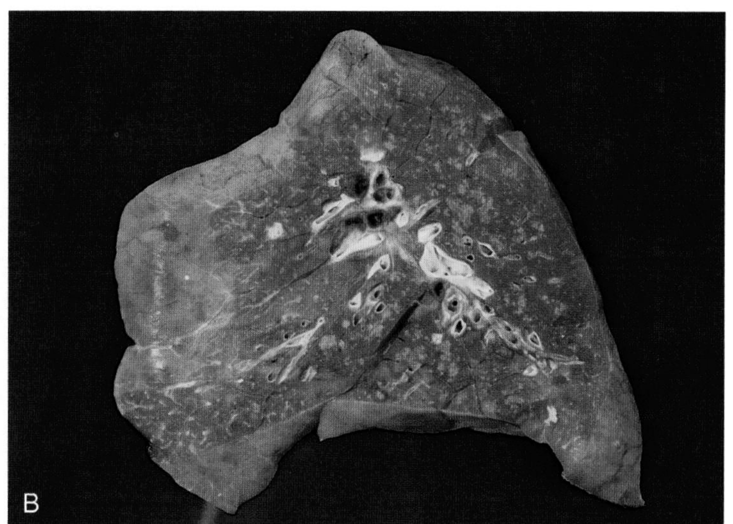

Mild viral pneumonias cause patchy consolidation of the lungs or mild diffuse interstitial inflammation along with acute congestion. Severe or fatal pneumonias result in more extensive lung injury that may be patchy or diffuse. Superimposed bacterial infection may modify the process. **A,** Organizing diffuse alveolar damage in cytomegalovirus pneumonia. **B,** Patchy necrosis due to adenovirus pneumonia.

LUNG DISEASE CAUSED BY INFECTIOUS AGENTS

VIRAL INFECTIONS

FIGURE 3-2

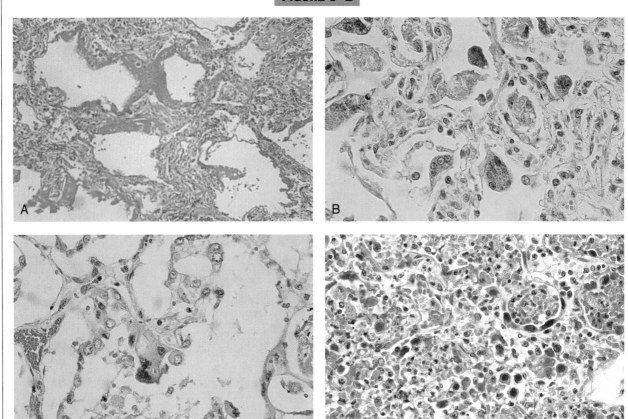

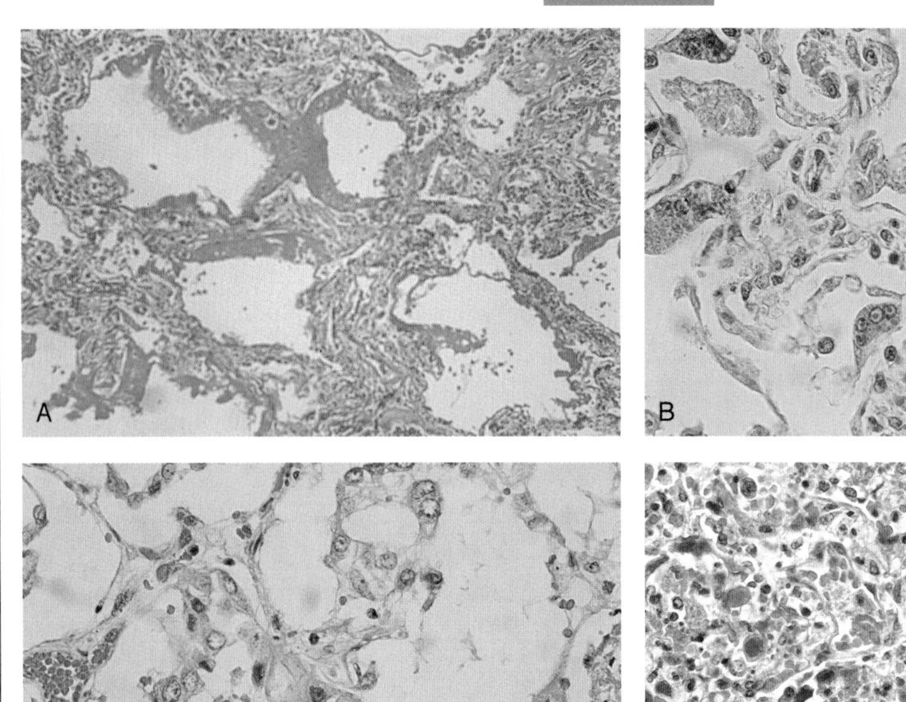

Light photomicrographs stained with hematoxylin and eosin (H & E), showing features of viral pneumonia. **A,** Influenza pneumonia showing diffuse alveolar damage with hyaline membranes. **B,** Measles giant cell pneumonia showing infected multinucleated cells with intranuclear eosinophilic inclusions and less distinct intracytoplasmic eosinophilic inclusions. **C,** Respiratory syncytial virus bronchiolitis in a lung transplant recipient. There is focal alveolar epithelial injury and a multinucleated (syncytial) cell. **D,** Adenovirus infection showing an area of inflammation and necrosis along with infected "smudge cells" with dense nuclear inclusions lacking a distinct halo.

Continued

LUNG DISEASE CAUSED BY INFECTIOUS AGENTS

VIRAL INFECTIONS

FIGURE 3–2

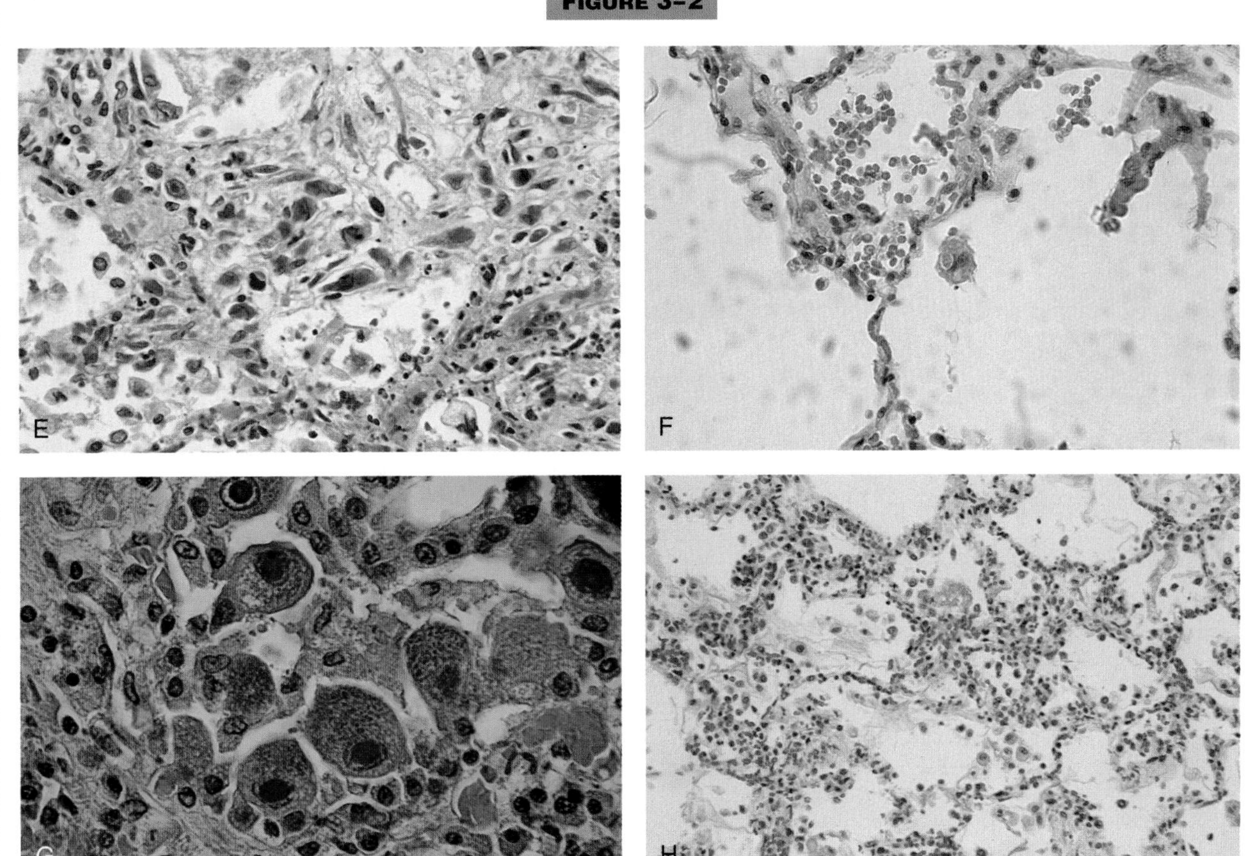

E, Herpes simplex virus pneumonia. Foci of acute necrosis contain virus-infected cells. The viral inclusions are intranuclear, eosinophilic with a ground-glass appearance, and frequently surrounded by a thin clear halo. **F,** Varicella-zoster infection characterized by inflammatory nodules and interstitial inflammation. The viral inclusions are similar to those seen in herpes simplex pneumonia. **G,** Cytomegalovirus pneumonia showing infected cells lining the alveoli and within the alveolar spaces. The cells show cytomegaly, large intranuclear amphophilic inclusions, and small basophilic cytoplasmic inclusions. **H,** Hantavirus infection leading to death in 3 days as a result of severe respiratory failure. At autopsy, the lungs showed early diffuse alveolar damage and interstitial infiltrates of lymphocytes.

LUNG DISEASE CAUSED BY INFECTIOUS AGENTS

VIRAL INFECTIONS

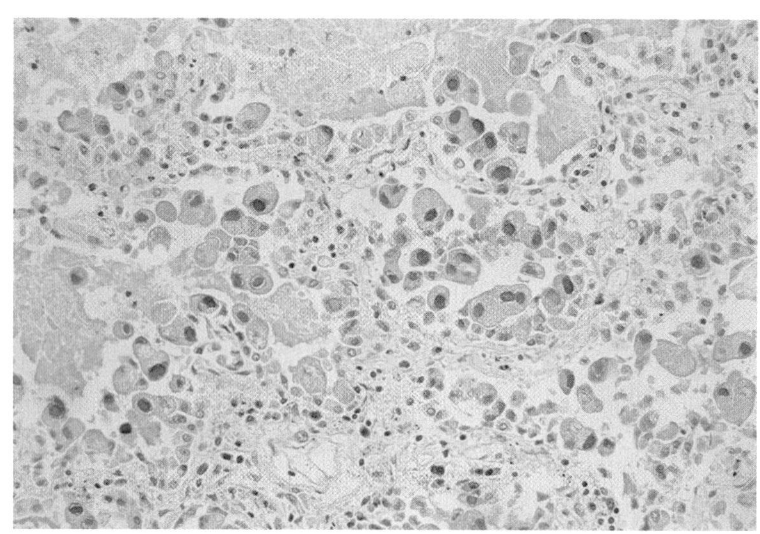

FIGURE 3–3

Immunocytochemical detection of cytomegalovirus in a patient with AIDS. The brown reaction product indicates the positive staining of cytomegalovirus antigen.

FIGURE 3–4

Electron microscopy in cytomegalovirus pneumonia. **A,** Cytomegalovirus-infected cell showing numerous intracytoplasmic membrane-bound virions. The nucleus contains filamentous material surrounded by a somewhat electron-lucent halo (×3300) **B,** High-power view of the nucleus demonstrates scattered intranuclear viral particles of about 140 nm (×55,000). (Courtesy of Robert Munn, University of California, Davis.)

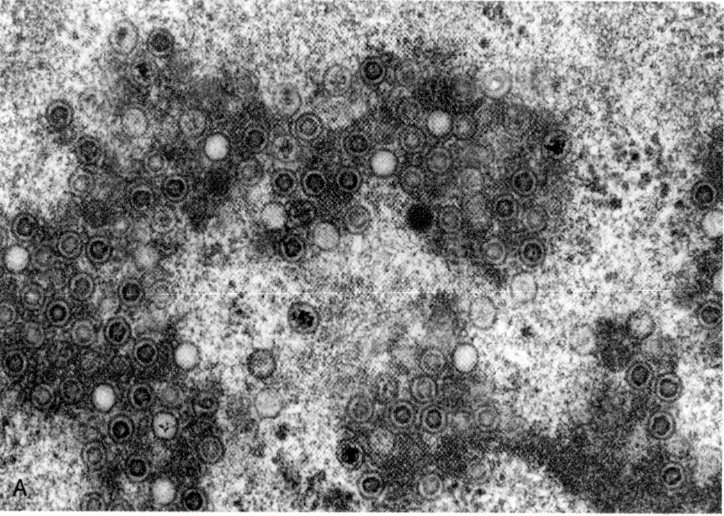

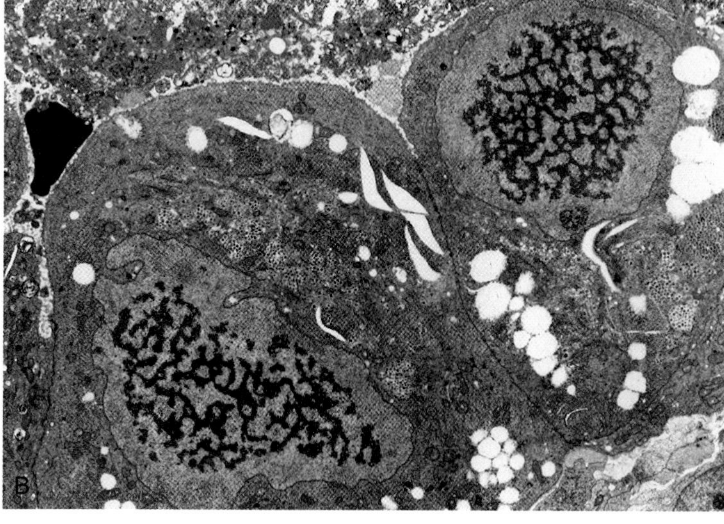

LUNG DISEASE CAUSED BY INFECTIOUS AGENTS

MYCOPLASMAL, CHLAMYDIAL, AND RICKETTSIAL INFECTIONS

Several mycoplasmal, chlamydial, and rickettsial organisms can infect the respiratory tract and cause important pathologic reactions (TABLE 3–5).

TABLE 3–5

Mycoplasmal, Chlamydial, and Rickettsial Organisms that Infect the Respiratory Tract

Organism	Major Pathologic Effects
Mycoplasma pneumoniae	Bronchiolitis; interstitial pneumonia; pleural effusions; hilar lymphadenopathy; rarely DAD
Chlamydia psittaci (psittacosis)	Bronchiolitis; interstitial pneumonia
Chlamydia pneumoniae	Bronchiolitis and peribronchiolar alveolitis
Chlamydia trachomatis	Interstitial pneumonia; occasionally bronchiolitis and intraalveolar inflammation
Rickettsia species	Alveolar edema; DAD; interstitial pneumonia; vasculitis
Coxiella burnetii (Q fever)	Ulcerative bronchiolitis and peribronchiolar alveolitis

DAD = diffuse alveolar damage.

BACTERIAL INFECTIONS

TABLE 3–6

Bacteria Associated with Lung Infection

Organism	Common Patterns of Lung Injury
COMMON PATHOGENS	
Gram-positive organisms	
– *Corynebacterium diphtheriae*	Acute tracheobronchitis
– *Streptococcus pneumoniae*	Lobar or bronchopneumonia
– Beta-hemolytic streptococci	Bronchopneumonia
– *Staphylococcus aureus*	Bronchopneumonia; lobar pneumonia; hematogenous spread; secondary infection after viral pneumonia; chronic pneumonia syndrome (botryomycosis)
– Anaerobes	Necrotizing aspiration pneumonia; colonization of bronchiectatic airways
Gram-negative organisms	
– *Bordetella pertussis* and *B. parapertussis*	Acute tracheobronchitis
– Enterobacteriaceae	
Escherichia coli	Bronchopneumonia
Klebsiella pneumoniae	Lobar pneumonia; aspiration pneumonia
Serratia marcescens	Necrotizing bronchopneumonia
Proteus species	Aspiration pneumonia
– *Haemophilus influenzae*	Lobar pneumonia or bronchopneumonia

continued

LUNG DISEASE CAUSED BY INFECTIOUS AGENTS

BACTERIAL INFECTIONS

TABLE 3-6

Bacteria Associated with Lung Infection *continued*

Organism	Common Patterns of Lung Injury
COMMON PATHOGENS *CONTINUED*	
- *Legionella* species	Lobar pneumonia or bronchopneumonia
- *Pseudomonas* species	Bronchopneumonia; hematogenous spread; airway colonization
- Anaerobes	Necrotizing aspiration pneumonia; colonization of bronchiectatic airways
UNUSUAL PATHOGENS	
Gram-positive organisms	
- *Bacillus anthracis*	Bronchial wall hemorrhage; hemorrhagic necrosis of hilar lymph nodes; hemorrhagic edema of lung
Gram-negative organisms	
- *Francisella tularensis*	Multifocal, nodular pneumonia that may become confluent (lobar pattern)
- *Moraxella catarrhalis*	Bronchopneumonia; sometimes lobar pneumonia
- *Yersinia pestis*	Primary pneumonic plague—necrotizing bronchopneumonia Secondary pneumonic plague—interstitial then necrotizing bronchopneumonia
Higher bacteria	
- *Actinomycetes* species	Multiple encapsulated abscesses
- *Nocardia asteroides*	Multiple encapsulated abscesses; bronchopneumonia; lobar pneumonia; fulminant necrotizing pneumonia; sometimes associated with alveolar proteinosis

FIGURE 3-5

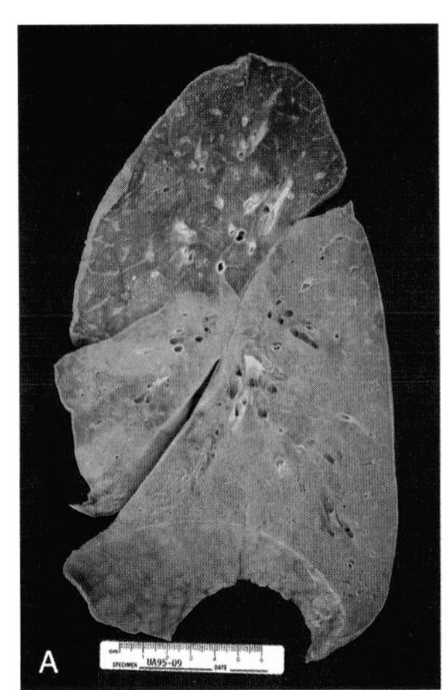

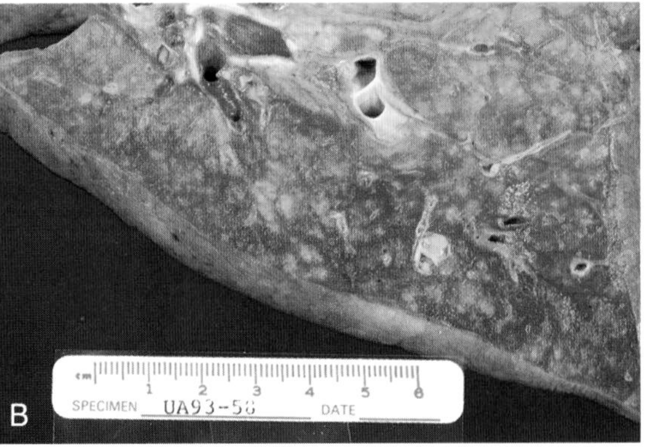

Bacterial organisms cause intra-alveolar exudation resulting in consolidation of the lung parenchyma. Traditionally, bacterial pneumonias have been classified anatomically according to whether the infection involves an entire lobe or segment of the lung diffusely (lobar pneumonia) or whether the infection is centered around the airways in a patchy distribution (bronchopneumonia). **A,** Lobar pneumonia. The entire right middle and lower lobes are inflamed, and the tissue is firm. **B,** Bronchopneumonia. There is patchy consolidation around small bronchi and bronchioles. The lesions are slightly elevated, dry, granular, and gray-red to yellow. In advanced cases, the lesions may become confluent resembling lobar pneumonia. (See Chapter 4, Radiography and Imaging.)

LUNG DISEASE CAUSED BY INFECTIOUS AGENTS

BACTERIAL INFECTIONS

FIGURE 3-6

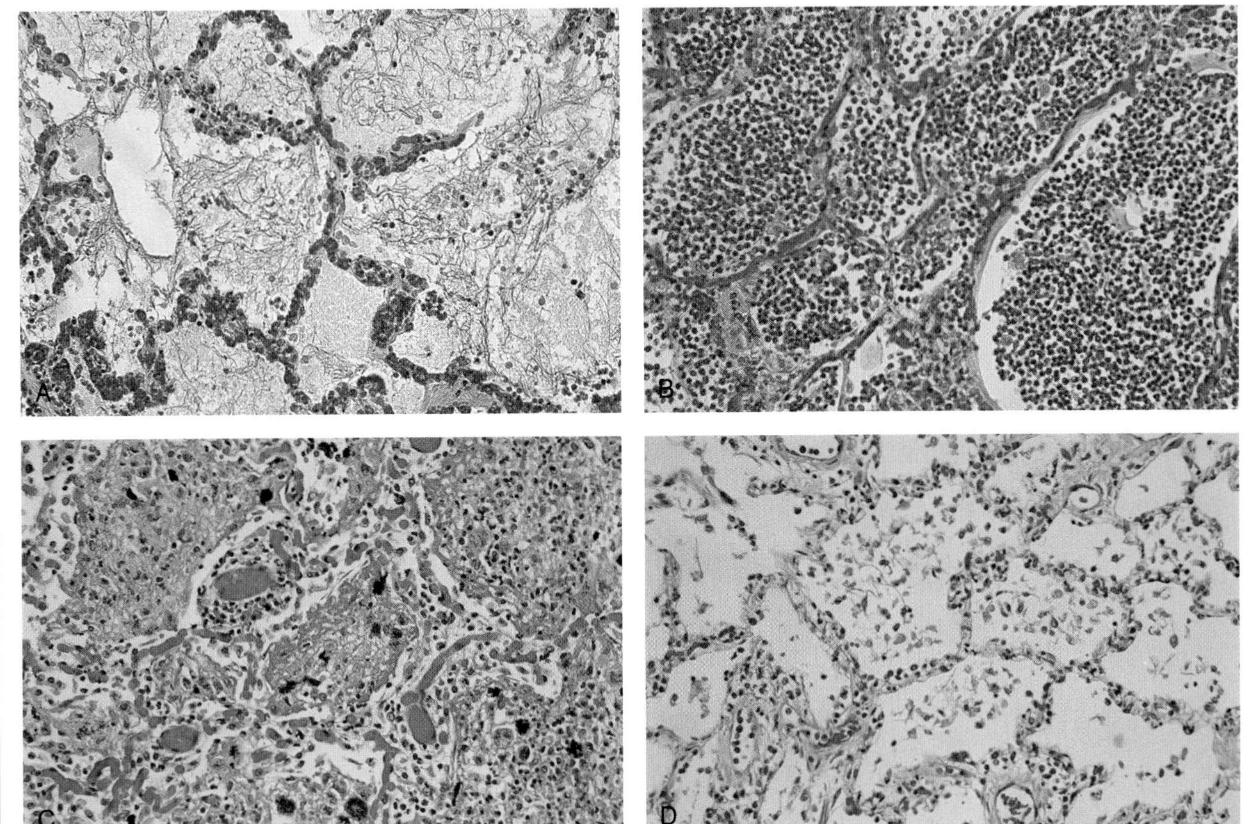

Classical histopathologic stages of untreated lobar pneumonia (H & E stain). **A,** Congestion (earliest finding)—there is prominent vascular engorgement and serous exudation. **B,** Red hepatization (days 1 to 3)—an infiltrate of neutrophils, fibrin, and extravasated red blood cells fills the airspaces. **C,** Gray hepatization (days 4 to 8)—the airspaces are replaced by a fibrinous network and degenerating white blood cells. **D,** Resolution (days 9 to 10)—there is dissolution of fibrin and clearing of the airspaces.

LUNG DISEASE CAUSED BY INFECTIOUS AGENTS

BACTERIAL INFECTIONS

FIGURE 3-7

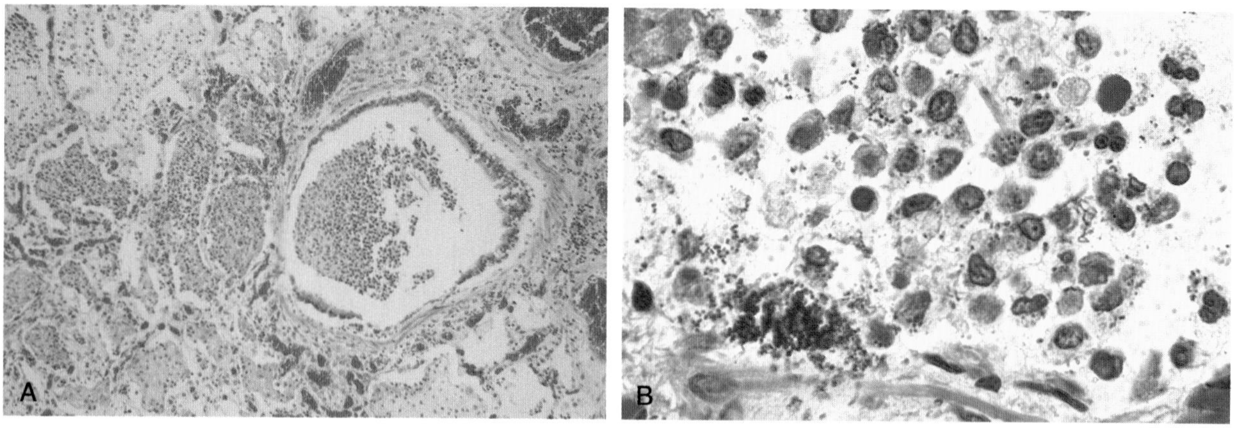

Histopathologic features of bronchopneumonia. **A,** The bronchiolar lumen and adjacent alveolar ducts and sacs are filled with neutrophils, fibrin, and macrophages (H & E stain). **B,** A Gram's stain identifies a mixed infection of gram-positive and gram-negative cocci and gram-negative rods.

FIGURE 3-8

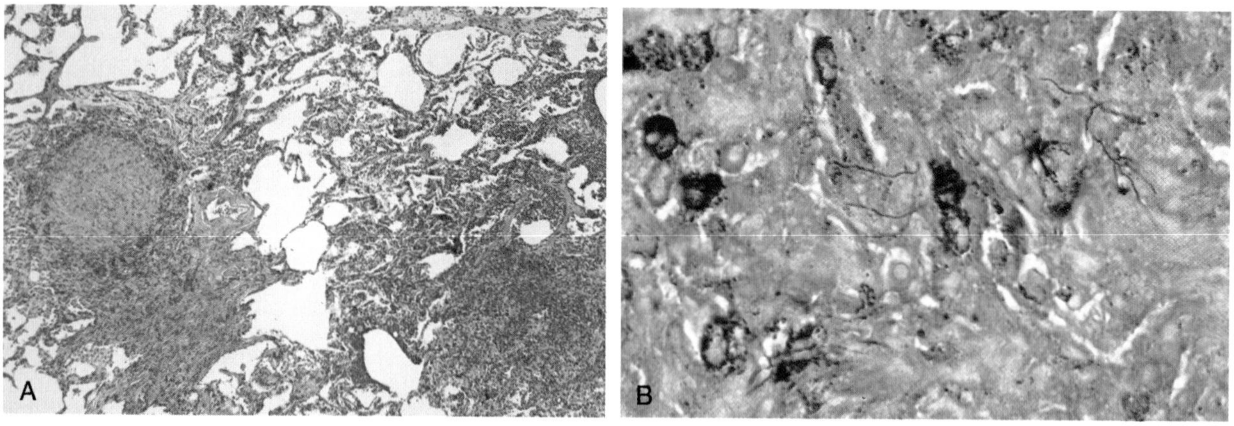

Pulmonary nocardiosis in a patient with recurrent pneumonia. **A,** An open lung biopsy demonstrated both acute and granulomatous inflammation (H & E stain). **B,** A Gomori methenamine silver (GMS) stain identifies a few fine filamentous organisms consistent with *Nocardia asteroides*.

LUNG DISEASE CAUSED BY INFECTIOUS AGENTS

BACTERIAL INFECTIONS

FIGURE 3-9

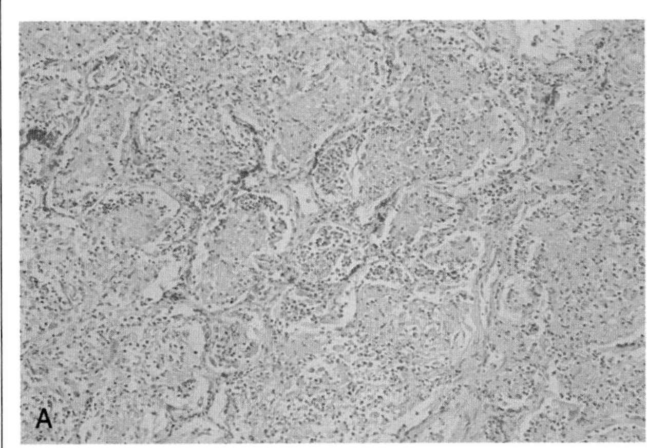

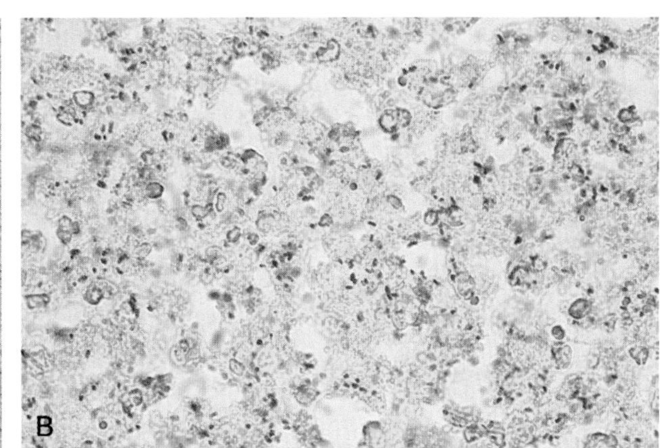

Legionnaire's disease may involve the lung as an acute lobar pneumonia or as a bronchopneumonia. In severe cases, diffuse alveolar damage may complicate the infection, as may necrosis and abscess formation. **A,** *Legionella* lobar pneumonia showing gray hepatization with early organization (H & E stain). **B,** The Dieterle technique stains the small, pleomorphic rods indicative of *Legionella* organisms black. Confirmation of a definitive diagnosis of Legionnaire's disease requires culture, using immunocytochemical or molecular techniques.

LUNG DISEASE CAUSED BY INFECTIOUS AGENTS

BACTERIAL INFECTIONS

TABLE 3–7

Complications of Bacterial Pneumonia

- Abscess formation
- Pleuritis, pleural effusion
- Empyema
- Organization
- Bacteremia
- Diffuse alveolar damage
- Bronchopleural fistula
- Bronchial damage leading to bronchiectasis
- Suppurative pericarditis (rare)

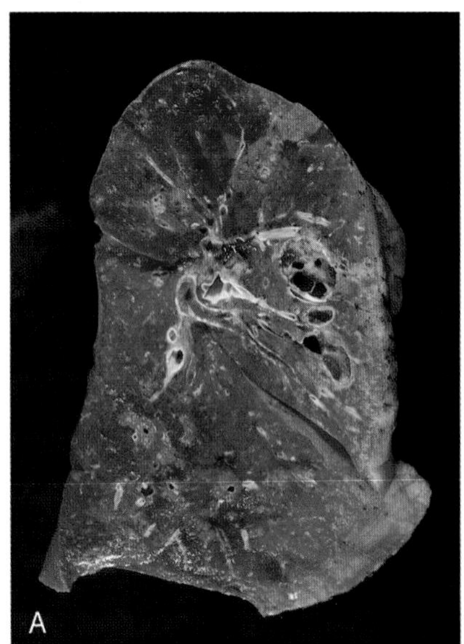

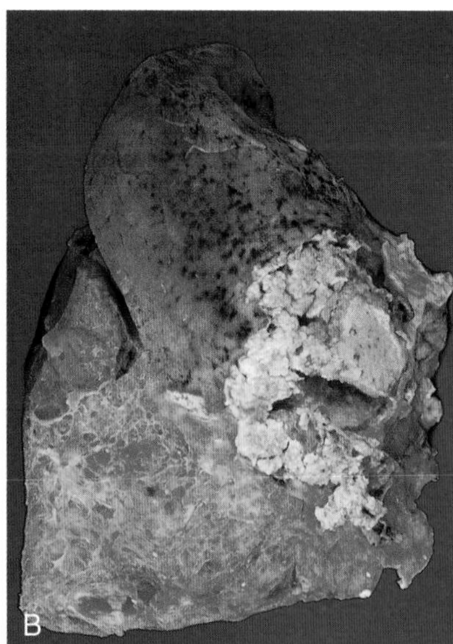

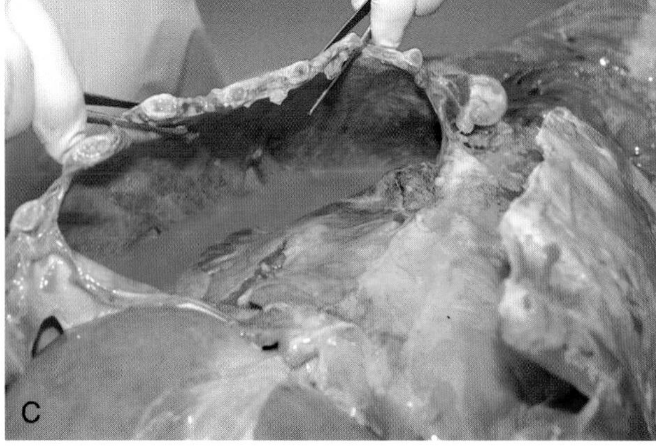

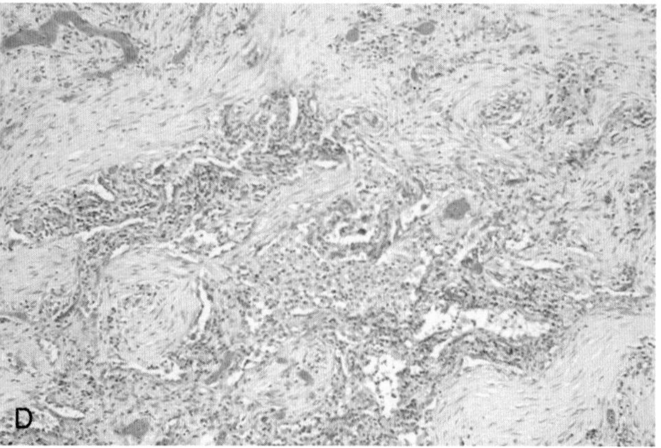

FIGURE 3–10

Complications of pneumonia. **A,** Abscess formation. The occurrence rate varies with the etiologic agent. This example shows necrotizing bronchopneumonia with multiple abscess cavities due to *Staphylococcus aureus.* **B,** Fibrinous pleuritis develops in approximately two thirds of cases. In this example of a mixed infection due to *Klebsiella oxytoca* and *Enterobacter cloacae,* there is extension of a necrotizing pneumonia through the left upper lobe visceral pleura and a marked acute pleuritis of the left lower lobe. **C,** Empyema occurs in 15 to 25% of cases of pneumonia. In this example, the right pleural cavity is partially filled with pus. **D,** With organization of the exudate (organizing pneumonia), fibroblasts are stimulated to produce collagen, plugging the airspaces with fibrous scar (H & E stain).

LUNG DISEASE CAUSED BY INFECTIOUS AGENTS

TUBERCULOSIS AND OTHER MYCOBACTERIAL INFECTIONS

TABLE 3-8

Mycobacteria Associated with Pulmonary Disease

Species	Comments
Mycobacterium tuberculosis complex	
- *M. tuberculosis*	Most common mycobacteria infecting humans
- *M. bovis*	Rare in North America
- *M. africanum*	Uncommon pathogen
Nontuberculosis mycobacteria	
- *M. avium* complex (MAC) (*M. avium; M. intracellulare-avium*)	Moderately common pathogens causing disseminated disease in the immunosuppressed, particularly those with AIDS; rare pulmonary infection in those with underlying lung disease
- *M. kansasii*	Moderately common pathogen
- *M. scrofulaceum*	Primarily lymph node disease but may involve lungs
- *M. fortuitum-chelonae* complex	Rapid growers; primarily cutaneous disease; chronic pulmonary disease resembles MAC
- *M. malmoense*	Rare; typically occurs with preexisting pneumoconiosis
- *M. simiae*	Rare; tuberculosis-like disease
- *M. szulgai*	Rare; tuberculosis-like disease
- *M. xenopi*	Chronic, subacute or acute pulmonary disease resembling MAC
Rarely pathogenic mycobacteria	
- *M. asiaticum* - *thermoresistible* - *M. nonchromogenicum* - *M. flavescens* - *M. shimoidei*	Positive cultures usually represent environmental contamination of specimens

LUNG DISEASE CAUSED BY INFECTIOUS AGENTS

TUBERCULOSIS AND OTHER MYCOBACTERIAL INFECTIONS

FIGURE 3–11

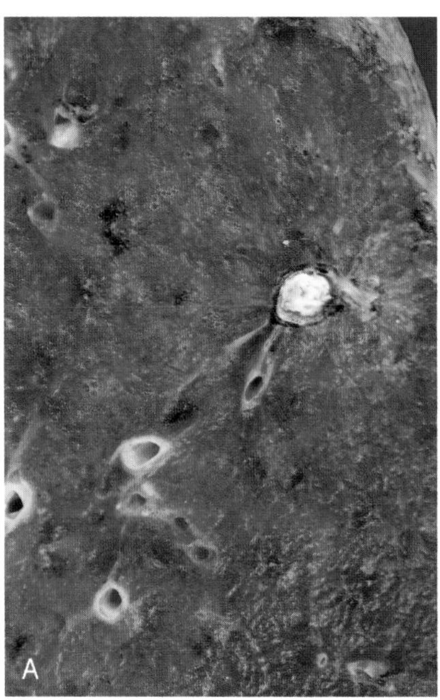

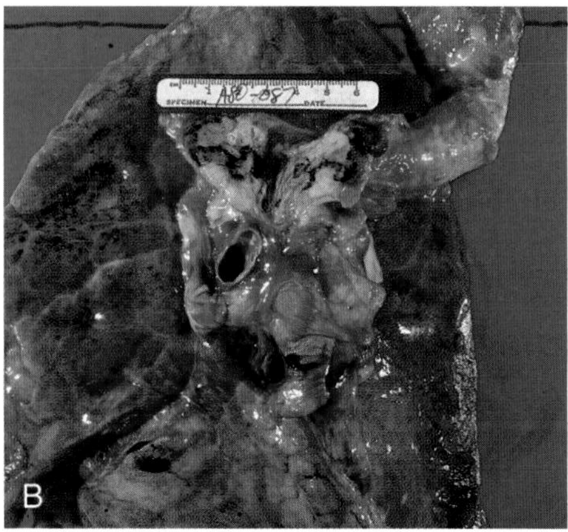

Mycobacterium tuberculosis causes millions of infections annually. Primary tuberculosis (TB) develops in previously unexposed, nonsensitized individuals. Inhaled bacilli implant in distal airspaces of the lower part of upper lobe or upper part of lower lobe. The cell wall lipids and carbohydrates of *M. tuberculosis* interfere with phagolysosomal fusion and allow intracellular survival of the organism. Initially, there is a nonspecific inflammatory reaction; delayed hypersensitivity (type IV) to the bacillus develops 2 to 4 weeks after the initial infection. The primary infection appears as a 1 to 1.5 cm gray-white area of consolidation and is called the Ghon focus. Drainage of bacilli, either free or within macrophages, to regional lymph nodes forms secondary areas of infection. The combination of the Ghon focus and nodal involvement is referred to as the Ghon complex. **A,** Primary site of TB infection (Ghon focus) in the lung periphery, exhibiting caseous necrosis. **B,** Caseous necrosis in regional hilar lymph nodes. With resolution, these lesions become fibrocalcific scars that may harbor viable organisms for years.

FIGURE 3–12

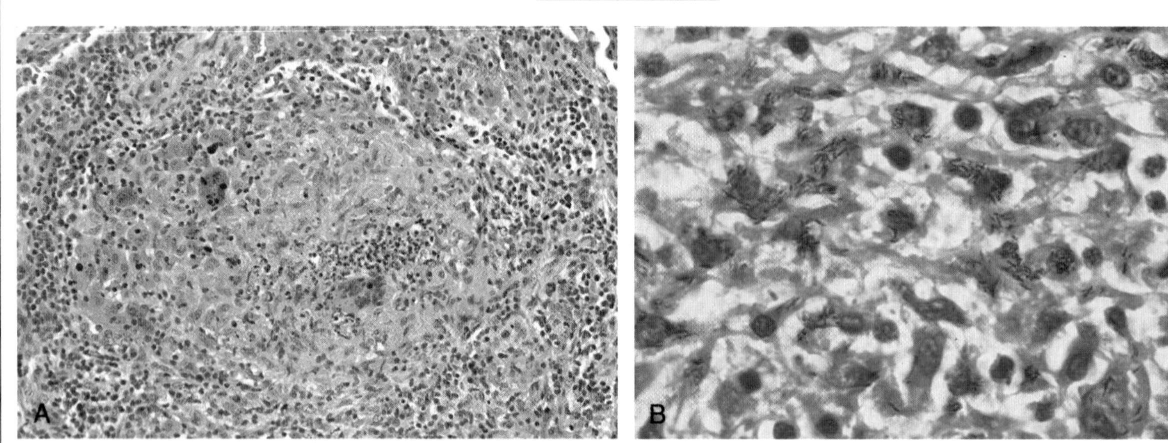

After sensitization, a nonspecific inflammatory reaction becomes granulomatous. The histopathologic features consist of a granulomatous inflammatory reaction forming both necrotizing and nonnecrotizing tubercles. **A,** This microscopic section shows an epithelioid cell granuloma with Langhans' giant cells surrounding a central area of early necrosis containing a collection of neutrophils (H & E stain). **B,** Necrotizing granulomatous inflammation containing acid-fast bacilli (acid-fast stain).

LUNG DISEASE CAUSED BY INFECTIOUS AGENTS

TUBERCULOSIS AND OTHER MYCOBACTERIAL INFECTIONS

FIGURE 3–13

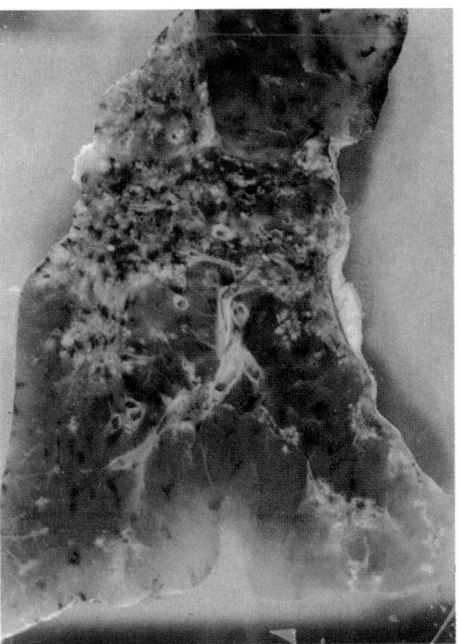

Progressive primary TB evolves from primary TB without interruption (<10% of TB infections) especially in children or when there is poor cell-mediated immunity due to debilitation or immunodeficiency. The infection progresses through direct extension, endobronchial spread (tuberculous pneumonia, "galloping consumption"), and lymphatic and hematogenous dissemination (miliary tuberculosis). This example shows a localized area of tuberculous pneumonia.

FIGURE 3–14

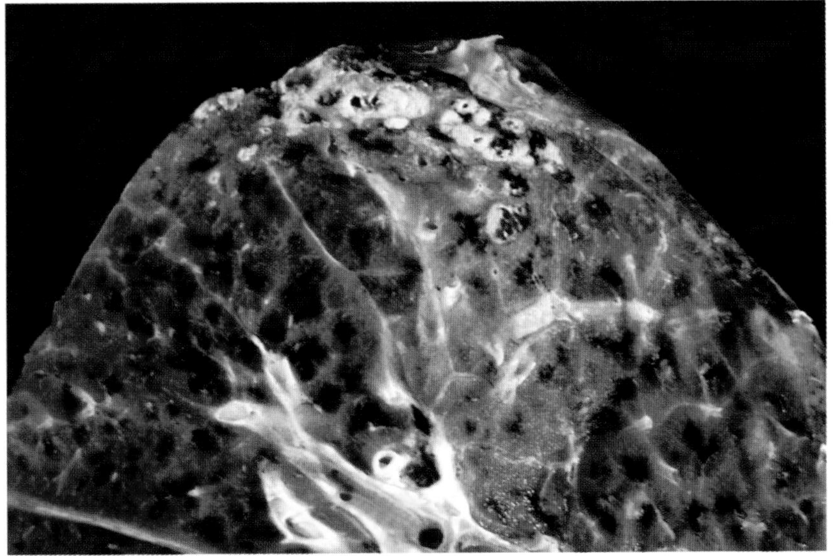

Secondary (reactivation, postprimary) TB arises in a previously sensitized host either from reactivation of dormant primary lesions or after reinfection with exogenous bacilli. Less than 5% of patients with primary TB develop secondary TB. Predisposing factors include diabetes mellitus, alcoholism, malnutrition, chronic lung disease (e.g., silicotuberculosis), and immunosuppression including HIV infection. Secondary TB is localized to the apices of upper lobes and typically consists of 1 to 2 cm areas of consolidation with central caseation and peripheral fibrotic reaction. Regional lymph nodes may be involved. Either spontaneously or with treatment, secondary lesions may resolve by progressive fibrous encapsulation and calcification. In unfavorable cases, the disease may persist and progress. This lung from a patient with diabetes mellitus, type II who was receiving corticosteroids for treatment of asthma developed progressive postprimary pulmonary tuberculosis. His lung contains multiple tubercles along with apical scarring and cavitation.

LUNG DISEASE CAUSED BY INFECTIOUS AGENTS

TUBERCULOSIS AND OTHER MYCOBACTERIAL INFECTIONS

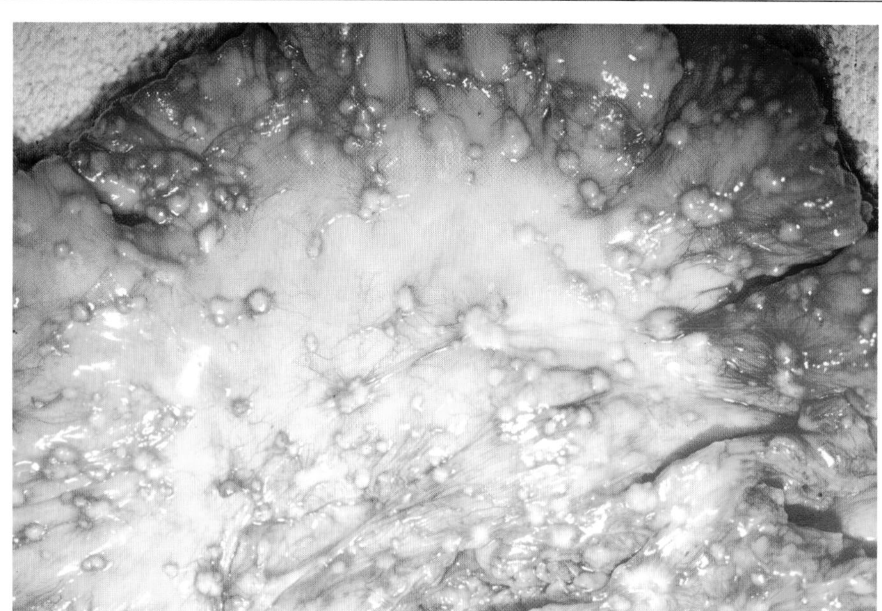

FIGURE 3-15

The favored sites of miliary (lymphohematogenous) spread of TB include lung, bone marrow, lymph nodes, liver, spleen, kidneys, adrenal gland, prostate, seminal vesicles, fallopian tubes, endometrium, meninges, and eyes. In this patient with progressive postprimary TB, autopsy showed miliary spread to the omentum, mesentery, and serosa of the small bowel.

TABLE 3-9

Complications of Tuberculosis

- Tuberculous bronchopneumonia
- Erosion into bronchi with seeding of airways (laryngeal, endobronchial, or tracheobronchial tuberculosis)
- Disseminated miliary tuberculosis
- Pleural involvement with effusion, secondary fibrosis, calcifications, and adhesions
- Tuberculous empyema
- Extensive fibrosis and distortion of lungs in advanced disease
- Intestinal tuberculosis
- Progressive, isolated-organ tuberculosis
- Amyloidosis

FIGURE 3-16

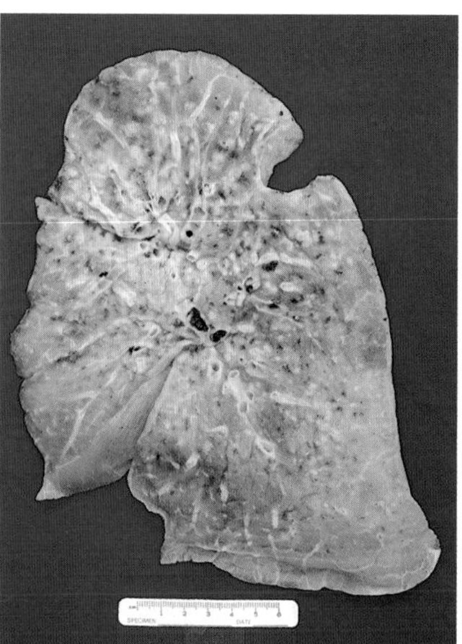

Infection with *Mycobacterium avium* complex. This patient with AIDS developed miliary spread of the organism throughout the lungs.

LUNG DISEASE CAUSED BY INFECTIOUS AGENTS

FUNGAL INFECTIONS

Fungi are obligate saprophytes or parasites with nutritional requirements similar to those of bacteria. Many pathogenic fungi affect only the skin; however, some also involve the viscera (deep mycoses), particularly the lung. The deep mycoses may occur in otherwise healthy individuals but most frequently occur as opportunistic infections during chronic diseases, during cancer chemotherapy or radiotherapy, prolonged antibiotic therapy, or immunosuppressive treatment. The type of lung disease produced by these agents varies from acute pneumonitis to chronic granulomatous infection similar to tuberculosis. Although fungi can sometimes be identified easily on routine hematoxylin and eosin stained slides, they are more readily seen using Gomori methenamine silver or periodic acid–Schiff stains.

TABLE 3–10

Characteristics of Major Pulmonary Fungal Infections

Disease	Organism	Demographics	Morphology	Immunocompetent Response
Aspergillosis	*Aspergillus fumigatus* *A. flavus* *A. niger*	Worldwide	Hyphae (3–6 μm wide); septate; 45-degree angle branching; occasional fruiting bodies in cavities	Tissue/vascular invasion; colonization; fungus balls
Blastomycosis	*Blastomyces dermatitidis*	North America, especially east of the Mississippi River	Broad-based budding yeast (8–15 μm); thick ("double-contoured") cell walls	Neutrophilic/granulomatous inflammation
Candidiasis	*Candida albicans* *C. krusei* *C. tropicalis* Other *Candida* species	Worldwide	Budding yeastlike (blastoconidia) forms (3–5 μm) and pseudohyphae (3–5 μm)	Respiratory space colonization; tissue invasion
Coccidioidomycosis	*Coccidioides immitis*	North American deserts	Spherules (15–60 μm); endospores (1–2 μm diameter)	Granulomatous inflammation
Cryptococcosis	*Cryptococcus neoformans*	Worldwide	Yeast (2–20 μm, but usually 4–10 μm); narrow-based budding; mucin capsule (immunocompetent); refractile center	Granulomatous inflammation
Histoplasmosis	*Histoplasma capsulatum* var. *capsulatum*	North and South America, especially Ohio and Mississippi River valleys	Small budding yeasts (2–4 μm)	Granulomatous inflammation
Paracoccidioidomycosis	*Paracoccidioidomyces braziliensis*	Central and South America	Yeast (3–30 μm) with multiple budding ("mariner's wheel")	Neutrophilic/granulomatous inflammation

continued

LUNG DISEASE CAUSED BY INFECTIOUS AGENTS

FUNGAL INFECTIONS

TABLE 3-10

Characteristics of Major Pulmonary Fungal Infections *continued*

Disease	Organism	Demographics	Morphology	Immunocompetent Response
Pneumocystis carinii pneumonia	*P. carinii*	Worldwide	Thick-walled cysts or spherules (4–7 μm) that collapse and assume cup shapes	Intra-alveolar foamy exudate; interstitial pneumonia; diffuse alveolar damage; occasionally granulomatous inflammation
Pseudallescheriasis	*Pseudallescheria boydii*		Hyphae (2–5 μm wide); septate; sometimes with prominent vesicles; sometimes ovoid conidia (5–10 μm) on short conidiophores	Tissue/vascular invasion
Sporotrichosis	*Sporotrichum schenckii*	Worldwide	Intracellular ovoid yeast (2–6 μm) with slight halo	Neutrophilic/granulomatous inflammation
Torulopsis infection	*Torulopsis glabrata*	Worldwide	Budding yeast (2–5 μm)	Parenchymal necrosis; abscess formation
Zygomycosis	*Mucor; Absidia; Rhizopus; Cunninghamella* and others	Worldwide	Hyphae, variably sized (5–30 μm wide); ribbon-like pauciseptate though septa rarely observed in tissue sections; 90-degree angle branching	Tissue/vascular invasion

Source: Modified from Cibas ES, Ducatman BS: Cytology: Diagnostic Principles and Clinical Correlates. Philadelphia, WB Saunders, 1996, pp 41–85.

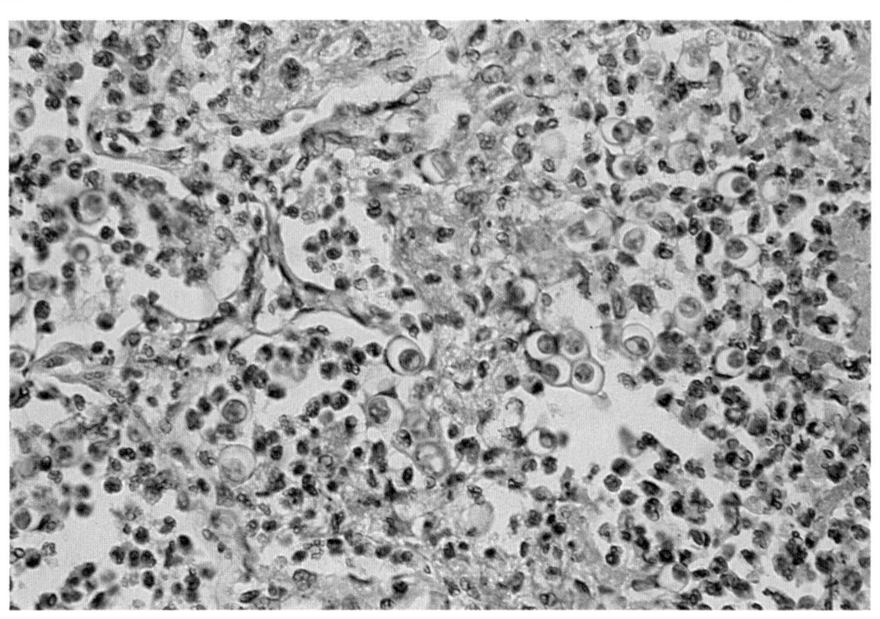

FIGURE 3-17

North American blastomycosis may cause asymptomatic pulmonary infection, progressive pulmonary disease, or rarely, miliary disease. It is endemic in the Mississippi River basin, the Great Lakes region, and in the southeastern United States. Round to oval yeast forms of *B. dermatitidis* are notable for their thick ("double contoured") walls and hematoxylinophilic nuclei. The cellular reaction contains neutrophils, macrophages, and necrotic cell debris (H & E stain).

LUNG DISEASE CAUSED BY INFECTIOUS AGENTS

FUNGAL INFECTIONS

FIGURE 3-18

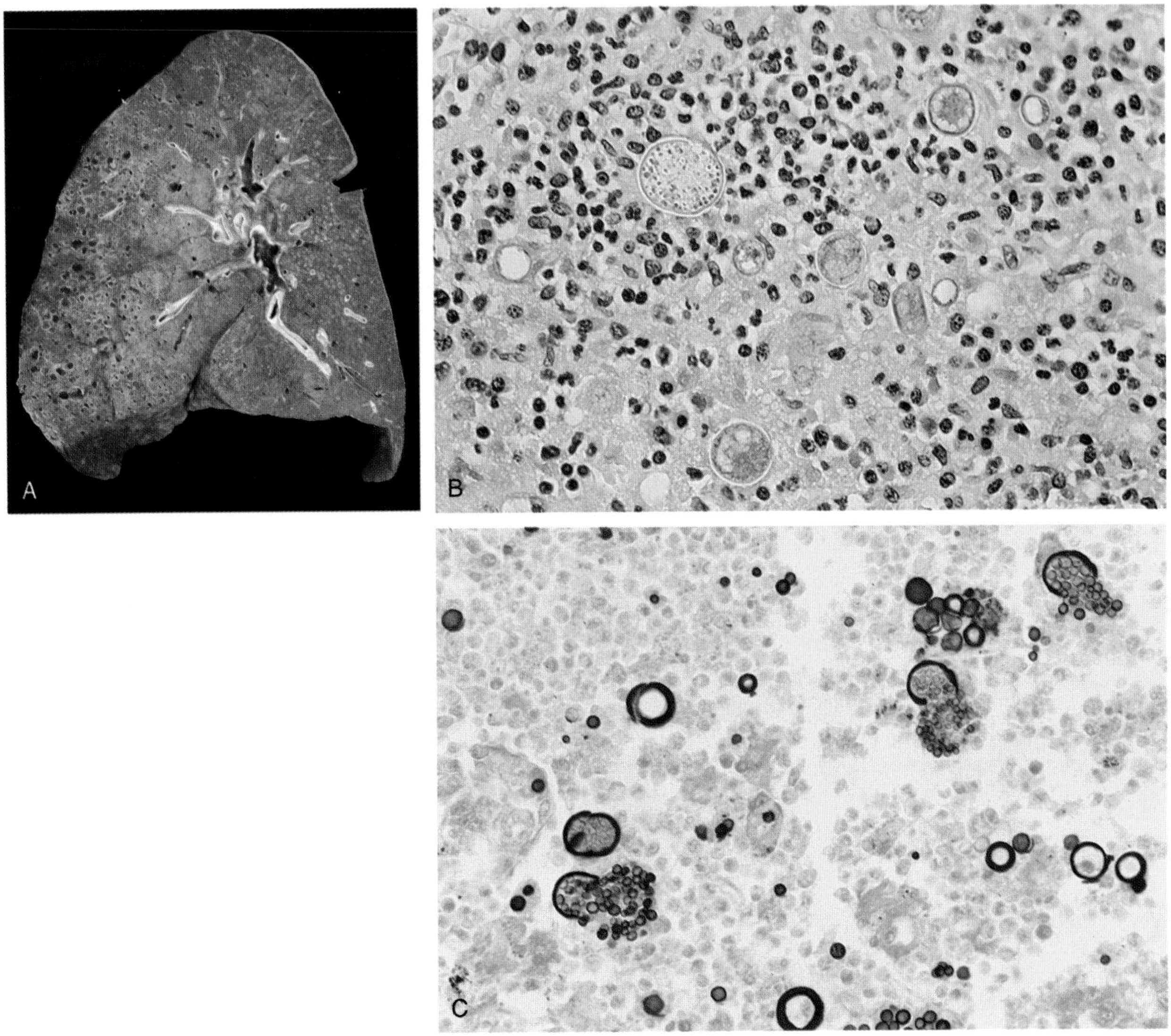

Coccidioidomycosis may cause asymptomatic pulmonary infection (60%), progressive pulmonary disease, or miliary disease. It is endemic in southwestern and far western United States, particularly the San Joaquin Valley (Valley Fever). **A,** Gross specimen from an autopsy of disseminated coccidioidomycosis that developed during pregnancy. The lung shows features of organized diffuse alveolar damage with cyst formation, but note the small necrotic nodules. **B,** The large number of spherules present within the lung tissue is easily seen with an H & E stain. **C,** A GMS stain showing spherules releasing their endospores.

LUNG DISEASE CAUSED BY INFECTIOUS AGENTS

FUNGAL INFECTIONS

FIGURE 3-19

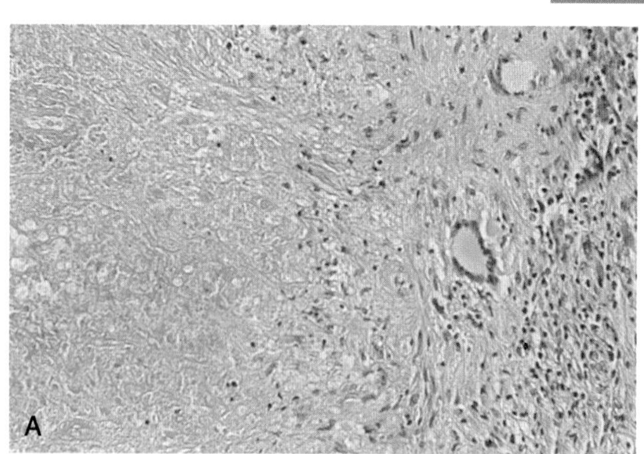

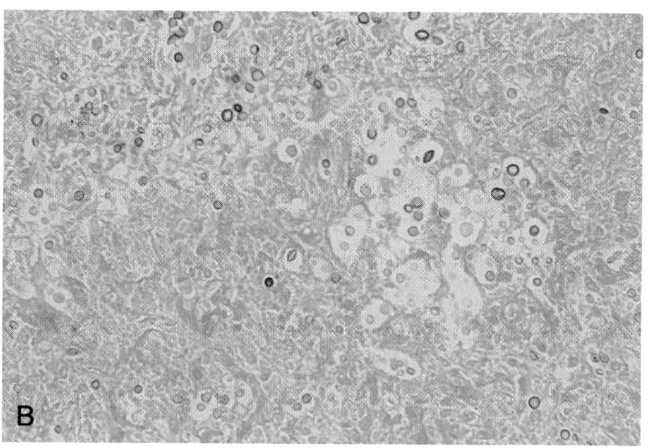

Cryptococcus rarely occurs in normal individuals; rather, it affects the immunocompromised host as a progressive pneumonia, which often disseminates to the meninges. It is not transmitted between humans but from pigeon droppings, which serve as the reservoir of infection. **A,** The pathologic reaction to *C. neoformans* is typically granulomatous but may be minimal in patients with severe immunodeficiencies (H & E stain). **B,** A GMS stain reveals the irregularly shaped organisms surrounded by a nonstaining capsule.

FIGURE 3-20

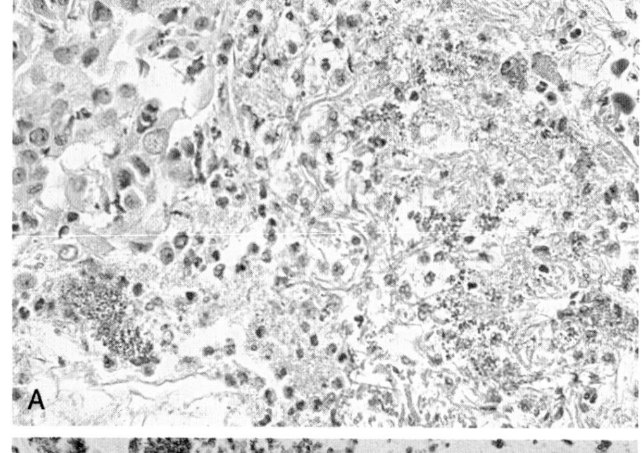

Histoplasmosis capsulati occurs in both normal and immunocompromised individuals and produces a disease similar to TB. It is endemic in the Ohio and central Mississippi River Valleys, Appalachian Mountains, and southeastern United States. **A,** A transbronchial biopsy shows reactivation infection occurring in a lung transplant recipient. The organisms can be identified within a focus of inflammation (H & E stain). **B,** Small yeast forms are present in the area of inflammation (GMS stain). **C,** The explant lung contained old hyalinized granulomas (H & E stain).

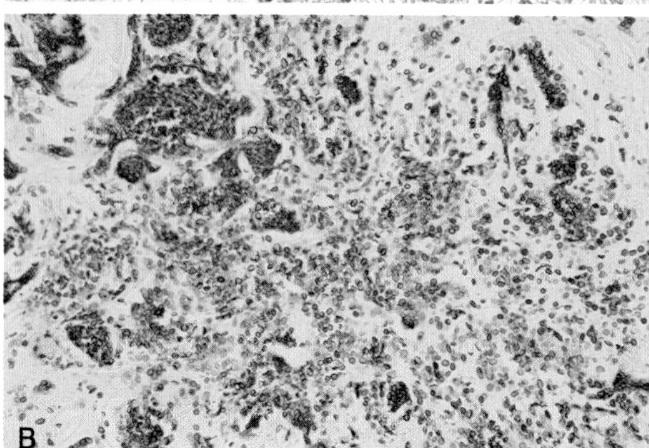

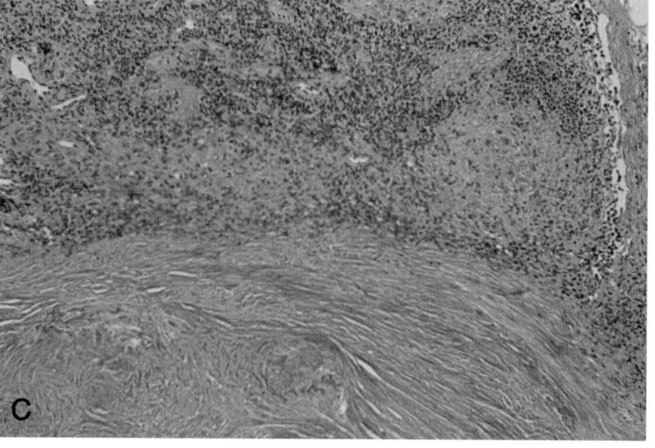

LUNG DISEASE CAUSED BY INFECTIOUS AGENTS

FUNGAL INFECTIONS

FIGURE 3-21

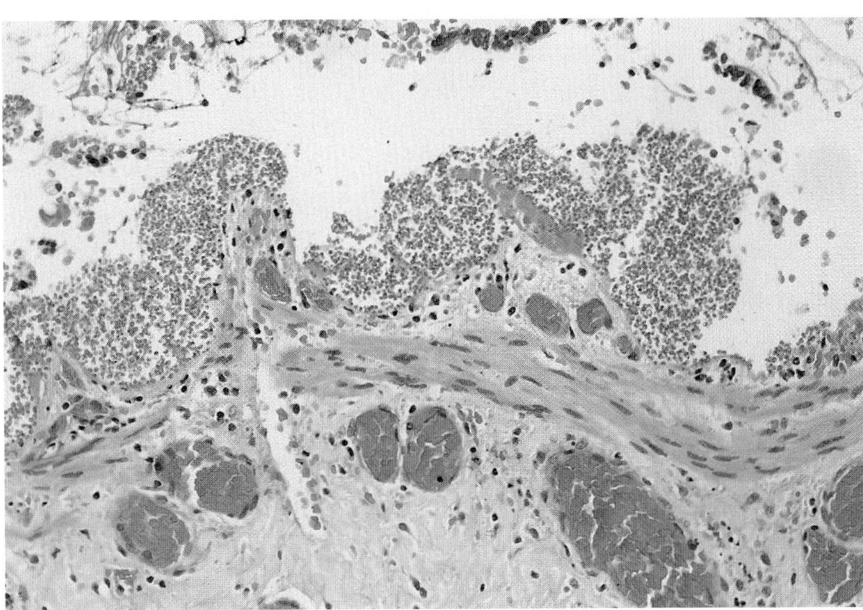

Among fungi, *Candida* species are the most common cause of disease. In the non-immunocompromised patient, candidiasis causes superficial infections of the epithelial surfaces of intertriginous areas of the skin, mouth, urinary tract, and vagina. In immunocompromised hosts it may involve the lungs, heart valves, kidney, liver, gastrointestinal tract and central nervous system. The lung is frequently involved in disseminated candidiasis following seeding of the lung during hematogenous spread or following aspiration from the upper respiratory tract. With aspiration, patchy lesions are seen in the lower lobes. Following hematogenous spread, the infection is often bilateral and miliary with extension to the pleura. In this immunosuppressed patient an acute, exudative tracheobronchitis developed. Microscopically, the yeast forms were seen invading the bronchial mucosa and eliciting an acute inflammatory reaction (H & E stain).

Aspergillosis lung disease may take on a number of different forms depending on a the status of the host's immune system, underlying lung disease, or the type of exposure.

TABLE 3-11

Forms of Aspergillus Lung Disease

Invasive aspergillosis
- Aspergillus pneumonia
- Necrotizing tracheobronchitis
- Necrotizing granulomatous inflammation
- Chronic necrotizing aspergillosis (semi-invasive aspergillosis)

Saprophytic infection
- Mycetoma (aspergilloma)

Hypersensitivity reaction
- Allergic bronchopulmonary aspergillosis

Source: Modified from Katzenstein A-L: Katzenstein and Askin's Surgical Pathology of Non-Neoplastic Lung Disease (3rd ed). Philadelphia, WB Saunders, 1997.

LUNG DISEASE CAUSED BY INFECTIOUS AGENTS

FUNGAL INFECTIONS

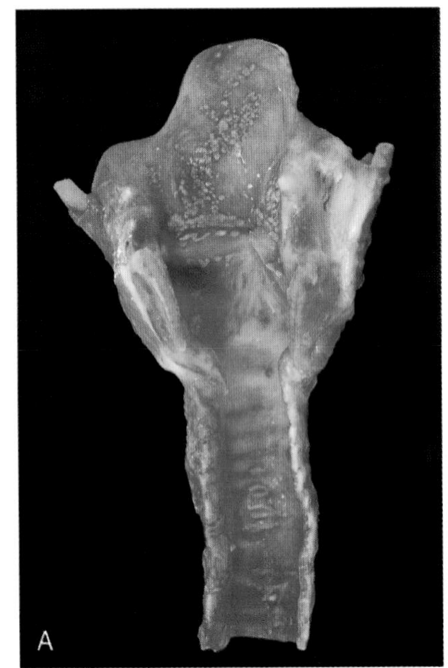
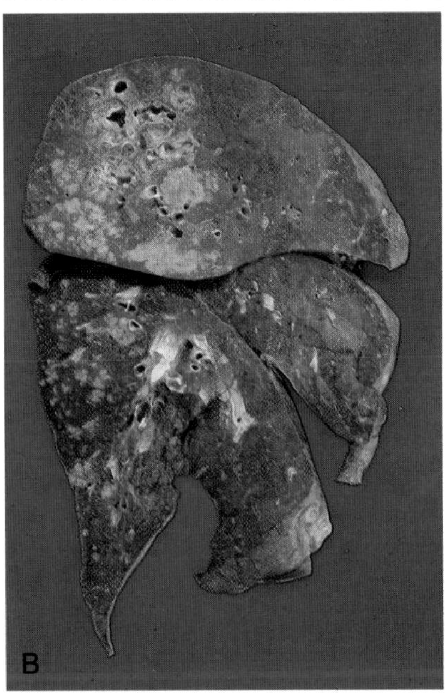
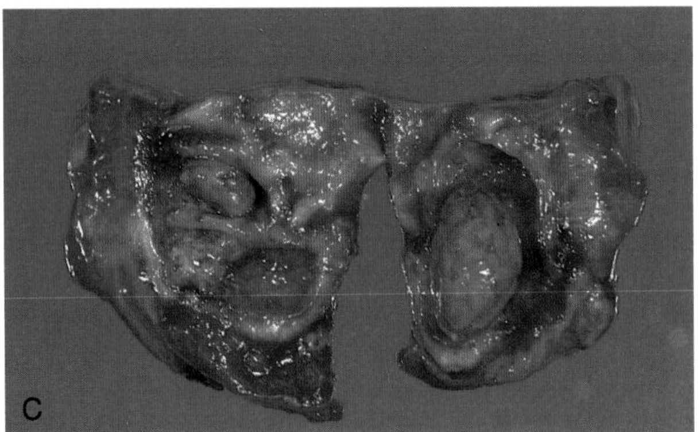
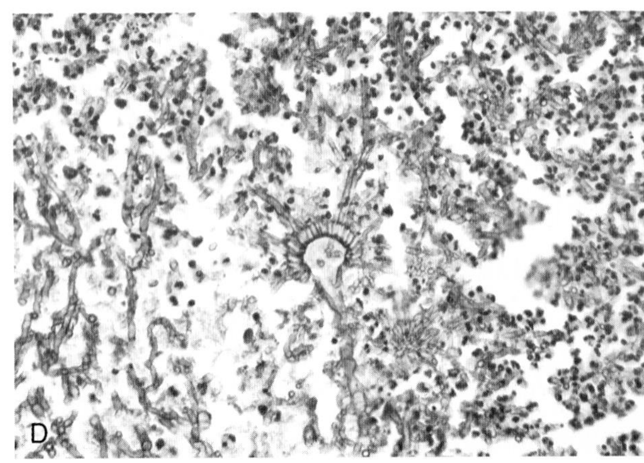
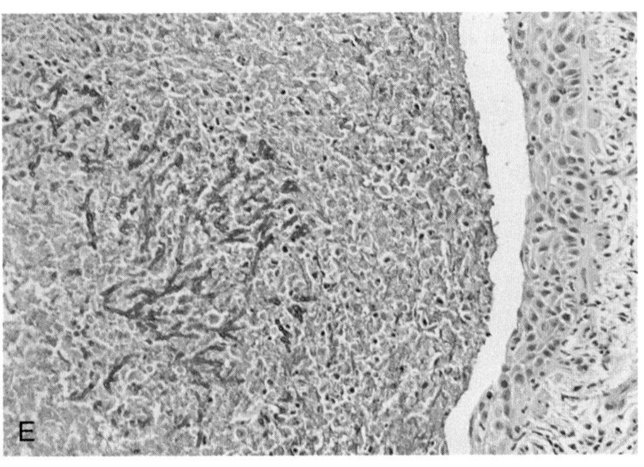

FIGURE 3-22

Some forms of aspergillosis. **A,** Necrotizing laryngotracheitis. **B,** Necrotizing aspergillus pneumonia with abscess formation in a patient with myelofibrosis. **C,** Aspergillus colonization of a lung cavity to form an aspergilloma. **D,** Conidial heads (fruiting bodies) of aspergillus seen here are rarely produced in tissue (H & E stain). They are most often seen in the aspergilloma in which the organism is exposed to air. **E,** Allergic bronchopulmonary aspergillosis manifesting as bronchocentric granulomatosis. The inflammation is centered on the airways, which have a metaplastic squamous epithelial lining. Aspergillus hyphae are present within the contents of the airway lumen (H & E stain).

LUNG DISEASE CAUSED BY INFECTIOUS AGENTS

FUNGAL INFECTIONS

FIGURE 3-23

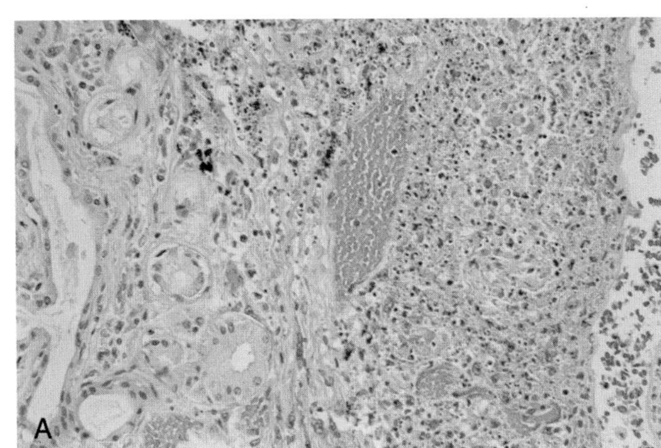

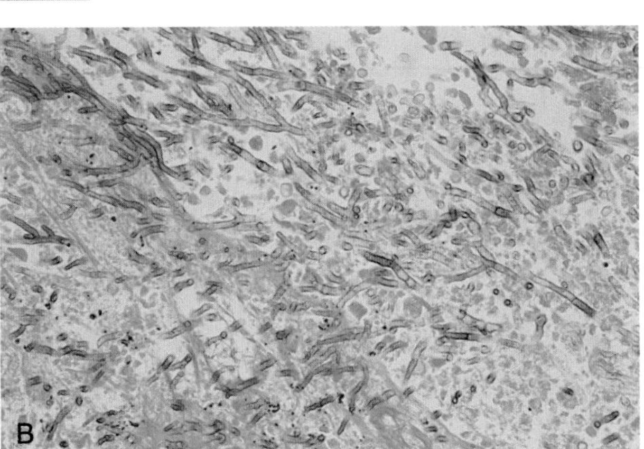

Pseudallescheriasis (maduromycosis) developing following chemotherapy for a malignant thymoma. The organisms cannot be distinguished from *Aspergillus* species on microscopic examination and require microbiologic confirmation. **A,** Acute and granulomatous inflammation of a bronchus (H & E stain). **B,** A GMS stain demonstrates branched, septated hyphae.

FIGURE 3-24

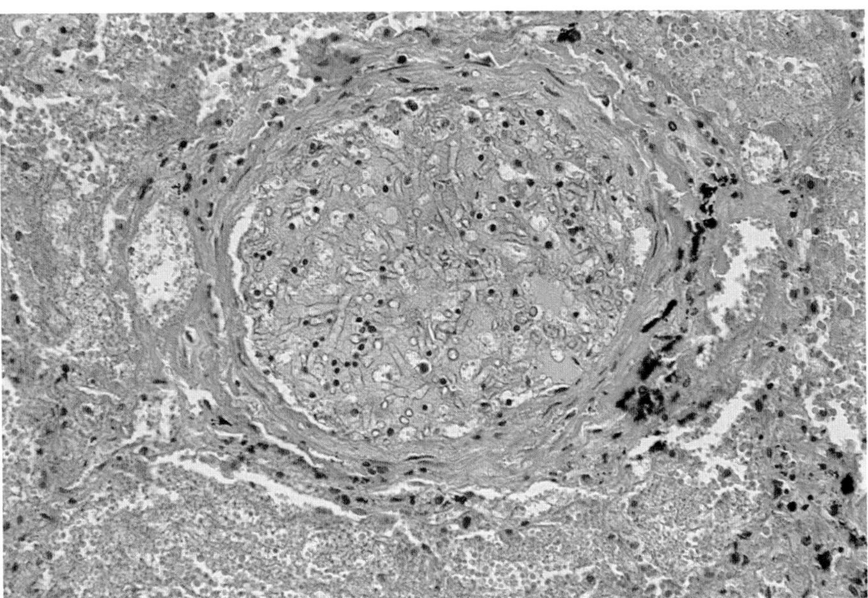

Zygomycosis (mucormycosis, phycomycosis) is caused by infection with fungi of the class Zygomycetes among which are *Rhizopus, Mucor, Absidia* species of the order Mucorales. These fungi cause invasive pneumonia in the immunosuppressed and endobronchial infection in the diabetic patient. The hyphae of mucoraceous zygomycetes are angioinvasive and result in infarcts. In this example, the broad, irregularly contoured and pleomorphic hyphae have penetrated a small pulmonary artery, causing thrombosis (H & E stain).

LUNG DISEASE CAUSED BY INFECTIOUS AGENTS

FUNGAL INFECTIONS

FIGURE 3-25

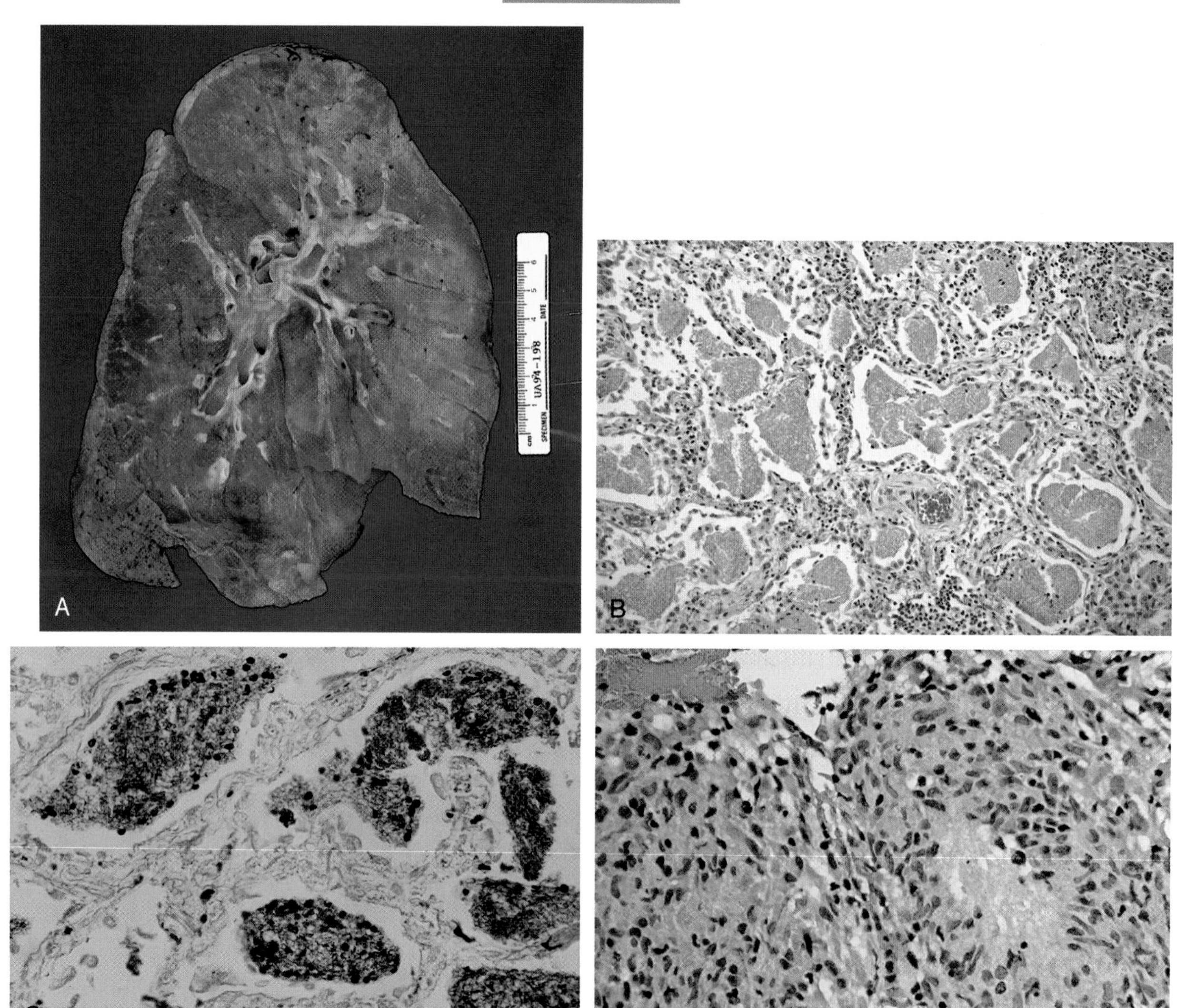

Pneumocystis carinii was formerly and sometimes still is classified as a protozoan. About 75% of people have serologic evidence of infection by early childhood. However, it causes symptomatic disease in the immunosuppressed. *Pneumocystis carinii* pneumonia (PCP) usually consists of interstitial lymphocytic or plasma cell pneumonitis with an intra-alveolar exudate. Diffuse alveolar damage, which tends to become organized, is a frequent complication. Coinfection with cytomegalovirus is found in 10% of patients, and bacterial coinfection may also occur. **A,** Organizing diffuse alveolar damage in a patient with AIDS and PCP. **B,** The most distinctive feature of PCP is the pink, foamy, or frothy intra-alveolar exudate (H & E stain). **C,** Special stains such as a GMS stain reveal the cup-shaped cysts walls. **D,** Granulomatous inflammation due to infection with *Pneumocystis carinii.* In approximately 10% of cases the organism may cause granulomatous inflammation (H & E stain). (See Chapter 5, Nuclear Medicine Techniques and Applications.)

LUNG DISEASE CAUSED BY INFECTIOUS AGENTS

PROTOZOAN AND HELMINTHIC INFECTIONS

Some protozoan and helminthic infections of the lung can produce major pathologic reactions.

TABLE 3-12

Pathologic Effects of Specific Protozoan and Helminthic Infections of the Lung

Organism	Disease	Pathologic Effects
PROTOZOAN INFECTIONS		
Amebae		
- *Entamoeba histolytica*	Amebiasis	Perforation of amebic abscess of liver through diaphragm causing empyema and lung abscess
Flagellates		
- *Leishmania* species	Visceral leishmaniasis	Rarely interstitial pneumonia
- *Trichomonas* species	Visceral leishmaniasis	Empyema and pneumonia following aspiration
Coccidia		
- *Toxoplasma gondii*	Toxoplasmosis	Interstitial pneumonitis progressing to parenchymal necrosis
- *Cryptosporidium*	Cryptosporidiosis	None, but in patients with gastrointestinal disease, the organisms may be found in sputum and may be associated with cough
Sporozoa		
- *Plasmodium falciparum*	Malaria	Acute pulmonary edema; diffuse alveolar damage
HELMINTHIC INFECTIONS		
Nematodes (roundworms)		
- *Strongyloides stercoralis*	Strongyloidiasis	Edema; hemorrhage; sometimes acute or granulomatous inflammation
- *Dirofilaria immitis*	Dirofilariasis (dog heartworm)	Spherical or lobulated peripheral nodules eliciting a granulomatous or nonspecific chronic inflammatory response, sometimes with prominent eosinophils
Cestodes (tapeworms)		
- *Echinococcus granulosus*	Hydatid disease	Circumscribed masses eliciting necrosis and granulomatosis inflammation with rupture
Trematodes (flukes)		
- *Paragonimus westermani* and other species	Paragonimiasis	Cystic cavity surrounded by eosinophilic and epithelioid histiocytic inflammatory infiltrate
- *Schistosoma* species	Shistosomiasis	Granulomatous inflammation

LUNG DISEASE CAUSED BY INFECTIOUS AGENTS

PROTOZOAN AND HELMINTHIC INFECTIONS

FIGURE 3–26

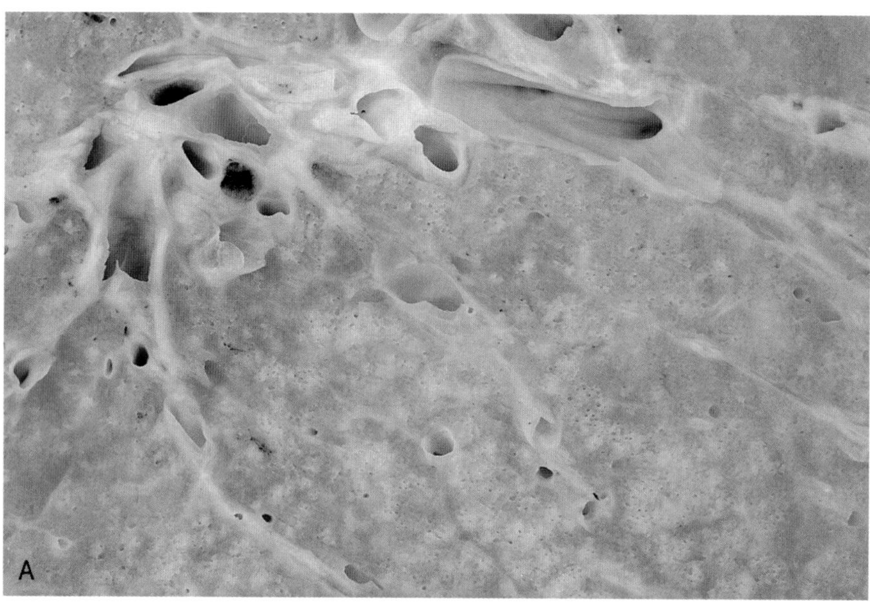

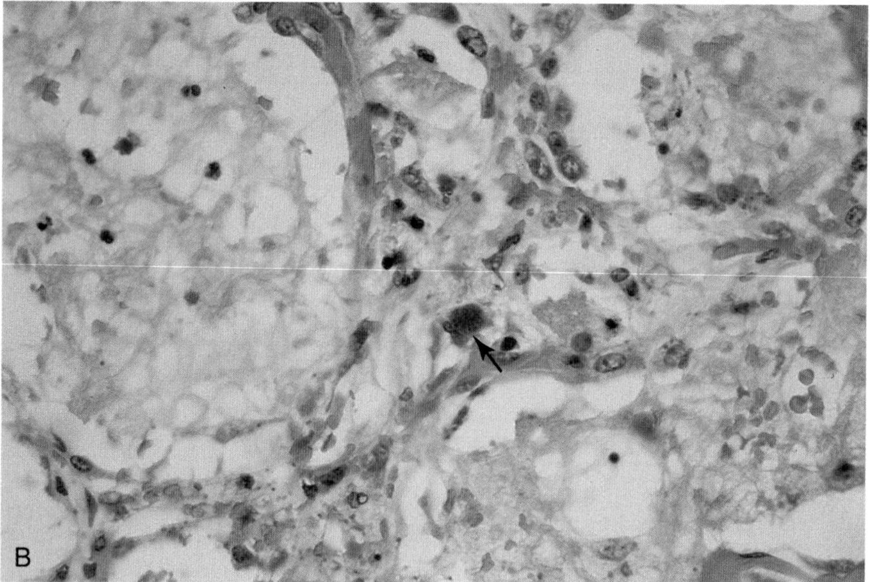

Toxoplasmosis in a patient with AIDS. **A,** The infection consists of multiple necrotic nodules in a miliary pattern. **B,** Microscopically, the lesions are characterized by foci of coagulative necrosis. *Toxoplasma gondi* cysts (*arrow*) and free organisms (tachyzoites) may be found within areas of necrosis (H & E stain).

CHRONIC OBSTRUCTIVE PULMONARY DISEASE

See Chapter 8, *Pulmonary Function Testing.*

EMPHYSEMA

FIGURE 3–27

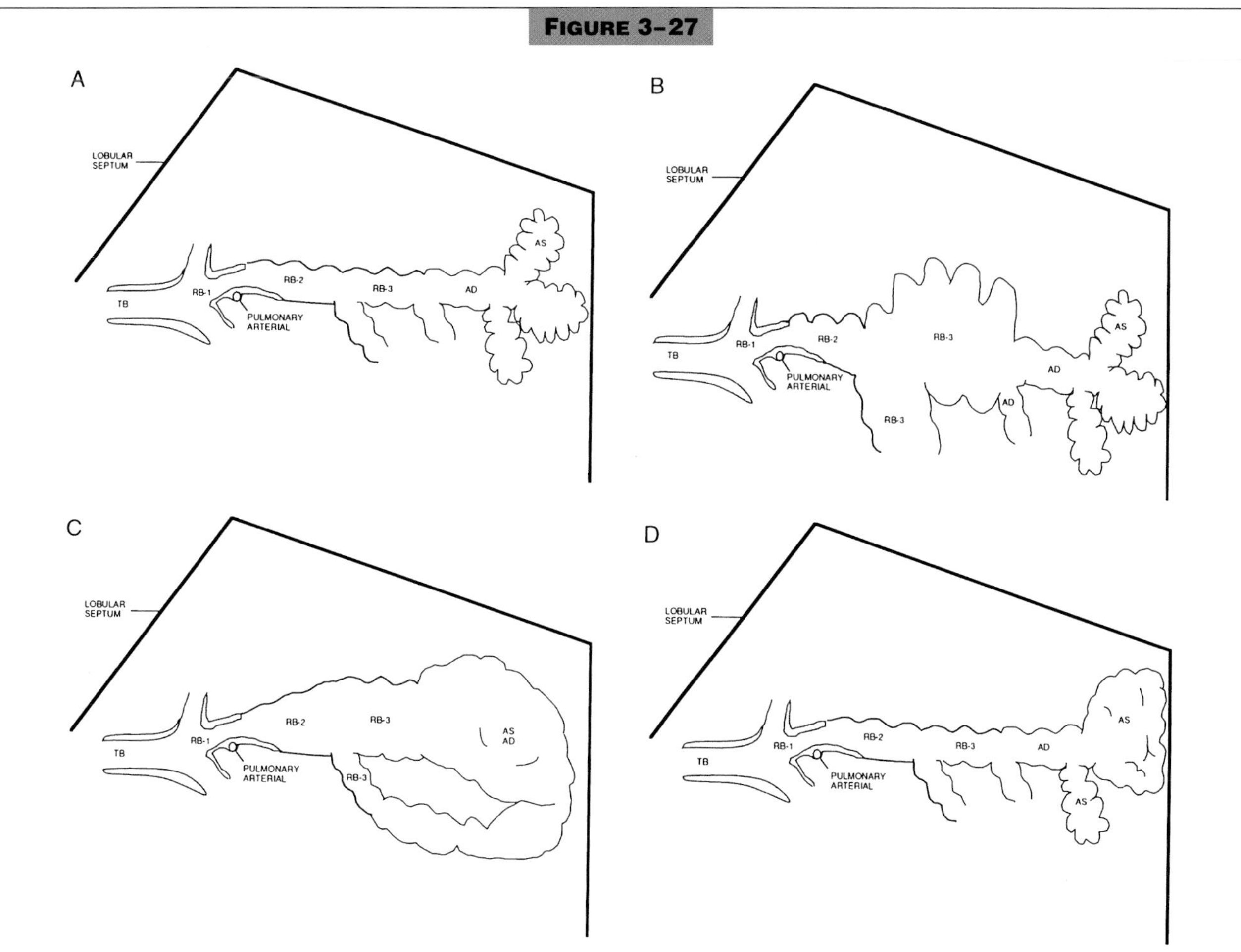

Emphysema, the enlargement of airspaces distal to the terminal bronchiole arising from destruction of their airspace walls can be classified by its anatomic distribution within the pulmonary acinus. **A,** Normal pulmonary acinus. The pulmonary acinus consists of the airspace structures that are derived from a single terminal bronchiole and include respiratory bronchioles, alveolar ducts, and alveolar sacs. **B,** Centriacinar emphysema (synonym: centrilobular emphysema). In this type of emphysema, the proximal portions of the acini (respiratory bronchioles) are affected and the distal portions of the acini (alveolar ducts and alveoli) are usually spared. In centriacinar emphysema the second- and third-order respiratory bronchioles are more severely affected than the first-order respiratory bronchiole. In severe centriacinar emphysema, the distal acinus may be involved making its differentiation from panacinar emphysema difficult. There is generally variation in the severity of centriacinar emphysema among acini and even within the same lobules. The lesions are more common and more severe in the upper lobes. Chronic inflammation of the airways supplying the emphysematous areas and chronic inflammation and fibrosis of the walls of emphysematous spaces can usually be seen. Centriacinar emphysema is the most common type of emphysema and is the type of emphysema associated with smoking. **C,** Panacinar emphysema (synonym: panlobular emphysema). In this type of emphysema the acini are more or less uniformly affected from the level of the respiratory bronchiole to the terminal alveoli. Panacinar emphysema tends to be more frequent in the lower zones of the lung. It is the type of emphysema associated with alpha-1-antitrypsin deficiency. It has also been found in 5 to 10% of random autopsies and in up to 20% in autopsies performed on persons over the age of 70. It may occur in combination with centriacinar emphysema, and in these cases, precise classification is difficult. **D,** Distal acinar emphysema (synonym: paraseptal emphysema) frequently occurs adjacent to areas of scarring, commonly adjacent to the pleura and along lobular septa and most frequently in the upper part of the lung. It may also be associated with panacinar emphysema, centrilobular emphysema, or chronic bronchitis. Distal acinar emphysema probably is the underlying cause in most cases of spontaneous idiopathic pneumothorax of young adults. This results from rupture of subpleural bullae (emphysematous spaces of more than 1 cm). (See Chapter 4, Radiography and Imaging.) AS = alveolar sac; AD = alveolar duct; RB = respiratory bronchiole; TB = terminal bronchiole. (Drawings after Thurlbeck WM: Chronic obstructive lung disease. *In* Sommers SC (ed): Pathology Annual, Vol. 3. New York, Appleton-Century-Crofts, 1968, pp. 367–398.)

CHRONIC OBSTRUCTIVE PULMONARY DISEASE

EMPHYSEMA

FIGURE 3-28

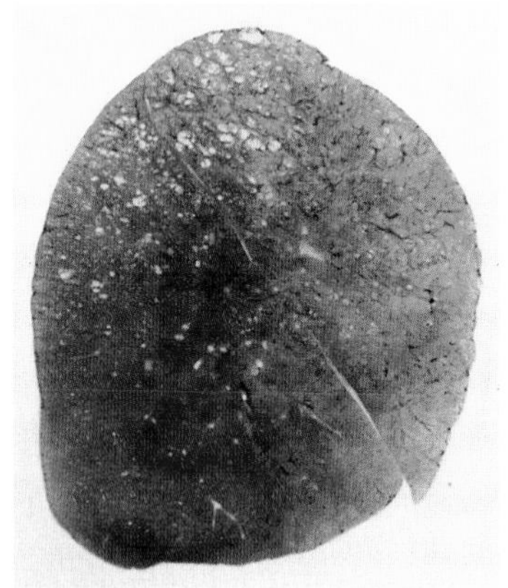

A paper mounted lung (Gough-Wentworth) section showing large centrilobular emphysematous spaces in the upper lobe of the lung of a chronic smoker.

FIGURE 3-29

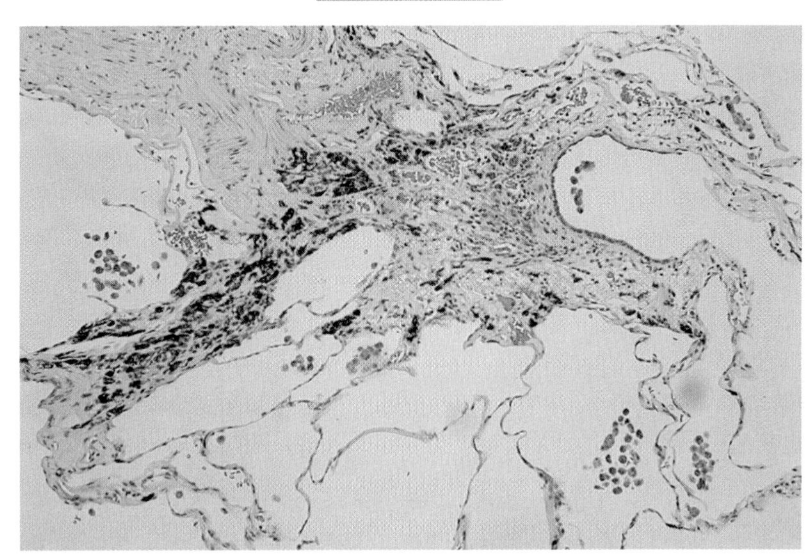

Respiratory bronchiolitis. Intra-alveolar macrophages containing smokers' pigment are present adjacent to respiratory bronchioles characterized by mild inflammation and fibrosis. Respiratory bronchiolitis occurs in the lungs of smokers. If this process becomes extensive, it can mimic infiltrative lung disease (respiratory bronchiolitis interstitial lung disease).

FIGURE 3-30

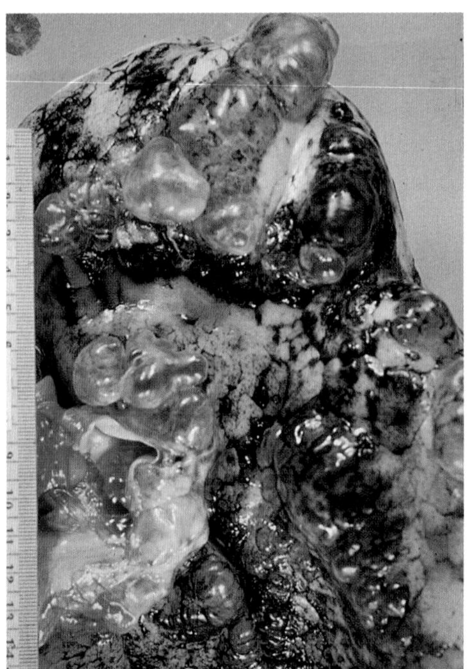

Bullae are emphysematous spaces more than 1 cm in diameter. Numerous thin-walled bullae project from the surface of this lung specimen. Abundant carbon has deposited within the lymphatics of the visceral pleura, causing the black discoloration (anthracosis).

CHRONIC OBSTRUCTIVE PULMONARY DISEASE

CHRONIC BRONCHITIS

FIGURE 3–31

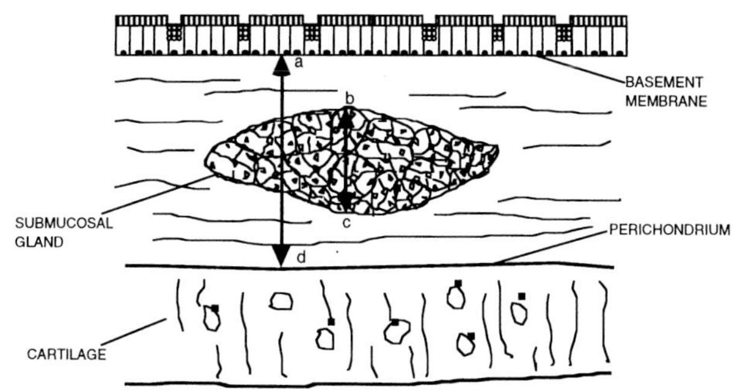

Chronic bronchitis is defined clinically as chronic excessive production of mucus in the airways not due to known specific causes (i.e., bronchiectasis, tuberculosis). In this definition "chronic" means on most days for more than 3 months a year for 2 or more successive years.[1] The pathologic finding that most consistently correlates with chronic bronchitis is enlargement of tracheobronchial submucosal glands and an increase in the number of surface goblet cells (goblet cell metaplasia). Hypertrophy and hyperplasia of the mucous secretory apparatus is associated with the increased sputum production so clinically apparent in this disease. Reid[2] described a simple light microscopic technique for measuring tracheobronchial gland enlargement. This measurement, now known as the Reid index, correlates well with the clinical presence of chronic bronchitis. The Reid index is obtained by determining the ratio of the thickness of the submucosal glands (the distance from b to c) to the distance between the perichondrium and the basal lamina of the bronchial lining epithelium (the distance from a to d). The mean Reid index in normal individuals is roughly one-third while in bronchitics it averages one-half. (Drawing after Thurlbeck WM: Chronic obstructive lung disease. *In* Sommers SC (ed): Pathology Annual, Vol. 3. New York, Appleton-Century-Crofts, 1968, pp. 367–398.)

FIGURE 3–32

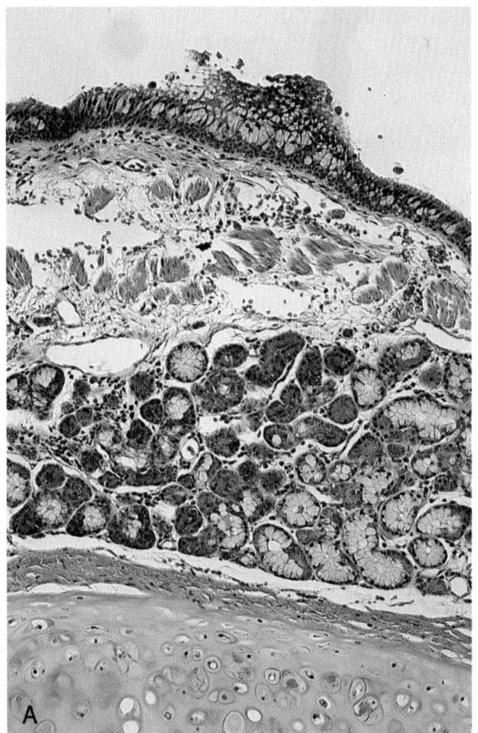

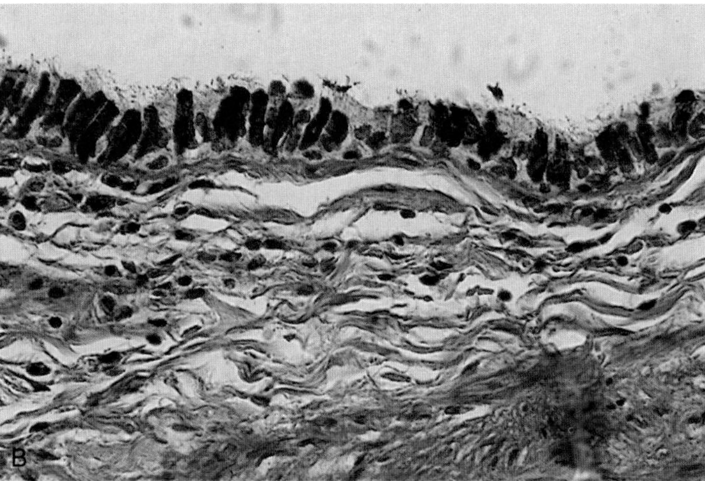

Histologic features of chronic bronchitis. **A,** The bronchial seromucous glands are enlarged, making up greater than half of the bronchial submucosa (H & E stain). **B,** The surface epithelium of a bronchiole shows considerable goblet cell hyperplasia (Alcian blue/periodic acid–Schiff stain pH 2.5).

CHRONIC OBSTRUCTIVE PULMONARY DISEASE

ASTHMA

Asthma is characterized by increased irritability of the tracheobronchial tree, potentiating paroxysmal narrowing of bronchial airways and airflow obstruction in response to varied stimuli. Asthma can be classified based on these stimuli or more traditionally, into two types: extrinsic (immunologic or allergic) and intrinsic (nonimmunologic or idiosyncratic). The types of asthma, precipitating factors, and pathogenic mechanisms are listed in TABLE 3–13.

TABLE 3–13

Types of Asthma and Related Characteristics

Types of Asthma	Stimuli	Pathogenic Mechanism
Extrinsic		
- Atopic (allergic) reaction	Specific allergens	Type I (IgE) immune (dusts, pollens, etc.)
Intrinsic		
- Nonatopic	Respiratory tract infection	Unknown; hyperreactive airways
- Occupational/irritants or allergens	Chemicals	Type I immune reactions; direct effects of irritant
- Drug-induced	Aspirin, NSAIDs, β-adrenergic antagonists, sulfites	Increased leukotrienes; decreased prostaglandins
- Infections	Viral (URI, bronchiolitis); allergic bronchopulmonary aspergillosis	Type I and III immune reactions

Key: NSAIDs = nonsteroidal anti-inflammatory drugs; URI = upper respiratory tract infection.

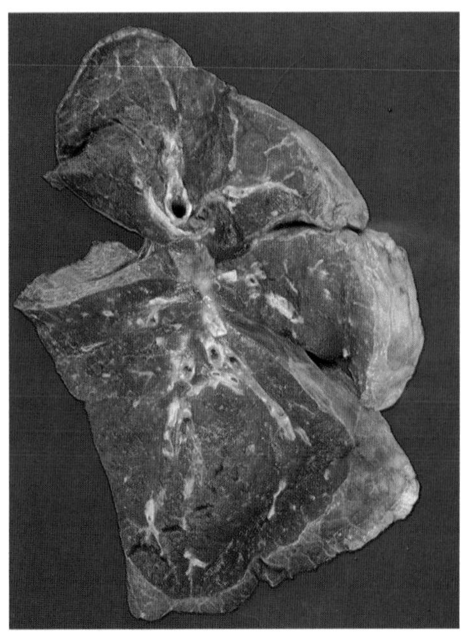

FIGURE 3–33

The gross appearance of lungs in patients dying of asthma usually shows a combination of hyperinflation and atelectasis, and the airways are occluded by mucous plugs. The autopsy specimen shown here came from a patient who had a fatal respiratory arrest following an acute asthma attack. At postmortem examination, the lungs were difficult to inflate and contained scattered mucous plugs in the small airways. The gross specimen shows irregular atelectasis but is not overdistended.

CHRONIC OBSTRUCTIVE PULMONARY DISEASE

ASTHMA

FIGURE 3-34

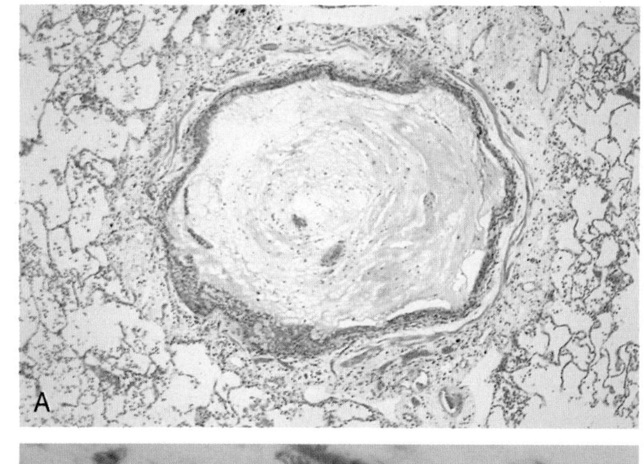

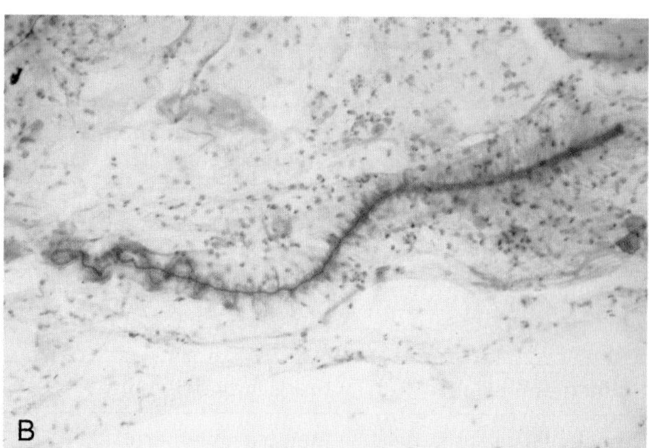

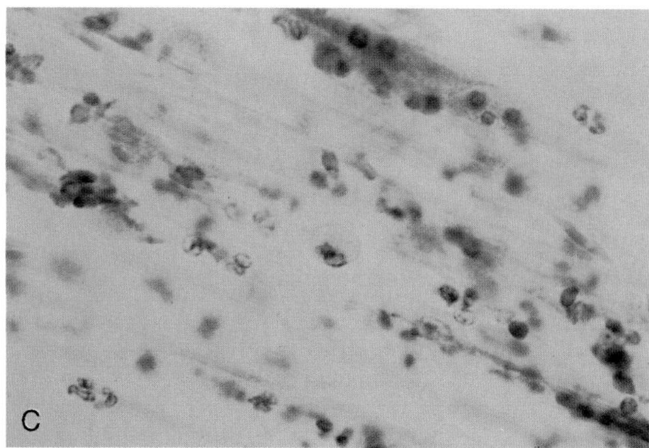

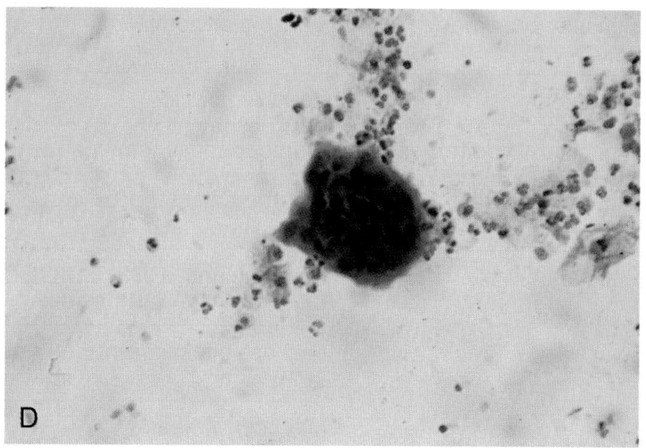

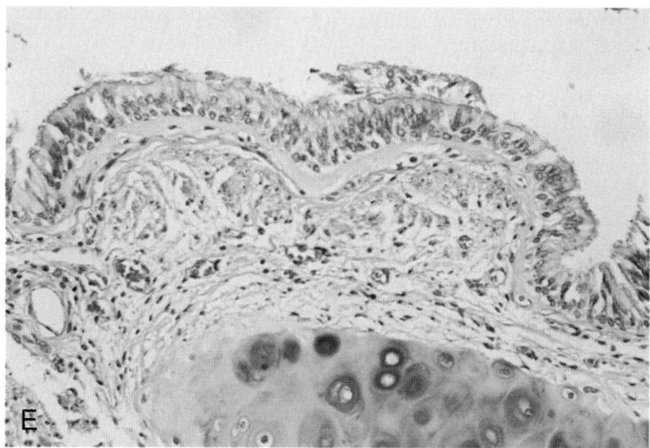

Histopathology of asthma (H & E stain unless indicated otherwise). The pathologic changes in asthma have been described primarily in patients dying of asthma. Nonfatal cases demonstrate similar if somewhat milder alterations. **A,** Mucous plugging is the most dramatic finding in asthma. Plugs of mucus occlude bronchi and bronchioles (shown here). **B,** Sputum from patients with asthma often contains mucous casts of the small airways (Curschmann's spirals) (Papanicolaou stain). **C,** The mucous plugs contain an inflammatory cell exudate in which eosinophils predominate and lipopolysaccharide secreted from eosinophils may form crystals (Charcot-Leyden crystals). **D,** Hyperplastic airway epithelium may be sloughed, and in sputum the sloughed bronchial or bronchiolar epithelial clusters may mimic carcinoma (Creola bodies) (Papanicolaou stain). **E,** Thickening of the "basement membrane" of the airway epithelium. Actually, the thickening occurs in the subepithelial collagen layer, which lies just under the basement membrane. This layer is usually 7.5 μm thick, but in asthma it averages 17.5 μm in thickness. The overlying epithelium may show basal cell hyperplasia, bronchial goblet cell hyperplasia, or squamous metaplasia. The airways may be edematous and inflamed. Airway smooth muscle is hyperplasic. Like chronic bronchitis, the airway secretory cells are prominent in asthma.

CHRONIC OBSTRUCTIVE PULMONARY DISEASE

ASTHMA

TABLE 3-14

Comparison of Chronic Bronchitis and Asthma

Feature	Chronic Bronchitis	Asthma
Airflow obstruction	• Progressive deterioration of lung function (? reversible component)	• Variable (± irreversible component)
Postmortem findings	• Excessive mucus (mucoid/purulent)	• Hyperinflation with airway plugs (exudate + mucus)
Sputum	• Macrophage/neutrophil (infective exacerbation)	• Eosinophilia • Metachromatic cells • Creola bodies
Surface epithelium	• Fragility undetermined	• Fragility/loss
Bronchiolar mucous cells	• Metaplasia/hyperplasia	• Mucous metaplasia is debated
Reticular basement membrane	• Variable or normal	• Homogeneously thickened and hyaline
Congestion/edema	• Variable/fibrotic	• Present
Bronchial smooth muscle	• Enlarged mass (small airways)	• Enlarged mass (large airways)
Bronchial glands	• Enlarged mass (increased acidic glycoprotein)	• Enlarged mass (no change in mucin histochemistry)
Cellular infiltrate	• Predominantly CD3, CD8, CD68, CD25 positive VLA-1 and HLA-DR positive	• Predominantly CD3, CD4, CD25 (IL-2R) positive
	• Mild eosinophilia (not degranulated?)	• Marked eosinophilia (EG2 positive) (degranulated)
	• Mast cell increase	• Mast cell increase (decrease in severe/fatal)
Cytokines (ISH)	• GM-CSF protein, IL-4 and IL-5 gene expression	• IL-4 + IL-5 but not IFN-γ gene expression (Th_2 profile)

Key: CD = cluster designation; CD3 = T lymphocytes; CD4 = T helper lymphocytes; CD8 = T cytotoxic/suppressor lymphocytes; CD25 = activated lymphocytes; CD68 = monocytes, histiocytes; EG2+ = activated eosinophils; GM-CSF = granulocyte macrophage-colony stimulating factor; IL = interleukin; HLA-DR = major histocompatibility complex class II antigen; IFN = interferon; Th_2 = T helper lymphocyte type 2; VLA-1 = late activation cells.

Source: Modified from Jeffry PK: Differences and similarities between chronic obstructive pulmonary disease and asthma. Clin Exp Allergy 29 (Suppl 2):14–26, 1999; Jeffry PK: Comparative morphology of the airways in asthma and chronic obstructive pulmonary disease. Am J Respir Crit Care Med 150:S6–S13, 1994.

CHRONIC OBSTRUCTIVE PULMONARY DISEASE

BRONCHIECTASIS

Bronchiectasis is a chronic necrotizing infection of the bronchi and bronchioles leading to or associated with abnormal dilation of these airways. Before the introduction of antibiotics and immunizations, bronchiectasis frequently developed during childhood as a complication of childhood infections. Today it is less common, but it remains clinically important in several conditions. Bronchiectasis occurs in a variety of diseases that have in common obstruction of airways, impaired mucociliary clearance, and persistent infection. In some cases, infection develops in bronchiectatic areas, and in others, infection is the precipitating cause of the airway injury and dilatation. The causes and specific pathogenetic mechanisms of bronchiectasis are listed in TABLE 3–15.

TABLE 3–15

Characteristics of Bronchiectasis

Causes	Pathogenesis
Postinfective (measles, pertussis, adenovirus, tuberculosis, suppurative pneumonias)	Impaired drainage of secretions
Congenital abnormalities	
- Intralobular sequestration	Recurrent infection
Hereditary conditions	
- Cystic fibrosis	Abnormal chloride secretion due to defective cystic fibrosis transmembrane regulatory (CFTR) protein leading to abnormal airway lining fluid and airway infection
- Primary ciliary dyskinesia (immotile cilia syndrome)	Impaired ciliary activity leading to impaired mucociliary clearance
- Immunodeficiency states (e.g., IgA deficiency)	Recurrent infection
- Congenital bronchiectasis	Defect in bronchial wall cartilage

FIGURE 3–35

Localized postinflammatory bronchiectasis. Bronchiectatic airways are dilated, sometimes up to four times normal size, and can usually be seen to reach the pleural surface.

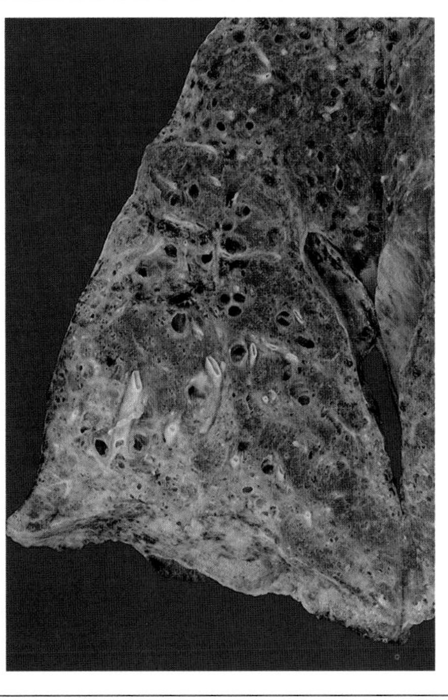

CHRONIC OBSTRUCTIVE PULMONARY DISEASE

BRONCHIECTASIS

FIGURE 3-36

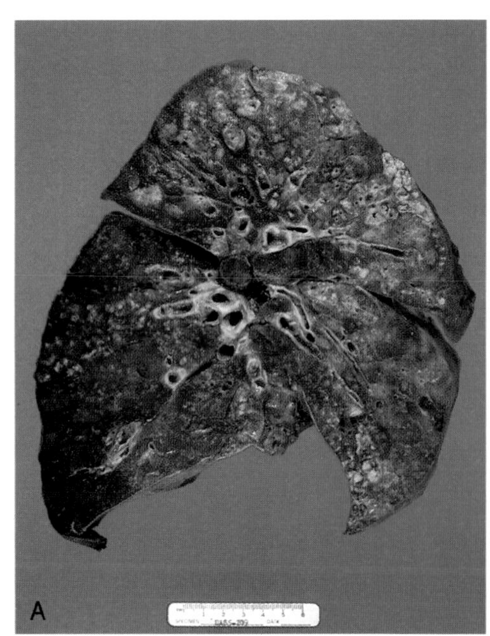

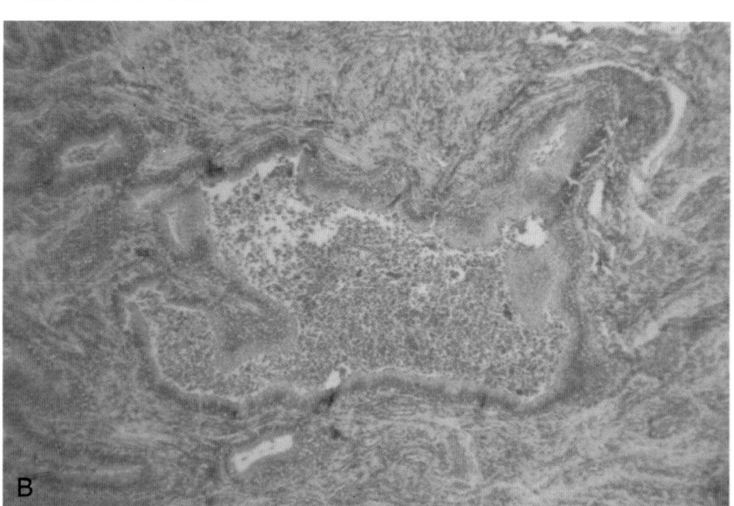

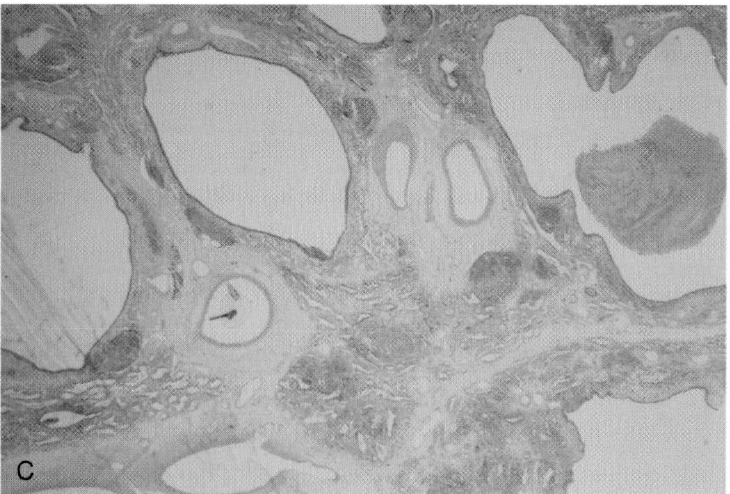

Cystic fibrosis. **A,** The gross specimen shows diffuse, purulent bronchiectasis, which is worse in the upper lobes. **B,** Bronchiectatic airways are filled with a suppurative exudate composed of acute and chronic inflammatory cells. There may be squamous metaplasia or pseudostratification of the remaining epithelium (H & E stain). **C,** With healing there may be regeneration of normal epithelium; however, dilatation and scarring persist (H & E stain). The adjacent lung parenchyma may show patchy emphysema, atelectasis, and fibrosis.

CHRONIC OBSTRUCTIVE PULMONARY DISEASE

BRONCHIECTASIS

FIGURE 3–37

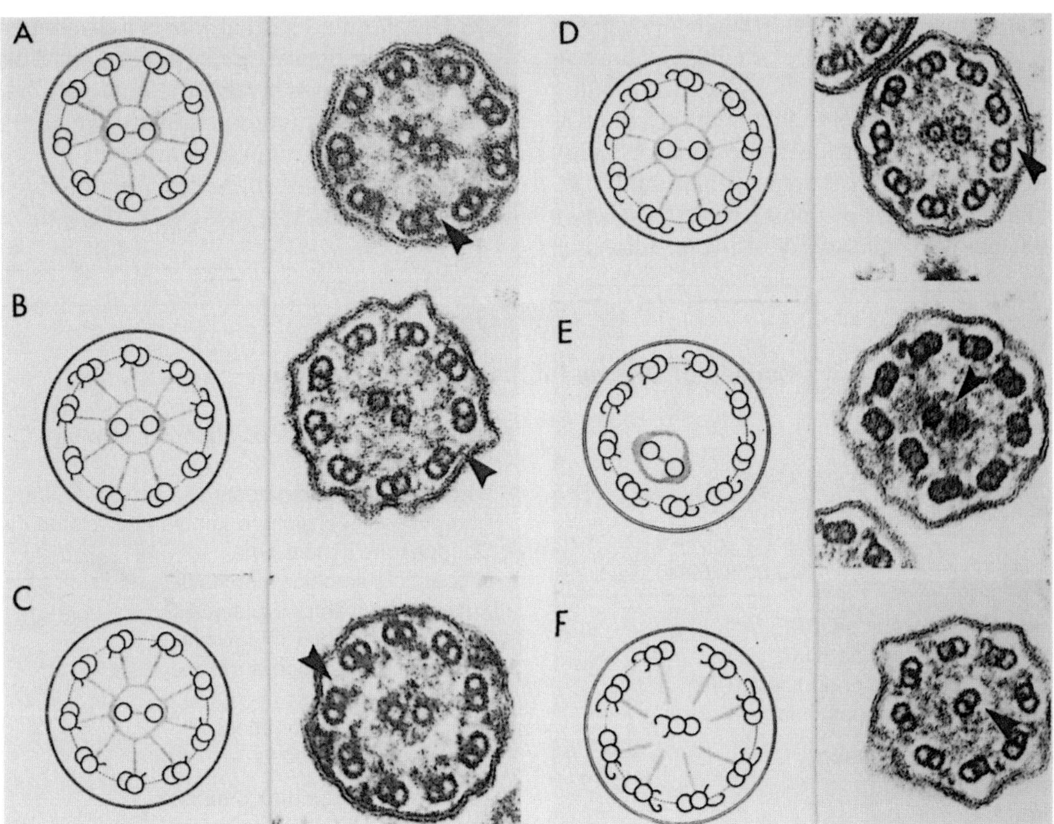

Primary ciliary dyskinesia. Transverse sections of cilium exhibiting ultrastructural defects are shown as diagrammatic representations on the left and in actual electron micrographs on the right. **A,** Complete dynein defect: the inner and outer dynein arms are lacking from the outer doublet microtubules. **B,** Partial dynein defect: most inner and outer dynein arms are defective. **C,** Outer dynein arm defect: the outer dynein arms are lacking, but inner dynein arms remain. **D,** Inner dynein arm defect: the inner dynein arms are defective, and outer dynein arms are present. **E,** Radial spoke defect: the radial spoke linkages cannot be distinguished, and the central core is eccentric. **F,** Microtubular transposition defect: the central core is lacking, and one outer microtubular doublet is transposed to the central axis, forming an 8 + 1 arrangement. (See normal cilia in Figure 2–18.) (From Sturgess JM: Ciliated cells in the lungs. *In* Massaro D (ed): Lung Cell Biology. New York, Marcel Dekker, 1989, pp. 115–151.)

DIFFUSE INFILTRATIVE (RESTRICTIVE) LUNG DISEASE

See Chapter 8, *Pulmonary Function Testing.*

Diffuse infiltrative lung disease is a term used to characterize a large group of lung diseases that share some common clinical and radiologic features. However, from the standpoint of etiology, pathogenesis, and pathologic anatomy, they often have little in common. These disorders often share dyspnea as the predominant clinical manifestation. Chest radiographs are characterized by diffuse "infiltration" of irregular linear, nodular, or diffuse ("ground glass") shadows. Laboratory studies reveal hypoxemia, impaired diffusing capacity, and in advanced stages of the diseases, decreased lung volumes and compliance. Despite the fact that this is a diverse group of diseases, their clinical similarities, the fact that pathologic abnormalities involve the lung periphery, and their contrasts with chronic obstructive lung diseases make their grouping convenient. Some important causes of diffuse infiltrative lung disease are listed in TABLE 3–16.

TABLE 3–16

Causes of Diffuse Infiltrative Lung Disease

1. Interstitial pneumonias
Acute
- Diffuse alveolar damage (DAD/ARDS)
- Acute interstitial pneumonia (AIP)

Subacute
- Bronchiolitis obliterans organizing pneumonia (BOOP)

Chronic
- Idiopathic pulmonary fibrosis (IPF)
- Usual interstitial pneumonia (UIP)
- Desquamative interstitial pneumonia (DIP)
- Nonspecific interstitial pneumonia

2. Connective tissue disease
- Rheumatoid arthritis
- Scleroderma
- Systemic lupus erythematosus
- Mixed connective tissue disease
- Other connective tissue diseases

3. Occupational and environmental diseases
- Allergic alveolitis (organic dusts)
- Asbestosis
- Berylliosis
- Silicosis (coal and graphite)
- Other silicates
- Hard metal pneumoconiosis (giant cell interstitial pneumonia)
- Toxic gases (NO_2, SO_2, Br_2, Cl_2)
- Fumes (toluene)
- Smoke inhalation

4. Drugs, toxins, and therapeutic agents
- Chemotherapeutic agents (busulfan, bleomycin)
- Antibiotics (nitrofurantoin)
- Other drugs (gold, penicillamine, amiodarone)
- Toxins (paraquot)
- Radiation
- Oxygen

5. Specific disorders of unknown etiology
- Sarcoidosis
- Wegener's granulomatosis
- Chronic eosinophilic pneumonia and related disorders
- Goodpasture's syndrome
- Idiopathic pulmonary hemosiderosis
- Pulmonary alveolar proteinosis
- Pulmonary alveolar microlithiasis
- Eosinophilic granuloma (histiocytosis X)
- Tuberous sclerosis
- Lymphangioleiomyomatosis
- Pulmonary amyloidosis

6. Pulmonary vascular diseases
- Vasculitis
- Pulmonary veno-occlusive disease
- Multiple/recurrent pulmonary embolism

7. Infections
- Miliary tuberculosis
- Fungal
- Viral

8. Neoplasms/lymphoproliferative disorders
- Leukemia
- Lymphoma
- Lymphocytic interstitial pneumonia (LIP)
- Adenocarcinoma-bronchioloalveolar type
- Metastatic carcinomatosis

9. Chronic obstructive pulmonary disease
- Respiratory bronchiolitis interstitial lung disease

10. Transplant-associated lung disease
- Acute lung rejection
- Chronic lung rejection
- Graft-versus-host disease

DIFFUSE INFILTRATIVE (RESTRICTIVE) LUNG DISEASE

Current hypotheses directed toward understanding the pathogenesis of diffuse interstitial lung diseases generally subscribe to the theory that injury to the lung, whether it is due to shock, toxic effects on cells, infectious agents, or immune-mediated mechanisms, causes alveolitis. The alveoli are composed of endothelial and epithelial cells, collagen fibers, elastic tissue, proteoglycans, fibroblasts, mast cells, and inflammatory cells. The resident inflammatory cells, as sampled by bronchoalveolar lavage (BAL), consist of macrophages (93%), lymphocytes (7%), and eosinophils and neutrophils (less than 1%) (TABLE 3–17). During alveolitis these inflammatory cells increase in number and change in their relative proportions. Mediators of inflammation, proteases, oxidants, and other cell products are released from these cells as well as from injured endothelial, epithelial, and mesenchymal cells. The net result is a perturbation of the delicate connective tissue framework of the lung. Continual injury may lead to progressive and irreversible scarring. Differential counts of inflammatory cells in BAL fluid are helpful in diagnosis of diffuse infiltrative lung disease and in monitoring response to therapy.

TABLE 3–17

Proportions of Cells in Diffuse Interstitial Lung Diseases

Disease	Proportions of Cells in Lavage Fluid
Idiopathic pulmonary fibrosis	Neutrophils and eosinophils increased
Sarcoidosis	Lymphocytes and T helper/suppressor ratio both increased
Hypersensitivity pneumonitis	Lymphocytes very increased; helper/suppressor ratio low; mast cells present
Histiocytosis X	Langerhans' cells increased

Source: Modified from Young JA: Cytopathology. *In* Brewis RAL, Corrin B, Geddes DM, Gibson GJ (eds): Respiratory Medicine. London, WB Saunders, 1995, pp. 352–356.

DIFFUSE ALVEOLAR DAMAGE (ADULT RESPIRATORY DISTRESS SYNDROME)

FIGURE 3–38

A, The lungs of patients dying during the early exudative stage of diffuse alveolar damage are heavy with firm, boggy, red parenchyma. **B,** Patients dying during the later proliferative stage have lungs with widespread organization, interstitial fibrosis, and sometimes cyst formation.

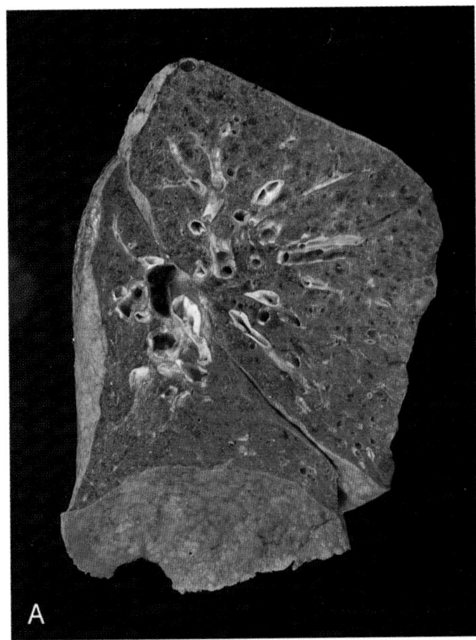

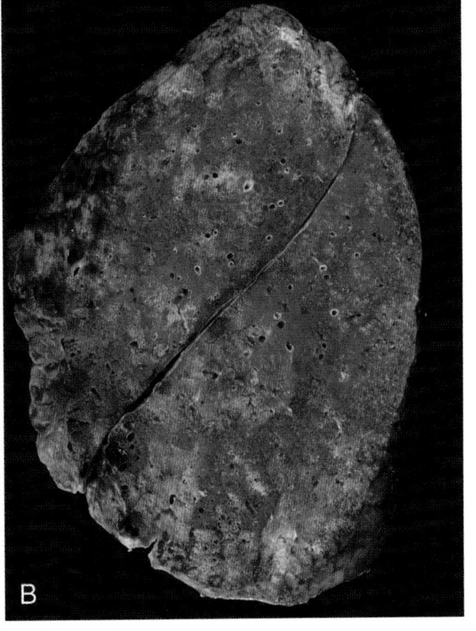

DIFFUSE INFILTRATIVE (RESTRICTIVE) LUNG DISEASE

DIFFUSE ALVEOLAR DAMAGE (ADULT RESPIRATORY DISTRESS SYNDROME)

FIGURE 3–39

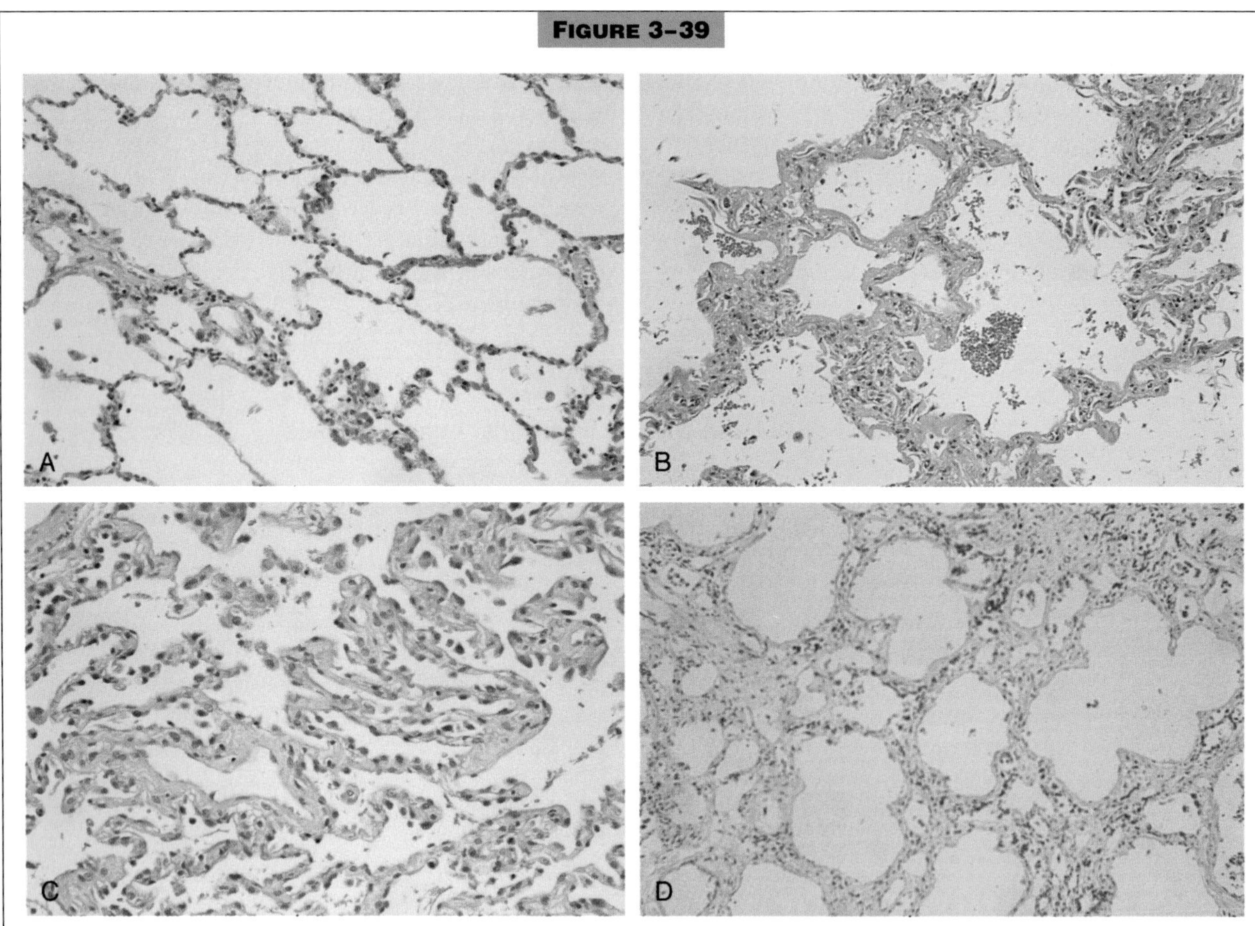

Microscopic pathology of diffuse alveolar damage. **A,** In the early stages, edema, congestion, and fibrin deposition are present. **B,** Twenty-four hours after injury, hyaline membranes become evident. They are composed of protein- and fibrin-containing edema fluid and cytoplasmic and lipid cellular debris from necrotic alveolar epithelial cells. Hyaline membranes increase in number for the next several days, but then begin to disappear at a somewhat variable rate. The loss of alveolar epithelial cells affects gas transport and surfactant production. With the loss of surfactant there is considerable atelectasis and this combined with the edema makes the lungs "stiff" or non-compliant. Additionally, the lung injury causes an inflammatory response. **C,** During the healing stage, if the cause of diffuse alveolar damage is removed, pulmonary edema resolves, type II pneumocytes proliferate and repair the alveolar lining, and atelectatic areas re-expand. **D,** However, with progression of the disease, there is organization of the fibrin exudate, and interstitial fibrosis develops.

DIFFUSE INFILTRATIVE (RESTRICTIVE) LUNG DISEASE

NONINFECTIOUS INTERSTITIAL PNEUMONIAS

Bronchiolitis obliterans organizing pneumonia (BOOP) or cryptogenic organizing pneumonia (COP) is a nonspecific acute injury pattern seen in the lung in a variety of settings. Numerous causes and associations have been identified, though many cases remain idiopathic. Some causes of BOOP are listed in TABLE 3–18.

TABLE 3–18

Causes of Bronchiolitis Obliterans Organizing Pneumonia

- Idiopathic (idiopathic BOOP or COP)
- Organizing infections (bacterial, fungal, viral, mycoplasma)
- Chronic aspiration of gastric contents
- Toxic fume inhalation
- Allergic reactions (allergic alveolitis, eosinophilic pneumonia)
- Organizing diffuse alveolar damage
- Drug toxicity
- Collagen vascular diseases (especially rheumatoid arthritis)
- Distal to bronchiectasis or large airway obstruction
- Nonspecific reaction at the periphery of an unrelated pathologic process
- Minor component of the pathologic reaction of other infiltrative lung diseases

Key: BOOP = bronchiolitis obliterans organizing pneumonia; COP = cryptogenic organizing pneumonia.

FIGURE 3–40

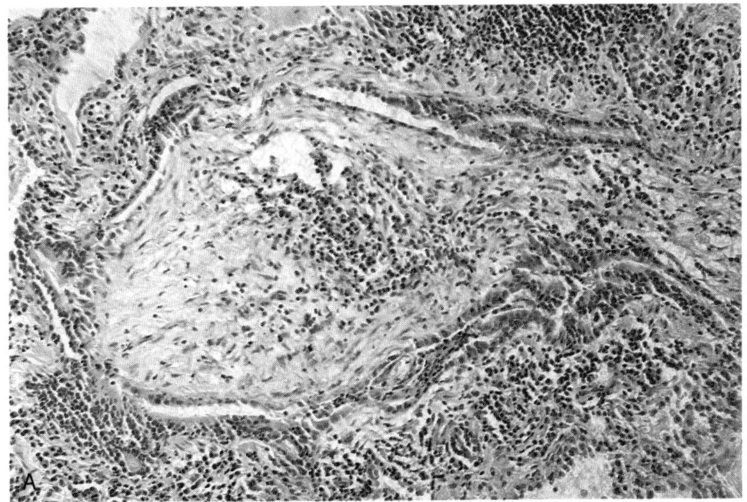

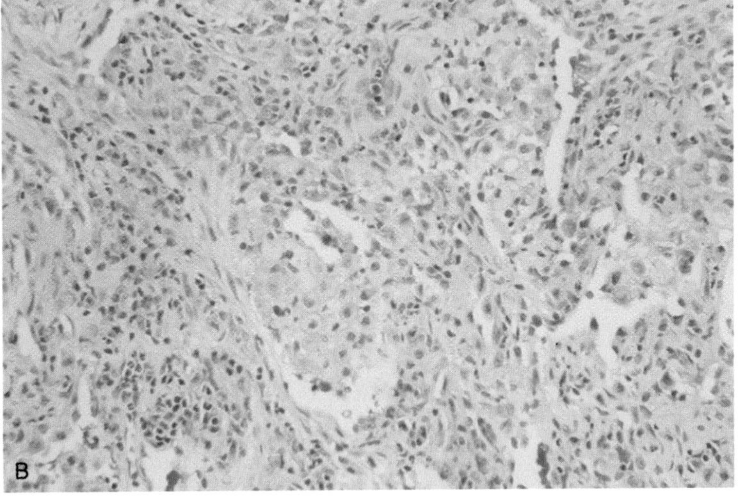

Microscopic pathology of BOOP (H & E stain). **A,** Edematous plugs of granulation tissue (Masson bodies) filling bronchioles and alveolar ducts. **B,** There is relative preservation of pulmonary parenchyma, although acute inflammation and fibrinous exudate within alveoli is present in a patchy distribution. Scattered interstitial infiltrate of lymphocytes and plasma cells and focal interstitial fibrosis concentrated in peribronchiolar regions are typical. Lipid-laden alveolar macrophages collect distal to airway obstruction.

DIFFUSE INFILTRATIVE (RESTRICTIVE) LUNG DISEASE

NONINFECTIOUS INTERSTITIAL PNEUMONIAS

FIGURE 3-41

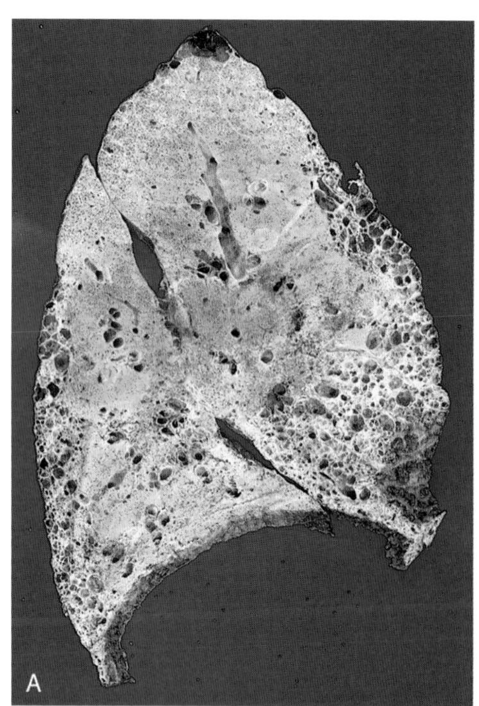

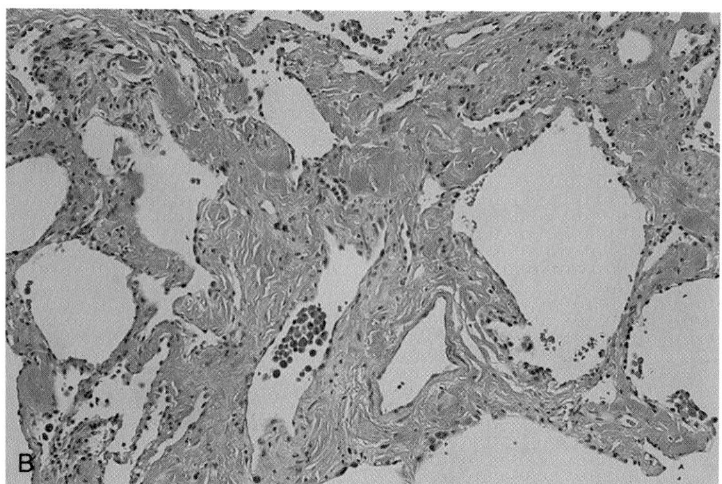

A, Usual interstitial pneumonia (UIP). Air-dried specimen shows fibrosis and end-stage architectural remodeling that has led to prominent cyst formation. **B,** Microscopically, there may be edema, hyperplasia of type II pneumocytes, and interstitial inflammation. With progression there is organization of the alveolar exudate and thickening of the interstitium due to inflammation and fibrosis (H & E stain).

FIGURE 3-42

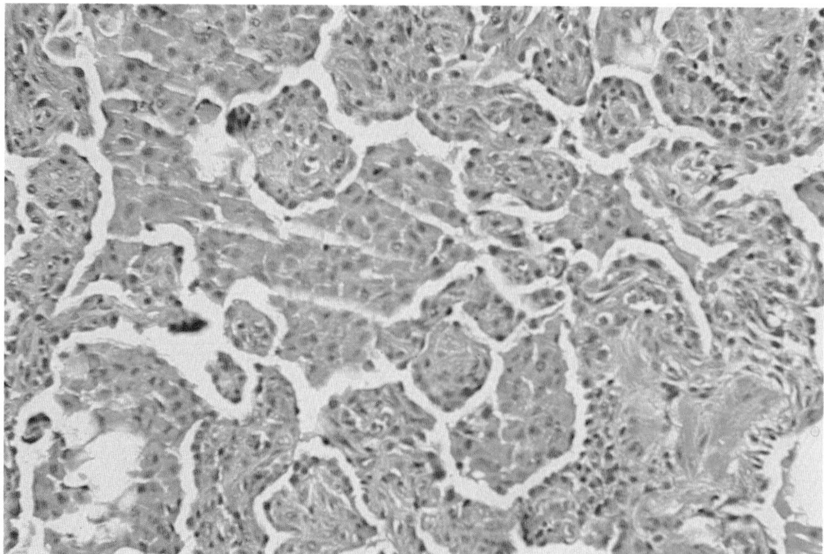

Desquamative interstitial pneumonia (DIP) has more uniform histology than UIP. Most notable is the presence of numerous intra-alveolar macrophages (H & E stain). Interstitial fibrosis is usually mild though the disease can progress to fibrosis with honeycombing.

DIFFUSE INFILTRATIVE (RESTRICTIVE) LUNG DISEASE

NONINFECTIOUS INTERSTITIAL PNEUMONIAS

FIGURE 3–43

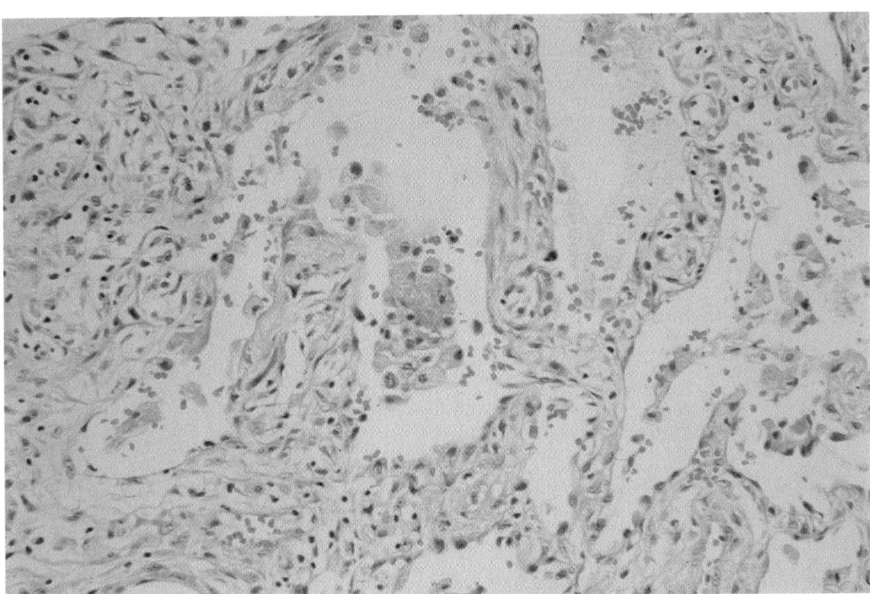

Acute interstitial pneumonia (Hamman-Rich disease). The histologic pattern is one of acute lung injury with organization (H & E stain).

DIFFUSE INFILTRATIVE (RESTRICTIVE) LUNG DISEASE

NONINFECTIOUS INTERSTITIAL PNEUMONIAS

TABLE 3-19

Contrasting Clinical and Pathologic Features of the Noninfectious Interstitial Pneumonias

	UIP	DIP/RBILD	AIP	NSIP	BOOP
CLINICAL FEATURES					
Onset	Insidious	Insidious	Acute	Insidious; occasionally subacute	Subacute
Prognosis	Poor	Fair (DIP); Good (RBILD)	Poor	Good	Good
Response to steroids	Poor	Good	Poor	Good	Good
PATHOLOGIC FEATURES					
Temporal appearance	Variegated	Uniform	Uniform	Uniform	Uniform
Interstitial inflammation	Scant	Scant	Scant	Usually prominent	Patchy
Fibroblast proliferation	Interstitial fibroblast foci prominent	No	Diffuse, interstitial	Occasional, diffuse, or rare fibroblast foci	Yes, loose, intraluminal
Honeycomb change	Yes	No	Yes	Rare	No
Intra-alveolar macrophage accumulation	Occasional, focal	Yes, diffuse (DIP) or peribronchiolar (RBILD)	No	Occasional, patchy	Yes, foamy macrophages common
Hyaline membranes	No	No	Occasional, focal	No	No
Bronchiolitis obliterans	No	No	No	Occasional, focal, rare	Yes

Key: AIP = acute interstitial pneumonia; DIP/RBILD = desquamative interstitial pneumonia/respiratory bronchiolitis interstitial lung disease; NSIP = nonspecific interstitial pneumonia; UIP = usual interstitial pneumonia; BOOP = bronchiolitis obliterans organizing pneumonia.

Source: Modified from Katzenstein A-L, Myers JL: Idiopathic pulmonary fibrosis: Clinical relevance of pathologic classification. Am J Respir Crit Care Med 157:1301–1315, 1998; Katzenstein A-L: Katzenstein and Askin's Surgical Pathology of Non-Neoplastic Lung Disease. Philadelphia, WB Saunders, 1997.

DIFFUSE INFILTRATIVE (RESTRICTIVE) LUNG DISEASE

NONINFECTIOUS INTERSTITIAL PNEUMONIAS

TABLE 3–20

Pleuropulmonary Lesions in Collagen Vascular Diseases

Pulmonary Lesions	Rheumatoid Arthritis	Juvenile Rheumatoid Arthritis	Lupus Erythematosus	Scleroderma	Dermatomyositis/ Polymyositis	Mixed Connective Tissue Disease
Pleural						
- Pleuritis, effusions	X	X	X	X	X	
Airway						
- Inflammation; lymphoid hyperplasia	X	X	X	X		
- Bronchiolitis obliterans	X					
Alveolar/ parenchymal						
- Diffuse alveolar damage	X		X	X	X	
- Hemorrhage		X	X	X		
- Chronic interstitial pneumonias (UIP, DIP, LIP, cellular interstitial pneumonia, lymphoid hyperplasia)	X	X	X	X	X	X
- Bronchiolitis obliterans organizing pneumonia	X		X	X	X	
- Eosinophilic pneumonia		X				
Vascular (hypertension, vasculitis)	X	X	X	X	X	X
Miscellaneous						
- Parenchymal nodules	X	X	X			
- Apical fibrobullous disease	X					

Key: DIP, desquamative interstitial pneumonia; LIP, lymphocytic interstitial pneumonia; UIP, usual interstitial pneumonia.

Source: Modified from Colby TV, Carrington CB: Interstitial lung disease. *In* Thurlbeck WM, Churg AM (eds): Pathology of the Lung. New York, Thieme Medical Publisher, 1995.

DIFFUSE INFILTRATIVE (RESTRICTIVE) LUNG DISEASE

NONINFECTIOUS INTERSTITIAL PNEUMONIAS

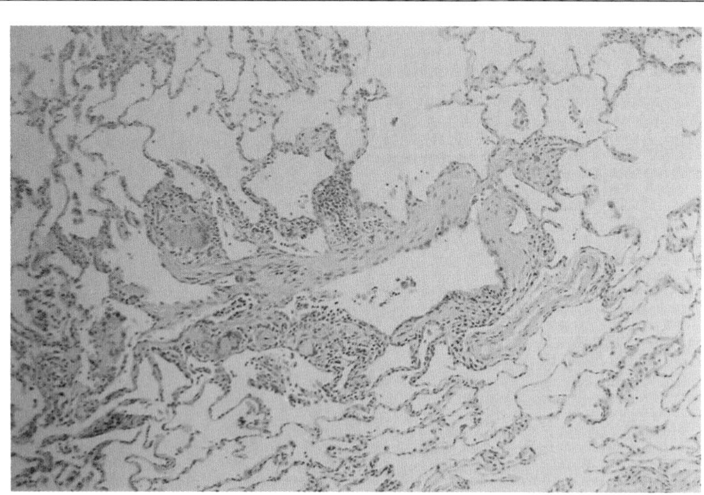

FIGURE 3-44

A wide array of antigens may cause a hypersensitivity pneumonitis (extrinsic allergic alveolitis) in the lung. Regardless of the inciting antigen, the pathologic reaction consists of a uniform, nonspecific chronic interstitial pneumonia. The majority of cases contain small, interstitial, nonnecrotizing granulomas (H & E stain).

FIGURE 3-45

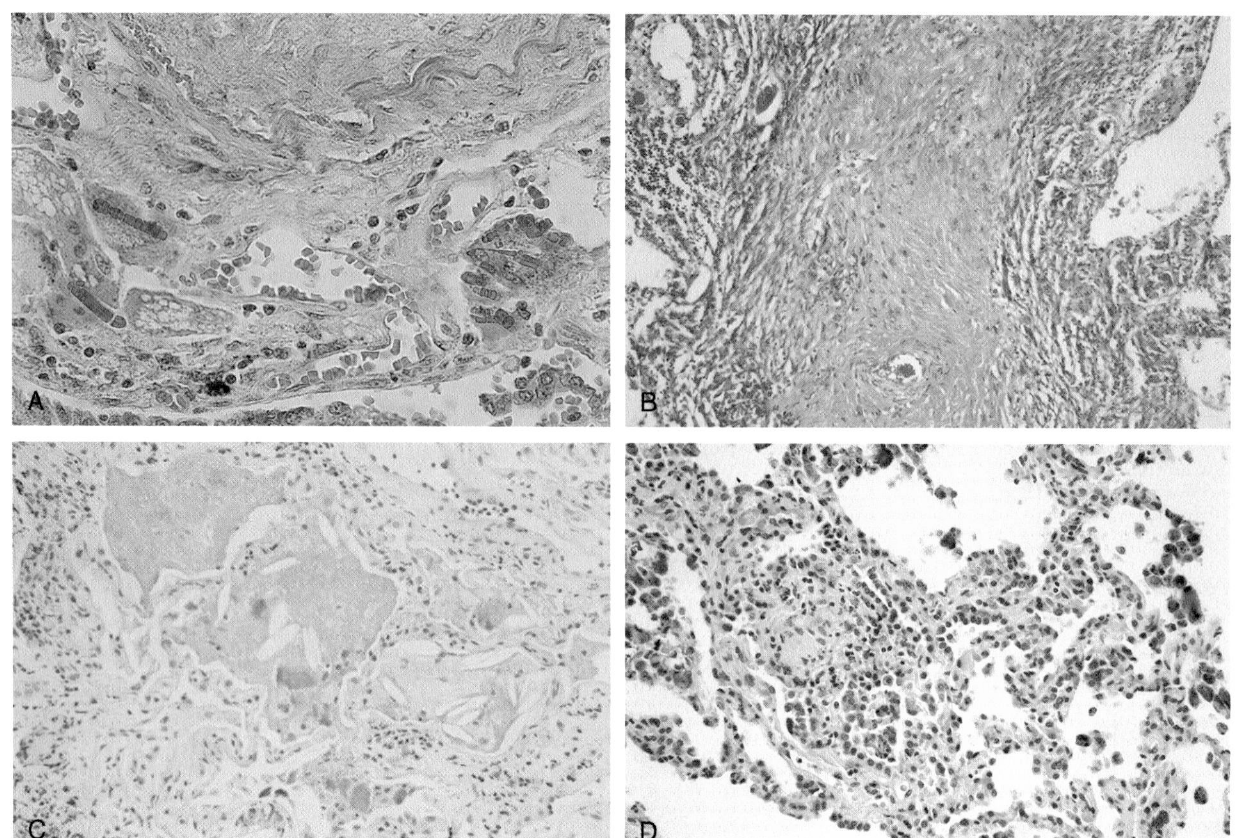

The pathology of the pneumoconiosis is quite variable; however, specific patterns of injury may allow the pathologist to identify the offending agent. **A,** Asbestosis. Diffuse fibrosis and the presence of iron encrusted particles (ferruginous bodies) are typical (H & E stain). **B,** Silicosis. Distinct nodules of laminated collagen and a histiocytic inflammatory reaction are seen in nodular silicosis (H & E stain). **C,** In acute silicosis, the injury causes alveolar proteinosis (acute silicoproteinosis) (periodic acid–Schiff stain). **D,** Berylliosis (H & E stain). The most common pattern of injury following respiratory exposure to beryllium is the development of non-necrotizing granulomas.

DIFFUSE INFILTRATIVE (RESTRICTIVE) LUNG DISEASE

NONINFECTIOUS INTERSTITIAL PNEUMONIAS

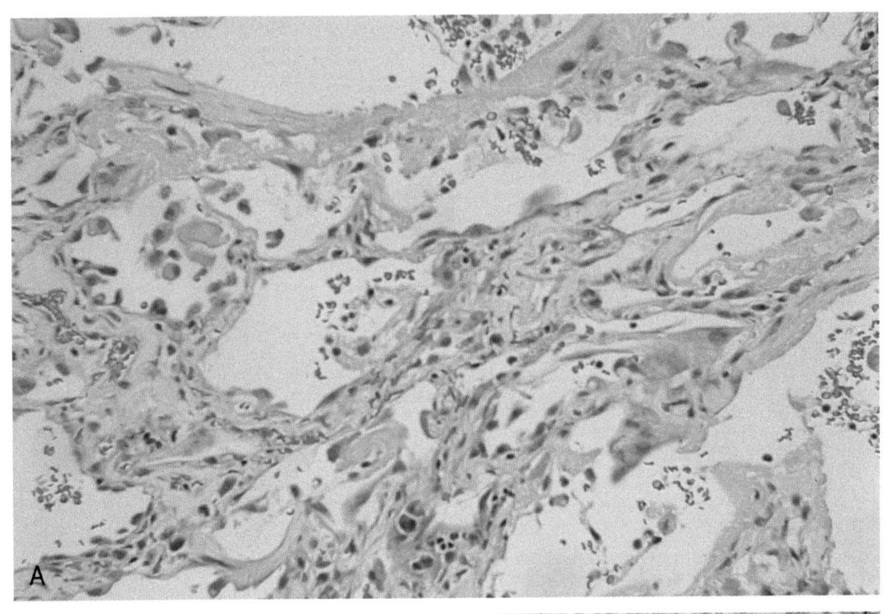

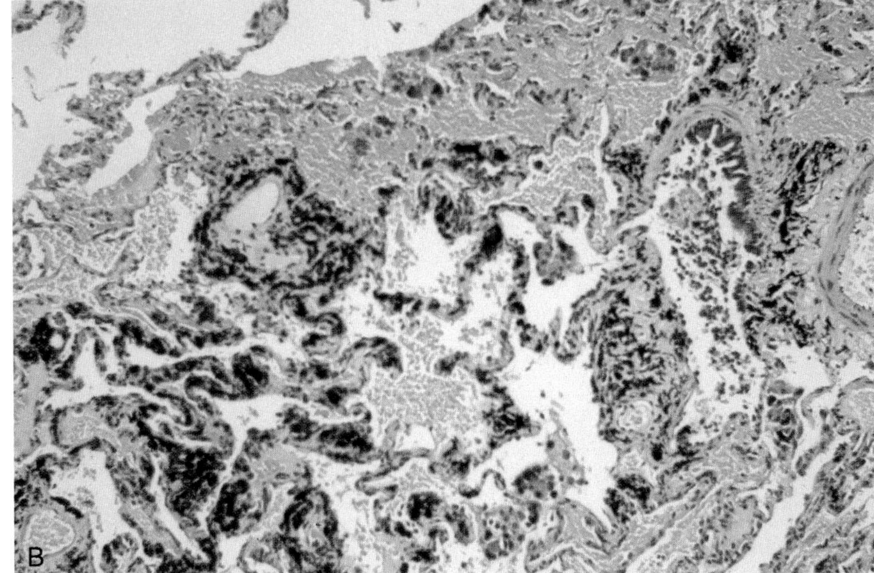

FIGURE 3–46

Many therapeutic and illicit drugs may cause injury to the lung and do so in a variety of ways. The resulting pathologic reactions include chronic interstitial pneumonia, diffuse alveolar damage, BOOP, eosinophilic pneumonia, pulmonary hemorrhage, pulmonary hypertension, pulmonary edema, pulmonary veno-occlusive disease and granulomatous inflammation. **A,** As a group, cytotoxic drugs probably are the most important drugs associated with lung toxicity. In this light microscopic photomicrograph of a patient with methotrexate pulmonary toxicity, there is diffuse alveolar damage and reactive hyperplasia of type II pneumocytes. **B,** Cocaine abuse may cause a chronic interstitial pneumonia, pulmonary edema, and medial hypertrophy of small muscular arteries or an acute reaction leading to respiratory distress from pulmonary edema, pulmonary hemorrhage, acute eosinophilic pneumonitis, or diffuse alveolar damage ("crack lung"). In this example of chronic cocaine pulmonary toxicity there is patchy interstitial pneumonitis with bronchiolar injury similar to that seen in BOOP along with medial hypertrophy of the small arteries. The alveoli contain macrophages filled with both hemosiderin and black pigment (H & E stain).

DIFFUSE INFILTRATIVE (RESTRICTIVE) LUNG DISEASE

SPECIFIC DISORDERS OF UNKNOWN ETIOLOGY

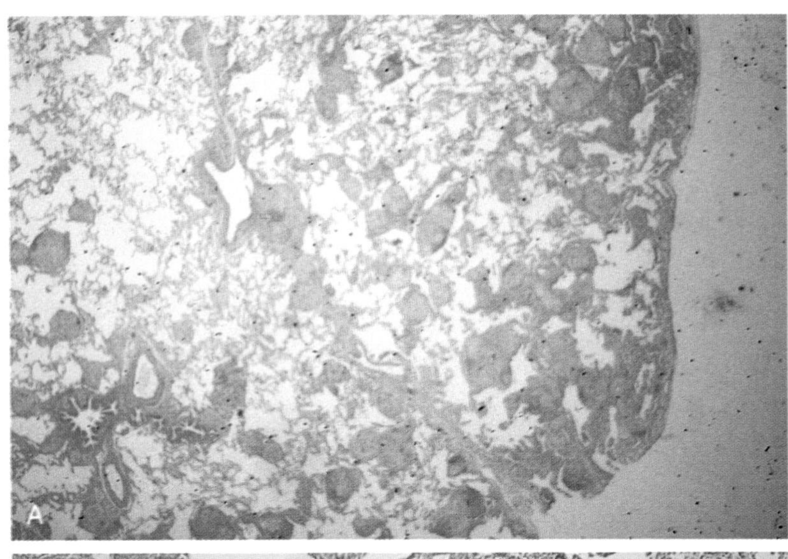

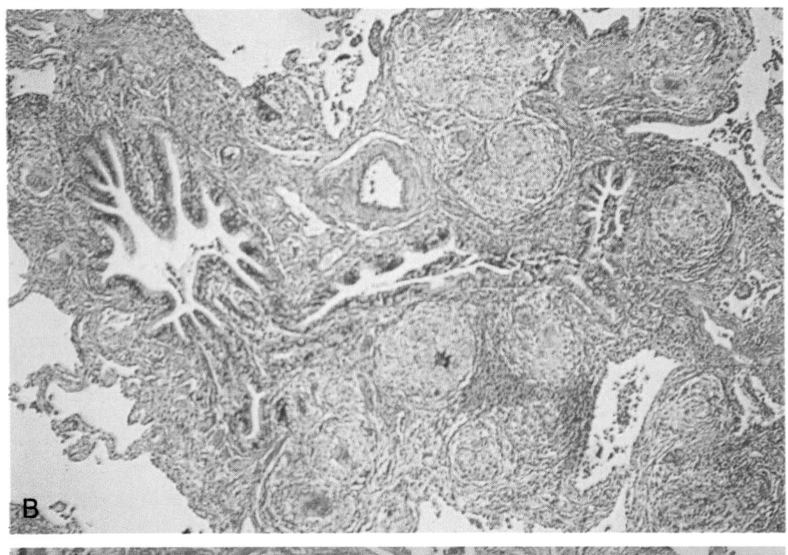

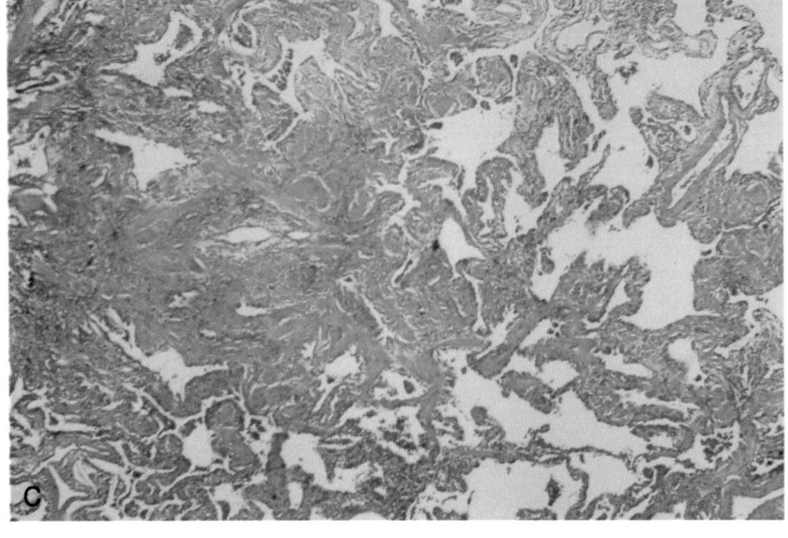

FIGURE 3-47

Sarcoidosis (H & E stains). **A,** Non-necrotizing granulomas are distributed along the lymphatic routes of the lung. **B,** Extensive sarcoidal reaction has narrowed this small airway. **C,** The disease may progress to interstitial fibrosis.

DIFFUSE INFILTRATIVE (RESTRICTIVE) LUNG DISEASE

SPECIFIC DISORDERS OF UNKNOWN ETIOLOGY

FIGURE 3-48

Eosinophilic pneumonia. The typical lesion of eosinophilic pneumonia is an extensive alveolar exudate, rich in eosinophils, creating pneumonic consolidation (H & E stain).

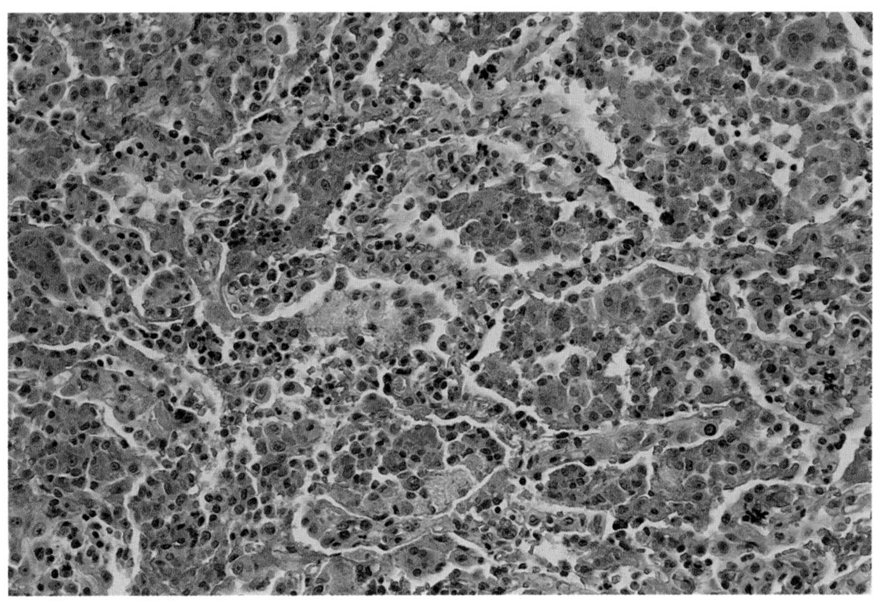

FIGURE 3-49

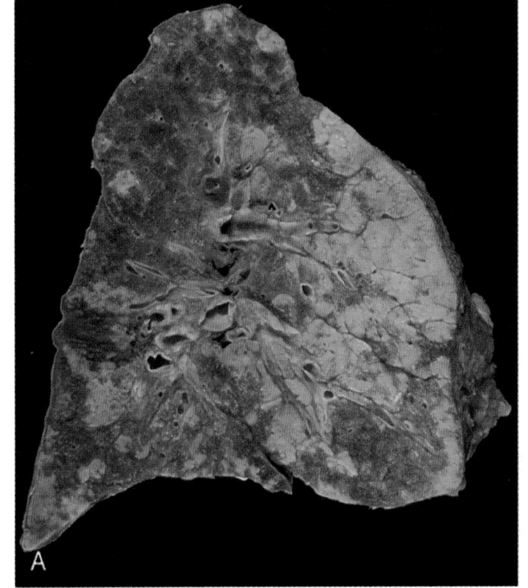

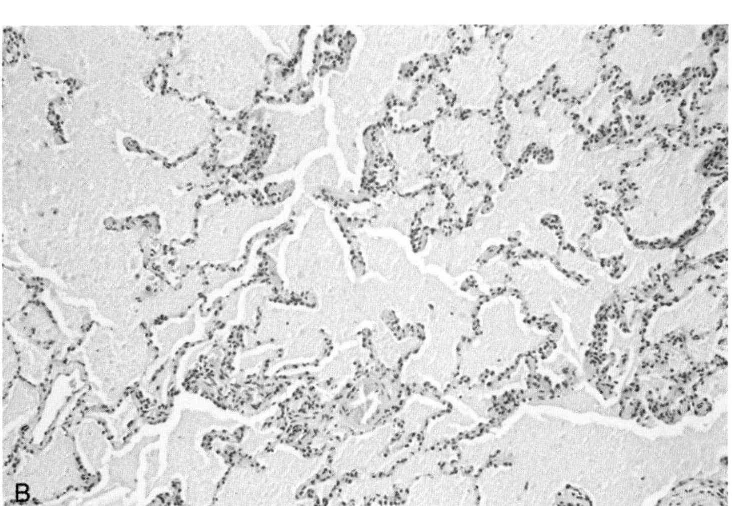

Pulmonary alveolar proteinosis. **A,** The gross pathology of a case of fatal primary pulmonary alveolar proteinosis shows firm yellow-tan areas of the lung parenchyma corresponding to where the alveoli are filled with proteinaceous fluid. **B,** Microscopy reveals the alveoli filled with granular eosinophilic material (H & E stain).

DIFFUSE INFILTRATIVE (RESTRICTIVE) LUNG DISEASE

SPECIFIC DISORDERS OF UNKNOWN ETIOLOGY

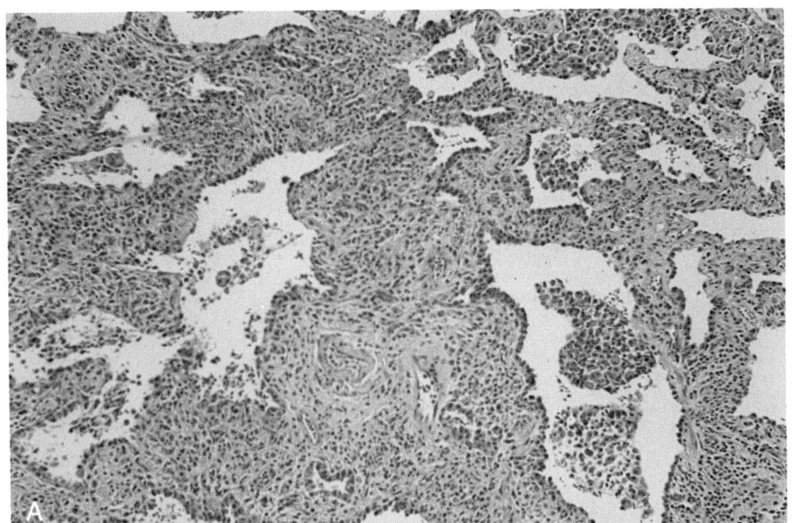

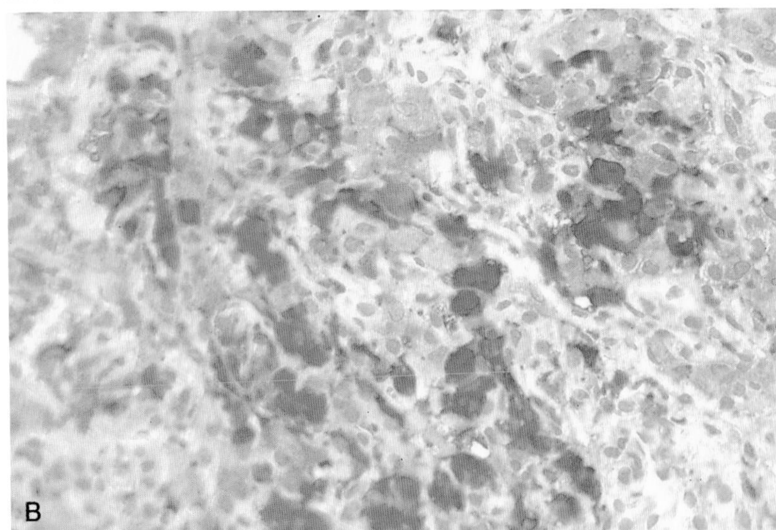

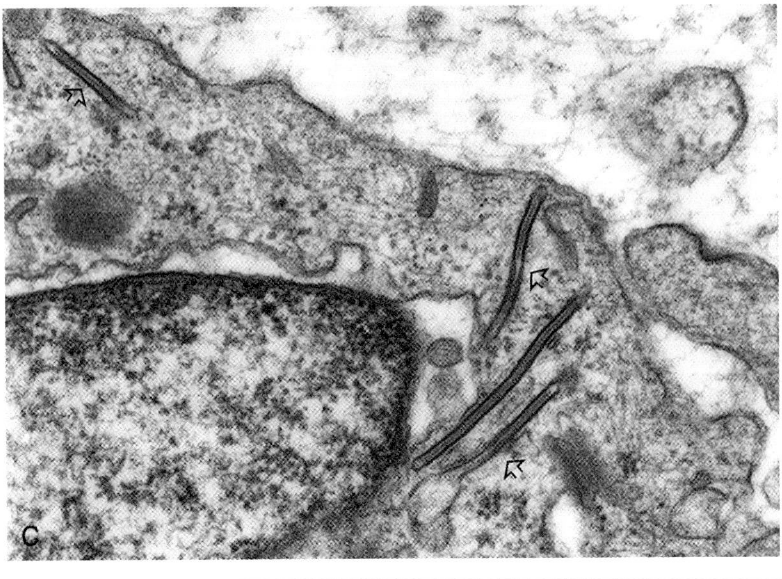

FIGURE 3-50

Histiocytosis X (eosinophilic granuloma). **A,** Light microscopy shows a stellate nodular lesion (H & E stain). **B,** Langerhans (histiocytosis X cells are identified with immunostaining for S-100 protein. **C,** Electron microscopy of a Langerhans cell from a patient with histiocytosis X shows numerous Langerhans cell granules (Birbeck granules, X bodies) within the cytoplasm of the cell. These are rod- or racquet-shaped cytoplasmic inclusions (*arrows*) that have a pentilaminar structure (×55,000). (Courtesy of Robert Munn, University of California, Davis.)

DIFFUSE INFILTRATIVE (RESTRICTIVE) LUNG DISEASE

SPECIFIC DISORDERS OF UNKNOWN ETIOLOGY

FIGURE 3-51

Lymphangio(leio)myomatosis. This rare disorder results in irregular proliferation of smooth muscle within the lung interstitium, creating thickened alveolar walls and cysts.

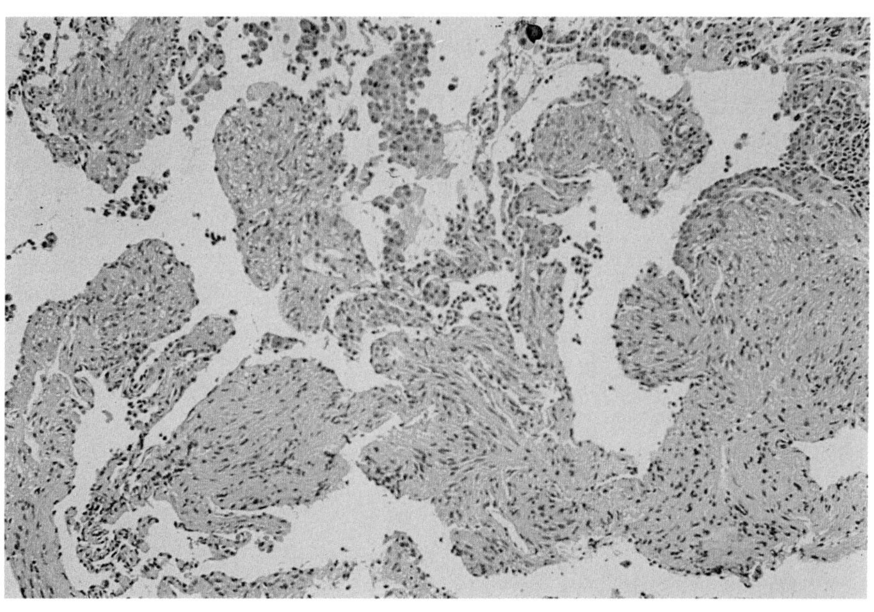

Diffuse pulmonary hemorrhage syndrome has many etiologies. In the immunocompromised, it may occur secondary to infection, malignancy, or hematologic alterations, most commonly thrombocytopenia. In the patient without obvious compromised immunity, the syndrome is frequently due to autoimmune disease, collagen vascular disease, or angiitis/granulomatosis, or may be idiopathic. Differentiating features of the most important diseases associated with diffuse pulmonary hemorrhage syndrome are listed in TABLE 3-21.

TABLE 3-21

Features of Diffuse Pulmonary Hemorrhage Syndrome Diseases

Disease	Necrotizing Capillaritis	Immunofluorescence	Immune Deposits (EM)	Helpful Laboratory Findings	Extrapulmonary Involvement
Goodpasture's syndrome	Occasional	Linear, epithelial basement membrane	No	Anti-GBM	Kidneys
Idiopathic pulmonary hemosiderosis	No	No	No	None	No
Systemic lupus erythematosus	Yes	Granular, endothelial basement membrane	Yes	ANA	Kidneys often Other organs sometimes
Wegener's granulomatosis	Yes	No	No	c-ANCA(60–90%)	Kidneys often Other organs often

Key: c-ANCA = antineutrophil cytoplasmic antibodies with cytoplasmic fluorescence; ANA = antinuclear antibodies; Anti-GBM = anti glomerular basement membrane antibodies; EM = electron microscopy.

Source: Modified from Katzenstein A-L: Katzenstein and Askin's Surgical Pathology of Non-Neoplastic Lung Disease. Philadelphia, WB Saunders, 1997.

DIFFUSE INFILTRATIVE (RESTRICTIVE) LUNG DISEASE

SPECIFIC DISORDERS OF UNKNOWN ETIOLOGY

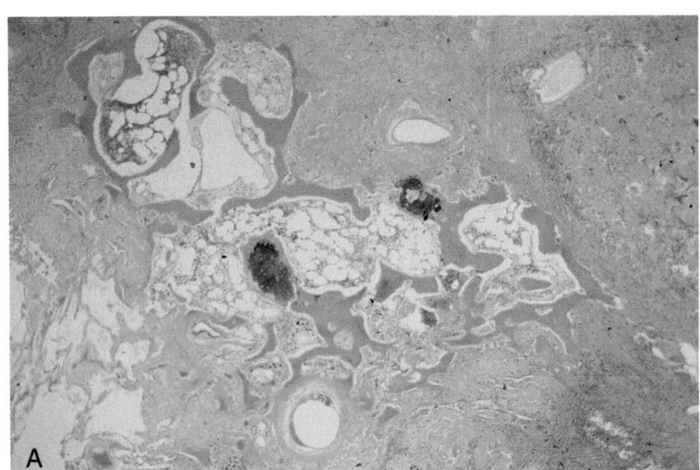

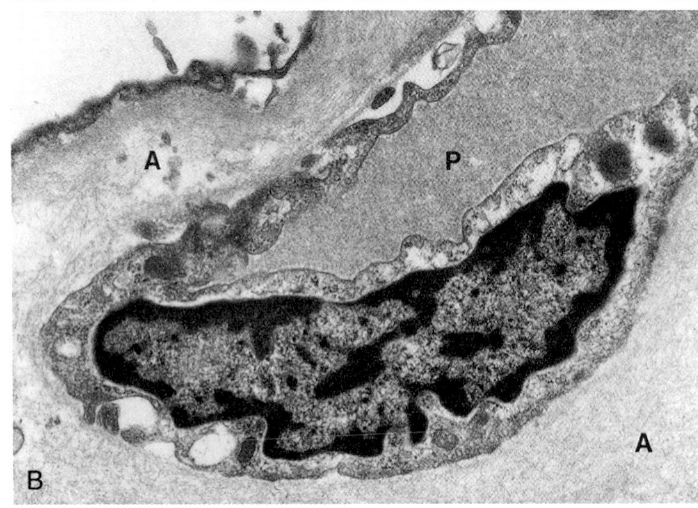

FIGURE 3-52

Pulmonary amyloid. Amyloidosis may take several forms in the lung: diffuse alveolar-septal amyloidosis, nodular amyloidosis, and tracheobronchial amyloidosis. **A,** Nodular amyloidosis with associated metaplastic bone formation (H & E stain). **B,** Electron microscopy of diffuse alveolar-septal amyloidosis showing fine nonbranching fibrils, 7.5 to 10 nm wide (A), characteristic of amyloid within an alveolar wall and surrounding a capillary lumen containing plasma (P). (Courtesy of Robert Munn, University of California, Davis.)

FIGURE 3-53

Recipients of bone marrow transplants are vulnerable to pulmonary infections, interstitial pneumonia, alveolar hemorrhage, and in about 10 percent of long-term survivors, constrictive bronchiolitis obliterans, which is probably related to graft-versus-host disease. The lesions in affected airways show epithelial ulceration, fibrosis, and peribronchiolar chronic inflammation (H & E stain).

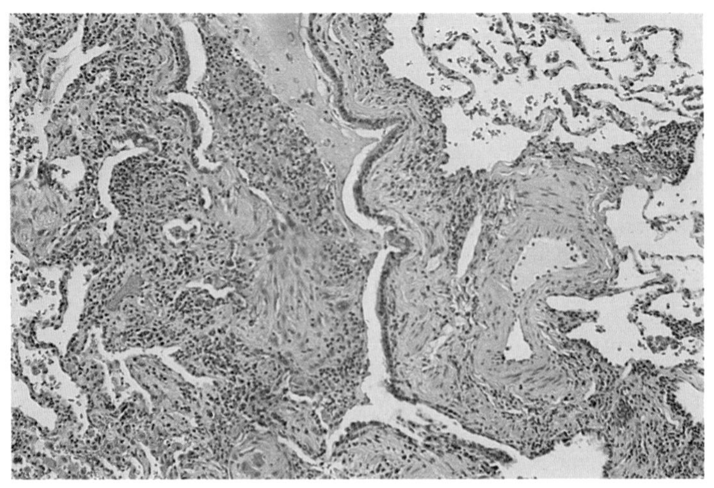

TABLE 3–22

Histologic Grading of Lung Transplant Rejection

Rejection Grade	Pathologic Features
A. Acute rejection	
0—none	
1—minimal	Rare perivascular inflammatory cell infiltrates
2—mild	Larger perivascular inflammatory cell infiltrates with subendothelial infiltration and endothelialitis
3—moderate	Perivascular inflammatory cell infiltrates extending into adjacent alveolar septa and airspaces; endothelialitis
4—severe	Grade 3 changes plus diffuse alveolar damage
B. Airway inflammation	Absence or severity of lymphocytic bronchitis/bronchiolitis graded
0—none	
1—minimal	Rare scattered mononuclear cells within submucosa of bronchi or bronchioles
2—mild	A circumferential band of mononuclear cells and occasional eosinophils within the submucosa of bronchi and/or bronchioles, unassociated with epithelial cell necrosis or significant transepidermal migration of lymphocytes
3—moderate	Dense band-like infiltrate of mononuclear cells in submucosa of bronchi and/or bronchioles accompanied by satellitosis of lymphocytes and marked lymphocyte transmigration through epithelium
4—severe	Dense band-like infiltrate of activated mononuclear cells in bronchi and/or bronchioles, associated with dissociation of epithelium from basement membrane, epithelial ulceration, fibrinopurulent exudates containing neutrophils, and epithelial necrosis
C. Chronic airway rejection	Constrictive obliterative bronchiolitis
D. Chronic vascular rejection	Fibrointimal thickening of arteries and veins

* Presence of combined large and small airway inflammation should be noted and recognized as a possible harbinger of bronchiolitis obliterans. Airway inflammation can be divided into five grades or simply designated as present or absent at the discretion of each institution.

Source: From Lung Rejection Study Group: Revision of the 1990 working formulation for the classification of pulmonary allograft rejection. J Heart Lung Transplant 1996; 15:1–15

DIFFUSE INFILTRATIVE (RESTRICTIVE) LUNG DISEASE

SPECIFIC DISORDERS OF UNKNOWN ETIOLOGY

FIGURE 3-54

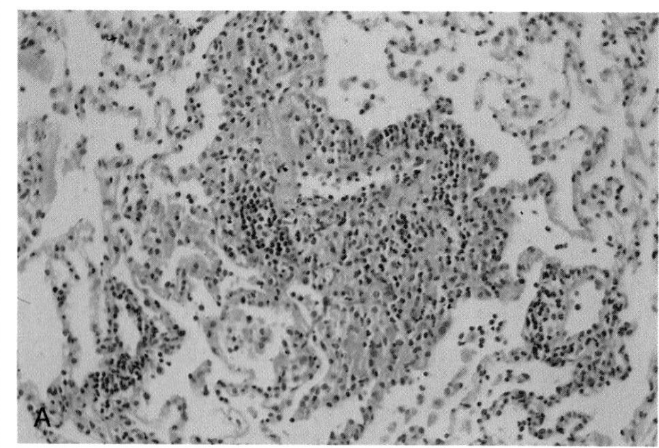

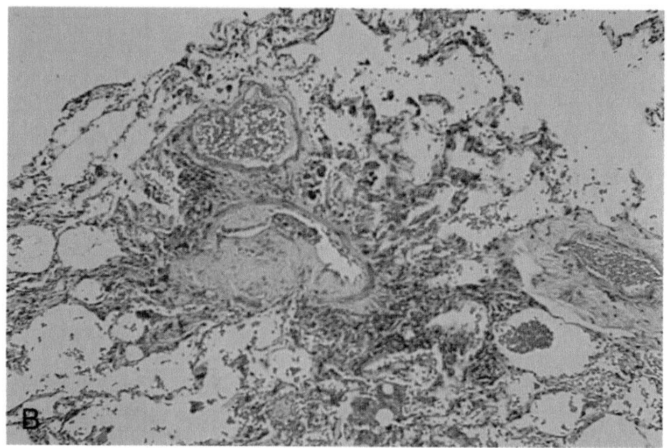

Pathology of lung transplant rejection (H & E stains). **A,** Mild and moderate (shown here) acute lung transplant rejection consists of perivascular, lymphocytic inflammation. **B,** Constrictive obliterative bronchiolitis in a lung transplant recipient (chronic lung transplant rejection).

FIGURE 3-55

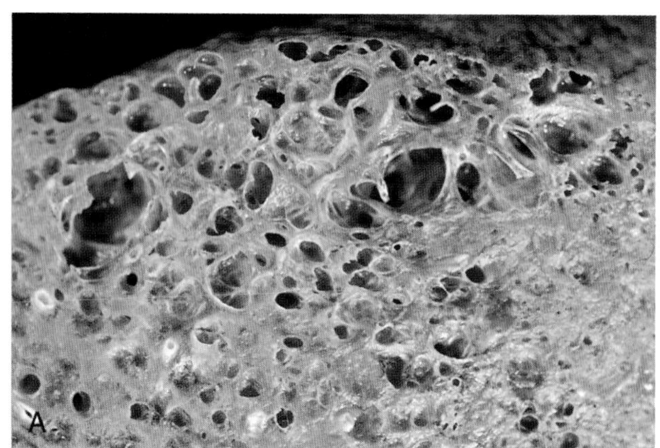

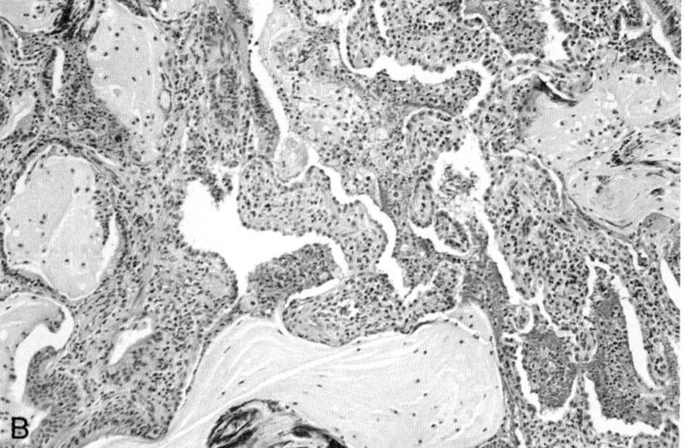

End-stage diffuse infiltrative lung disease (honeycomb lung). As diffuse infiltrative lung disease progresses, there is extensive scarring and remodeling of the lung parenchyma. At this stage, it may be difficult or impossible to make a diagnosis of the underlying disease on pathologic grounds alone. **A,** Gross pathology—the lung is composed of multiple small cysts resembling honeycombs. The lung tissue is firm and the pleural surface is irregular and nodular. **B,** Microscopic pathology (H & E stain)—there is extensive interstitial fibrosis and scarring with remodeling of airspaces. Some of these spaces may be filled with accumulations of mucoid secretions. The thickened interstitium may contain lymphoid aggregates. Pulmonary arteries tend to have hyperplastic intima.

DISEASES OF PULMONARY VESSELS

See Chapter 8, *Pulmonary Function Testing.*

PULMONARY THROMBOEMBOLI

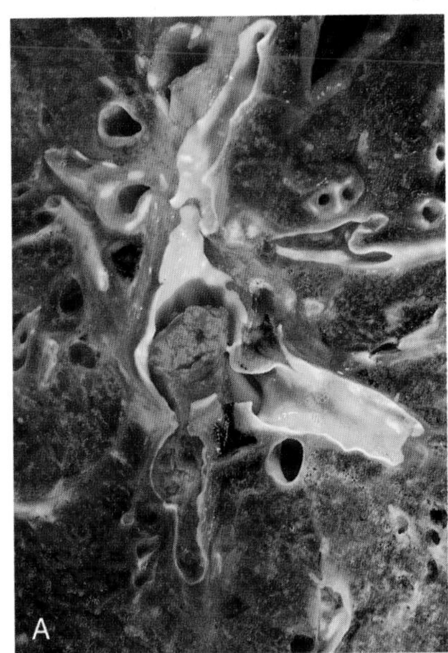

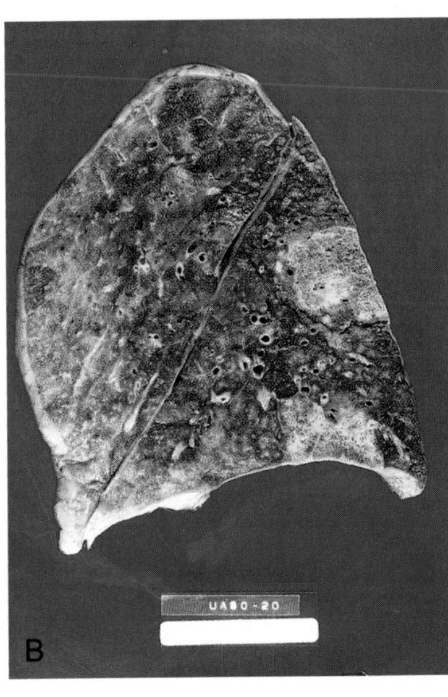

FIGURE 3–56

Pulmonary thromboembolism remains a common cause of death in hospitalized patients though only about one third are diagnosed premortem. **A,** A large fatal pulmonary thromboembolus can be seen obstructing the main pulmonary artery. **B,** Recent infarcts are wedge-shaped lesions extending to the visceral pleura. The pale yellow-tan appearance indicates that these infarcts are a few days old. (See Chapter 5, Nuclear Medicine Techniques and Applications.)

PULMONARY HYPERTENSION

The histopathologic lesions of pulmonary hypertension are not particularly specific. The grading scheme of Heath and Edwards[3] has been used to classify the pathologic changes present in the pulmonary vasculature accompanying pulmonary hypertension. Grade I and II changes are usually reversible; however, Grade III and VI changes accompany severe hypertension and are not usually reversible. TABLE 3–24 lists the six grades for pulmonary hypertension.

TABLE 3–23

Classification of Pulmonary Hypertension

Site	Causes
Precapillary	• Congenital heart disease • Chronic pulmonary embolism • Primary (idiopathic) pulmonary hypertension
Capillary	• Alveolar destruction (e.g., from emphysema or fibrosis)
Postcapillary	• Pulmonary veno-occlusive disease • Pulmonary capillary hemangiomatosis

TABLE 3–24

Grading of Pulmonary Hypertension

Heath-Edwards Grade	Pathologic Findings
Grade I	Muscular extension into arterioles
Grade II	Medial hypertrophy with intimal cellular proliferation
Grade III	Progressive intimal fibrosis and occlusion
Grade IV	Plexiform lesions and dilation of arteries
Grade V	Chronic dilatation lesions with veinlike arteries
Grade VI	Arterial necrosis and arteritis

DISEASES OF PULMONARY VESSELS

PULMONARY HYPERTENSION

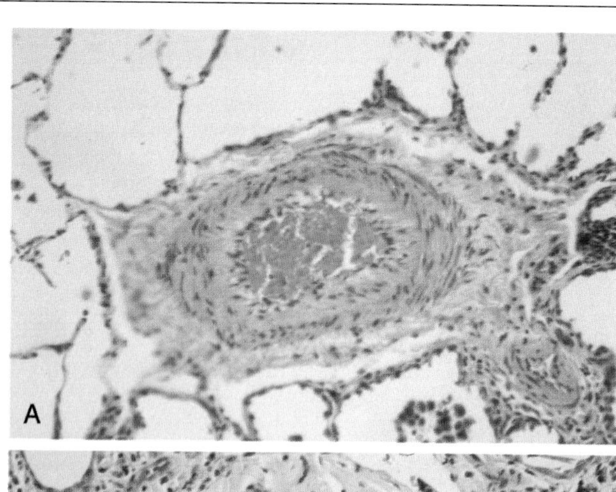

FIGURE 3–57

Examples of vascular histopathologic changes due to pulmonary hypertension (H & E stains). **A,** Muscularized pulmonary arteriole. **B,** Muscularized pulmonary arteriole with concentric laminar intimal fibrosis. **C,** Plexiform lesion.

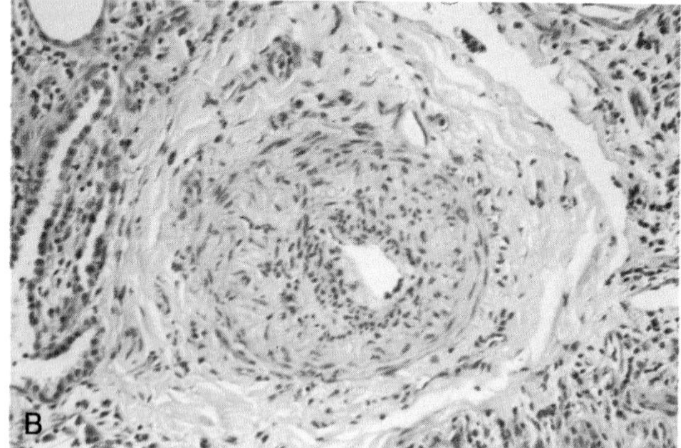

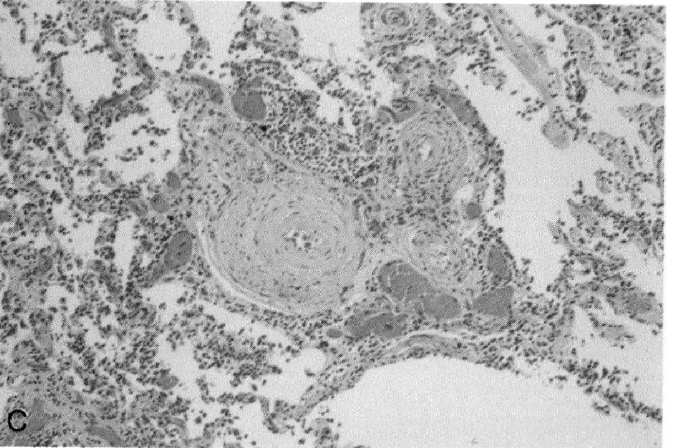

FIGURE 3–58

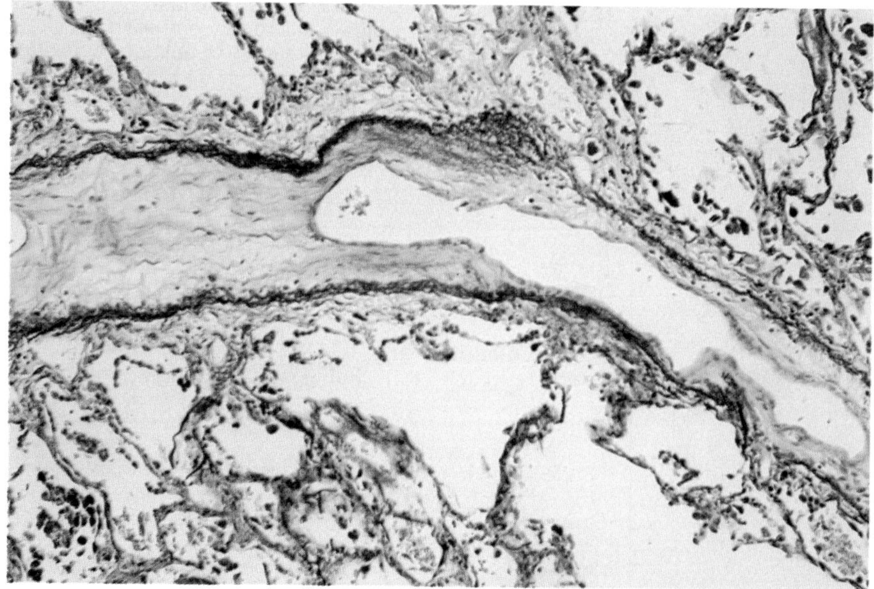

Pulmonary veno-occlusive disease is a rare cause of pulmonary hypertension. The primary lesion is obliteration of small pulmonary veins (elastic van Giesen stain).

DISEASES OF PULMONARY VESSELS

PULMONARY ANGIITIS AND GRANULOMATOSIS

The category of pulmonary angiitis and granulomatosis includes a number of diseases characterized by a variable combination of inflammation of blood vessels and destruction of pulmonary parenchyma often associated with a granulomatous inflammatory pattern. Some contrasting clinical and pathologic features are listed in TABLE 3-25.

TABLE 3-25

Features of Pulmonary Angiitis and Granulomatosis

Feature	WG	AAG	NSG	BCG	LYG
Extrapulmonary involvement	Yes	Rare	No	No	Occasional
Laboratory findings					
- Eosinophilia	No	Yes	No	Frequent	No
- ANCA	Yes (c-ANCA 60–90%)	Sometimes (p-ANCA)	No	No	No
Asthma	No	Yes	No	Frequent	No
Pathologic features					
- Nature of infiltrate	Inflammatory	Inflammatory	Inflammatory	Inflammatory	Lymphoproliferative
- Composition of infiltrate					
Necrotizing granulomas	Yes	Yes	Yes	Yes	No
Nonnecrotizing granulomas	No	No	Yes	Occasional	No
Multinucleated giant cells	Yes	Occasional	Occasional	Occasional	No
Neutrophils	Yes	Occasional	No	Frequent	No
Eosinophils	Not usually	Yes	No	Frequent	No
Atypical lymphoid cells	No	No	No	No	Yes
- Necrotizing vasculitis	Yes	Yes	Occasional	No	No

Key: AAG = allergic angiitis and granulomatosis; ANCA = antineutrophil cytoplasmic antibodies; c-ANCA = c(cytoplasmic staining pattern)-ANCA; p-ANCA = p(perinuclear staining pattern)-ANCA; BCG = bronchocentric granulomatosis; LYG = lymphomatoid granulomatosis; NSG = necrotizing sarcoid granulomatosis; WG = Wegener's granulomatosis.

DISEASES OF PULMONARY VESSELS

PULMONARY ANGIITIS AND GRANULOMATOSIS

FIGURE 3-59

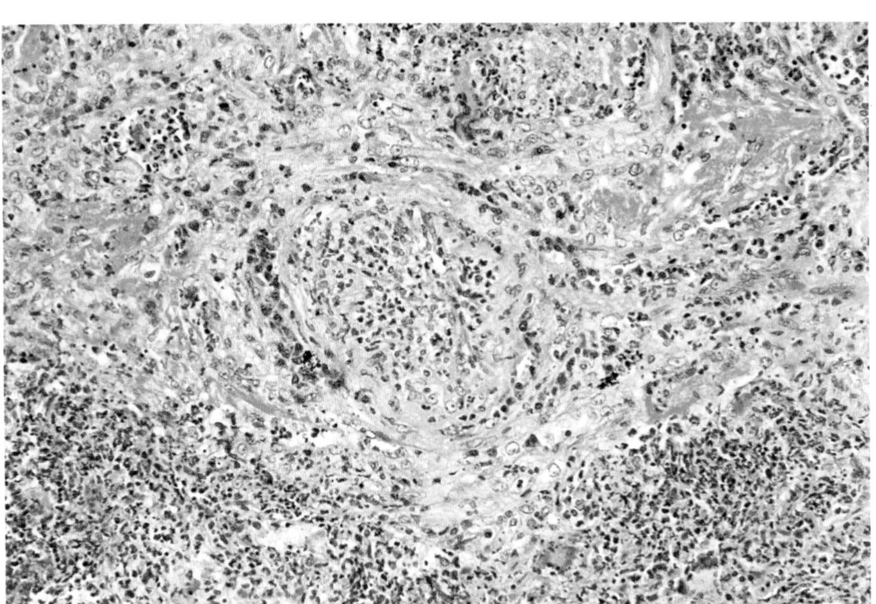

Wegener's granulomatosis. Necrotizing vasculitis is present (H & E stain).

FIGURE 3-60

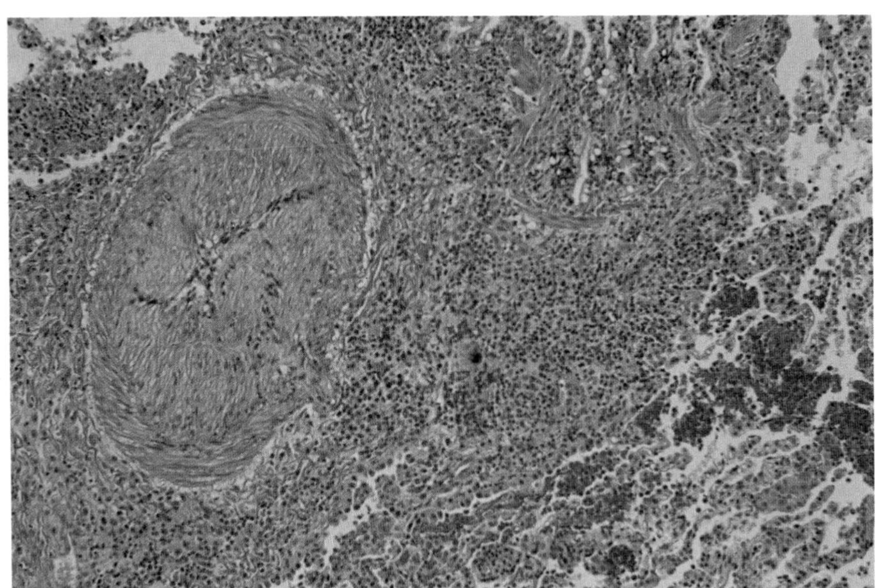

Allergic angiitis and granulomatosis (Churg-Strauss disease). A focus of eosinophilic pneumonia surrounds a small pulmonary artery obliterated by an eosinophilic vasculitis.

NEOPLASIA OF THE LUNG

BRONCHOGENIC CARCINOMA

Cancer of the epithelial cells of the lung is usually referred to as "bronchogenic carcinoma" despite the fact that not all lung carcinomas arise in the bronchi. Over 90% of tumors of the lung are included in this group, and they are all malignant. The remaining lung tumors consist of a variety of benign and malignant tumors arising from both epithelial and mesenchymal tissues. Lung tumors exert clinical effects locally through obstruction or invasion and distantly due to metastasis or paraneoplastic syndromes. The four major histopathologic types of lung cancer are listed in TABLE 3–26. In recent surveys, adenocarcinoma is increasing in frequency and squamous cell carcinoma is decreasing. (See Chapter 4, Radiography and Imaging, and Chapter 5, Nuclear Medicine Techniques and Applications.)

TABLE 3–26

Characteristics of the Four Histopathologic Types of Lung Cancer

Type	Frequency (%)	Gross Features	Microscopic Features
Squamous cell carcinoma	25–40	Gray, yellow, white masses, predominantly central (90% in segmental or larger bronchi), may cavitate	Stratification of cells when well differentiated, keratinization, intercellular bridges; tonofilaments and desmosomes by EM
Adenocarcinoma	25–40	Gray or white mass, peripheral, rarely cavitates but may become necrotic	Gland formation in well-differentiated carcinomas, demonstrable mucin by histochemistry; junctional complexes with tight junctions, microvilli, intracellular lumina and secretory vesicles by EM
Neuroendocrine carcinoma (small cell type)	10–15	Gray to white masses, generally arising centrally	Small cells about 1.5–2 times the diameter of a lymphocyte; easily crushed during microscopic processing causing diagnostically useful artifact; positive for neuroendocrine markers by IHC; membrane-bound dense-core neurosecretory granules by EM
Large cell carcinoma	20–25	Soft, gray or tan, frequently necrotic, 50% central, 50% peripheral	Lacks differentiated features

Key: EM = electron microscopy; IHC = immunocytochemistry.

NEOPLASIA OF THE LUNG

BRONCHOGENIC CARCINOMA

FIGURE 3–61

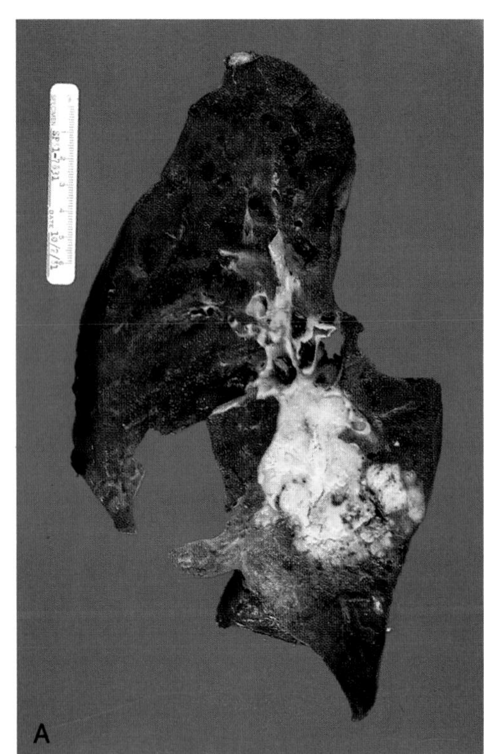

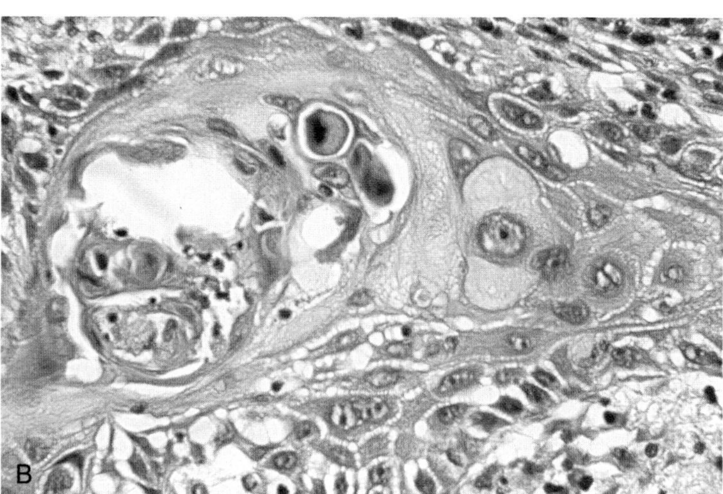

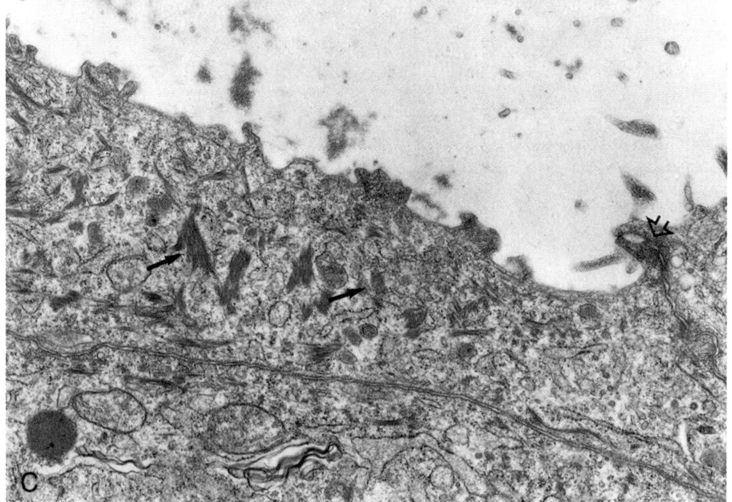

Squamous cell carcinoma. **A,** A large tumor extends from the right lower lobe bronchus to the visceral pleural surface of the lower lobe. **B,** Light microscopic photomicrograph showing a well-differentiated squamous cell carcinoma demonstrating keratin pearls. Intercellular bridges can be seen between the tumor cells (H & E stain). **C,** Electron microscopy shows abundant intracellular keratin filaments (*arrows*) and a junctional complex (*open arrow*) (×20,000). (Courtesy of Robert Munn, University of California, Davis.)

NEOPLASIA OF THE LUNG

BRONCHOGENIC CARCINOMA

FIGURE 3–62

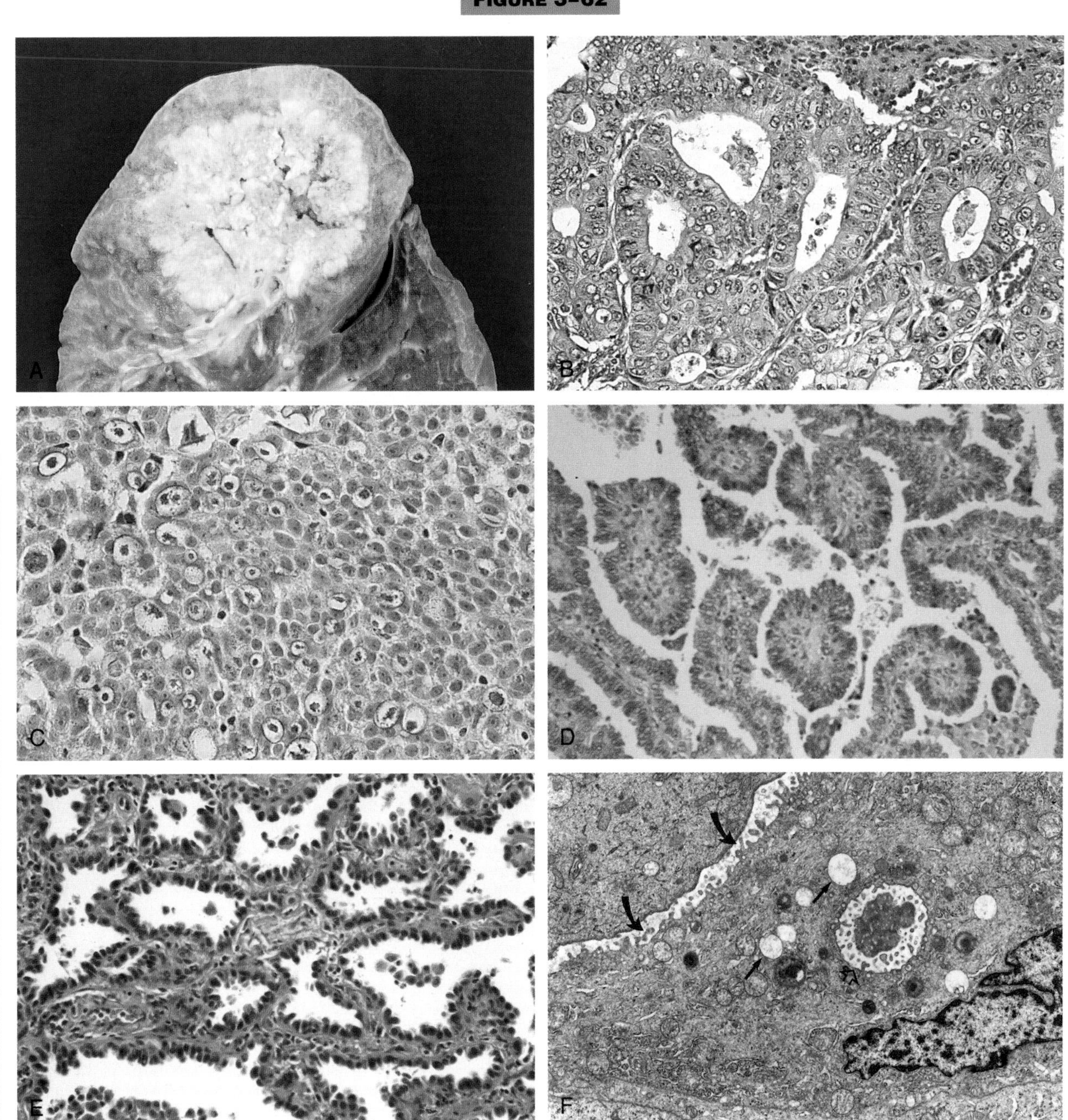

Adenocarcinoma. **A,** A large bulky tumor of the upper lobe is evident. **B,** Well-differentiated adenocarcinomas are recognized by the formation of glandular structures (H & E stain). **C,** Poorly differentiated, solid adenocarcinomas can be recognized by histochemical stains for mucin (mucicarmine stain). **D,** A papillary variant contains a predominance of papillary structures. **E,** Bronchioloalveolar carcinomas consist of tall columnar cells that grow along the alveolar septae (H & E stain). **F,** Electron microscopy of adenocarcinomas demonstrates short microvilli (*curved arrows*) and intracellular lumen (*open arrow*) and secretory granules (*small arrows*) (×9200). (Courtesy of Robert Munn, University of California, Davis.)

NEOPLASIA OF THE LUNG

BRONCHOGENIC CARCINOMA

FIGURE 3-63

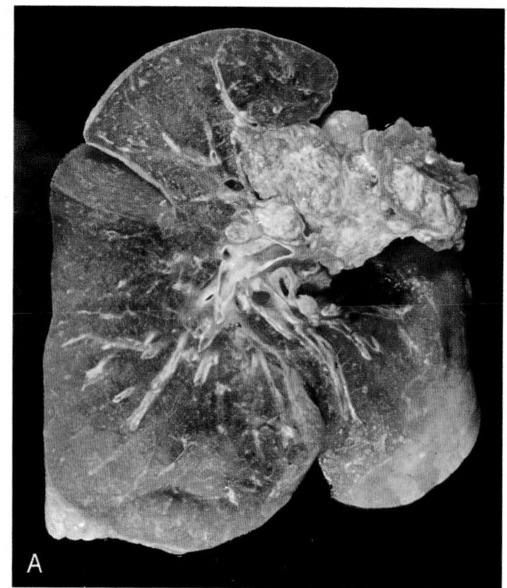

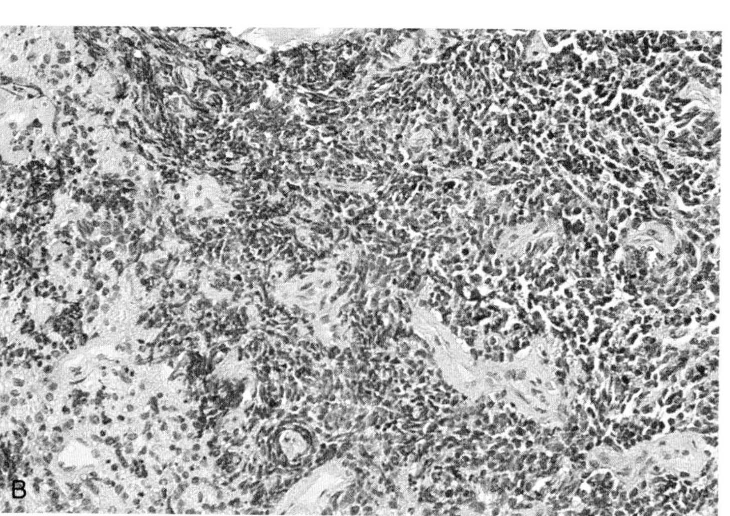

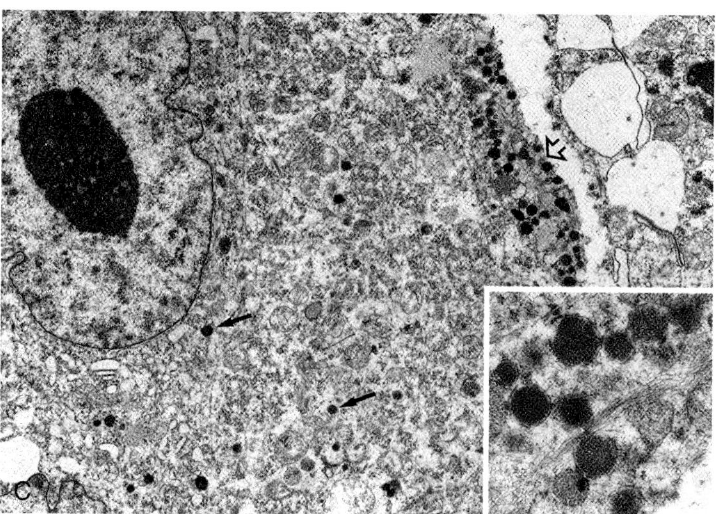

Small cell neuroendocrine carcinoma. **A,** A large gray and white tumor arising near the hilum infiltrates into the upper lobe and adjacent hilar structures. **B,** Classical small oat cell carcinomas are very cellular. The cells are small and have little cytoplasm. The cells often show a crush artifact (H & E stain). **C,** Electron microscopy shows a tumor cell containing a cluster of neurosecretory granules (*open arrow*) and scattered individual granules (×8250). *Inset,* High magnification demonstrates the double membrane of the neurosecretory granules or vesicles (×33,000). The granules typically range from 100 to 300 nm. (Courtesy of Robert Munn, University of California, Davis.)

NEOPLASIA OF THE LUNG

BRONCHOGENIC CARCINOMA

FIGURE 3–64

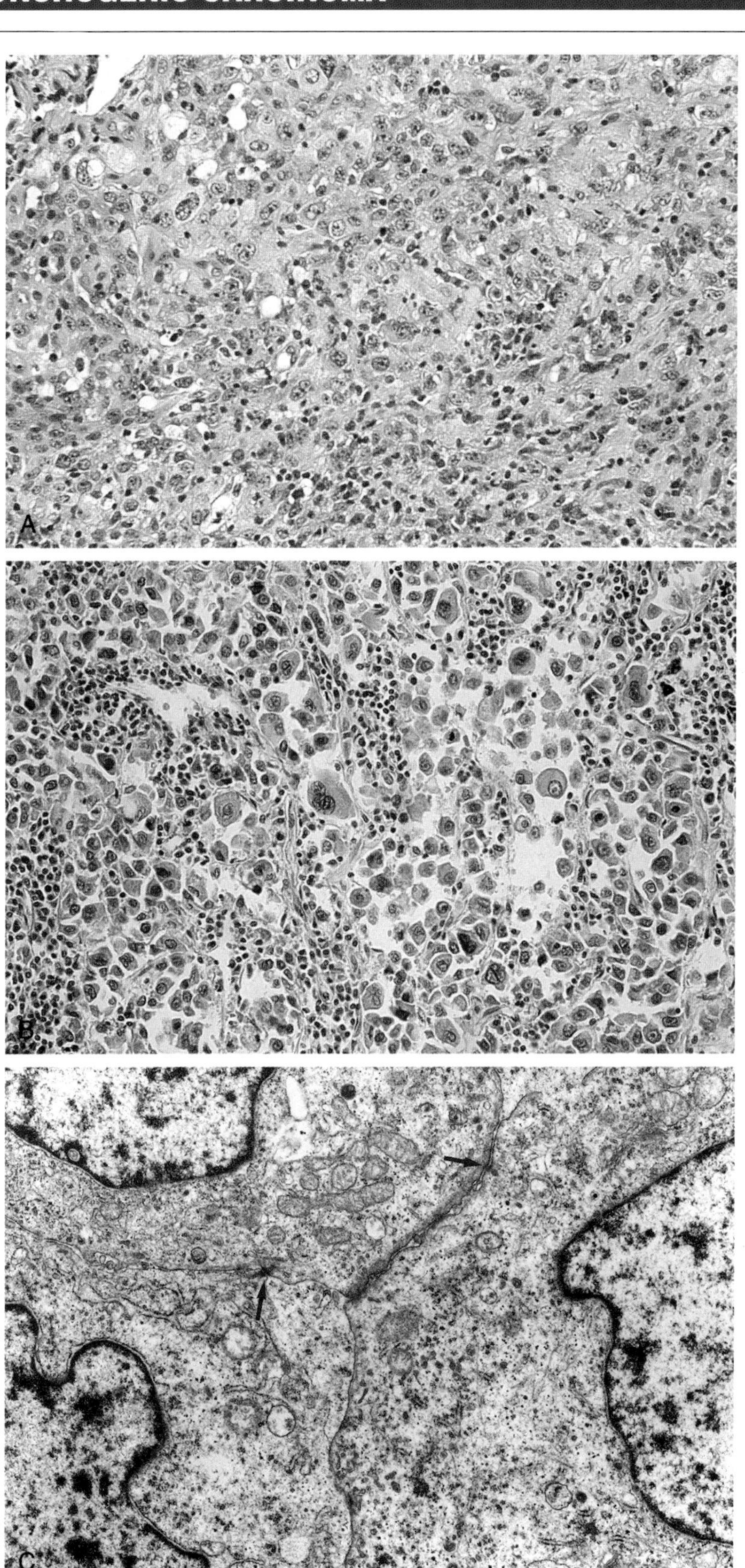

Large cell carcinoma. **A,** The light microscopic findings of large cell carcinoma show rudimentary epithelial features but no glandular or squamous cell differentiation (H & E stain). **B,** Giant cell carcinoma variant is composed of highly pleomorphic, and often multinucleated, tumor giant cells (H & E stain). **C,** Ultrastructure of large cell carcinomas show only features of undifferentiated epithelial cells such as desmosomes (*arrows*) (×15,400). (Courtesy of Robert Munn, University of California, Davis.)

NEOPLASIA OF THE LUNG

OTHER LUNG NEOPLASMS

FIGURE 3-65

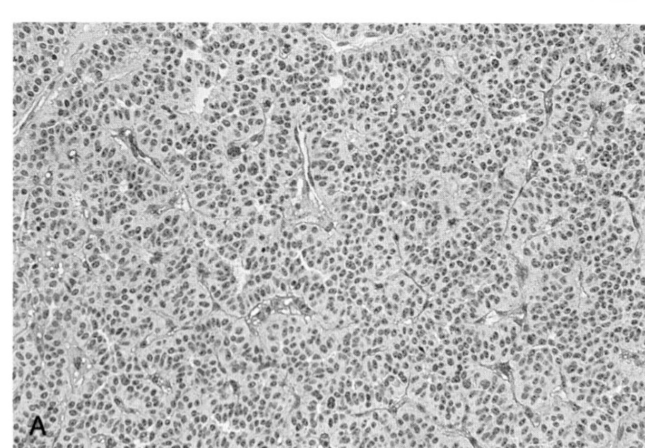

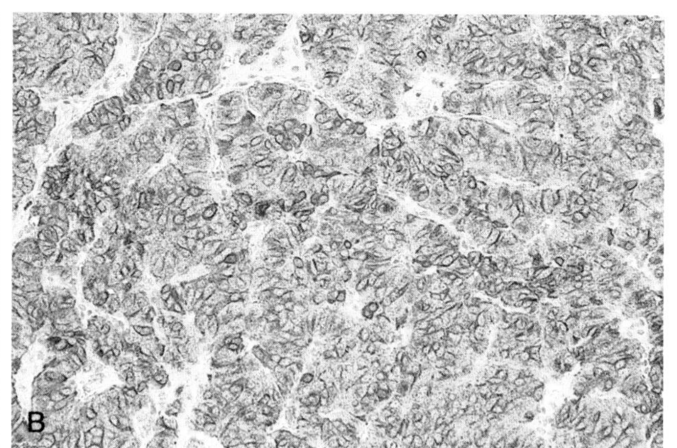

Carcinoid tumors (neuroendocrine carcinoma). These tumors make up about 5% of all lung neoplasms. They arise in bronchial mucosa from neuroendocrine argentiffin cells (Kulchitsky cells). They contain dense-core neurosecretory granules in their cytoplasm and may secrete hormonally active polypeptides. They may be locally aggressive and are capable of undergoing metastasis. Carcinoid tumors are related to small cell carcinomas, and both fall into the "neuroendocrine carcinoma" group. **A,** Microscopically, carcinoid tumors are arranged in a trabecular type pattern though variants may show spindle-shaped cells (H & E stain). **B,** Immunoperoxidase staining for chromagranin A is positive indicating neuroendocrine differentiation.

FIGURE 3-66

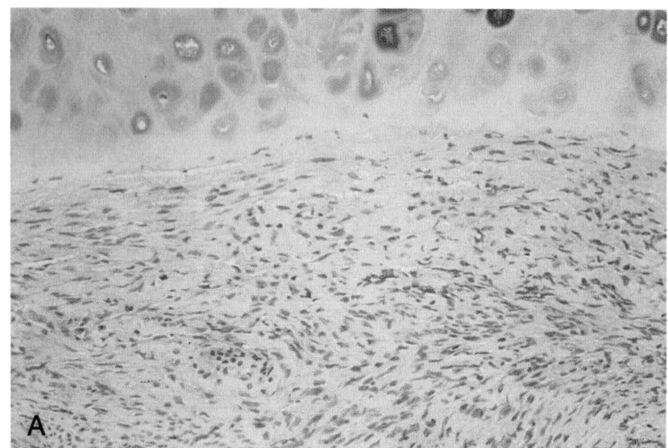

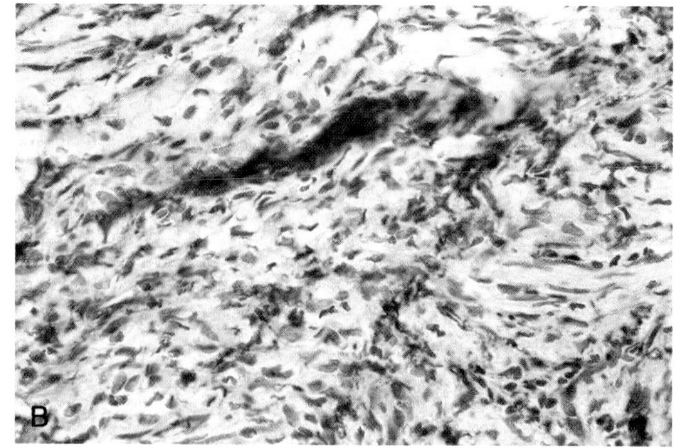

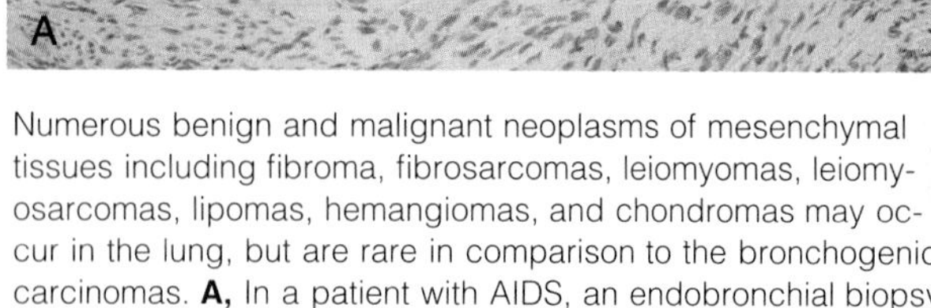

Numerous benign and malignant neoplasms of mesenchymal tissues including fibroma, fibrosarcomas, leiomyomas, leiomyosarcomas, lipomas, hemangiomas, and chondromas may occur in the lung, but are rare in comparison to the bronchogenic carcinomas. **A,** In a patient with AIDS, an endobronchial biopsy shows the spindle cells of Kaposis's sarcoma infiltrating the bronchial wall (H & E stain). **B,** Staining with the lectin *Ulex europaeus* demonstrates the endothelial nature of the spindle cells.

NEOPLASIA OF THE LUNG

OTHER LUNG NEOPLASMS

FIGURE 3-67

Benign and malignant neoplasms of lymphoreticular cells including lymphomas, may arise in the lung. **A,** Diffuse low-grade lymphoma that presented as interstitial infiltrates on a chest radiograph shows prominent infiltration of a vessel (H & E). **B,** Positive immunoperoxidase staining for CD74 indicates B-lymphocyte origin. **C,** Immunoperoxidase staining for a T-lymphocyte marker (CD3) is negative.

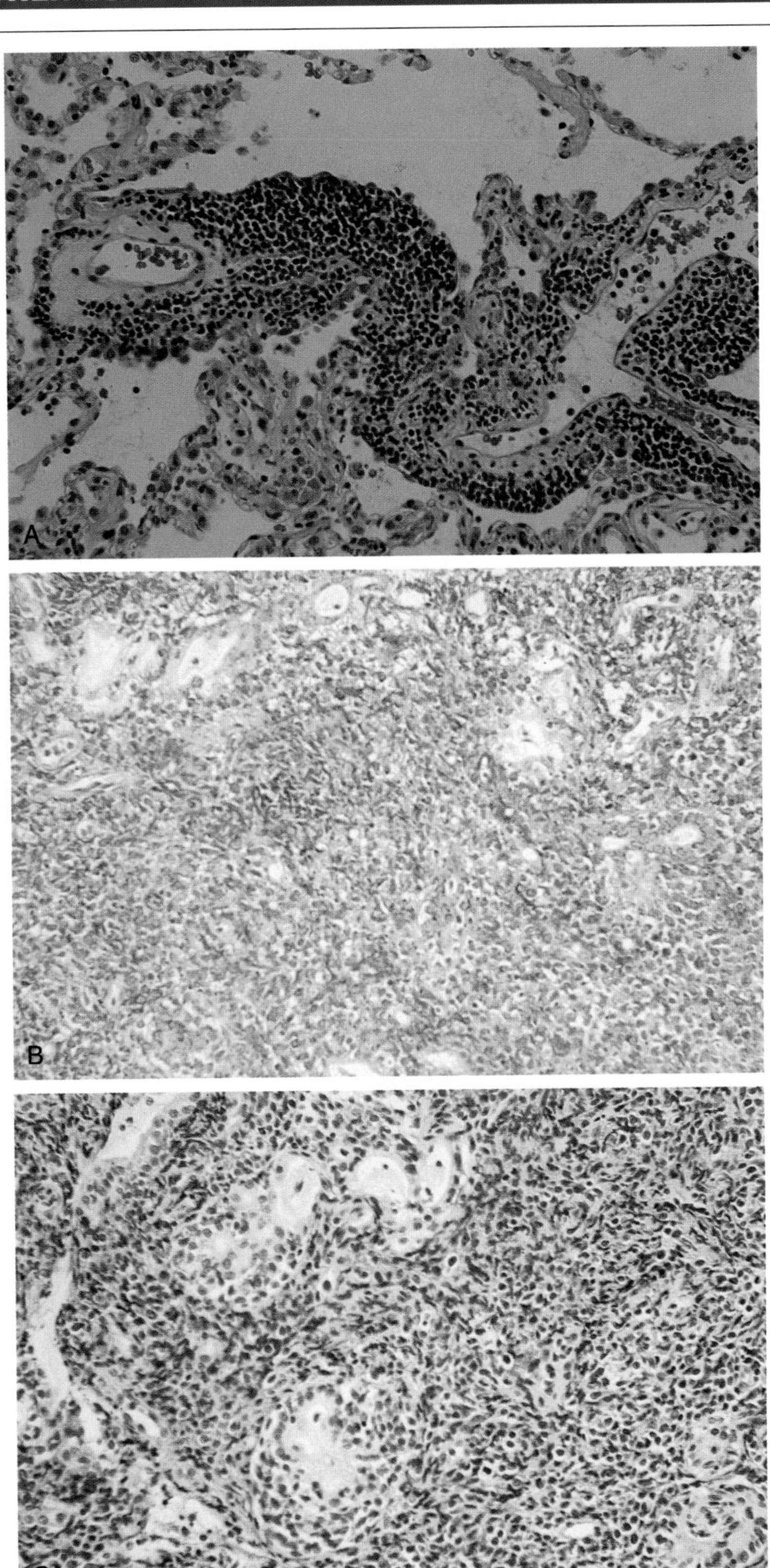

NEOPLASIA OF THE LUNG

OTHER LUNG NEOPLASMS

FIGURE 3–68

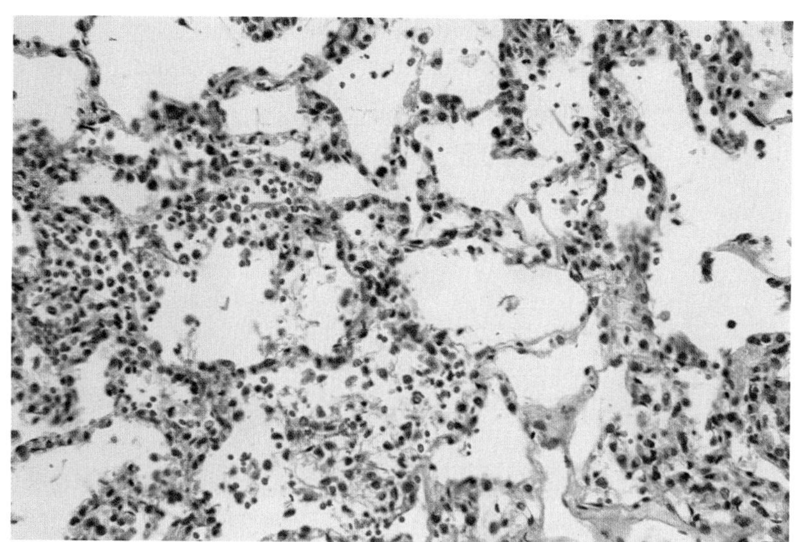

Clinically significant involvement of the lung in acute and chronic leukemia is uncommon but can occur. This example shows extensive infiltration of acute myelogenous leukemia cells into the alveolar walls with a few cells entering the alveolar spaces (H & E stain).

FIGURE 3–69

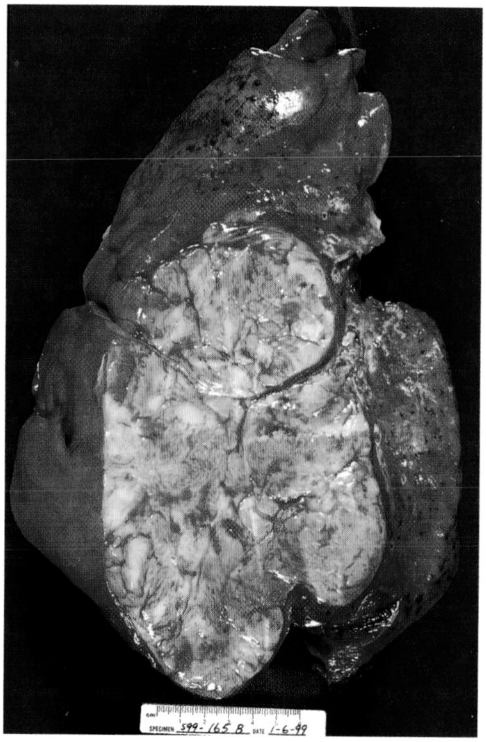

Metastatic tumors. The lung is a frequent site of metastases. Generally metastatic growths form multiple discrete nodules scattered throughout all lobes. Cancers metastatic to the lung may also spread through the lung lymphatics diffusely infiltrating the lung parenchyma (lymphangitic spread). In this example a single metastasis from a malignant germ cell tumor has reached tremendous size and involves a large portion of the left lung.

DISEASES OF THE PLEURA

Non-neoplastic pleural diseases are often secondary to inflammatory or neoplastic diseases of the lung, or due to congestive heart failure (see TABLE 3–27). (See Chapter 4, Radiography and Imaging.)

TABLE 3–27

Pathologic Conditions Associated with Non-Neoplastic Pleural Diseases

Benign Pleural Disease	Associated Pathologic Conditions
Pleural effusion	Lung or pleural infection or neoplasms; pulmonary infarcts; congestive heart failure
Pleuritis	Lung inflammation; sarcoidosis; collagen vascular disease; ruptured pleural blebs
Reactive mesothelial hyperplasia	Inflammation; infections; neoplasia
Fibrosis	Infections, collagen vascular disease; drug reactions; asbestos exposure
Rounded atelectasis	Following hemothorax or empyema; uremia
Pleural plaque	Postinflammatory; asbestos exposure

FIGURE 3–70

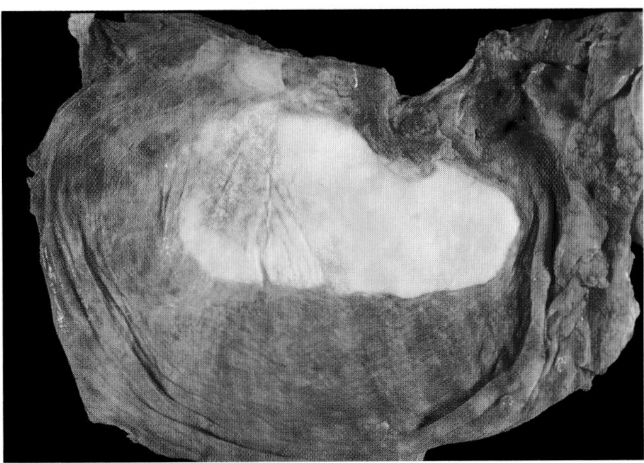

Pleural plaques are raised fibrous lesions of the parietal pleura found in the lower lung zones or on the superior surface of the diaphragm such as shown here. They are found in association with asbestos exposure but also occur following resolution of hemothorax, empyema, or traumatic injury.

DISEASES OF THE PLEURA

Localized tumors of the pleural include both benign and malignant varieties. Diffuse neoplasms of the pleura are primarily mesothelium-derived malignant mesotheliomas. Diffuse pleural mesotheliomas show a tremendous amount of heterogeneity in their microscopic features. Thus, the differential diagnosis is quite broad, and distinguishing pleural mesothelioma from metastatic pleural cancer can be quite difficult. One histologic classification of pleural neoplasms is listed in TABLE 3–28.

TABLE 3–28

Histologic Classification of Pleural Neoplasms

Benign
- Localized benign fibrous tumor
- Benign cystic mesothelioma

Malignant
- Localized malignant fibrous tumor
- Well-differentiated papillary mesothelioma
- Diffuse malignant mesothelioma
  - Epithelial
    Tubulopapillary
    Adenomatoid/microcystic
    Epithelioid/solid
  - Sarcomatoid
  - Mixed/biphasic
  - Poorly differentiated/undifferentiated
  - Unusual variants
    Small cell
    Lymphohistiocytoid
    Deciduoid

FIGURE 3–71

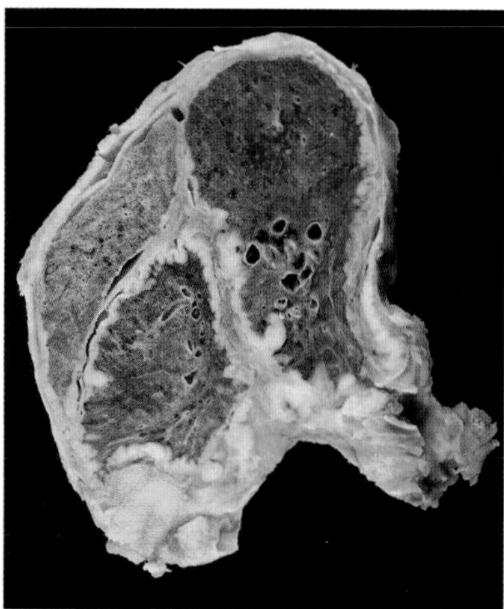

This malignant mesothelioma had encased the lung diffusely.

DISEASES OF THE PLEURA

FIGURE 3–72

Histopathology of malignant mesothelioma (H & E stains). **A,** Epithelial type malignant mesothelioma. **B,** Sarcomatoid malignant mesothelioma. The tumor cells are spindled.

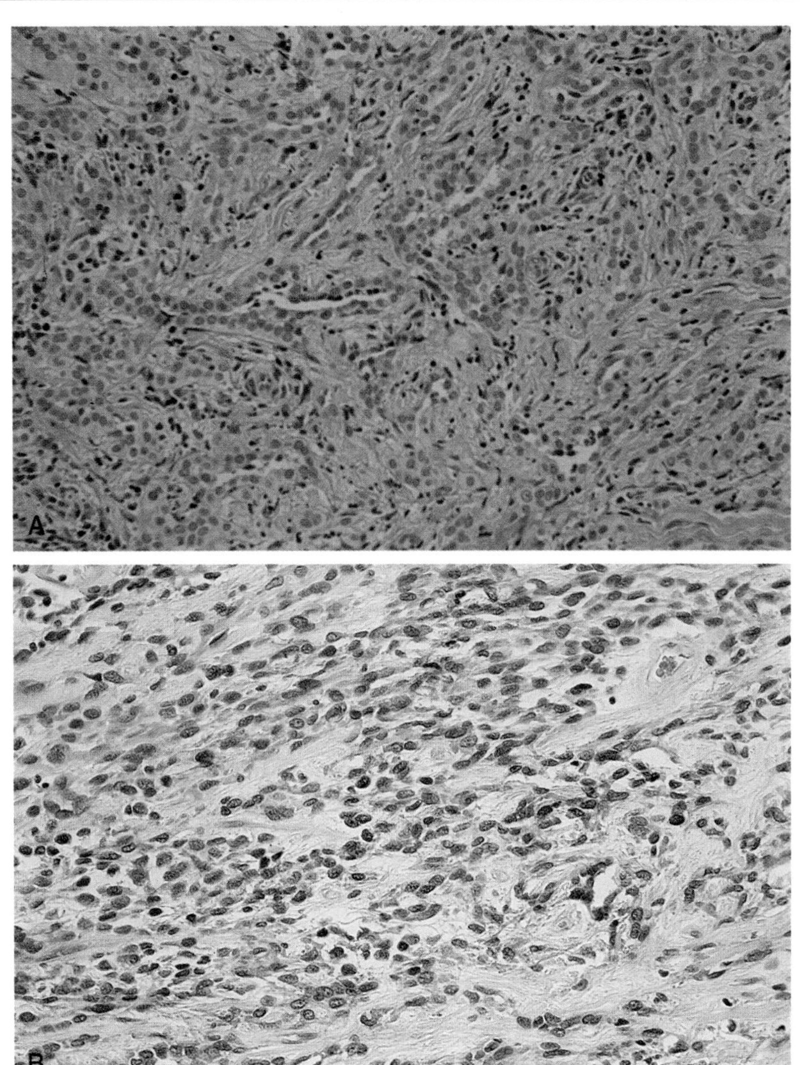

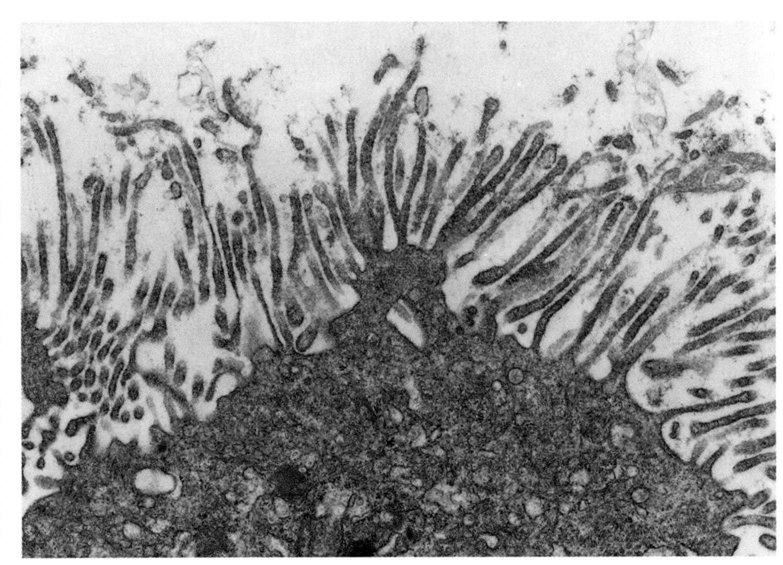

FIGURE 3–73

Electron photomicrograph of a pleural malignant epithelial mesothelioma (×20,000). The distinguishing feature of epithelial mesotheliomas is the long, thin, curved and branching microvilli (compare to the shorter, straighter microvilli of the adenocarcinoma shown in Figure 3–62F. Length to diameter ratios (LDR) greater than 15 support a diagnosis of mesothelioma because adenocarcinomas typically have an LDR of 10 or less.[4]

REFERENCES

1. Fletcher CM: Chronic bronchitis, its prevalence, nature, and pathogenesis. Am Rev Respir Dis 80:483–494, 1959.

2. Reid L: Measurement of the bronchial mucous gland layer: A diagnostic yardstick in chronic bronchitis. Thorax 15:132–141, 1960.

3. Heath D, Edwards JE: The pathology of hypertensive pulmonary vascular disease. A description of six grades of structural changes in the pulmonary arteries with special reference to congenital cardiac septal defects. Circulation 18:533–547, 1958.

4. Warhol M, Hickey WF, Corson JM: Malignant mesothelioma: Ultrastructural distinction from adenocarcinoma. Am J Surg Pathol 6:307–314, 1982.

CHAPTER

4

Radiography and Imaging

David L. Levin, M.D., Ph.D.,

and

W. Richard Webb, M.D.

INTRODUCTION

GENERAL

- Imaging is essential for the clinical evaluation of many patients with pulmonary disease.
- Radiologic studies of value in chest diagnosis are varied and reflect a rapidly changing technology.
- This chapter will discuss and provide examples of some of the more common techniques of evaluation.

HISTORY

Roentgen and Others

- The first public demonstration of x-rays took place in 1896 in Würzburg.
- News of "a light that, for the purpose of photography, will penetrate wood, flesh and most other organic substances" had already been widely reported.
- At the demonstration, Wilhelm Roentgen invited anatomist Albert von Kölliker to have his hand photographed using x-rays.
- This first public display sparked an explosion in the use of x-rays to evaluate the human body.

Chest Atlas

- By the turn of the century, it was already postulated that "systematic and skilled use" of fluoroscopy would become as common a method of examination as auscultation of the chest.
- By 1901, an atlas of chest radiographs made with exposure times of less than 1 second had been published.
- By 1905, radiographs demonstrating tubercles the size of a pinhead within the lung parenchyma had been reported.

Fluoroscopy

- Rosenfeld published the first chest radiograph in 1897. Initially, however, radiologic evaluation of the thorax was almost exclusively performed using fluoroscopy.
- Francis Williams presented an image of the normal lungs and thoracic structures in 1897 at the meeting of the Association of American Physicians.
  - Changes in diaphragmatic position with respiration were reported for both normal subjects and patients with tuberculosis.
  - Williams concluded that in most cases of pulmonary tuberculosis, fluoroscopic examination provided the best method of assessment of the disease.
  - Fluoroscopic observations were also reported for pleural effusions, pneumothorax, pulmonary edema, and pneumonia.

Routine Radiography

- During the next decade there were many technical improvements, with changes in the design of transformers, cathode tubes, and intensifying screens, as well as x-ray shielding of equipment.
- Eastman produced the first single emulsion x-ray film in 1914, which enabled radiographic diagnosis of pulmonary disease to become increasingly more commonplace.
- By 1917, criteria for the diagnosis of tuberculosis were established, being based largely upon radiographic appearance.
- Shortly thereafter, radiographic standards for the evaluation of pneumoconioses were developed.
- By the mid-1920s, the classic radiographic appearance of many pulmonary diseases had been described.

INTRODUCTION

HISTORY

Computed Tomography

• The development of computed tomography (CT) is largely attributed to Godfrey Hounsfield, who shared the 1979 Nobel Prize in Medicine and Physiology with Allen M. Cormack for this achievement.
• The CT scanner was developed as a means to verify his calculations.
• Cormack had produced similar work earlier as part of his research in the distribution of x-rays within the body during radiation therapy.
• Unknown to both men, Johann Radon had described the mathematics of projection imaging in 1917 while producing equations relating to his interest in the physics of gravity.
• The first clinical CT scanner was installed in London in 1971 for evaluation of the head. Data acquisition took over 2 minutes per image, with a reconstruction time of nearly 1 minute. The resolution of the image was on the order of 3 mm per pixel; despite this, the initial results were well received.
• Technical improvements came rapidly and the first whole-body scanner was installed at the University of Minnesota in 1973. This unit, however, still required long acquisition times, and imaging of the thorax was severely compromised by respiratory motion.
• The second generation of scanners reduced acquisition times to less than 20 seconds per slice, permitting greatly improved imaging of the body.
• Current CT scanners can evaluate the entire thorax within a single breathhold.

Nuclear Magnetic Resonance Spectroscopy

• The first papers demonstrating nuclear magnetic resonance (NMR) were independently published by groups headed by Felix Bloch at Stanford and Edward Purcell at Harvard in 1946. These two investigators shared the Nobel Prize for Physics in 1952.
• The first human NMR spectrum came from Bloch's finger. Not to be outdone, Purcell later obtained a spectrum from his head.
• Although NMR spectroscopy was used to evaluate living systems, it was limited by the 5-cm bore of the early spectrometers.
• Raymond Damadian showed a change in tissue relaxation constants in excised malignant rat tumors, as compared with normal tissue, in 1971.
• By 1980, spectrometers with bores large enough to accommodate extremities were available, and high-resolution spectra of extremities were obtained in both normal and diseased limbs.

Nuclear Magnetic Resonance Images

• The creation of images using NMR was a more complex issue.
• The first proton NMR image was published by Paul Lauterbur in 1973, which showed a cross-sectional image of two capillary tubes of water.
• Lauterbur termed this imaging process "zeugmatography."

Magnetic Resonance Imaging

• The first image of a live animal was published by Damadian, and coworkers, in 1976, with the first human image produced a year later by the same group. Early images were quite limited in resolution and required long exposure times, but established the feasibility of NMR imaging.
• Rapid advancements occurred at many centers with a dramatic improvement in image resolution and decrease in image acquisition times.
• By the mid-1980s, MRI became the imaging examination of choice for the evaluation of the brain and spine. MRI also gained rapid acceptance in the imaging of the extremities.
• MRI is generally of limited use in the imaging of the thorax. When used, it is far more commonly employed to evaluate the heart and the great vessels. However, this application is changing as new methods to evaluate the lung parenchyma itself are developed.

GENERAL RADIOGRAPHY

PLAIN RADIOGRAPHS

- Plain radiographs are fundamental to the radiographic assessment of many chest diseases, and are often sufficient for radiographic diagnosis.
- Several plain radiographic projections and techniques can be used in chest diagnosis, and familiarity with each, including their uses and limitations, is important for understanding their value and determining which studies to obtain in different clinical settings.
- Obtaining good chest radiographs can be technically difficult, and their interpretation can be quite subtle.
- Minor alterations in radiographic technique can significantly change how an x-ray looks, can produce confusing appearances, and can significantly affect diagnostic accuracy.
- A knowledge of how various radiographic studies are performed and what findings to look for is very important in recognizing technical artifacts and artifacts of patient positioning, and forms the basis for recognizing significant abnormalities.
- Knowing how specific abnormalities manifest themselves radiographically is also of obvious importance.

Technique

- A routine chest examination consists of upright posteroanterior (PA) and lateral views (FIGURE 4–1).
- Proper technique is essential for optimizing diagnostic information.
- The examination should be obtained with respiration suspended at end-inspiration, which is about 95% of total lung capacity in most people.[1]
- Plain radiographs are useful in assessing a wide variety of thoracic abnormalities.

FIGURE 4–1

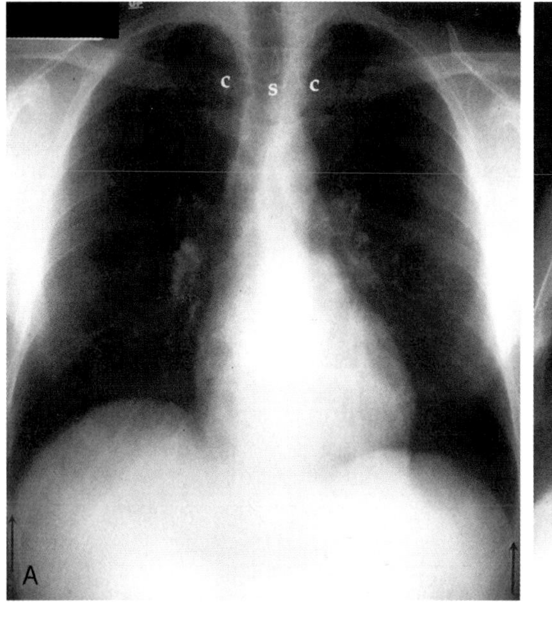

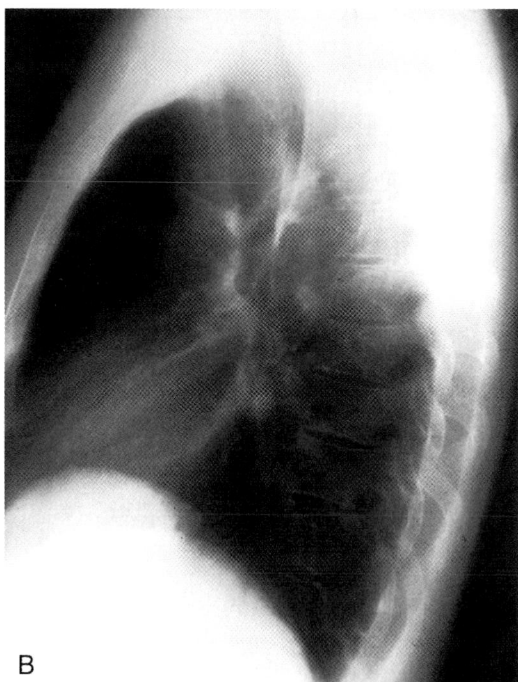

Normal chest radiograph. **A,** Upright, posteroanterior (PA) view. **B,** Left lateral view. On a properly positioned PA view of the chest, the spinous process (s) lies midway between the clavicular heads (c) and the patient is centered so that both costophrenic angles (*arrows*) are visible. On a properly positioned left lateral film **(B),** the posterior ribs are offset slightly, and the right ribs project slightly more posteriorly than the left ribs. If the radiograph is adequately exposed, vertebral bodies should be visible throughout the thorax and upper abdomen.

GENERAL RADIOGRAPHY

PLAIN RADIOGRAPHS

Attenuation

- The difference in attenuation of the x-ray beam by lung and mediastinum[2] can vary by up to a factor of 10. This difference can result in underexposure of the mediastinum when the lungs are optimally exposed or, conversely, overexposure of the lungs when technique is optimized for showing the mediastinum.
- Attempts to improve radiographic technique have been based on the use of high kVp (kilovolt peak) technique and wide latitude film.[3, 4]
- kVp refers to the peak voltage applied across the x-ray tube in the production of the x-ray beam.
  - A high kVp technique (greater than 90 kVp) allows a wider range of densities (e.g., bone and lung) to be imaged on a single radiograph.
  - Exposure times are also shorter with high kVp, which decreases motion artifact.
  - The use of high kVp technique results in decreased contrast between different tissues (such as lung, vessels, or mediastinum) and a "flatter" image.

Latitude

- Film latitude is a measure of the range of x-ray exposures of which a film is capable.
- A wide latitude film allows for improved visualization of the mediastinum without overexposure of the lung parenchyma.
- Film latitude, however, varies inversely with film contrast. The improvement in visualization of the mediastinal and retrocardiac structures on wide latitude film comes at a loss in contrast within the lung parenchyma. Less contrast may decrease the ability to detect subtle nodules or interstitial disease.[3]
- There is no single optimal technique for chest radiographs. This problem has led some to suggest that film should be replaced as an x-ray detector by other media (see Digital Radiography, later in this chapter).

GENERAL RADIOGRAPHY

PORTABLE CHEST RADIOGRAPHS

Equipment

- Portable radiographs are used commonly for imaging patients with limited mobility but have several disadvantages[4, 5] (FIGURE 4–2).
- Portable studies are produced using a low kVp technique that provides less latitude, often resulting in poor visualization of the lungs, especially in the retrocardiac regions, or poor visualization of mediastinal structures.
- The maximum mA (tube current in milliamperes) produced by portable equipment is less that that used for routine chest radiography and thus requires longer exposure times, leading to increased motion artifact.
- The distance between the x-ray source and the film is shorter, resulting in magnification of the cardiac silhouette and mediastinal structures.
- Furthermore, portable radiographs are usually performed without grids, which are generally used for routine radiographs and serve to reduce scattered radiation reaching the film.

FIGURE 4–2

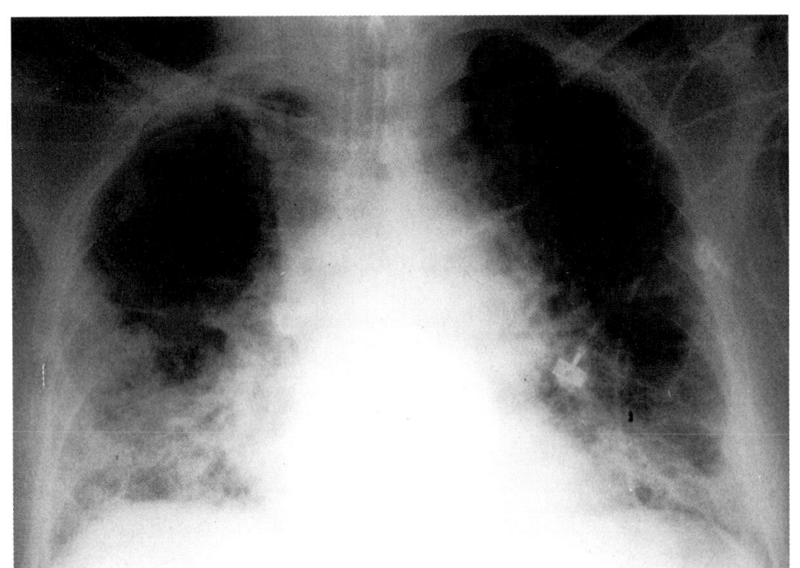

Portable chest radiograph. Usually obtained in the anteroposterior (AP) position, instead of PA, which results in magnification of the heart shadow. Because the patient is supine or semierect, it is difficult to identify a pleural effusion or pneumothorax. Because the degree of inspiration rarely approaches that of an upright position, the radiographic density is increased at the lung bases, which makes it difficult to detect subtle focal abnormalities. Increased pulmonary blood flow in the supine posture makes the upper lobe vessels more prominent than in PA films.

Position

- Portable radiographs are usually obtained in the anteroposterior (AP) position instead of PA, resulting in magnification of the heart shadow.
- The patient is often positioned supine or semierect, making it more difficult to identify a pleural effusion or pneumothorax.
- Regardless of patient position, the degree of inspiration rarely approaches that of an upright film.
  - This reduced inspiration increases the radiographic density of the lung parenchyma, especially at the lung bases, and makes detection of subtle focal abnormalities difficult.
  - The increase in pulmonary blood flow associated with the supine position makes the upper lobe vessels more prominent.

Lateral Views

- Lateral films are rarely performed in portable studies.
  - They have the same technical limitations as AP portable radiographs,
  - They generate radiation exposure to nearby patients and medical personnel.

Portable studies are common, but because of their limitations should be requested only when patients are unable to travel to the radiology department.

GENERAL RADIOGRAPHY

CLINICAL EXAMPLES

(See examples of pathology in Chapter 3.)

Pneumonia

- PA and lateral radiographs are often sufficient for the radiographic evaluation of acute lung disease, such as pneumonia.
- In a patient with bacterial pneumonia, PA and lateral radiographs show focal increased opacity in the right middle lobe (FIGURE 4–3).
- The silhouette sign can be an important clue to the presence of subtle airspace consolidation, and can help to identify the location of the parenchymal abnormality.[6] The silhouette sign is particularly useful when only a frontal radiograph is available for interpretation.
- Invisibility or obscuration of the right or left hemidiaphragm is seen with lower lobe disease; obscuration of the right or left border of the heart reflects consolidation in the right middle lobe or lingula; and obscuration of the aortic arch or the superior vena cava is seen, respectively, with left upper lobe or right upper lobe consolidation.
- Often, the parenchymal consolidation will increase the radiographic contrast between gas within the airways and the surrounding lung, producing an "air bronchogram," a common feature of bacterial pneumonia.

FIGURE 4–3

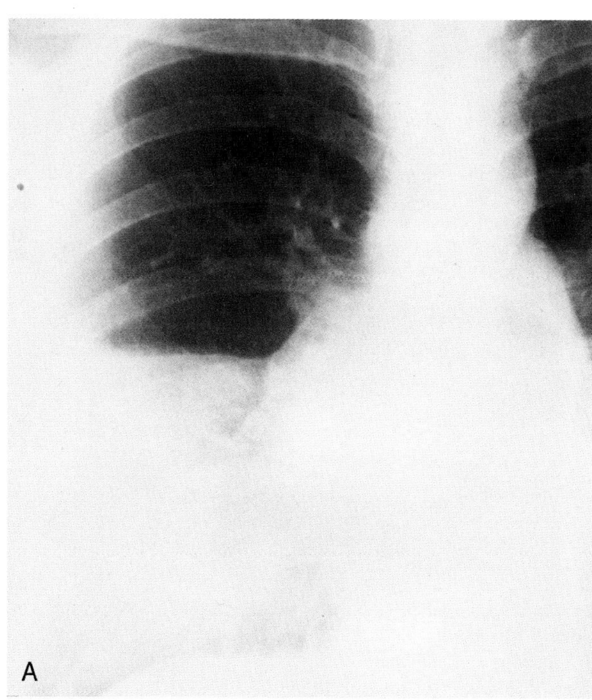

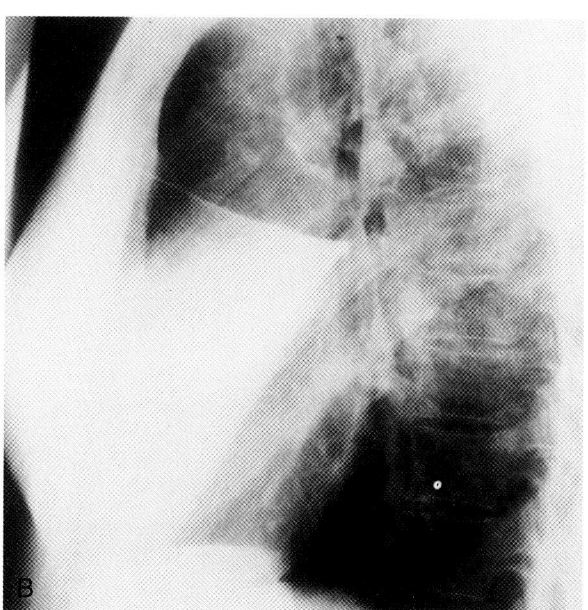

Pneumonia. **A,** Bacterial pneumonia in the right middle lobe (RML) resulting in parenchymal consolidation, which appears as a relatively homogeneous increased opacity in the RML, which obscures the normal interface between the right border of the heart and the right lung (silhouette sign) in the PA radiograph.[6] **B,** In the lateral film, the consolidation is localized between the major fissure, inferiorly, and the minor fissure, superiorly, localizing the opacity to the middle lobe.

GENERAL RADIOGRAPHY

CLINICAL EXAMPLES

Congestive Heart Failure

- Chest radiograph in a patient in congestive heart failure shows a generalized increase in the radiographic density of the lungs (FIGURE 4–4).
- The radiographic features are typical of the combined interstitial and airspace abnormalities commonly seen in patients with cardiogenic pulmonary edema.
- There is enlargement of the cardiac silhouette and loss of definition of the margins of the pulmonary veins.
- The loss of definition of the hilar pulmonary vessels is often termed "perihilar haze," and is another common finding in pulmonary edema.
- Multiple septal lines (Kerley's B lines) are present and are typically located at the periphery of the lung bases with a horizontal orientation. Usually 2 to 3 cm in length, these lines represent fluid within the interlobular septa.
- Although most commonly seen with cardiogenic pulmonary edema, Kerley's B lines can also be seen with lymphangitic spread of carcinoma, pulmonary hemorrhage, sarcoidosis, pulmonary Kaposi's sarcoma, and viral pneumonia.[7, 8]
- An airspace abnormality is indicated by consolidation, which is often patchy in appearance, with obscuration of the pulmonary vessels. Occasionally, air bronchograms are present, but they are more commonly a feature of noncardiogenic pulmonary edema.
- The radiographic distinction between cardiogenic and noncardiogenic pulmonary edema is difficult.
- Features that are felt to be more common in cardiogenic edema include:
  - Redistribution pulmonary blood flow
  - A homogeneous distribution of edema within the lungs
  - Increased width of the mediastinal great vessels (vascular pedicle)[9]

FIGURE 4–4

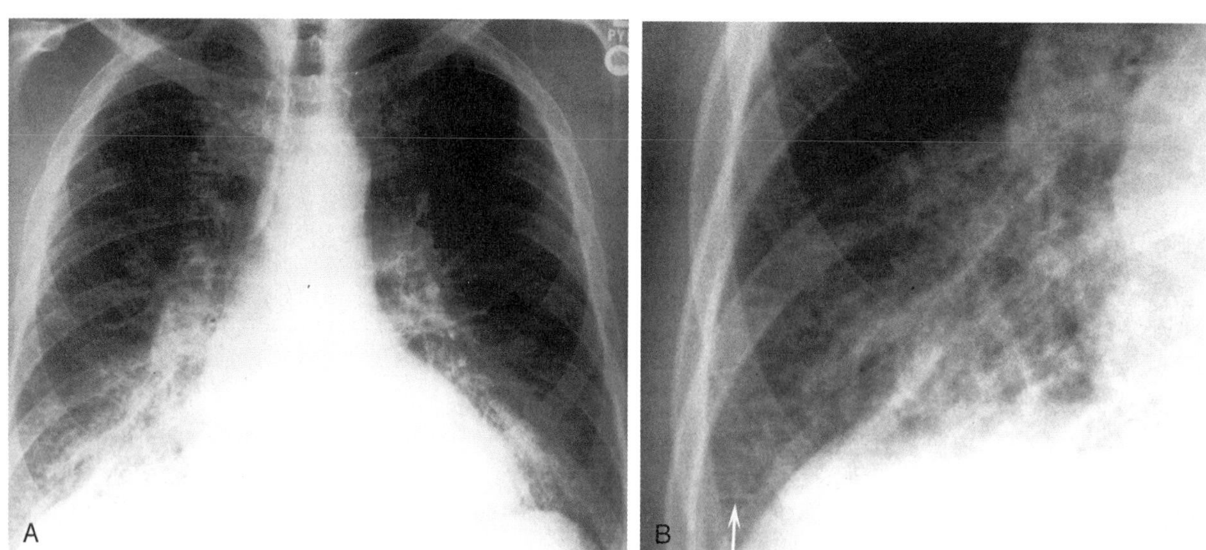

Congestive heart failure. **A,** There is generalized increase in the radiographic density of the lungs, enlargement of the cardiac silhouette, and loss of definition of the margins of the pulmonary veins in the PA view. The loss of definition of the hilar pulmonary vessels is often termed "perihilar haze." **B,** Kerley's B lines (*arrow*).

GENERAL RADIOGRAPHY

CLINICAL EXAMPLES

Chronic Obstructive Pulmonary Disease

(See results of Nuclear Medicine Techniques and Applications in Chapter 5.)

- In chronic obstructive pulmonary disease (COPD) there is generalized hyperinflation, indicated by
  - Flattening of the hemidiaphragms
  - Increased AP diameter of the chest
  - Increased retrosternal clear space
- Diaphragmatic flattening is most reliable sign in the diagnosis of hyperinflation.[10]
- The hyperinflation is often appreciated as a generalized lucency.
- Reduction in the size of pulmonary vessels is associated with emphysema.

Chronic Obstructive Pulmonary Disease; Other Findings

- Relative narrowing of the tracheal air column on the frontal film, known as a "saber-sheath" deformity, commonly associated with COPD.[11]
- Enlargement of the central pulmonary arteries with pruning of the distal vessels may develop as a result of pulmonary hypertension.
- Bullae may also be seen, especially at the apices Often only a portion of the bulla wall is visible, and clear demarcation from the surrounding lung is difficult.
- In some patients with emphysema and chronic bronchitis, increased linear opacities will be present, most prominently at the lung bases. These opacities most likely reflect chronic bronchial wall inflammation, atelectasis, and scarring.

FIGURE 4–5

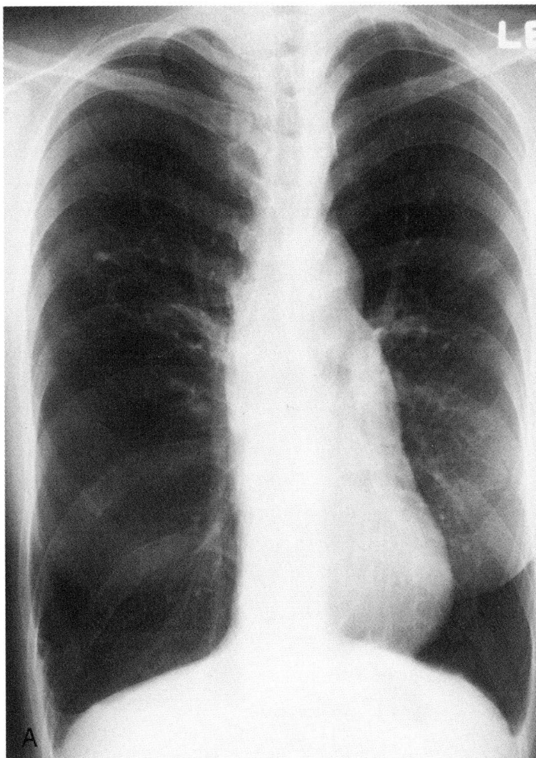

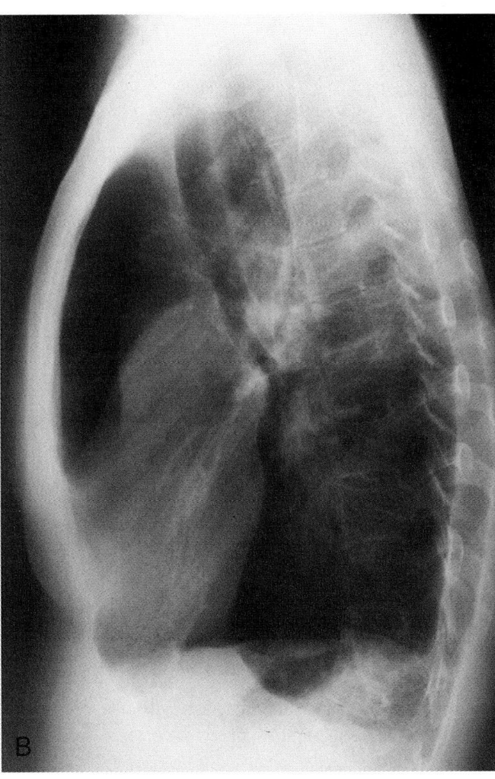

Chronic obstructive pulmonary disease. Generalized hyperinflation, characterized by a flattening of the hemidiaphragms, an increase in the AP diameter of the chest, and an increase in the retrosternal clear space are seen in PA **(A)** and lateral **(B)** views.

GENERAL RADIOGRAPHY

CLINICAL EXAMPLES

Right Upper Lobar Collapse

- The inferior and lateral margins of the right upper lobe opacity (FIGURE 4–6) have a sharp interface with the adjacent lung (*arrows*).
  - This border represents the minor fissure, which is displaced from its normal location because of right upper lobe collapse.
  - The combination of increased opacity and volume loss signifies atelectasis or collapse.
- Other signs include elevation of the ipsilateral hemidiaphragm, ipsilateral shift of the mediastinum, and crowding of ipsilateral ribs.
- In this example, the minor fissure also curves around a mass in the right hilum. This focal convexity of the medial fissure in association with upward displacement of the lateral fissure is termed the "S sign of Golden" because of the sigmoid shape of the fissure. As in this case, it usually results from bronchogenic carcinoma.

FIGURE 4–6

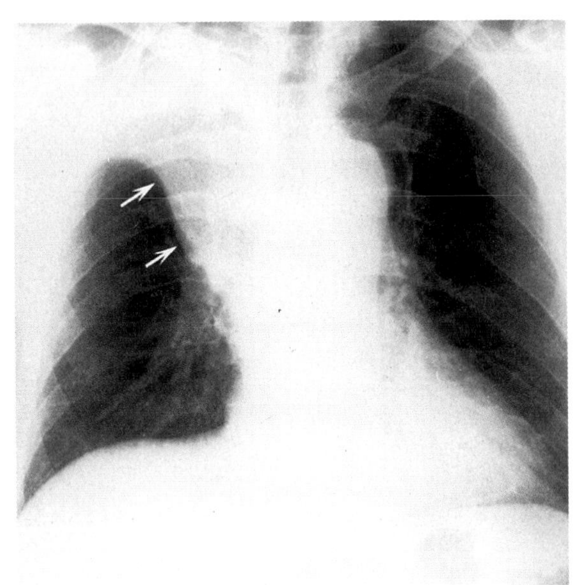

Right upper lobe collapse. The inferior and lateral margins of the right upper lobe opacity have a sharp interface with the adjacent lung (*arrows*). In this example, the minor fissure also curves around a mass in the right hilum. This focal convexity of the medial fissure in association with upward displacement of the lateral fissure is termed the "S sign of Golden" because of the sigmoid shape of the fissure.

Interstitial Lung Disease

- Diffuse peripheral reticular pattern, which consists of a meshwork of fine lines surrounding small holes 5 to 10 mm in diameter, indicates interstitial lung disease (FIGURE 4–7).
- This pattern is most prominent in the lung periphery.
- The stacking of one small hole upon another is often termed "honeycombing."

FIGURE 4–7

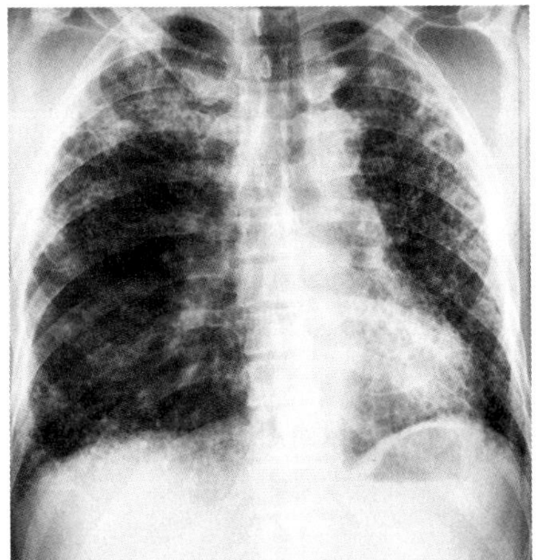

Interstitial lung disease.

Idiopathic Lung Fibrosis

- A peripheral reticular pattern can be seen with many forms of diffuse lung fibrosis, but the most common cause of this pattern is idiopathic pulmonary fibrosis.[12] This type is most often predominantly basilar in location and is associated with an overall decrease in lung volume.
- A similar appearance is seen with fibrosis resulting from collagen vascular diseases, such as rheumatoid arthritis or scleroderma. In this case, the fibrosis involves the upper and lower lobes equally; additionally, the lung volumes are preserved. These described features are more typical of the fibrosis that accompanies chronic extrinsic allergic alveolitis.[13]

(See pulmonary function test results of the preceding clinical examples in Chapter 8, Pulmonary Function Testing.)

GENERAL RADIOGRAPHY

CLINICAL EXAMPLES

Nodules

- Frontal radiograph shows multiple, small, well-defined nodules (FIGURE 4–8*A*).
- The nodules are roughly 3 to 5 mm and are distributed in a homogeneous fashion throughout the lungs.
- This pattern is commonly referred to as a miliary pattern.
  - The sharply defined borders of the nodules suggest a location within the pulmonary interstitium, as opposed to the distal airways.
  - Additional support for this comes from the lack of consolidation, even in regions where there is a profusion of nodules.
- A CT image (FIGURE 4–8*B*) in this patient confirms that these nodules are sharply defined, homogeneously distributed, and roughly 3 to 5 mm.
- The radiographic differential diagnosis for nodules with a miliary pattern of distribution consists of metastatic and granulomatous diseases.
  - The malignancies that most typically present with this pattern include thyroid and renal carcinomas, melanoma, and choriocarcinoma, although other primary malignancies have been reported to demonstrate miliary spread.[14]
  - More typically, granulomatous infections, such as tuberculosis or fungal disease, result in this appearance.
  - Noninfectious granulomatous diseases, such as eosinophilic granuloma and sarcoidosis, as well as pneumoconioses, especially silicosis, can also present with this radiographic pattern.
- In this immunocompromised patent, a specific diagnosis was made only following a wedge resection.
  - The excised lung parenchyma demonstrated multiple necrotizing granulomas with fibrosis.
  - With special stains, *Pneumocystis carinii* organisms were identified within the granulomas and no additional organisms were identified.

FIGURE 4–8

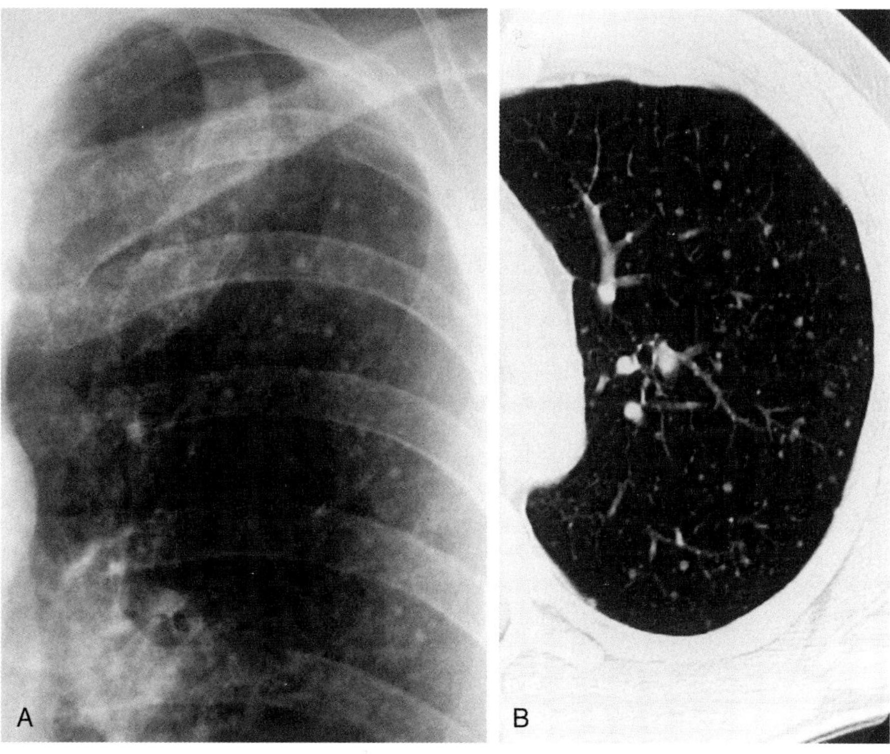

Nodules. **A,** Chest radiograph (frontal) shows 3 to 5-mm nodules distributed in a homogeneous miliary pattern. **B,** CT image in the same patient confirms the presence of sharply defined, homogeneously distributed nodules 3 to 5 mm in diameter.

GENERAL RADIOGRAPHY

CLINICAL EXAMPLES

Pleural Disease

- Chest radiographs are valuable in diagnosing pleural disease (FIGURE 4–9).
- A frontal radiograph in this patient demonstrates a large right hydropneumothorax.
- The underlying disease process in this example was *coccidioidomycosis* in a patient with acquired immunodeficiency syndrome (AIDS).

FIGURE 4–9

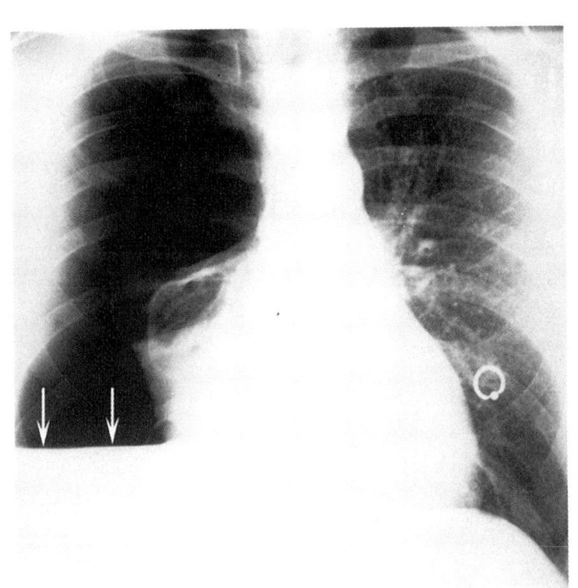

Right hydropneumothorax. A large pleural effusion is present, which demonstrates a straight superior border (*arrows*), characteristic of a hydropneumothorax. The edge of the collapsed right lung is seen medially, adjacent to the right border of the heart. There is no shift of the mediastinum, which would be expected if a tension pneumothorax were present. This patient had acquired immunodeficiency syndrome (AIDS) complicated by *coccidioidomycosis*.

GENERAL RADIOGRAPHY

CLINICAL EXAMPLES

Pleural Effusion

• A lateral decubitus radiograph is a frontal view of the chest taken while the patient is lying on his or her side (FIGURE 4–10).

• The lateral decubitus view demonstrates small effusions more readily than an upright frontal view of the chest. Blunting of the costophrenic angle on a frontal view of the chest requires 250 to 300 mL of fluid, but as little as 25 mL of fluid may be detected using a lateral decubitus view.[15]

• Although the lateral decubitus view is usually centered on the dependent side to assess pleural fluid, evaluation of the nondependent hemithorax can be used to demonstrate pneumothoraces, especially in patients who are unable to be placed in an upright position.

Special Views

• The apical lordotic position (FIGURE 4–11) projects the clavicles and the first costochondral joints above the apex of the lung, allowing improved visualization of the apical parenchyma.

• Special views, such as the apical lordotic or the shallow oblique, have been largely supplanted by CT.

FIGURE 4–10

Pleural effusion. A lateral decubitus film shows a freely flowing effusion layer dependently within the pleural space, which is seen as a stripe of increased density between the chest wall and the lung (*arrows*).

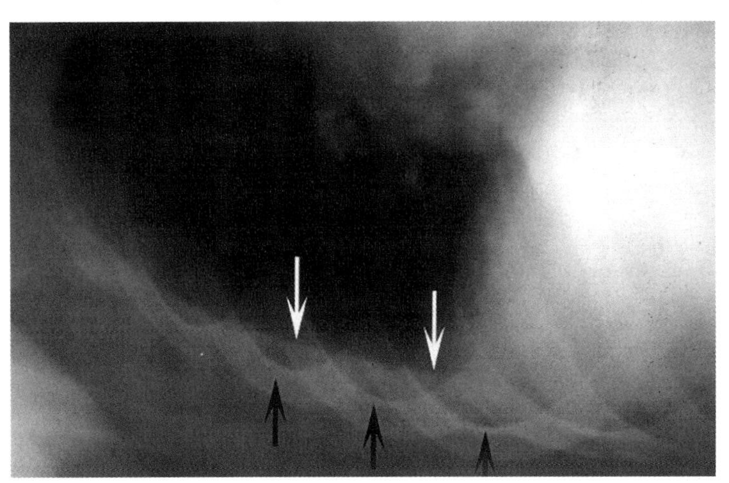

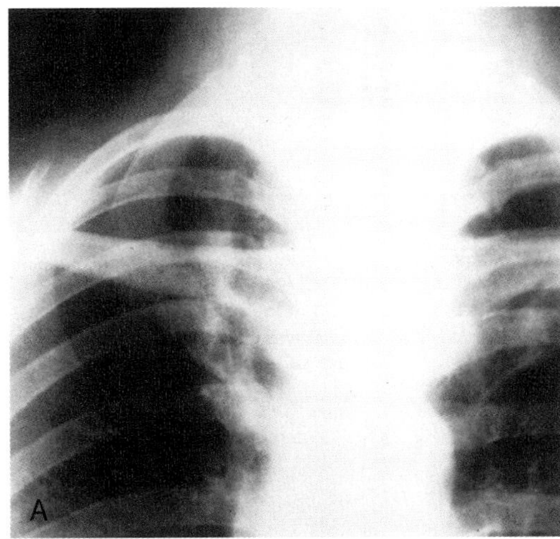

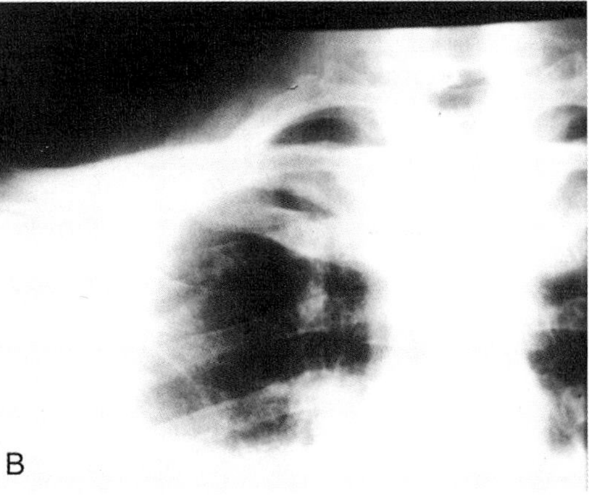

FIGURE 4–11

Apical lordotic position. **A**, PA chest radiograph. A lung nodule is covered by the first costochondral joint on the right. **B**, Apical lordotic view to visualize the apical parenchyma clearly demonstrates a spiculated lesion, later found to be a primary non–small cell carcinoma.

DIGITAL RADIOGRAPHY

- The term digital radiography (FIGURE 4–12) can be applied to any system that uses an array of numbers to represent the original analog x-ray signal.
- With conventional radiography, the film serves three separate functions:
  1. Detects the incoming x-rays
  2. Displays the image
  3. Acts as a permanent record of the examination
- With digital radiography, each of these functions is performed by a separate element of the imaging system.

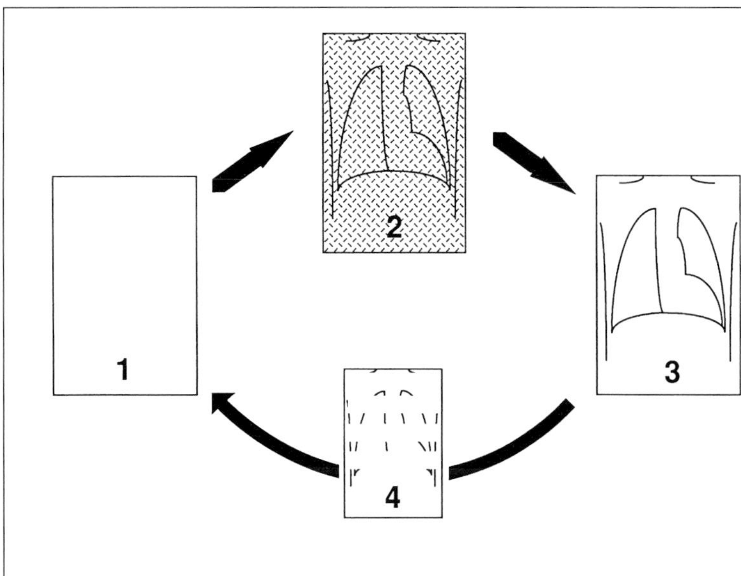

FIGURE 4–12

Digital radiography system, image detection. Several methods can be used to detect the incoming x-ray signal:

- Standard film-screen combination can be used to produce a radiograph, and then digitize this image.
- Nonfilm detectors, such as a photostimulable phosphor, can also be used, in a four-step process.
  1. The image receptor, in this case, is a plate covered with a storage phosphor.
  2. The energy of the x-ray photons that strike the plate raises electrons within the phosphor into a metastable state, which produces a "latent image."
  3. Scanning the plate with a laser beam subsequently captures the image information.
  4. Once this data is obtained, the phosphor plate is erased by exposure to light and reused to acquire new images.

IMAGE DISPLAY

FIGURE 4–13

Digital radiography image display.

- After the digital image information is acquired, it can be transferred to film for image display or routed through a picture archiving and communications system (PACS) (FIGURE 4–13).
- Images within a PACS are usually viewed on high-resolution monitors that can provide images to anyone connected to the system.
  - For example, a patient's study might be viewed simultaneously, and at different locations, by radiologists, emergency room physicians, and primary care physicians.
  - PACS can also display images acquired from other sources: e.g., computed tomography, magnetic resonance imaging, and nuclear medicine.
  - When integrated with a radiology information system (RIS), physicians can view images and reports simultaneously.

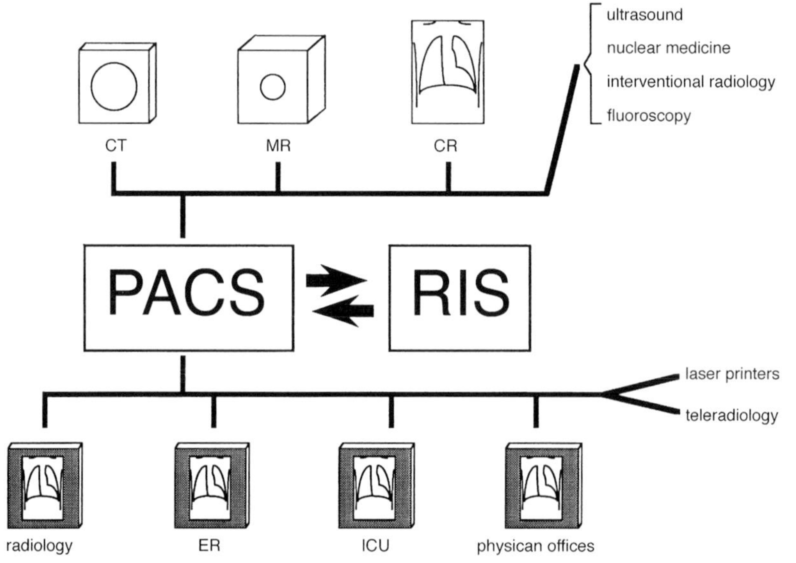

Image Storage and Analysis

- The PACS can also be used to store the digital information that makes up an examination.
- Archiving of the digital image within a PACS allows for rapid access to all studies for a patient, from any location.
- A laser printer can be used to transfer the image onto film, which can also act as the storage format.
- The PACS can be integrated with a teleradiology system to allow for remote viewing and interpretation of images.

DIGITAL RADIOGRAPHY

IMAGE MANIPULATION

- Digital images can be manipulated after their acquisition to enhance image contrast or edge detail (FIGURE 4–14).
- The digital image has the same basic appearance as that of conventional film.
- The analog information of a conventional radiograph, however, is represented by an array of numbers (pixels) that define spatial location and gray-scale intensity.

FIGURE 4–14

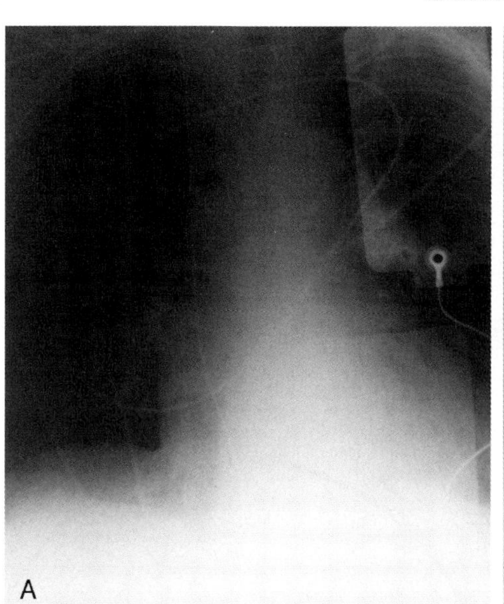

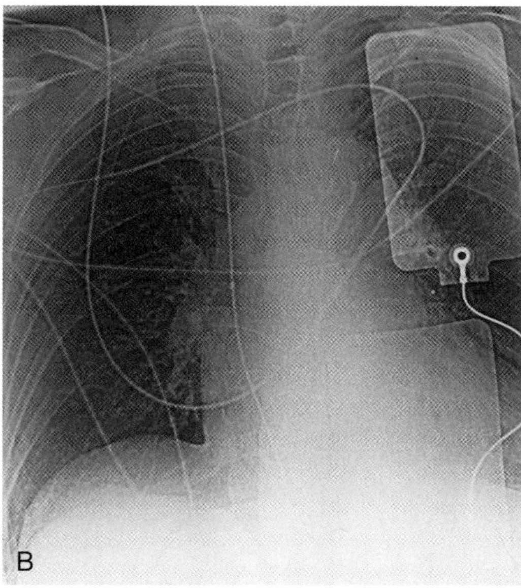

Image manipulation. Original image **(A)** did not demonstrate pulmonary interstitial markings. After the image data were manipulated **(B),** lung parenchyma was clearly demonstrated and significant pneumothorax could be excluded.

LIMITATIONS

Digital radiography currently suffers from several limitations.

- Spatial resolution is generally less than that of a conventional radiograph.
- Signal-to-noise ratio is also lower.[16, 17]

These limitations will likely decrease as the technology improves. It is unclear, however, whether digital radiography will need to equal the resolution of conventional film to be clinically useful.

ADVANTAGES

- The inherent advantage of digital radiography is the ability to adjust the appearance of the image after it has been obtained.
  - The global image density can be altered to emphasize different portions of the film, such as the mediastinum and hila.
  - Specific features of an image can be improved.
  - Edge enhancement can be obtained by suppressing low spatial frequencies using unsharp masking.[18, 19] This increases the detection of pneumothoraces[16] and enhancement can be useful in the evaluation of central venous catheters and endotracheal tubes.
  - Unsharp masking, however, decreases the detection of interstitial disease, lung nodules, and emphysema.[18, 19]
- Image enhancement is performed after data acquisition, and therefore does not require additional radiation exposure of the patient.
- In FIGURE 4–14, the original image did not demonstrate the pulmonary interstitial markings clearly (A). The image data was manipulated (B) to demonstrate more clearly the lung parenchyma and to exclude a significant pneumothorax.

COMPUTED TOMOGRAPHY

GENERAL

- A CT scanner functions by passing a collimated x-ray beam through a selected thickness of tissue from multiple angles, detecting the transmitted x-ray photons electronically, and reconstructing an image using a computer (FIGURE 4–15).[20]
- When the x-ray beam passes through the body, its intensity decreases due to interactions (absorption or scattering) within tissue.
- The final intensity of the beam reflects the sum of all the interactions along its path.
- By knowing the transmitted x-ray intensity from all the projections through a plane of tissue, the two-dimensional distribution of the x-ray attenuation coefficients can be calculated using an image reconstruction algorithm.
- The calculated x-ray attenuation coefficient is compared to that of water to give each pixel in the image a CT number, which is measured in Hounsfield units (H).
  - Water is assigned a value of 0.
  - Tissues, such as soft tissue and bone, which attenuate an x-ray beam to a greater extent, will have positive numbers.
  - Air and fat, which attenuate an x-ray beam to a lesser extent, will have negative numbers.

The CT image is formed by assigning a level of gray to a small region of tissue based upon its Hounsfield unit, with brighter shades used for the higher values:
- Parenchyma is black.
- Skeletal structures are white.

FIGURE 4–15

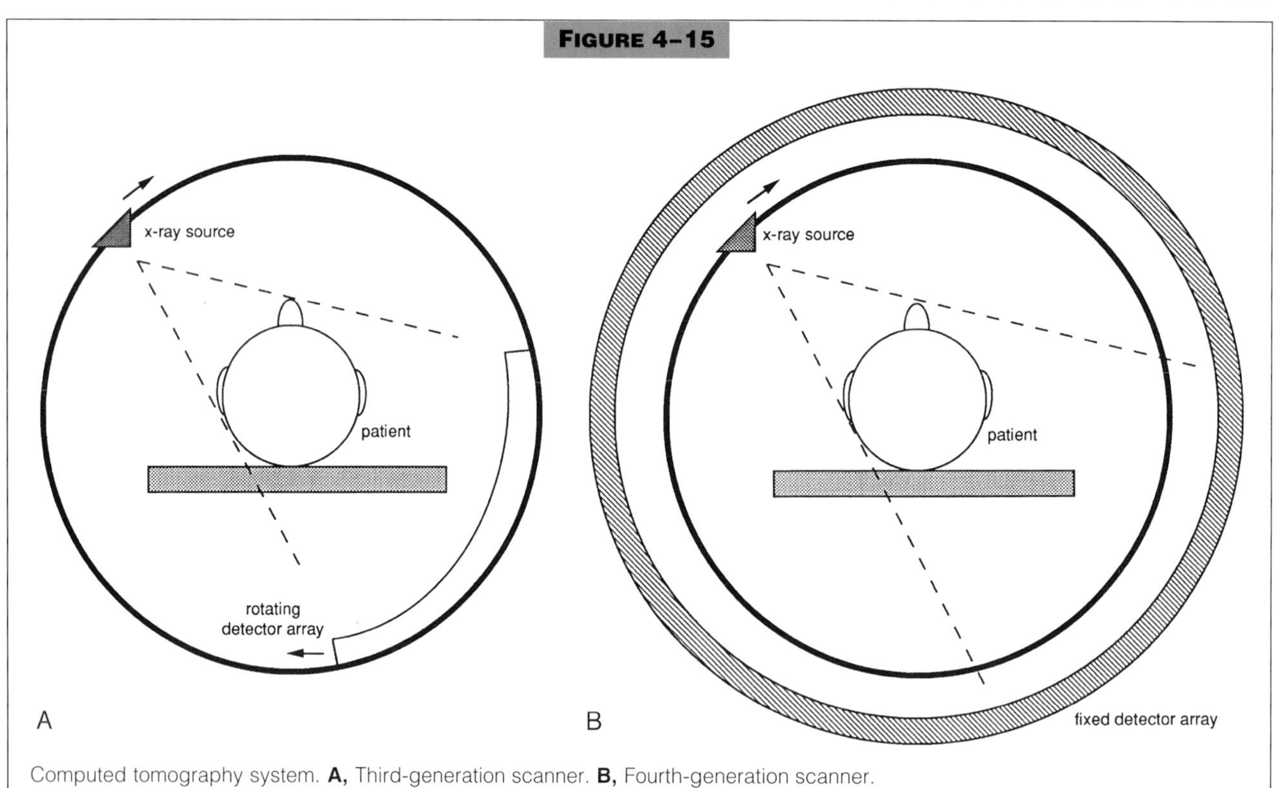

Computed tomography system. **A,** Third-generation scanner. **B,** Fourth-generation scanner.

COMPUTED TOMOGRAPHY

CT SCANNERS

- Two basic configurations of CT scanners are used most commonly (FIGURE 4–15).
- In a third-generation scanner (FIGURE 4–15*A*), the patient lies on the scanner table while both the x-ray source (x-ray tube) and the detector, contained within the scanner gantry, rotate around the patient.
- In a fourth-generation scanner (FIGURE 4–15*B*), the x-ray source moves around the patient while the x-ray beam is detected by a ring of stationary detectors.
- These differences are relatively minor, and at the most basic level, both systems serve to project an x-ray beam through a plane of tissue from multiple angles, and the images produced are the same.

CALCULATIONS AND SLICE THICKNESS

- The calculations assume that the imaged plane has no appreciable thickness.
- In reality, a slice thickness of 1 mm to 10 mm is usually evaluated to produce one CT image.
- A partial volume artifact may be produced if there are substances of differing x-ray attenuation within the volume of tissue being examined (voxel), because the calculated Hounsfield number will reflect an average of those values. Thus, if a voxel of lung tissue contained air and a small, soft-tissue nodule, an average Hounsfield value equal to fat might be observed, even though no fat was actually present within the voxel.
- To minimize this partial volume artifact, CT scanning is best performed with the thinnest possible slice thickness.[21]

ELECTRON-BEAM AND CINE CT

- A different approach is used for electron-beam (ultrafast or cine) CT.
- In a conventional CT scanner, the x-rays are produced in an x-ray tube by electrons that bombard a small tungsten target, and the tube moves around the subject.
- In an electron-beam scanner, a magnetic field is employed to deflect an electron beam, which can be scanned rapidly to strike a tungsten ring (target) that surrounds the patient. This approach produces a fan of x-rays that moves around the patient and strikes fixed detectors.
- Because there is no physical motion of an electron-beam scanner gantry, the x-ray beam can be made to rotate very quickly, and images can be produced in as little as 50 msec (compared with 0.8 to 1 second for a third- or fourth-generation scanner).
- The electron-beam CT method allows for rapid imaging of dynamic processes.

COMPUTED TOMOGRAPHY

CONVENTIONAL CT SCANNER

- The difference between helical CT and conventional CT stems from how the x-ray source moves with respect to the patient (FIGURE 4–16).
- Conventional scanning alternates patient movement with data acquisition.
  - The scanner obtains image data from one tissue plane and then moves the patient into position to obtain the next image (FIGURE 4–16*A*). This is termed incremental scanning.
- The data acquisition for a single image might take 1 to 2 seconds with an additional 2 to 3 seconds required to move the patient into position for the next image.
- This time requirement means that a patient cannot hold his or her breath for an entire study.

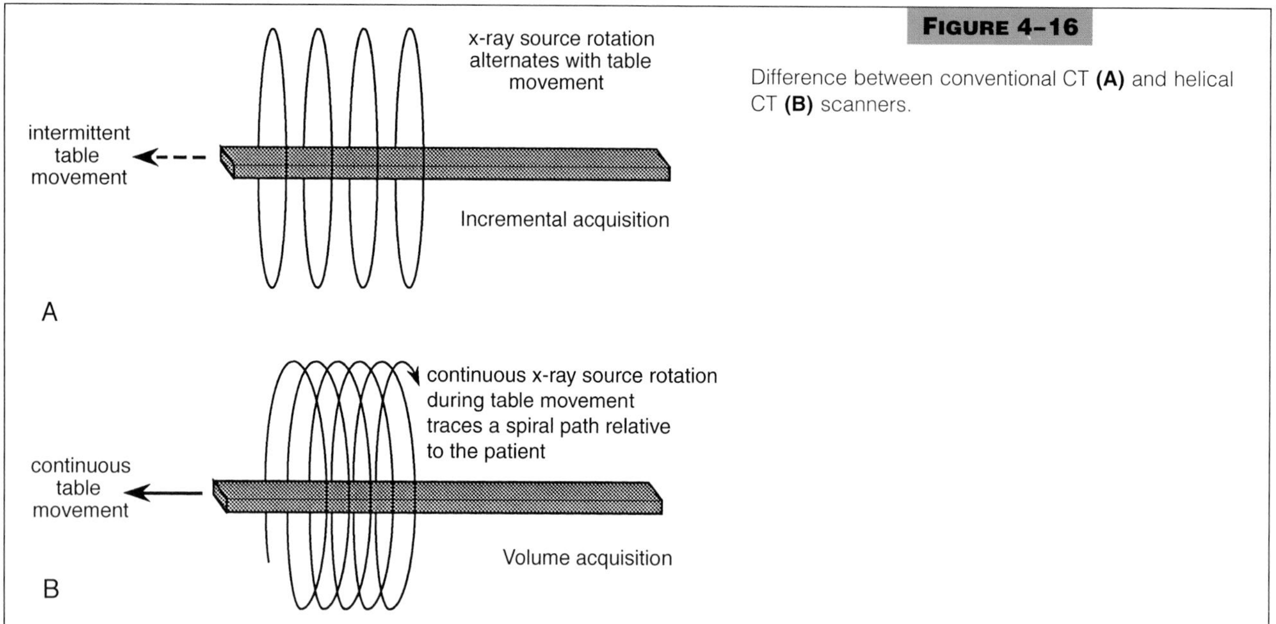

FIGURE 4–16

Difference between conventional CT **(A)** and helical CT **(B)** scanners.

HELICAL (SPIRAL) CT

- With helical CT (also referred to as spiral CT) (FIGURE 4–16), the patient moves continuously while image data is acquired continuously (FIGURE 4–16*B*).[22]
- This process is referred to as a "volume acquisition."
- There are several advantages to helical CT:
  - Study can be completed during a single breath-hold.
  - Can be timed to obtain images during peak contrast opacification of vessels.
  - Less contrast is needed for an adequate examination.
  - Contrast can be injected more rapidly if dense vascular opacification is desired.

Two technical advances were needed to change from conventional to helical CT:

1. Slip rings are used to connect the x-ray source with the power supply. The use of slip rings eliminates electrical cables and allows the x-ray source to rotate continuously.
2. Image interpolation algorithms were developed to reconstruct data despite patient motion. Thus, as the image data is obtained for a volume of tissue, images can be constructed in any plane, and with any slice thickness.

COMPUTED TOMOGRAPHY

ADJUSTMENT OF GRAYSCALE

- The grayscale display of the CT image can be adjusted to better evaluate different portions of the image (FIGURE 4–17).
- The CT window refers to the range of Hounsfield numbers that are displayed in the image.
- A *wide* window setting spreads the levels of gray of the image over a large range of Hounsfield numbers. This setting provides a broad range of tissue types, but offers less discrimination between tissues of relatively similar x-ray attenuation.
- A *narrow* window differentiates better between two tissues of similar x-ray attenuation, but demonstrates a smaller range of tissue types.
- The CT level refers to where the window is centered.
- The CT window and level are similar to the contrast and brightness controls on a black and white television.
- In practice, each image from a patient's study is evaluated at several standardized settings of window and level.

FIGURE 4–17

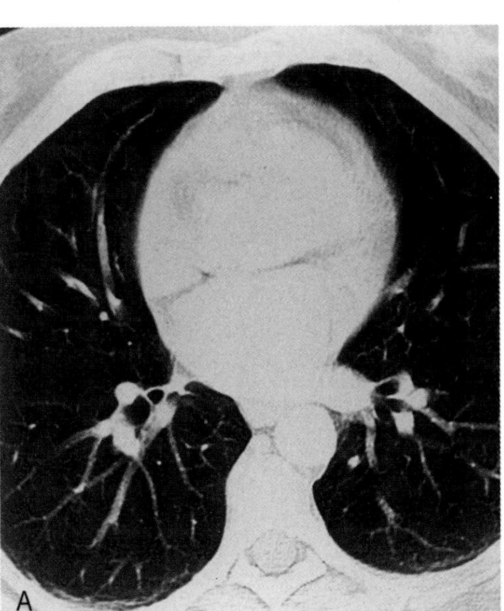

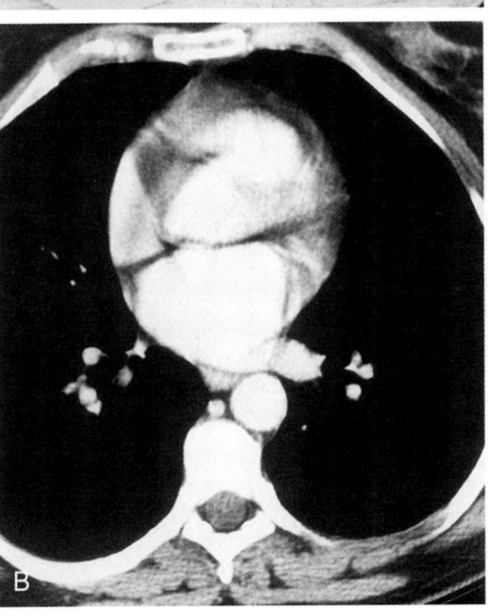

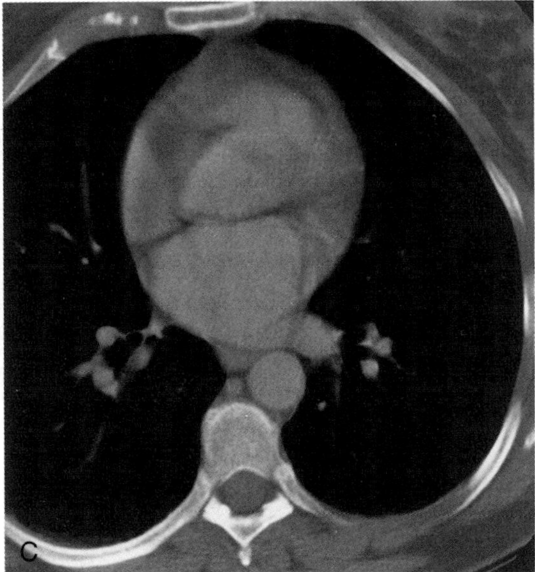

The three images are all at the same anatomic location. **A,** Standard lung window uses a level of −600 to −700 with a window width of 1000 to 1500 Hounsfield units. This window shows the lung parenchyma and bronchi well, but most of the detail of the mediastinum is lost. **B,** Mediastinal window. This window provides better discrimination of the mediastinal structures, but the lung parenchyma is not visualized. **C,** Bone window. On occasion this window may be used to improve detection of cortical destruction or fractures.

COMPUTED TOMOGRAPHY

CLINICAL EXAMPLES

Enhancement with Contrast Material

Contrast-enhanced CT demonstrates normal mediastinal anatomy with excellent detail (FIGURE 4–18).

FIGURE 4–18

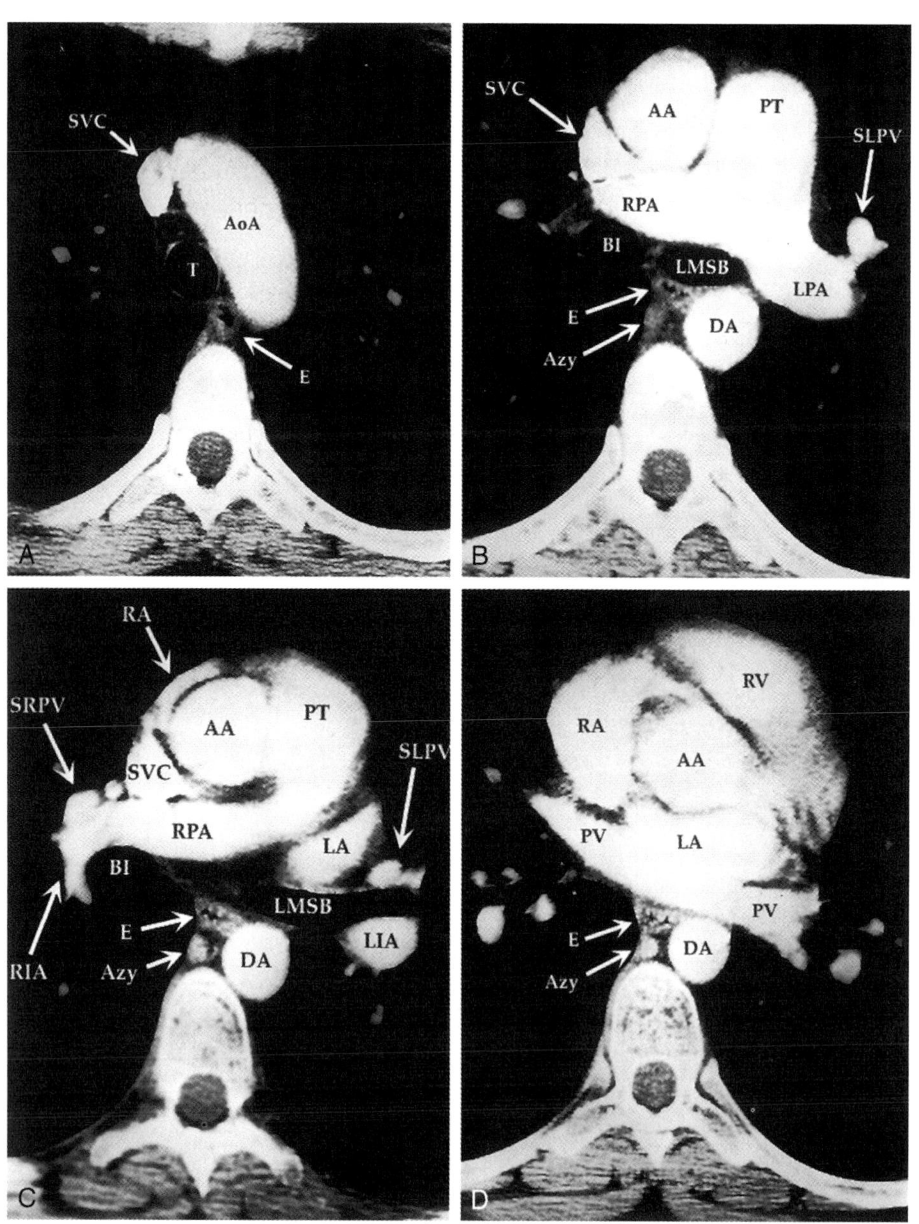

Contrast-enhanced CT. Key: AA, ascending aorta; AoA, aortic arch; Azy, azygos vein; BI, bronchus intermedius; DA, descending aorta; E, esophagus; LA, left atrium; LIA, left interlobar pulmonary artery; LMSB, left main-stem bronchus; LPA, left pulmonary artery; PT, pulmonary trunk; PV, pulmonary vein (confluence); RA, right atrium; RIA, right interlobar pulmonary artery; RPA, right pulmonary artery; RV, right ventricle; SLPV, superior left pulmonary vein; SRPV, superior right pulmonary vein; SVC, superior vena cava; T, trachea.

COMPUTED TOMOGRAPHY

CLINICAL EXAMPLES

Pulmonary Nodules

- Pulmonary nodules can be characterized by their morphologic appearance and attenuation.
- Images from three patients were obtained using a 1-mm slice collimations are illustrated in FIGURE 4–19.

FIGURE 4–19

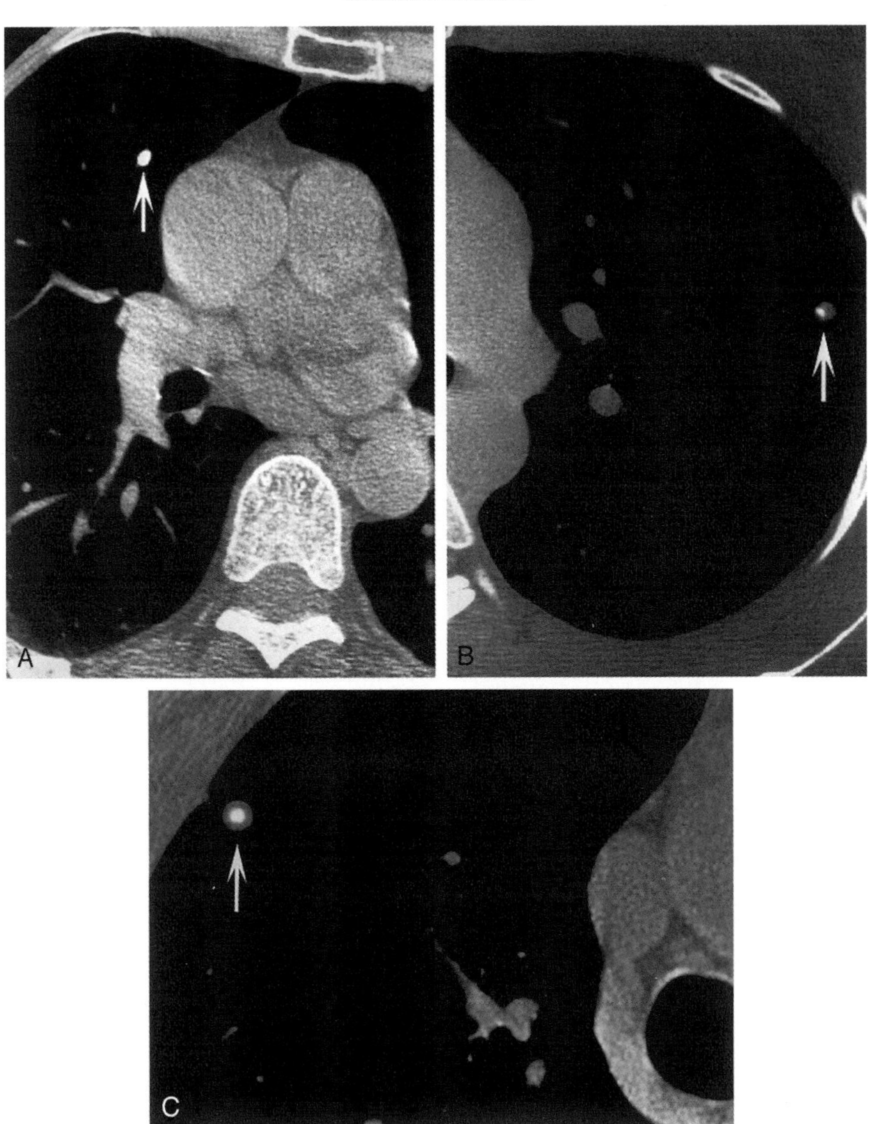

Pulmonary nodules. Pulmonary nodules can be characterized by their morphologic appearance and attenuation. Images from three different patients obtained using 1-mm slice collimation are illustrated. **A,** A nodule is seen in the right middle lobe (*arrow*). The nodule has the same density as bone and represents a calcified granuloma; no further evaluation is required.[21] **B,** Nodule within the left upper lobe (*arrow*). Only a small focus of calcification is seen and has an eccentric location. This pattern is not clearly benign, so the nodule should be either evaluated by other means (e.g., biopsy) or followed closely, as clinically indicated.[21, 23, 24] **C,** RUL nodule (*arrow*) contains a dense central calcification. The pattern of central calcification is benign and is seen usually following histoplasmosis infection.[21]

COMPUTED TOMOGRAPHY

CLINICAL EXAMPLES

Primary Lung Carcinoma

- CT is of great value in the assessment of primary lung carcinoma (FIGURE 4–20).
- Spiculation is also a common feature of malignancy; in one study, 88% of lesions demonstrating spiculated margins were malignant.[23]
- Other features associated with malignancy include size greater than 3 cm, age greater than 50 years old, and a history of smoking.[21, 23, 24]
- A central location is common with squamous and small cell carcinoma, whereas a peripheral location is typical of adenocarcinoma.[25]

FIGURE 4–20

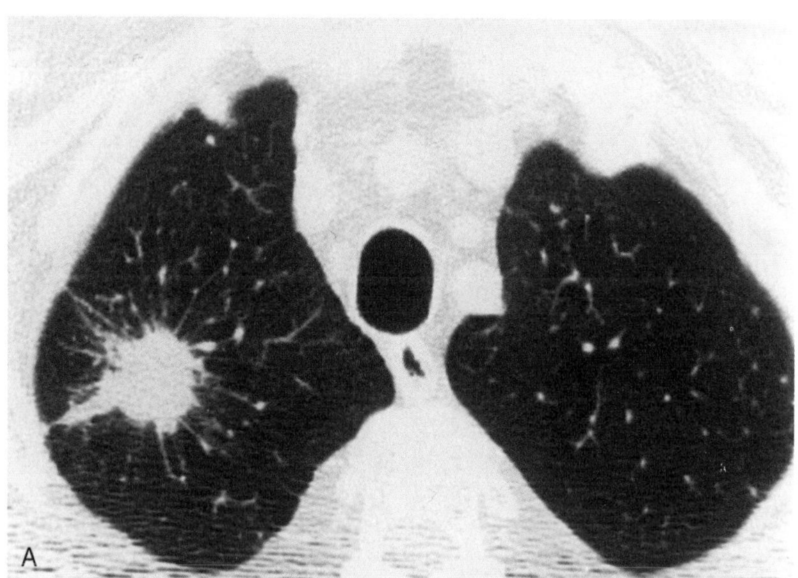

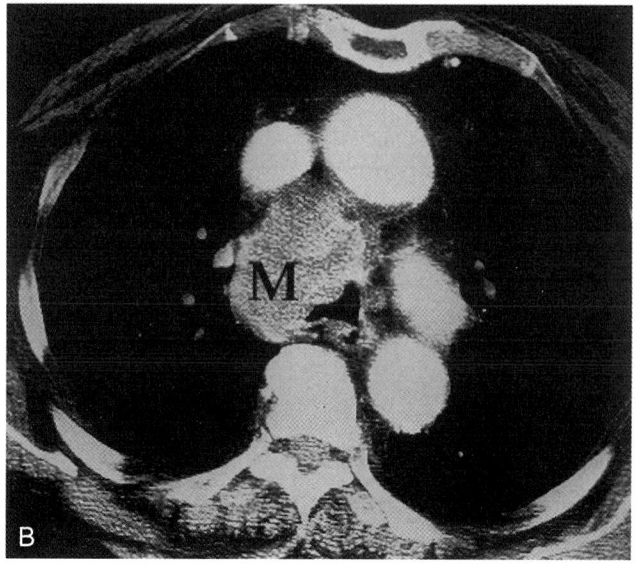

Primary lung carcinoma. **A,** A single image from a noncontrast CT demonstrates a right apical adenocarcinoma. Margins of the mass are spiculated, and the soft tissue windows did not demonstrate calcification. The peripheral location is typical of adenocarcinoma. (The patient's plain radiographs are shown in FIGURE 4–11.) **B,** An image from another patient, who presented initially with hemoptysis, shows a large, central, squamous cell carcinoma extending through the tracheal wall and into its lumen. Tumor (m) is centered in the pretracheal region. A central location is common with squamous and small cell carcinoma.

COMPUTED TOMOGRAPHY

CLINICAL EXAMPLES

Vascular Problems

• CT angiography (FIGURE 4–21) is useful in the diagnosis of vascular abnormalities such as pulmonary embolism (FIGURE 4–21*A*) and aortic dissection (FIGURE 4–21*B*).
• The increased speed of imaging with helical CT means that a series of scans can be obtained during peak vascular contrast enhancement.
• In the chest, this technique is used most frequently to evaluate the pulmonary arteries and the aorta.

Pulmonary Embolism

• CT angiography of the pulmonary arteries is highly sensitive in the detection of central pulmonary emboli (main, lobar, or segmental arteries) (FIGURE 4–21*A*).
• In one study, 132 of 135 emboli identified with angiography were demonstrated using CT by observers blinded to the result of the angiographic study.[26] In two cases CT results were considered inconclusive, and in only one case was an embolus missed.
• Specificity in this group was also very high (99%).
• CT angiography demonstrated 56 of 63 peripheral emboli.
• Although the detection of subsegmental emboli using CT is certainly less than for central emboli, the frequency of isolated subsegmental emboli was only 5%.

Aortic Dissection

• CT is often the only imaging study performed in the evaluation of suspected dissection (see FIGURE 4–21*B*).
• The CT diagnosis of aortic dissection is made by identifying two opacified lumens or an intimal flap.[27] Often the differential flow in the true and false channels is seen as a difference in the density of contrast medium in the two lumens.
• The reported sensitivity of CT in detecting dissection ranges from 90% to 100%, with associated specificities of 87% to 100%.[28, 29]
• The diagnostic accuracy of CT is the same as, or better than, that of aortography in the detection of aortic dissection, and CT offers the advantage of evaluating the mediastinum, pleural cavity, and pericardial spaces.
• False negative examinations are often related to technique, with motion, streak artifacts, or poor contrast opacification leading to the lack of visualization of a flap.[30]
• When the axial images do not clearly define the anatomy, three-dimensional reconstructions may help evaluate dissection.[31]

FIGURE 4–21

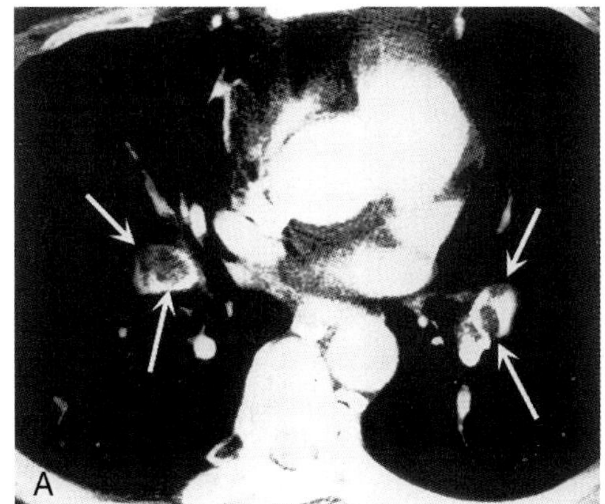

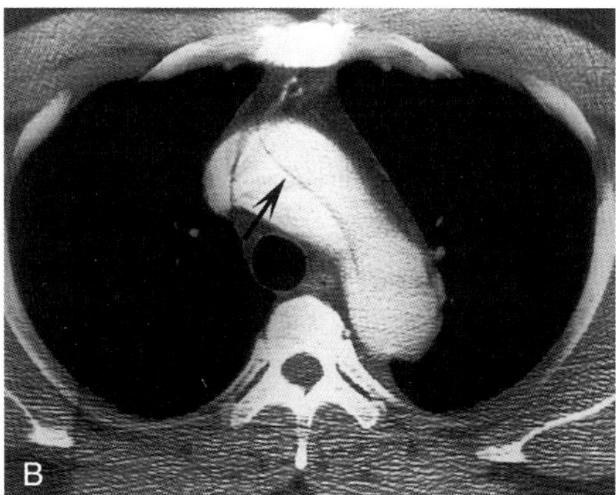

Vascular problems. **A,** Pulmonary embolism. A single image from a CT pulmonary angiogram in a patient with pulmonary embolism is shown. Dense contrast opacification of the vessels is present. Pulmonary emboli are identified within the left and right interlobar pulmonary arteries (*arrows*). Contrast material is seen surrounding the emboli, which confirms an intravascular location. **B,** Aortic dissection. CT angiogram of the aorta in a patient with dissection demonstrates a thin, curvilinear density extending through the arch. This is the intimal flap, surrounded by contrast material in the true and the false lumina. Extension of the dissection into the ascending aorta in this patient classifies this as a type A dissection.

COMPUTED TOMOGRAPHY

CLINICAL EXAMPLES

Polychondritis

Dynamic CT demonstrates focal collapse of the trachea in a patient with polychondritis (FIGURE 4–22).

FIGURE 4–22

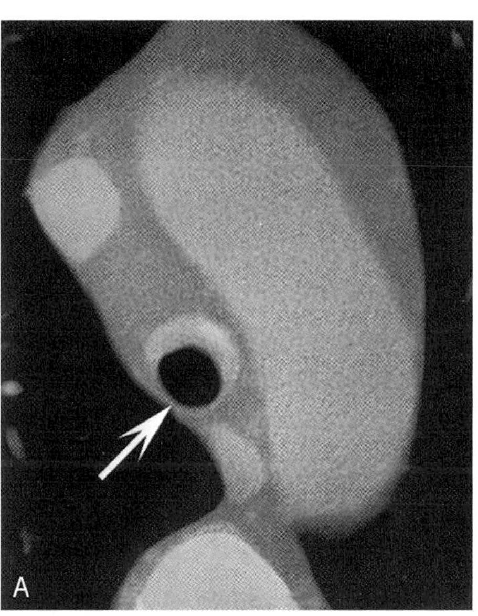

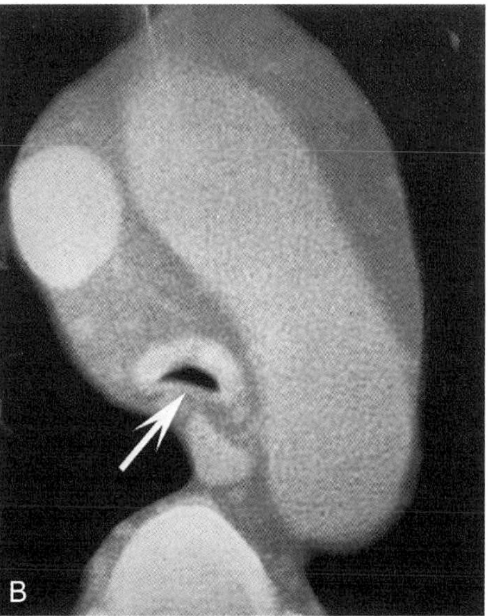

Polychondritis. Dynamic CT demonstrates focal collapse of the trachea in a patient with polychondritis. Using the cine mode of a helical CT scanner, images can be obtained every second at one anatomic level. In this example, 12 consecutive images were obtained during forced expiration. **A,** Image obtained at the beginning of expiration. **B,** Image obtained at end-expiration. The trachea (*arrow*) is seen to collapse with expiration, with near complete obliteration of the lumen. Both images were obtained at the level of the aortic arch. Although poorly visualized at this level and window setting, the anterior wall of the trachea is thickened, a finding commonly seen with polychondritis.[32]

COMPUTED TOMOGRAPHY

HIGH RESOLUTION CT

- HRCT provides images at spaced intervals (TABLE 4–1).
- A typical HRCT protocol images a 1-mm thick slice of lung at 20-mm intervals with the patient in both supine and prone positions.
- HRCT images assess only 10% of the lung parenchyma, at best.
- Usually HRCT is obtained to assess suspected diffuse lung disease, and the basic assumption is that representative abnormalities will be visible at one or more of the levels studied.
- One-millimeter thick images cannot be obtained contiguously throughout the lungs because of the danger of excessive radiation exposure to the patient.
- Focal lung disease is usually assessed using a standard CT or a few HRCT slices through the lesions.

Conventional versus HRCT Techniques

HRCT provides improved visualization of small structures and detailed anatomic features (FIGURE 4–23). A comparison of conventional and high-resolution techniques is provided in TABLE 4–1. Advantages and uses of these techniques are also highlighted in the following clinical examples.

TABLE 4–1

Comparison of Conventional and High Resolution CT

Characteristic	Conventional CT	High Resolution CT
Slice thickness	7 mm	1 mm
Spacing	Contiguous images	Every 20 mm
CT algorithm	Standard	High spatial frequency (e.g., bone)
Patient position	Supine	Supine and prone
Intravenous contrast material	Optional	No
Amount of lung imaged	100%	5–10%

FIGURE 4–23

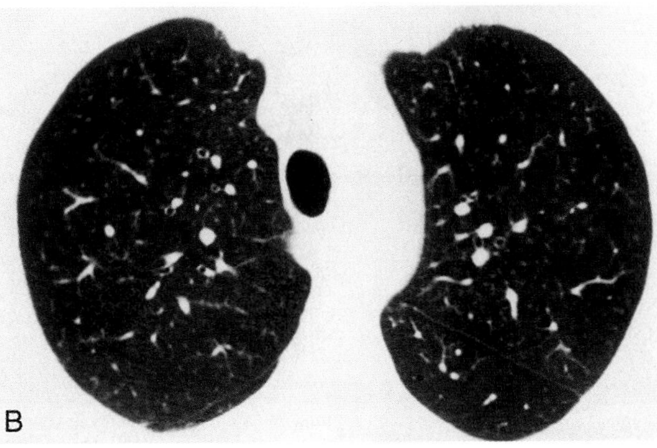

High-resolution computed tomography (HRCT). HRCT provides improved visualization of small structures and detailed anatomic features. The two images were obtained at the same level in the same patient using both conventional **(A)** and high-resolution **(B)** techniques. The HRCT image demonstrates bronchial walls and fissures with much greater clarity than conventional CT. There is also a better visualization of small vessels.

COMPUTED TOMOGRAPHY

HIGH RESOLUTION CT

Clinical Examples

Pulmonary Fibrosis

- The morphologic details of interstitial abnormalities can be demonstrated clearly with HRCT.
- HRCT images in three patients with pulmonary fibrosis are illustrated in FIGURE 4–24.

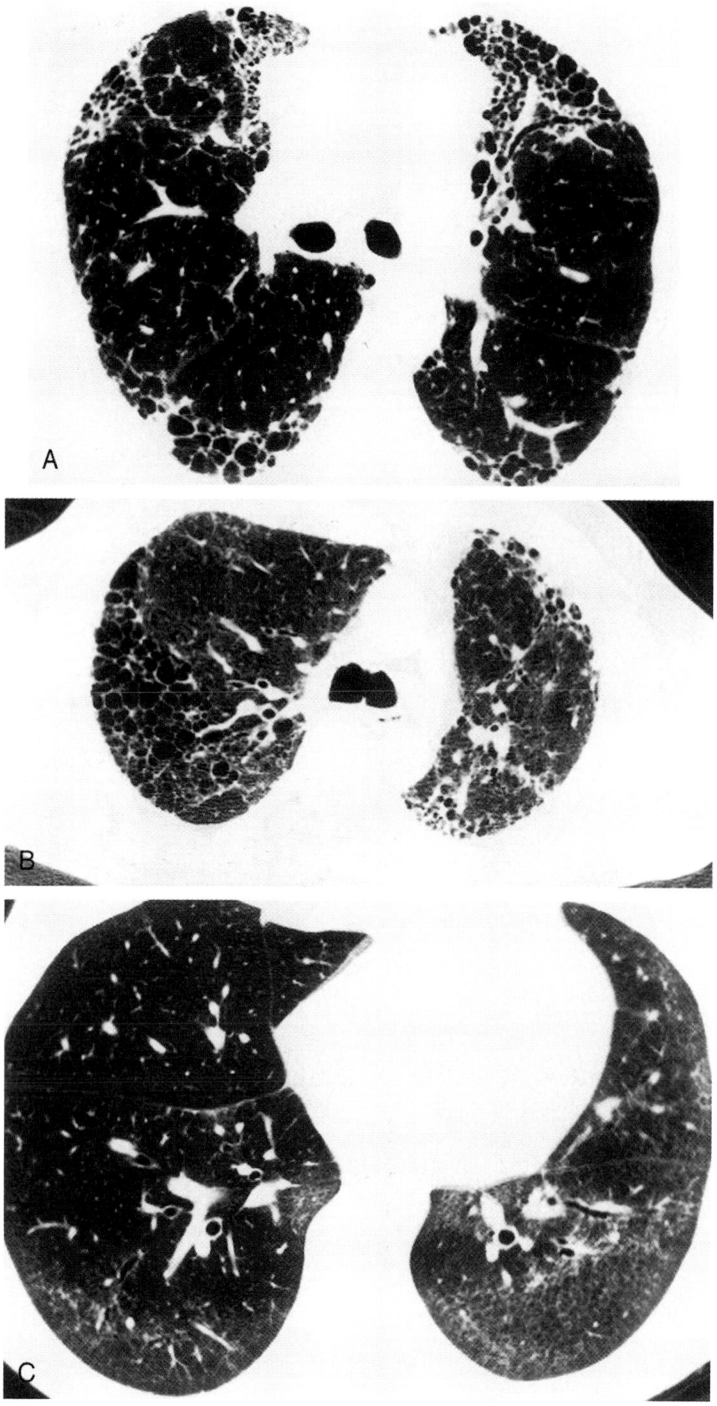

A

B

C

FIGURE 4–24

HRCT in pulmonary fibrosis. HRCT can clearly demonstrate the morphologic appearance of interstitial abnormalities. HRCT images are shown from three patients with pulmonary fibrosis. **A,** Idiopathic pulmonary fibrosis. Subpleural honeycombing is present. A dilated bronchus is seen within the lingula, consistent with traction bronchiectasis. Other images in this patient demonstrated similar findings. A basilar predominance was present. **B,** Chronic extrinsic allergic alveolitis. Peripheral honeycombing and traction bronchiectasis are present. Relatively equal involvement of the lung apices and lung bases. (The patient's plain radiographs are shown in Figure 4–7.) **C,** Early fibrosis in collagen vascular disease. A fine reticular pattern is seen within the lung bases, most prominently on the left. Associated with this is a generalized increase in parenchymal attenuation. This does not obscure the pulmonary vessels, and is termed ground-glass opacity. This finding suggests an active parenchymal inflammatory process when it is not associated with traction bronchiectasis.[33] HRCT is often used to assess disease activity in patients with known or suspected inflammatory disease by demonstrating the presence or absence of ground-glass opacity. The location of the increased attenuation also helps to guide lung biopsy, if necessary.

COMPUTED TOMOGRAPHY

HIGH RESOLUTION CT

Clinical Examples

Parenchymal Nodules

- HRCT can characterize patterns of lung involvement in patients with parenchymal nodules (FIGURE 4–25).
- The ability to define basic patterns of disease gives HRCT an improved diagnostic accuracy compared with plain films and conventional CT.[34]
- FIGURE 4–25*A* shows multiple parenchymal nodules.
  - These demonstrate a patchy distribution, which follows the bronchovascular bundles.
  - Nodules are also seen along the major fissures and in a subpleural location.
  - There is also thickening of the bronchial walls.
  - These features are typical of sarcoid,[35, 36] which was proved on transbronchial biopsy in this patient.
  - The primary radiographic differential for this appearance is lymphangitic carcinomatosis.[37]

FIGURE 4–25*B* also demonstrates multiple parenchymal nodules.

- In contrast with *A,* these nodules are uniformly distributed throughout the lungs.
- Nodules are seen along the fissures and in subpleural locations.
- This random distribution of nodules is commonly seen with hematogenous spread of infection, as occurs in tuberculosis, as in this patient, or malignancy.

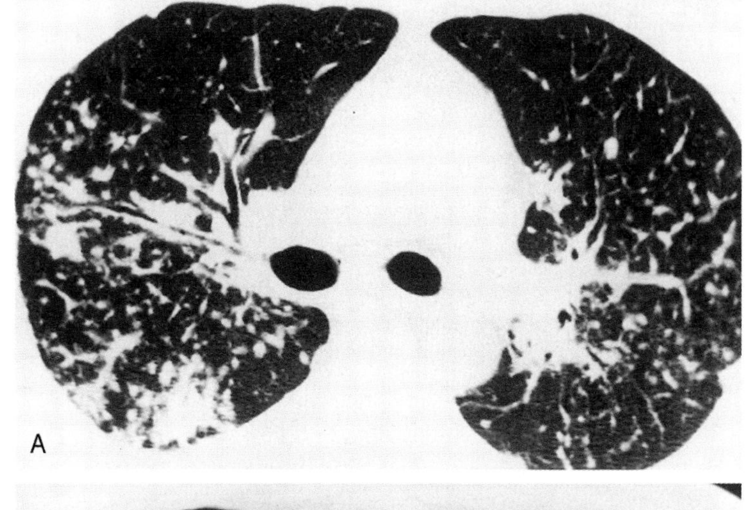

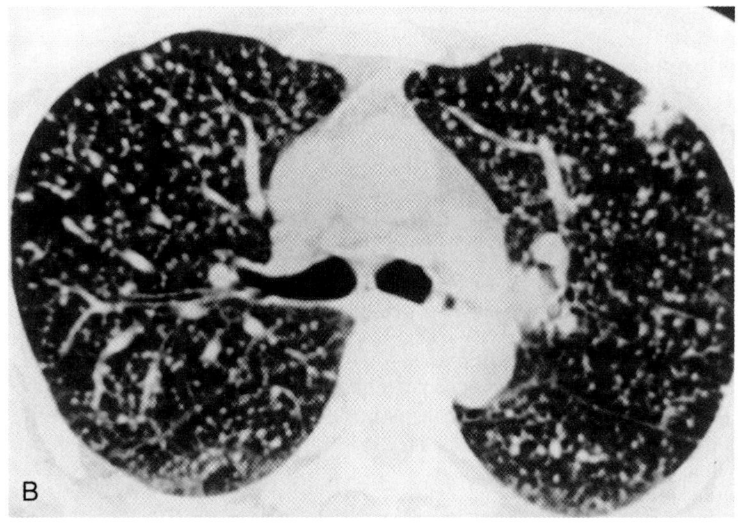

FIGURE 4–25

HCRT for parenchymal nodules. **A,** Multiple parenchymal nodules demonstrate a patchy distribution, which follows the bronchovascular bundles. Nodules are also seen along the major fissures and in a subpleural location. There is also thickening of the bronchial walls. These features are typical of sarcoid. **B,** Multiple parenchymal nodules. In contrast with the image shown in *A,* these nodules are uniformly distributed throughout the lungs. Nodules are seen along the fissures and in subpleurel locations. This random distribution of nodules is commonly seen with hematogenous spread of infection, such as tuberculosis, as in this patient, or malignancy.

COMPUTED TOMOGRAPHY

THREE-DIMENSIONAL RECONSTRUCTIONS

Clinical Examples

- CT image data can be manipulated to provide a three-dimensional representation of the scan volume (FIGURE 4–26).
- Although the reconstructed images do not contain any additional information, the change in format can be helpful in selected cases.

FIGURE 4–26

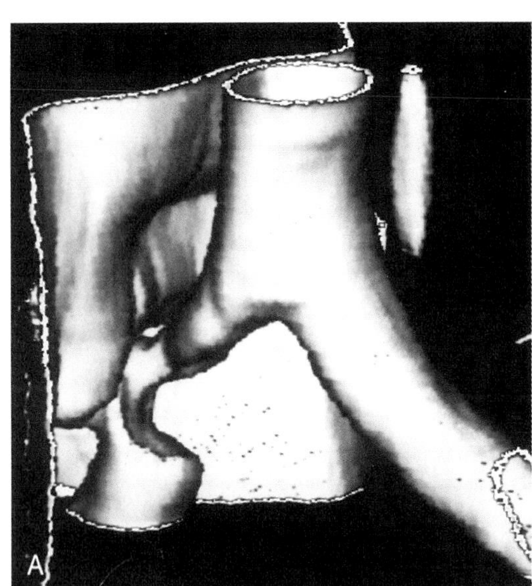

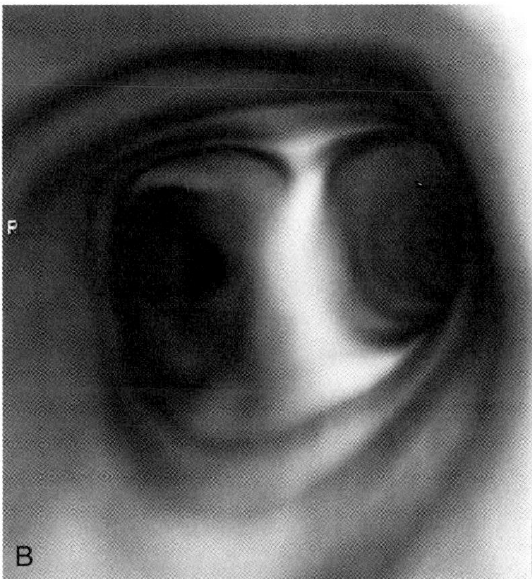

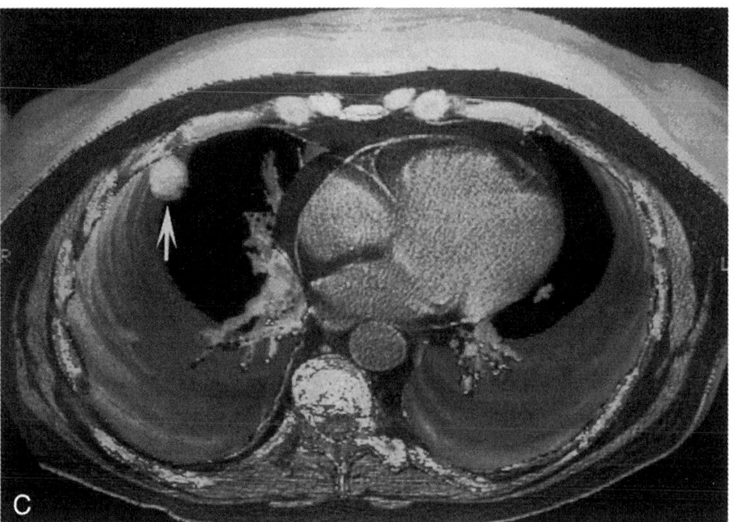

Three-dimensional reconstruction. **A,** Reconstruction of the trachea in a patient with an endobronchial carcinoid tumor. The image is a shaded surface reconstruction of the tracheal air column. A large irregularity is seen on the right, at the level of the bifurcation of the right main-stem bronchus to the right upper lobe bronchus and the bronchus intermedius. This represents the outline of the tumor. **B,** Reconstruction of the CT data provides a simulated bronchoscopic view. The carina is seen with the bifurcation into the right and left main-stem bronchi. The image is created by selecting a position within the lumen, determining the direction of view, and displaying a surface when there is a change in the Hounsfield number (from air to soft tissue). The point of view is arbitrary and can even be from beyond a lesion looking back. **C,** Three-dimensional reconstruction of 20-cm of image data from a conventional CT. The image is viewed from below. A partially calcified nodule within the RML (*arrow*).

MAGNETIC RESONANCE IMAGING

GENERAL

- Magnetic resonance imaging (MRI) can be used as a primary imaging modality in the thorax in some cases, or as an adjunct to other studies (TABLE 4–2).
- If MRI offers information that is only equivalent to CT, then CT is usually the more appropriate test owing to its greater availability and lower cost.
- Advantages of MRI relate to:
  - Ability to image in nontransaxial planes
  - A better distinction between different types of tissues
  - Imaging of vessels without the use of iodinated contrast material[38]

TABLE 4–2

MRI Used as a Primary or Secondary Modality

Primary Modality	Secondary Modality
Chest wall or mediastinal invasion by tumor	Diagnosis of mediastinal or hilar mass
Evaluation of superior sulcus tumor	Vascular invasion by mediastinal or hilar mass
Posterior mediastinal mass	Lung cancer staging
Differentiation of fibrosis and mass	Cardiac mass
Aortic dissection and aneurysm	Upper extremity venous thrombosis
Congenital anomalies of the great vessels	—
Paracardiac mass	—
Mediastinal venous obstruction	—
Brachial plexopathy	—

CLINICAL EXAMPLES

Lung Cancer

- In patients with primary lung cancer, MRI may be used to diagnose chest wall or mediastinal invasion (FIGURE 4–27).
- The extent of chest wall invasion may be shown better by MRI than by CT because of increased contrast between the tumor and the chest wall fat and muscle.[39]
- Imaging in the sagittal or coronal plane may also help to demonstrate chest wall or mediastinal invasion, particularly of superior sulcus tumors, for which involvement of the subclavian artery or brachial plexus may be poorly demonstrated on transaxial images.[40]
- MRI has been shown in small numbers of patients to be more accurate than CT in the detection of mediastinal and vascular invasion by lung carcinoma.[41]

FIGURE 4–27

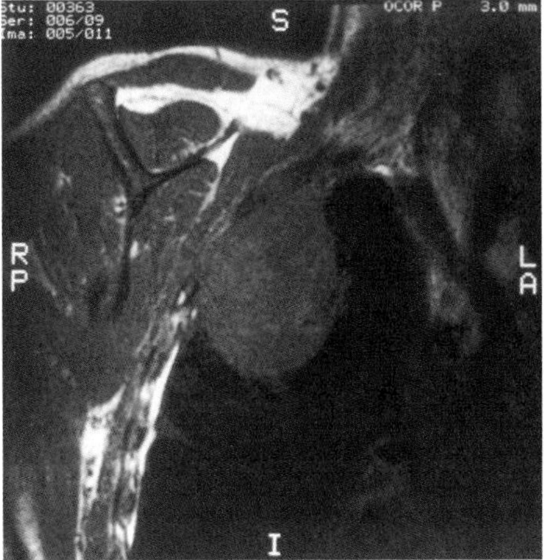

Magnetic resonance imaging (MRI) in lung cancer. A T_1-weighted coronal image demonstrates invasion of the chest wall by a bronchogenic carcinoma. The high signal from the extrapleural fat is seen inferiorly, but is obliterated at the level of the tumor.

MAGNETIC RESONANCE IMAGING

CLINICAL EXAMPLES

Parenchymal Lesions

- MRI is of limited value in the diagnosis of pulmonary parenchymal lesions because of its poorer spatial resolution and the lack of strong signal from the lung parenchyma.[42]
- This problem can be surmounted by the use of ultrashort echo sequences. Even these, however, generally provide less information than comparable CT images.

Mediastinal Lesions

- MRI can be useful in diagnosing mediastinal lesions (FIGURE 4–28).
- In the diagnosis of mediastinal and hilar masses, transaxial T_1- and T_2-weighted sequences are usually obtained.
- MRI is rarely the initial imaging choice, but it may be useful in evaluation of suspected vascular lesions, duplication cysts, and patients who are unable to tolerate contrast material.[38]
- MRI is very useful in the evaluation of posterior mediastinal and paravertebral masses.[43]
  - MRI is better than CT to evaluate extension of these masses into the spinal canal and cord involvement.
  - The ability to image in sagittal and coronal planes is also especially useful in characterizing these masses.

FIGURE 4–28

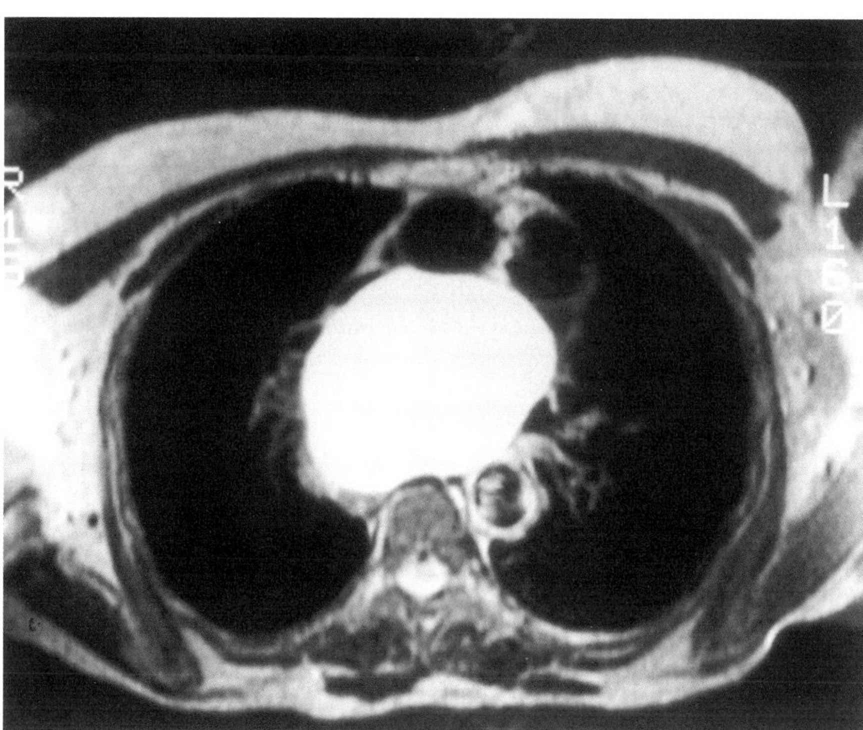

MRI in mediastinal lesions. A transaxial MRI demonstrates a large, subcarinal mass of high signal intensity. The high signal intensity on this T_2-weighted sequence is characteristic of a fluid-filled mass. The mass in this patient was a bronchogenic cyst.

MAGNETIC RESONANCE IMAGING

CLINICAL EXAMPLES

Aortic Dissection

- MRI offers several advantages over CT in the evaluation of suspected aortic dissection (FIGURE 4–29):
  - Ability to image in both transaxial (FIGURE 4–29*A*) and sagittal (FIGURE 4–29*B*) or coronal planes.
  - Ability to image without intravenous contrast medium administration.
  - Ability to detect aortic insufficiency and left ventricular function using cine MRI.
- MR imaging, however, is usually limited to the evaluation of hemodynamically stable patients, as the study takes longer to perform, and patients cannot be readily monitored during the study.
- Reported accuracy approaches 100%.[28, 44]
- Mediastinal, pericardial, and pleural spaces can also be evaluated in the same study.
- The key to diagnosis is the identification of an intimal flap.
- As an additional finding, the signal intensity within the false lumen on "bright-blood" sequences may be less than that of the true lumen due to a slower flow velocity.
- These differences can also be detected with velocity-sensitive sequences.
- The presence of thrombosis within the false channel is often best demonstrated using gradient echo sequences.
- MRI is also of value in the evaluation of the aorta following surgical repair for dissection.[45]

FIGURE 4–29

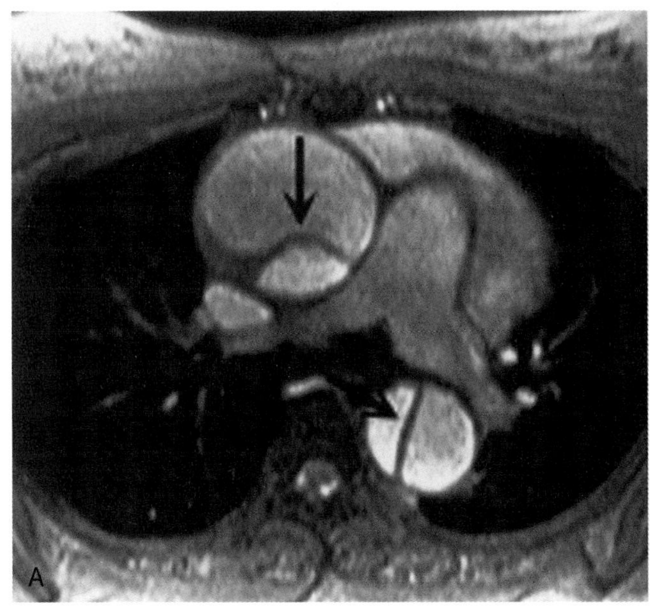

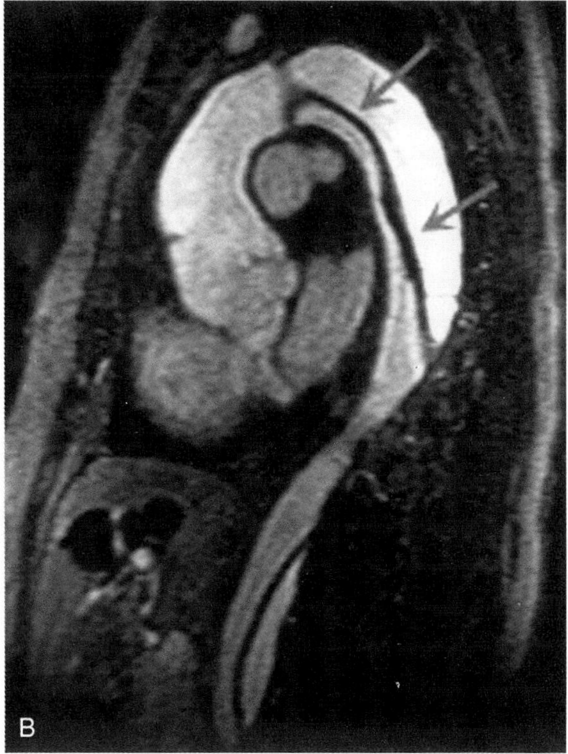

MRI in aortic dissection. Images can be presented in both the transaxial **(A)** and sagittal **(B)** or coronal planes. The key to diagnosis is the identification of an intimal flap (*arrows*). As an additional finding, the signal intensity within the false lumen on "bright-blood" sequences may be less than that of the true lumen because of a slower flow velocity. These differences can also be detected with velocity-sensitive sequences. The presence of thrombosis within the false channel is often best demonstrated using gradient echo sequences.

MAGNETIC RESONANCE IMAGING

CLINICAL EXAMPLES

Regional Ventilation

- MRI can be used to assess regional lung ventilation (FIGURE 4–30).
- Inhaled laser polarized xenon and helium gases have been used to provide sufficient signal from the airways.[46] However, these gases are expensive to produce and have a narcotic effect at high concentration.
- Inhaled oxygen has been used as the contrast agent[47] and has several advantages;
  - Molecular oxygen contains two unpaired electrons, which makes it weakly paramagnetic.
  - The inhaled oxygen dissolves within the lung parenchyma and pulmonary capillary bed.
  - The paramagnetic effect of the dissolved oxygen can be detected using specialized MRI sequences.

The image demonstrates the change in signal intensity in the lungs of a normal volunteer following the inhalation of 100% oxygen for 30 seconds.

- The enhancement is a function of both regional ventilation and the movement of oxygen from the alveolus to the capillary.
- Further development of this technique may allow for noninvasive assessment of region lung function using MRI.

FIGURE 4–30

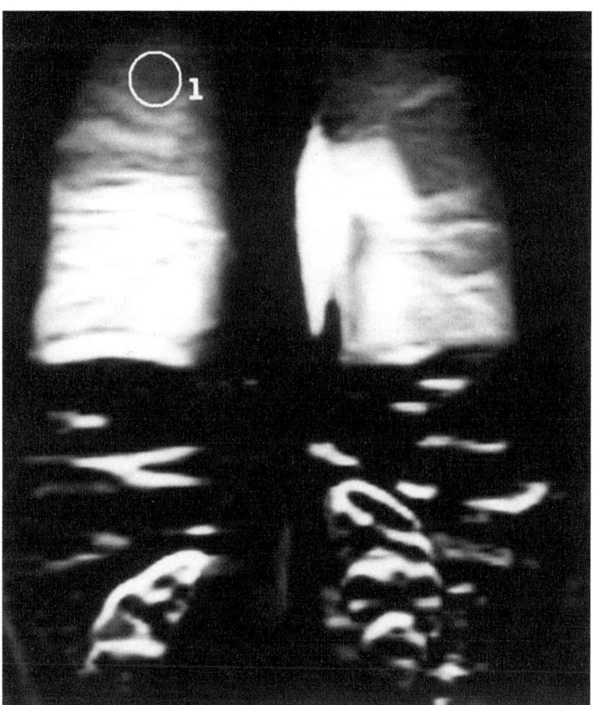

MRI in regional ventilation. The paramagnetic effect of the dissolved oxygen can be detected using specialized MR sequences. The image demonstrates the change in signal intensity in the lungs of a normal volunteer following the inhalation of 100% oxygen for 30 seconds. The enhancement is a function of both regional ventilation and the movement of oxygen from the alveolus to the capillary.

REFERENCES

1. Crapo R, Montague T, Armstrong J: Inspiratory lung volume achieved on routine chest films. Invest Radiol 14: 137–140, 1979.

2. Wandtke J: Newer imaging methods in chest radiography. J Thorac Imag 5:1–9, 1990.

3. Logan P, Tunney T, McCoy CT, Masterson J: Comparison of a new dual characteristic film-screen system (Insight) with a standard film-screen system for chest radiology. Br J Radiol 67:162–165, 1994.

4. MacMahon H, Vyborny C: Technical advances in chest radiography. Am J Radiol 163:1049–1059, 1994.

5. Wiener M, Garay S, Leitman B, et al: Imaging of the intensive care patient. Clin Chest Med 12:169–195, 1991.

6. Felson B, Felson H: Localization of intrathoracic lesions by means of the postero-anterior roentgenogram: The silhouette sign. Radiology 55:363–73, 1950.

7. Felson B: A new look at pattern recognition of diffuse pulmonary disease. Am J Radiol 133:183–189, 1979.

8. Gruden J, Huang L, Webb W, et al: AIDS-related Kaposi sarcoma of the lung: Radiographic findings and staging system with bronchoscopic correlation. Radiology 195: 545–552, 1995.

9. Milne E, Pistolesi M, Miniati M, Giuntini C: The radiologic distinction of cardiogenic and noncardiogenic edema. Am J Radiol 144:879–894, 1985.

10. Nicklaus T, Stowell D, Christiansen W, Renzetti A Jr: The accuracy of the roentgenologic diagnosis of chronic pulmonary emphysema. Am Rev Respir Dis 93:889–899, 1966.

11. Greene R: "Saber-sheath" trachea: Relation to chronic obstructive pulmonary disease. Am J Radiol 130:441–445, 1978.

12. Miller J Jr: Chest radiographic evaluation of diffuse interstitial disease. Review of a dying art: Thoracic imaging. Soc Thorac Radiol p 335–341, 1996.

13. Cook P, Wells I, McGavin C: The distribution of pulmonary shadowing in farmer's lung. Clin Radiol 39:31–47, 1988.

14. Fraser R, Paré J: Synopsis of Diseases of the Chest. 2nd ed. Philadelphia, WB Saunders, 1994, pp. 521–530.

15. Blackmore C, Black W, Dallas R, Crow H: Pleural fluid volume estimation: A chest radiograph prediction rule. Acta Radiol 3:103–109, 1996.

16. Aberle D, Hansell D, Huang H: Current status of digital projection radiography of the chest. J Thorac Imag 5:10–20, 1990.

17. Fuhrman C, Gur D, Schaetzing R: High-resolution digital imaging with storage phospors. J Thorac Imag 5: 21–30, 1990.

18. Goodman L, Foley W, Wilson C, et al: Pneumothorax and other lung diseases: Effect of altered resolution and edge enhancement on diagnosis with digitized radiographs. Radiology 167:83–88, 1988.

19. MacMahon J, Vyvorny C, Sabeti V, et al: The effect of digital unsharp masking on the detectability of interstitial infiltrates and pneumothoraces. Proceedings of the International Society of Optical Engineers 555:246–252, 1985.

20. Boyd D, Parker D, Goddsitt M: Principles of computed tomography. *In* Moss A, Gamsu G, Genant H (eds): Computed tomography of the body with magnetic resonance imaging. 2nd ed. Philadelphia, WB Saunders, 1992, pp. 1355–1383.

21. Webb W: Radiologic evaluation of the solitary pulmonary nodule. Am J Radiol 154:701–708, 1990.

22. Heiken J, Brink J, Vannier M: Spiral (helical) CT. Radiology 189:647–656, 1993.

23. Siegelman S, Khouri N, Leo F, et al: Solitary pulmonary nodules: CT assessment. Radiology 160:307–312, 1986.

24. Midthun D, Swenson S, Jett J: Approach to the solitary pulmonary nodule. Mayo Clin Proc 68:378–385, 1993.

25. Rosado-de-Christenson M, Templeton P, Moran C: Bronchogenic carcinoma: Radiologic pathologic correlation. Radiographics 14:429–446, 1994.

26. Remy-Jardin M, Remy J, Deschild F, et al: Diagnosis of pulmonary embolism with spiral CT: Comparison with pulmonary angiography and scintigraphy. Radiology 200: 699–706, 1996.

27. Higgins C: Thoracic Aortic Disease. New York, Lippincott, 1992.

28. Cigarroa J, Isselbacher E, DeSanctis R, Eagle K: Diagnostic imaging in the evaluation of suspected aortic dissection. N Engl J Med 328:35–43, 1993.

29. Sommer T, Fehske W, Holzknecht N, et al: Aortic dissection: A comparative study of diagnosis with spiral CT, multiplanar transesophageal echocardiography, and MR imaging. Radiology 199:347–352, 1996.

30. Silverman P, Cooper C, Wietman A, Zeman R: Helical CT: Practical considerations and potential pitfalls. Radiographics 15:25–36, 1995.

31. Zeman R, Berman P, Silverman P, et al: Diagnosis of aortic dissection: Value of helical CT with multiplanar reformation and three-dimensional rendering. Am J Radiol 164:1375–1380, 1995.

32. Eng J, Sabanthan S: Airway complications in relapsing polychondritis. Ann Thoracic Surg 51:686–692, 1991.

33. Remy-Jardin M, Giraud F, Remy J, et al: Importance of ground-glass attenuation in chronic diffuse infiltrative lung disease: Pathologic-CT correlation. Radiology 189: 693–698, 1993.

34. Mathieson J, Mayo J, Staples C, Muller N: Chronic diffuse infiltrative lung disease: Comparison of diagnostic accuracy of CT and chest radiography. Radiology 171:111–116, 1989.

REFERENCES

35. Miller B, Rosado-de-Christenson M, McAdams H, Fishback N: Thoracic sarcoidosis: Radiologic-pathologic correlation. Radiographics 15:42–437, 1995.

36. Nishimura K, Itoh H, Kitaichi M, et al: Pulmonary sarcoidosis: Correlation of CT and histopathologic findings. Radiology 189:105–109, 1993.

37. Corcoran H, Renner W, Milstein M: Review of high-resolution CT of the lung. Radiographics 12:917–939, 1992.

38. Webb A, Sostman H: Clinical applications of magnetic resonance to thoracic disease. *In* Cutillo A (ed): Application of magnetic resonance to the study of the lung. New York, Futura Publishing, 1996, pp. 439–475

39. Haggar A, Pearlberg J, Froelich J, et al: Chest wall invasion by carcinoma of the lung: Detection by MR imaging. J Radiol 148:1075–1078, 1987.

40. Webb W, Jensen BG, Gamsu G, Sollitto R, Moore E: Coronal magnetic reonance imaging of the chest: Normal and abnormal. Radiology 153:729–735, 1984.

41. Webb A, Gatsonis C, Zerhouni E, et al: CT and MR imaging in staging non–small cell bronchogenic carcinoma: Report of the Radiologic Diagnostic Oncology Group. Radiology 178:705–713, 1991.

42. Müller N, Gamsu G, Webb W: Pulmonary nodules: Detection using magnetic resonance and computed tomography. Radiology 155:687–690, 1985.

43. Weinreb J, Naidich D: Thoracic magnetic resonance imaging. Clin Chest Med 12:33–54, 1991.

44. Nienaber C, Von Kodolitsch Y, Nicolas V, et al: The diagnosis of thoracic aortic dissection by noninvasive imaging procedures. N Engl J Med 328:1–9, 1993.

45. Slavotinek J, Kendall S, Flower C, et al: Radiological evaluation of the ascending aorta following repair of type A dissection. Cardiovasc Intervent Radiol 16:293–296, 1993.

46. Albert M, Cates C, Driehuys B, et al: Biological magnetic resonance imaging using laser-polarized ^{129}Xe. Nature 370:199–207, 1994.

47. Edelman R, Hatabu H, Tadamura E, et al: Non-invasive assessment of regional ventilation in the human lung using oxygen-enhanced magnetic resonance imaging. Nature Med 2:1236–1239, 1996.

Nuclear Medicine Techniques and Applications

David C. Price, M.D.

NUCLEAR MEDICINE APPLICATIONS

INTRODUCTION

Kinetic Studies of Radioactive Gases

- Knipping et al. introduced multiprobe detector methods for kinetic studies of pulmonary function using radioactive gases in 1955.[1]
- West et al. extended these studies with positron-emitters ^{11}CO (carbon monoxide), ^{13}N (nitrogen), and ^{15}O (oxygen) at Hammersmith in 1962.[2]
- David Bates and his group studied ^{133}Xe (xenon) in Montreal in 1962.[3]
- These investigators were limited to analysis of data derived from regional probes.

ADVANCES IN INSTRUMENTATION

- Greater diversity of radiotracer techniques for pulmonary imaging was made possible by three major advances:
  - The rectilinear scanner by Ben Cassen in 1951.[4]
  - The scintillation camera by Hal Anger in 1958.[5]
  - The more recent addition of state-of-the-art minicomputers utilizing the digitizable analog output of Anger's scintillation camera (FIGURE 5–1).

Commercial development of solid-state detector cameras led to improved energy and spatial resolution in more compact detectors.
- Continued improvement in positron-emission tomographic (PET) scanners led to their much broader introduction into standard diagnostic imaging for routine applications.

FIGURE 5–1

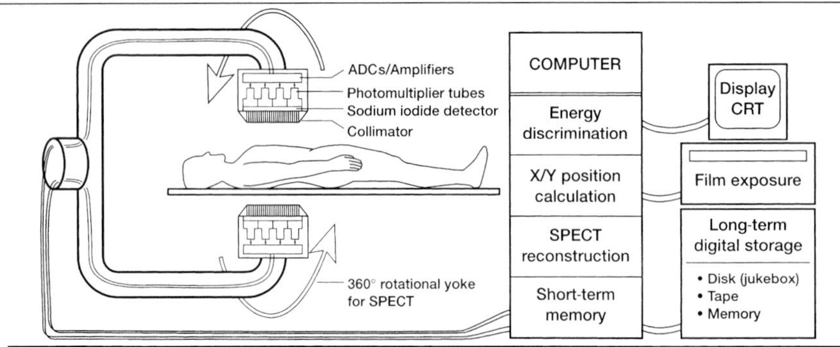

A

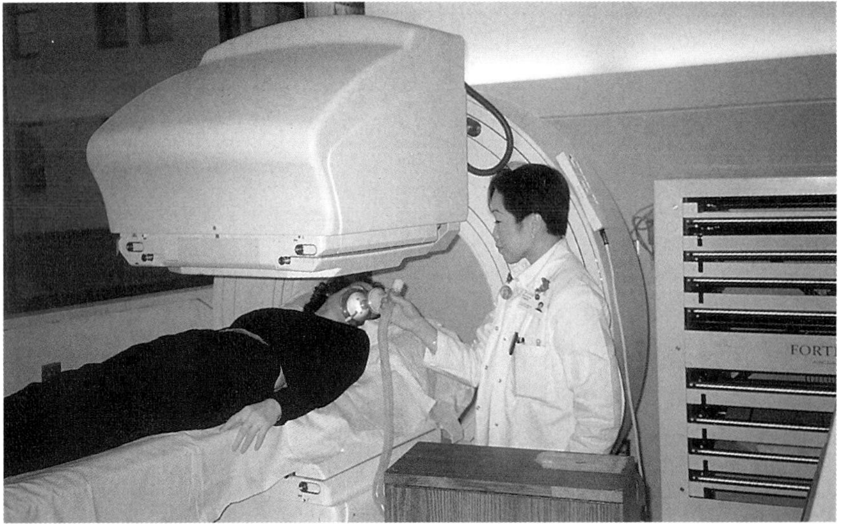

B

A, Equipment system components involved in the acquisition, image processing, and image display of pulmonary ventilation and perfusion scans, including single photon emission computed tomography (SPECT) images (ADC, analog-to-digital convertor). **B,** Photograph of a ^{133}Xe ventilation scan under way using a state-of-the-art dual-headed scintillation camera and a closed rebreathing system for the radioxenon.

NUCLEAR MEDICINE APPLICATIONS

ADVANCES IN INSTRUMENTATION

Recent Advances in Radiopharmaceuticals

- Initial studies used radioactive gases to evaluate ventilatory function.
- In 1964 Taplin developed macroaggregated human serum albumin (MAA) labeled with ^{131}I (iodine) and subsequently ^{99m}Tc (technetium) for pulmonary perfusion imaging.[6]
- ^{99m}Tc-MAA has remained the standard pulmonary perfusion agent for diagnostic imaging for many years.
- Improved ventilatory radiopharmaceuticals have been developed, including:
  - Radiolabeled aerosols in kit form (generally utilizing ^{99m}Tc-DTPA [diethylene triaminepenta-acetic acid] as the tracer)
  - ^{81}Rb-^{81m}Kr (krypton) generators for multiview pulmonary inhalation imaging
  - ^{99m}Tc pertechnetate gas generators for a different approach to inhalation imaging using dry radiolabeled particulates

LUNG SCAN

GENERAL INDICATIONS

- Clinical assessment for acute pulmonary embolism is the most common reason to request a lung scan in a diagnostic nuclear medicine department.
- A lung scan is also useful to diagnose massive pulmonary embolism.[7]

DEVELOPMENT OF SOPHISTICATED ALGORITHMS

- Sophisticated algorithms have been developed to integrate pulmonary perfusion, pulmonary ventilation, and the chest radiograph into probability ranges for acute pulmonary embolism.
- Barbara McNeil developed the first fully comprehensive algorithm in 1976.[8]
- Biello et al. used an early meta-analysis to refine this algorithm.[9] TABLE 5–1 summarizes different probability data derived from the Biello data.
- The PIOPED (NIH Prospective Investigation of Pulmonary Embolism Diagnosis) study created the most advanced form of the algorithm.[10–12] TABLE 5–2 summarizes different probability data from the PIOPED study.

LUNG SCAN

DEVELOPMENT OF SOPHISTICATED ALGORITHMS

TABLE 5-1

The Biello Criteria for the Probability of Acute Pulmonary Embolism

High Probability (87–92%)

- One or more large segmental perfusion defects (>75% of the volume of a segment) with normal regional ventilation and x-ray (p = 92%)
- Two or more moderate-sized segmental perfusion defects (25–75% of the volume of a segment) with normal regional ventilation and chest radiograph (p = 92%)
- Either of the above with a radiographic abnormality substantially larger than the perfusion defect(s) (p = 87%)

Intermediate Probability (20–33%)

- One moderate-sized subsegmental perfusion defect with normal ventilation and x-ray (p = 33%)
- One or more large or two or more moderate-sized segmental/subsegmental perfusion defects with normal ventilation and matching x-ray abnormalities (p = 20%)
- One or more large or two or more moderate-sized segmental/subsegmental perfusion defects with diffuse severe airway disease (p = 20%)

Low Probability (0–10%)

- One or more small subsegmental perfusion defects (<25% of the volume of a segment) (p = 5%)
- One or more moderate or large perfusion defects with x-ray abnormalities substantially larger than the defects in each case (p = 10%)
- One or more moderate or large perfusion defects with focal V/Q matches and a normal x-ray (p = 5%)

Very Low Probability (<1%)

- Completely normal perfusion scan (p = <1%)

TABLE 5-2

The PIOPED Criteria for the Probability of Acute Pulmonary Embolism

High Probability

- Two or more large segmental perfusion defects (>75% of the volume of a segment) with normal regional ventilation and chest radiograph
- Two or more large segmental perfusion defects substantially larger than corresponding ventilation or x-ray abnormalities
- Two or more moderate subsegmental perfusion defects (25–75% of a segment) and one large segmental perfusion defect with normal regional ventilation and x-ray
- Four or more moderate subsegmental perfusion defects with normal regional ventilation and x-ray

Intermediate Probability

- Not in the normal, very low, low, or high categories
- Borderline high or borderline low
- Difficult to classify in one of the other categories

Low Probability

- One or more perfusion defects in the otherwise high or intermediate categories, but associated with a substantially larger x-ray abnormality
- Four or more subsegmental perfusion defects (<25% of the volume of a segment) with a normal x-ray
- One to four moderate or large segmental perfusion defects in one lung, or one to three such defects in one lung region, associated with matching or larger ventilation defects and normal x-ray or substantially smaller x-ray regional abnormalities
- One or more small nonsegmental perfusion defects (e.g., elevated hemidiaphragm, prominent pulmonary hilum, small pleural effusion, cardiomegaly) (one moderate subsegmental perfusion defect with normal ventilation and x-ray: subsequent studies showed p = 33%)

Very Low Probability

- None to three small subsegmental perfusion defects with a normal x-ray

Normal

- Completely normal perfusion scan
- Uniform perfusion scan outline exactly matching the pulmonary outline on a current chest radiograph

NORMAL LUNG SCAN

ANATOMY OF LUNG LOBES AND SEGMENTS

- To identify segmental versus subsegmental or nonsegmental perfusion defects in these algorithms, it is essential to know lung segmental anatomy.
- FIGURE 5–2 illustrates the lobar and segmental anatomy of the lungs.
- FIGURES 5–3 and 5–4 illustrate the patterns of normal ventilation (^{133}Xe) and normal perfusion (^{99m}Tc-MAA), respectively, in one normal subject.
- In the ventilation study, a 30-second image is obtained following inhalation of a single breath of radioxenon.
- Then, a 30-second image is obtained after 1 to 3 minutes of rebreathing in a closed system.
- Finally, a sequence of 30-second images is obtained during at least 3 minutes while room air is inhaled to wash out the xenon-labeled air.

FIGURE 5–2

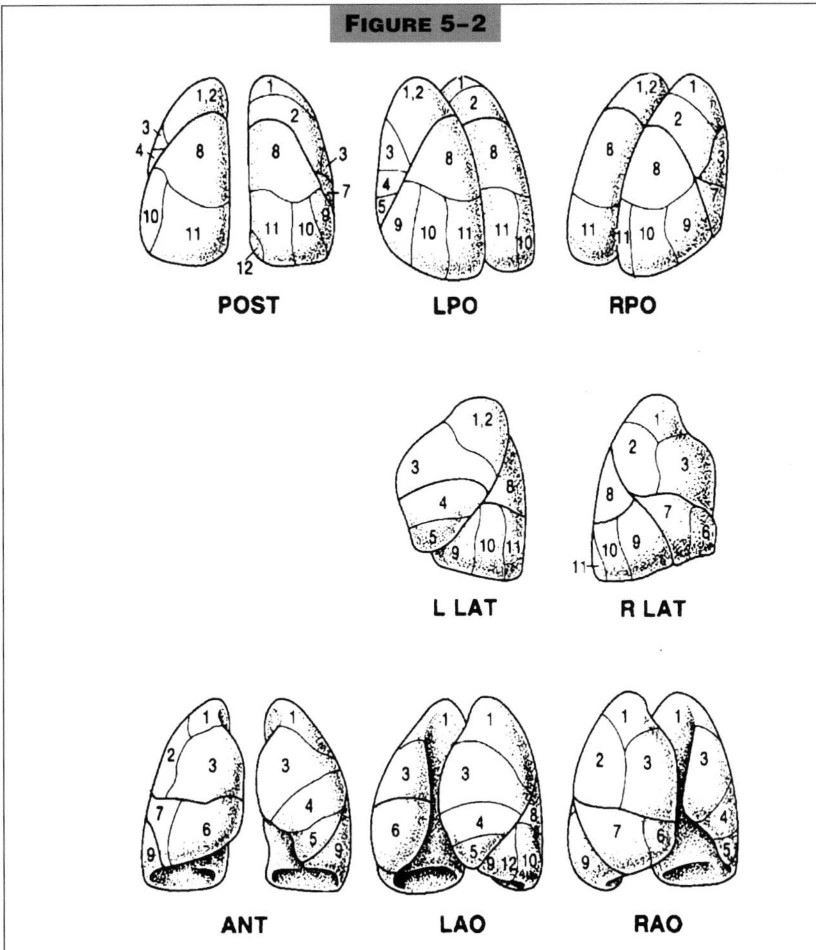

Segmental anatomy of the lungs. Upper lobes: 1, Apical segment. 2, Posterior segment. 3, Anterior segment. Lingula: 4, Superior segment. 5, Inferior segment. Right middle lobe: 6, Medial segment. 7, Lateral segment. Lower lobes: 8, Superior segment. 9, Anterior basal segment. 10, Lateral basal segment. 11, Posterior basal segment. 12, Medial basal segment (generally not visible on planar scintigraphy). POST, Posterior; LPO, Left posterior oblique; RPO, right posterior oblique; L LAT, left lateral; R LAT, right lateral; ANT, anterior; LAO, left anterior oblique; RAO, right anterior oblique. (From Spies WG: Ventilation/perfusion scintigraphy. *In* Henkin RE et al: Nuclear Medicine. St. Louis, Mosby, 1966, p 1398.)

NORMAL LUNG SCAN

ANATOMY OF LUNG LOBES AND SEGMENTS

FIGURE 5–3

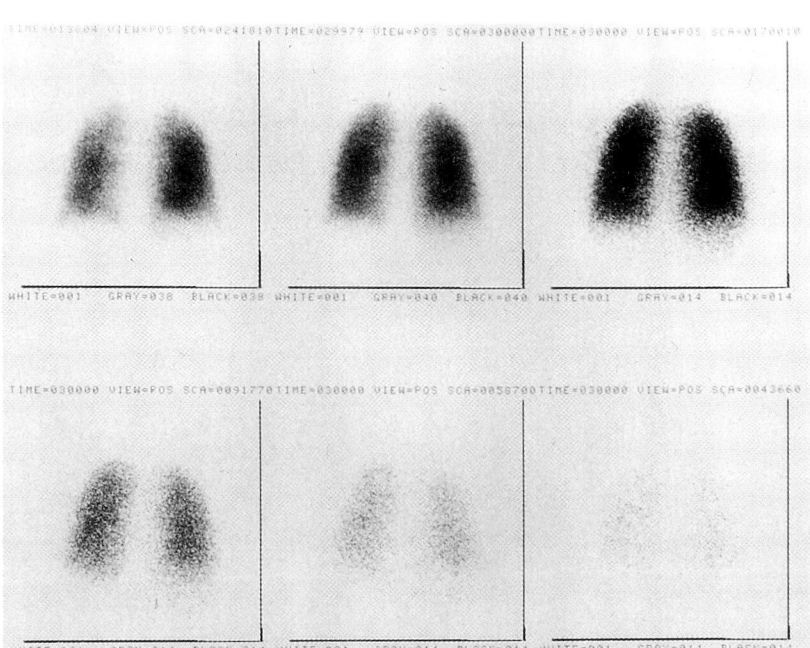

Normal posterior ^{133}Xe pulmonary ventilation scan in one normal subject. In this study, a 30-second image was obtained following inhalation of a single breath of radioxenon. Then, a second image was obtained after 1 to 3 minutes of rebreathing in a closed system. Finally, a sequence of 30-second images was obtained over at least 3 minutes during a washout phase as room air was inhaled to replace the xenon-labeled air. (Images progress from upper left to lower right.)

NORMAL LUNG SCAN

ANATOMY OF LUNG LOBES AND SEGMENTS

FIGURE 5–4

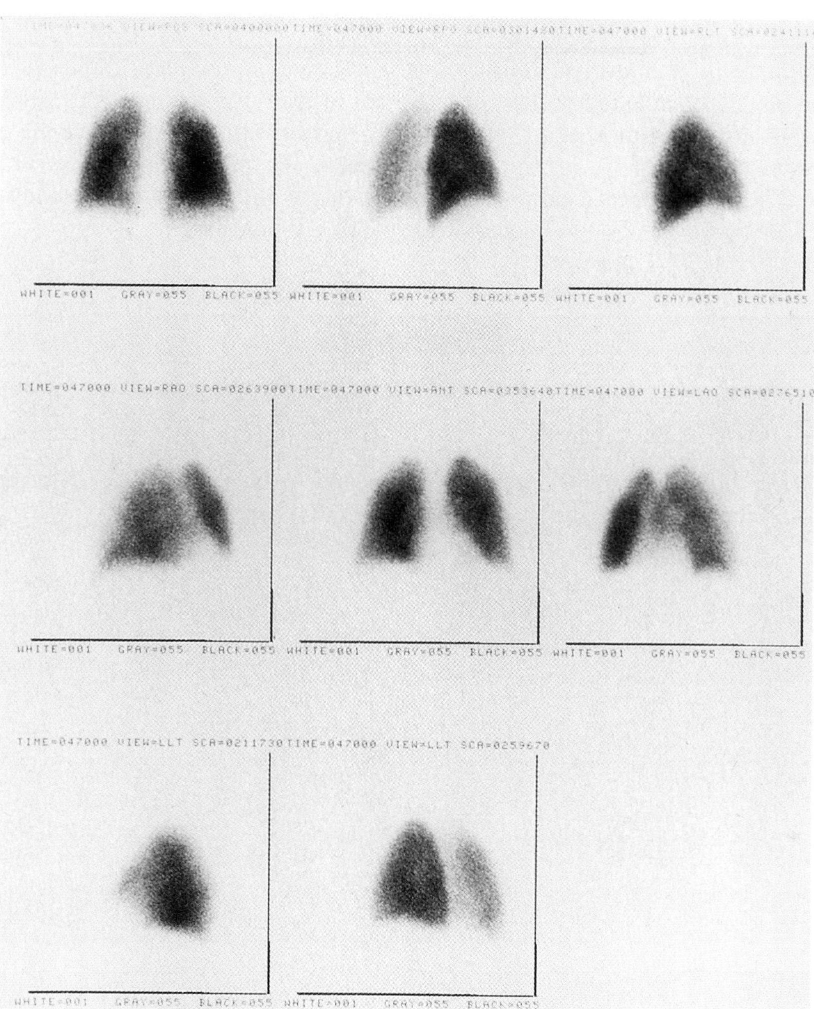

Normal planar pulmonary perfusion images with ^{99m}Tc-macroaggregated albumin in the same normal subject studied in FIGURE 5–3. The image sequence (from upper left to lower right) is posterior, right posterior oblique, right lateral, right anterior oblique, anterior, left anterior oblique, left lateral, and left posterior oblique.

SINGLE-PHOTON EMISSION COMPUTED TOMOGRAPHY

- Imaging provided by single-photon emission computed tomography (SPECT) permits better characterization of lobes and segments than planar imaging of the lungs.
- Radioxenon SPECT imaging of pulmonary ventilation is achievable only with special rapid-acquisition cameras or scanners because proper SPECT acquisition takes several minutes. These rapid-acquisition scanners are not widely available.

ABNORMAL LUNG SCAN

SINGLE-PHOTON EMISSION COMPUTED TOMOGRAPHY

Perfusion Defects

- Ventilation/perfusion (V/Q) SPECT studies, conducted by a small number of laboratories, utilize ^{99m}Tc-DTPA aerosols for the ventilation portion of the scan because of its slow dynamics, and ^{99m}Tc-MAA for the perfusion scan.
- FIGURES 5–5*A* and *B* (transverse slices), 5–6*A* and *B* (coronal slices), and 5–7*A* to *D* (sagittal slices) illustrate a positive SPECT pulmonary V/Q study with correlated images.
- However, all the algorithms in current use with V/Q SPECT studies (see TABLES 5–1 and 5–2) have evolved from planar imaging of the lungs. There is insufficient data to be certain if the same criteria for the different probability categories apply to SPECT images.

FIGURE 5–5A

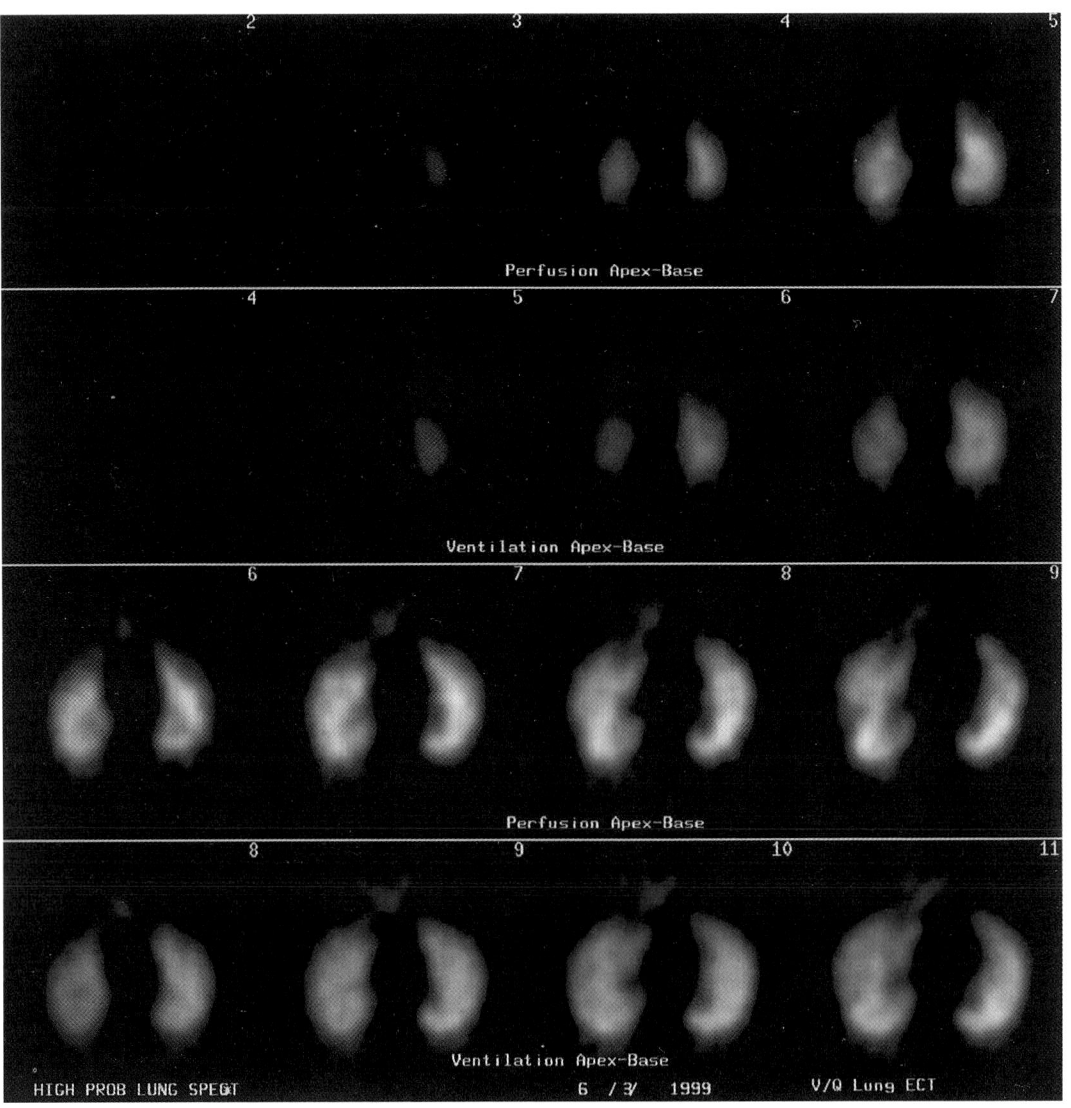

A

(A and **B).** Transverse matching perfusion (^{99m}Tc-MAA, first and third rows) and ventilation (^{99m}Tc-DTPA aerosol, second and fourth rows) SPECT images extending from apex to base (*upper left to lower right*) in a patient with a high probability scan based upon unmatched segmental perfusion defects in the lateral basal segments of the right lower lobe (*short arrows*) and the left lower lobe (*long arrow*). (Images courtesy of Dr. John Seitz and Mr. Wes Wooten of St. Agnes Hospital, Fresno, CA.)

(continued)

ABNORMAL LUNG SCAN

SINGLE-PHOTON EMISSION COMPUTED TOMOGRAPHY

Perfusion Defects

FIGURE 5–5B

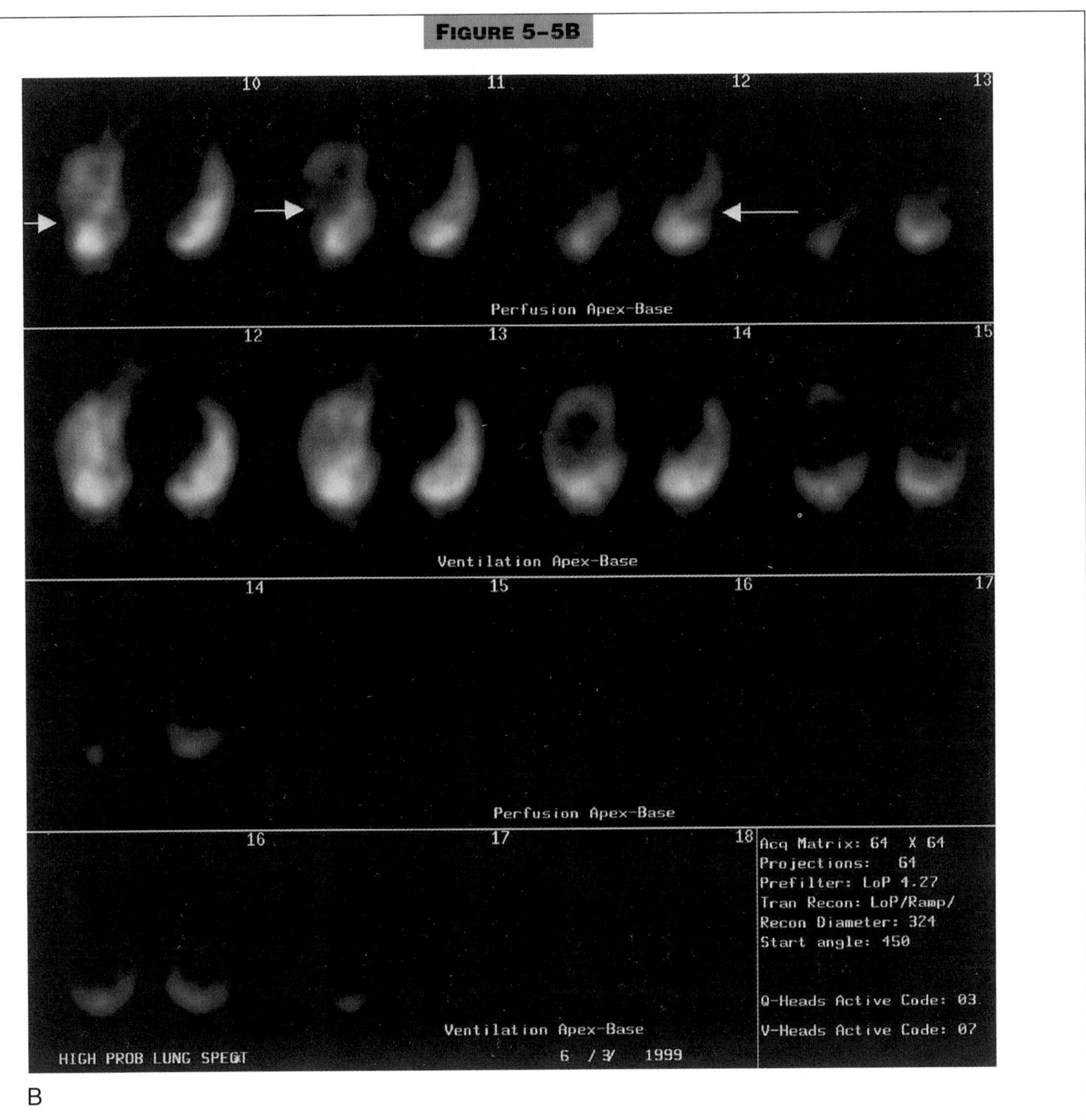

B

See legend on facing page

ABNORMAL LUNG SCAN

SINGLE-PHOTON EMISSION COMPUTED TOMOGRAPHY

Perfusion Defects

FIGURE 5–6A

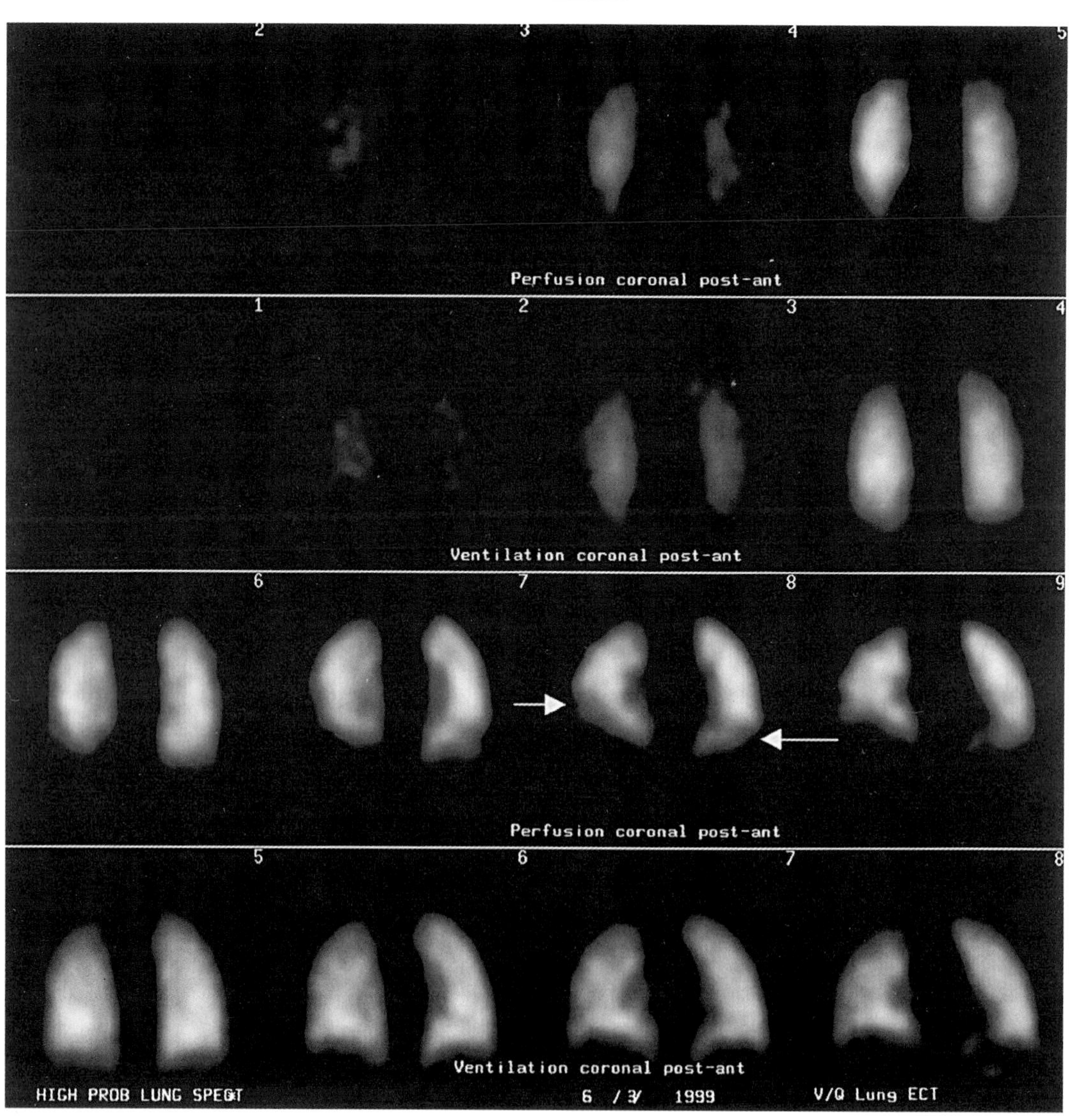

A

(A and **B).** Coronal SPECT slices of the same high probability pulmonary ventilation and perfusion scan as in FIGURE 5–5, extending from posterior (*upper left*) to anterior (*lower right*) (Images courtesy of Dr. John Seitz and Mr. Wes Wooten of St. Agnes Hospital, Fresno, CA.)

(continued)

ABNORMAL LUNG SCAN

SINGLE-PHOTON EMISSION COMPUTED TOMOGRAPHY

Perfusion Defects

FIGURE 5–6B

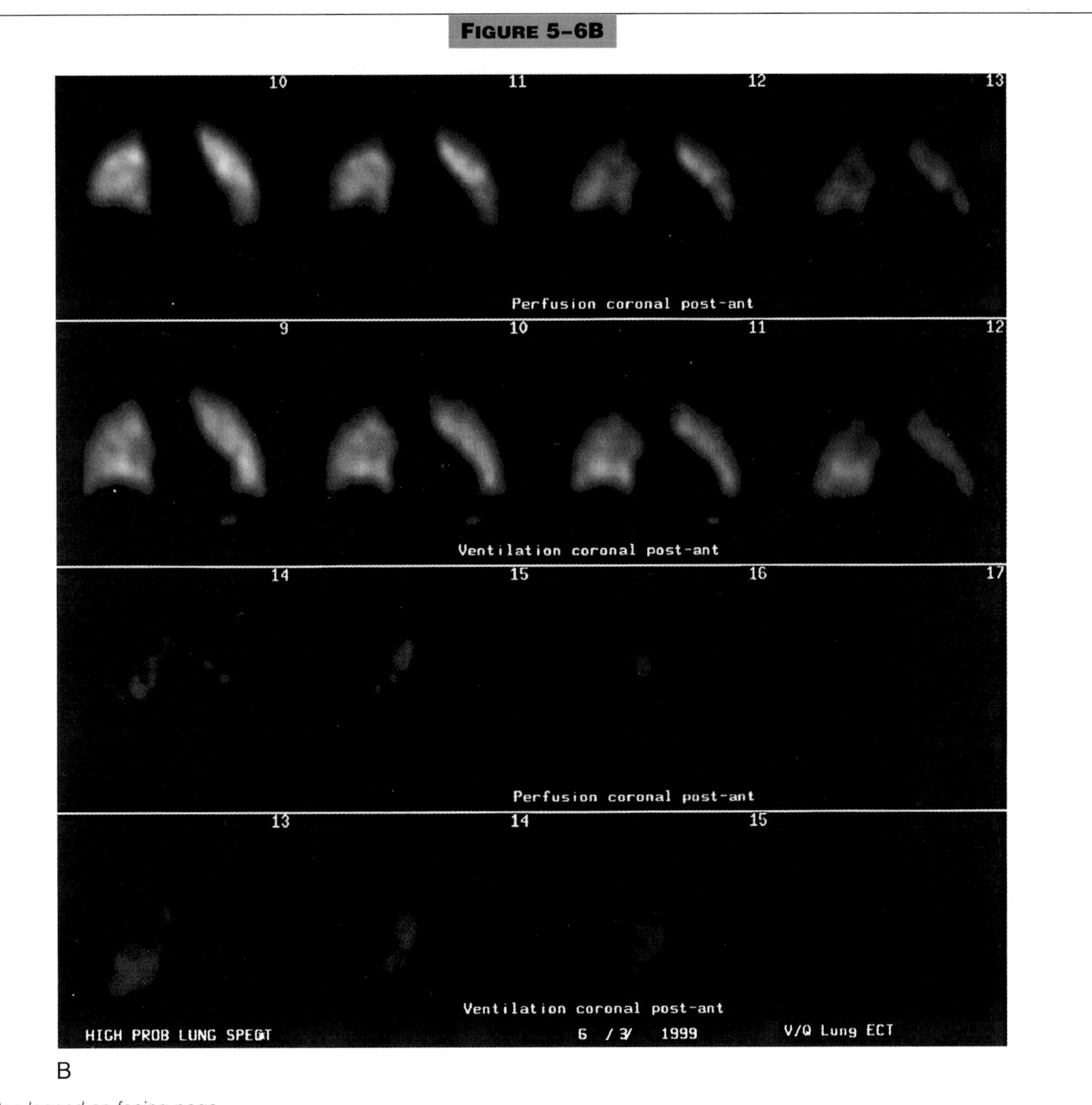

B

See legend on facing page

ABNORMAL LUNG SCAN

SINGLE-PHOTON EMISSION COMPUTED TOMOGRAPHY

Perfusion Defects

FIGURE 5–7A

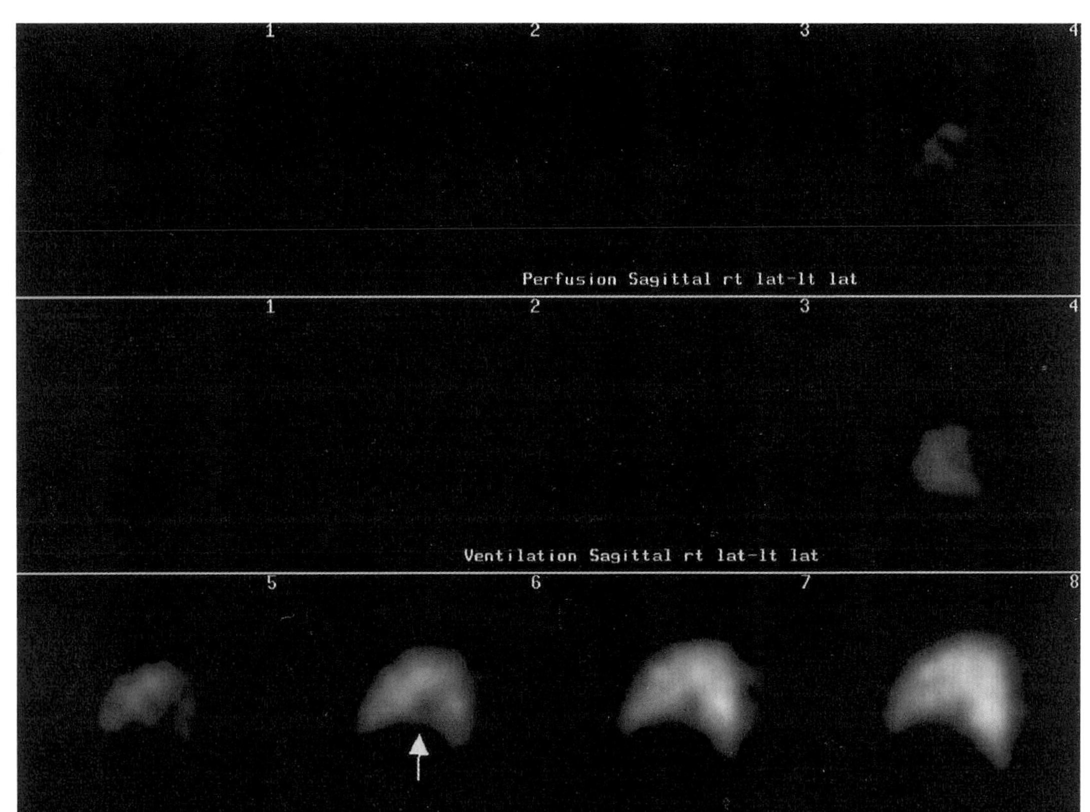

A

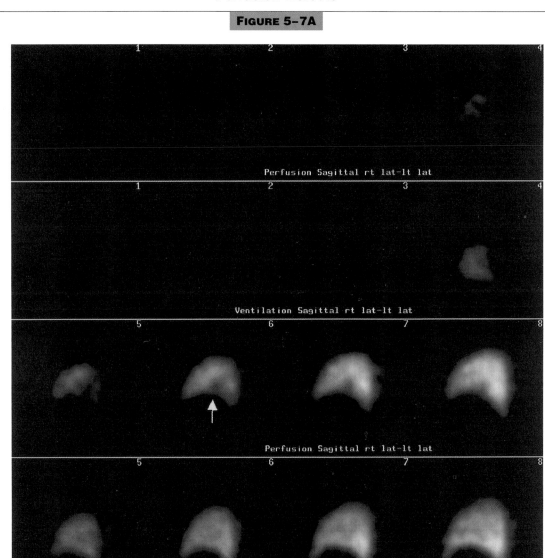

(A to **D). A** and **B,** right lung; **C** and **D,** left lung. Arrows as in FIGURE 5–5. Sagittal SPECT slices in the same patient illustrated in FIGURES 5–5 and 5–6, extending from the lateral aspect of the right lung (**A,** *upper left*) to the lateral aspect of the left lung (**D,** *lower right*). (Images courtesy of Dr. John Seitz and Mr. Wes Wooten of St. Agnes Hospital, Fresno, CA.)

(continued)

ABNORMAL LUNG SCAN

SINGLE-PHOTON EMISSION COMPUTED TOMOGRAPHY

Perfusion Defects

FIGURE 5–7B

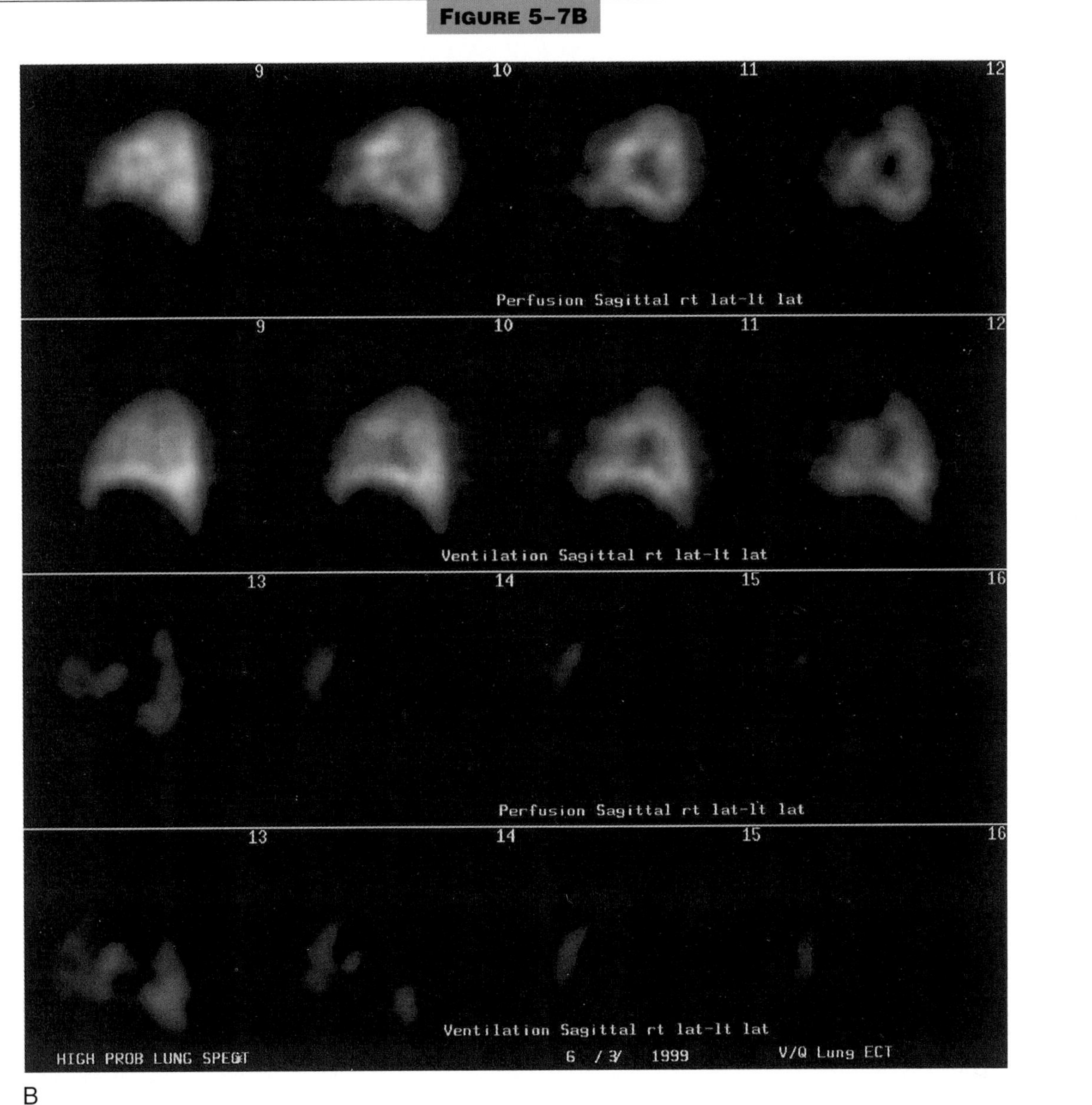

B

See legend on facing page

(continued)

ABNORMAL LUNG SCAN

SINGLE-PHOTON EMISSION COMPUTED TOMOGRAPHY

Perfusion Defects

FIGURE 5-7C

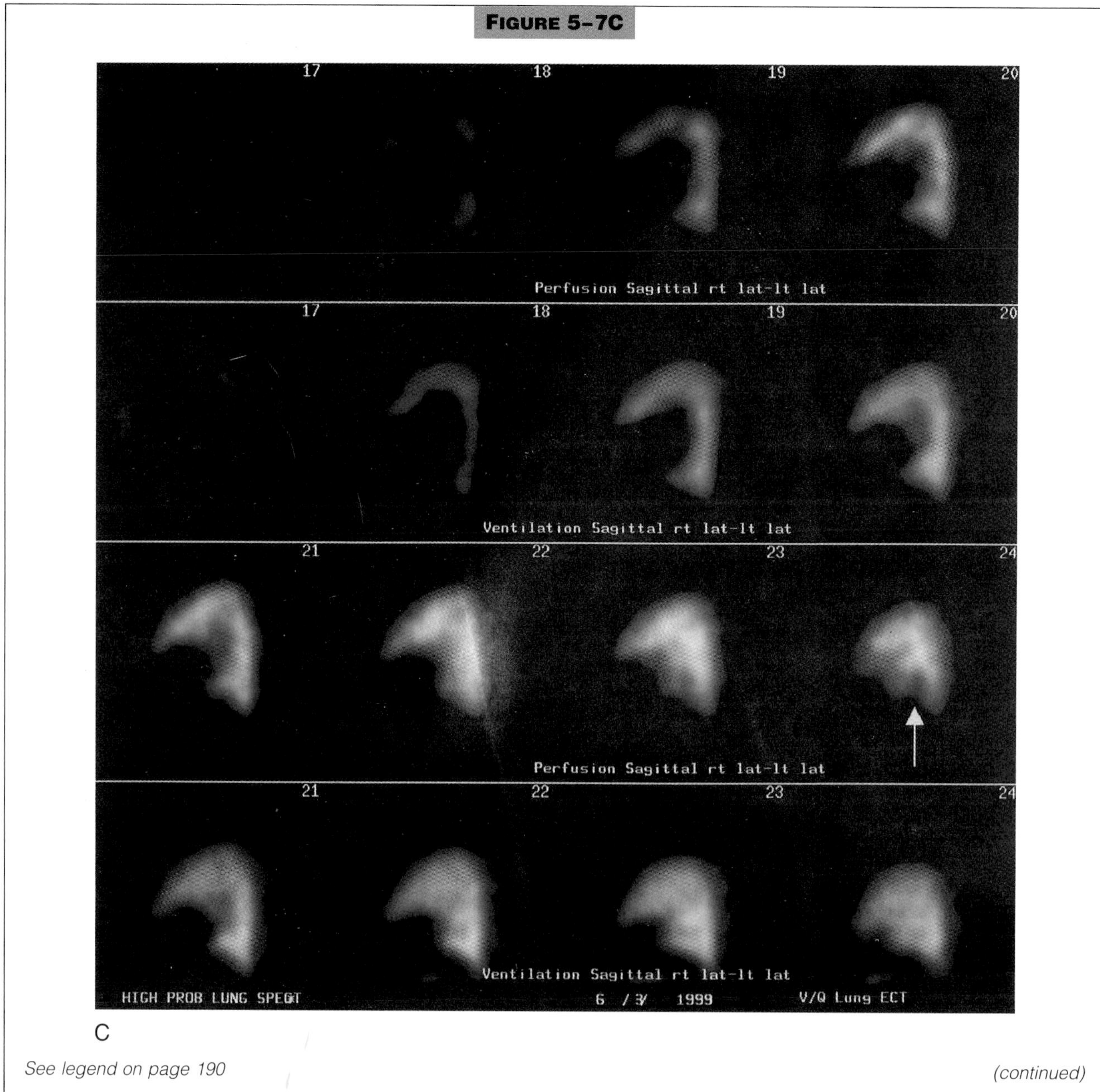

C

See legend on page 190

(continued)

ABNORMAL LUNG SCAN

SINGLE-PHOTON EMISSION COMPUTED TOMOGRAPHY

Perfusion Defects

FIGURE 5–7D

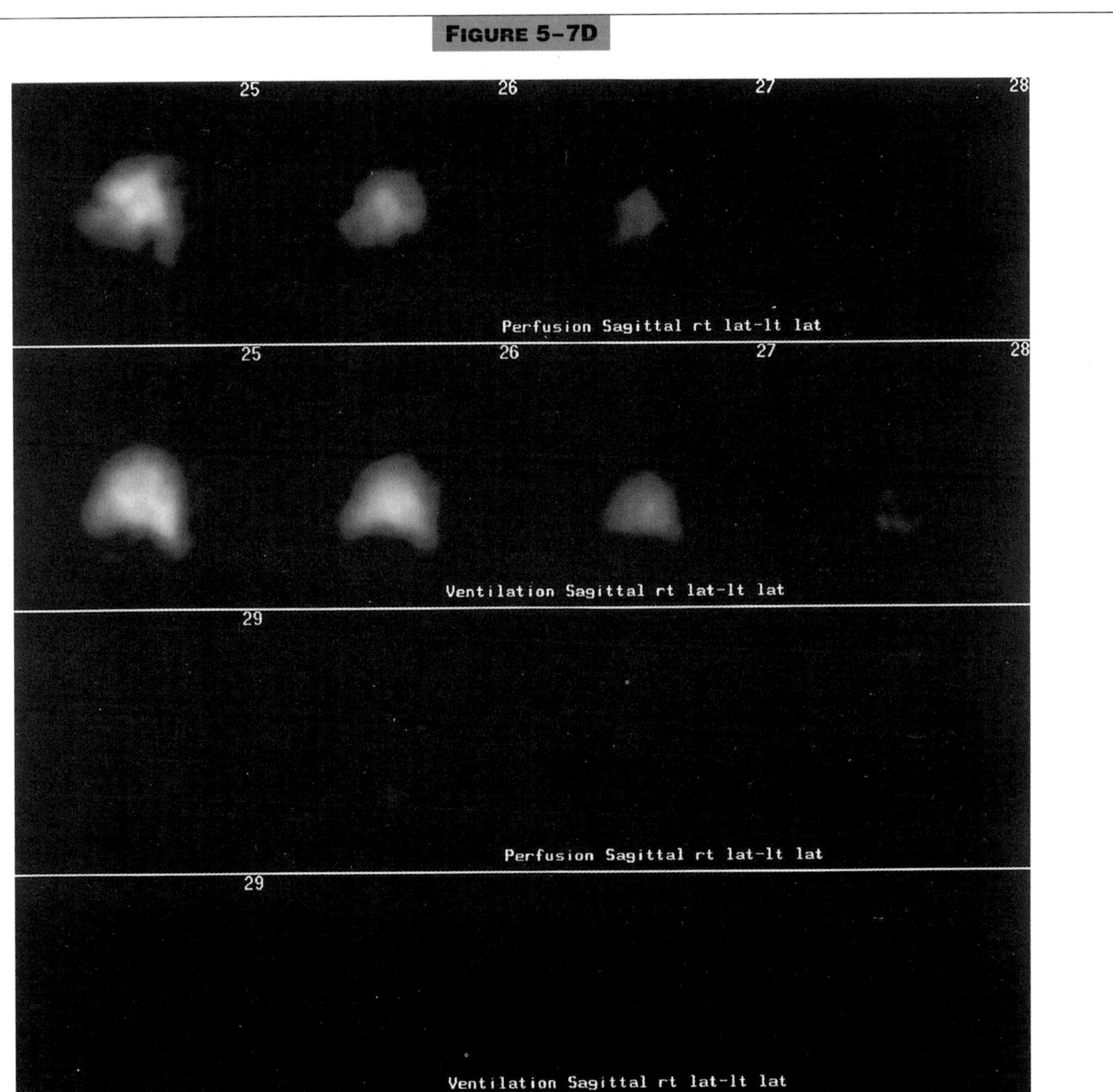

D

See legend on page 190

ABNORMAL LUNG SCAN

KRYPTON-81m PULMONARY SCINTIGRAPHY

- The energy of ^{81m}Kr gamma emission (190 KeV, 65% abundance) is sufficiently above that of ^{99m}Tc to permit imaging of ventilation after the perfusion portion of the scan.
- This sequence allows the ventilation images to be obtained in multiple projections, which best identify the Tc-MAA perfusion defects.
- Because the physical half-life of ^{81m}Kr is only 13 seconds, continuous imaging in each projection results in a pure inhalation image of high counts and high quality.
- The short half-life of the parent ^{81}Rb (rubidium, 4.7 hours) requires daily delivery of the ^{81}Rb-^{81m}Kr generators. The cost is prohibitive for routine clinical use and to maintain continuous availability for emergency scans.

Segmental Defects

- Morrell et al.[13] imaged ^{81m}Kr pulmonary patterns in the lungs of normal volunteers, then imaged the same subjects during temporary balloon occlusion of specific lung segments to assess the sizes and locations of such segmental defects, thus mimicking segmental perfusion defects.
- FIGURES 5–8 and 5–9 illustrate segmental perfusion defects involving the lateral basal segment of the left lower lobe and the posterior basal segment of the right lower lobe, respectively.
- These studies document the unexpectedly small segmental defect that is more characteristic of those two segments in vivo in humans than those portrayed in the drawings of FIGURE 5–2.
- FIGURE 5–2 is an idealized drawing of lung segments; thus, there can be substantial variation from this pattern in vivo.
- Unusually small true segmental defects lead to significant clinical underestimation of the size and number of segments involved in the clinical setting and thus to underestimation of the probability of acute pulmonary embolism in many patients.[14]

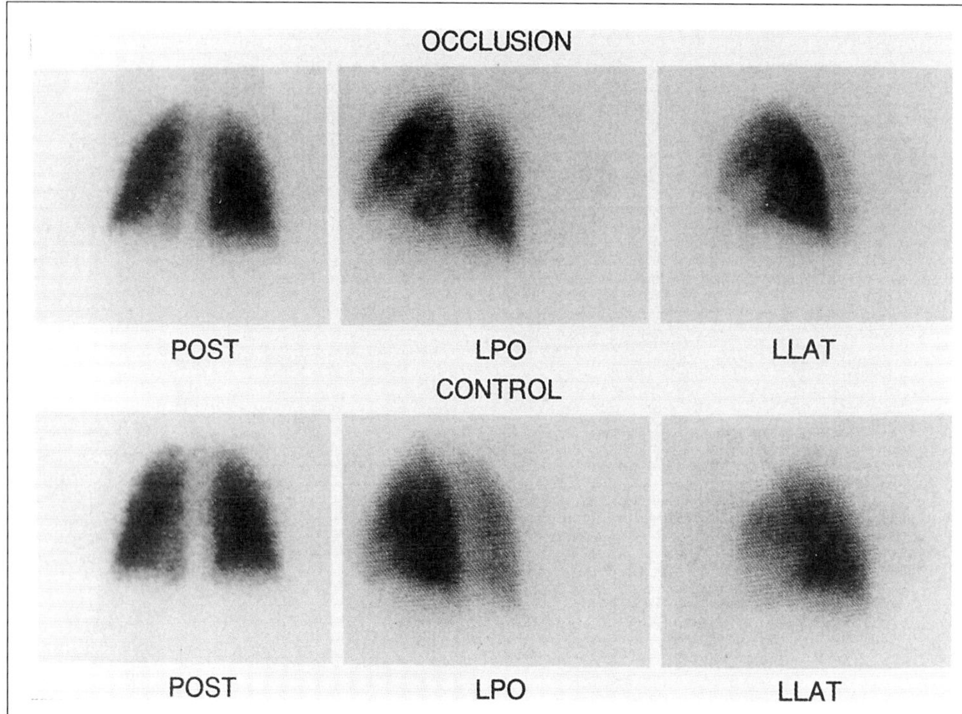

FIGURE 5–8

A clinical experiment with ^{81m}Kr was performed in a human volunteer with a segmental defect involving the lateral basal segment of the left lower lobe. These images illustrate the extent to which such segmental defects can be considerably underestimated in vivo (in contrast to the prominent segmental outlines suggested in traditional anatomic drawings, such as in FIGURE 5–2). (From Morrell N, Roberts C, Jones B. The anatomy of radioisotope lung scanning. J Nucl Med 33:676–683, 1992.)

ABNORMAL LUNG SCAN

KRYPTON-81m PULMONARY SCINTIGRAPHY

Segmental Defects

FIGURE 5–9

Clinical study corresponding to the subject in FIGURE 5–8 demonstrating a full segmental defect involving the posterior basal segment of the right lower lobe. (From Morrell N, Roberts C, Jones B: The anatomy of radioisotope scanning. J Nucl Med 33: 676–683, 1992.)

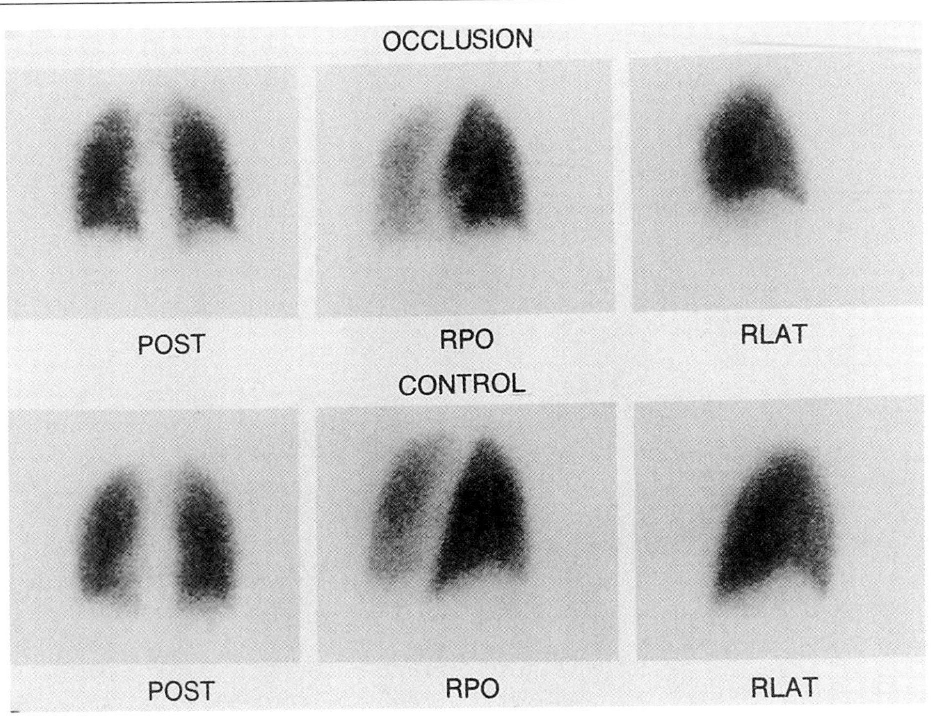

CLINICAL EXAMPLES

ACUTE PULMONARY EMBOLISM

- FIGURES 5–10 and 5–11 are the normal ventilation and markedly abnormal perfusion study of an otherwise healthy 43-year-old woman who began birth control pills 3 months prior to presenting with acute shortness of breath and a normal chest radiograph.
- Multiple bilateral segmental and subsegmental perfusion defects are clearly evident (high probability for acute pulmonary embolism—92% probability by Biello criteria).
- FIGURES 5–12 and 5–13 illustrate the relatively normal ventilation and single-segment perfusion defect scan (lateral segment of right middle lobe) in a 69-year-old male patient with a normal chest x-ray and consequent intermediate probability for acute pulmonary embolism (33% probability according to Biello criteria). In this particular case a pulmonary angiogram was done and was positive.
- FIGURES 5–14 and 5–15 show major matching ventilation and perfusion defects at the right lung base, which were associated with an exactly matching radiographic infiltrate in the same location, a triple match. Intermediate probability for acute pulmonary embolism. (See also Chapter 3, Pathology; Chapter 4, Radiography and Imaging; and Chapter 8, Pulmonary Function Testing.)

FIGURE 5–10

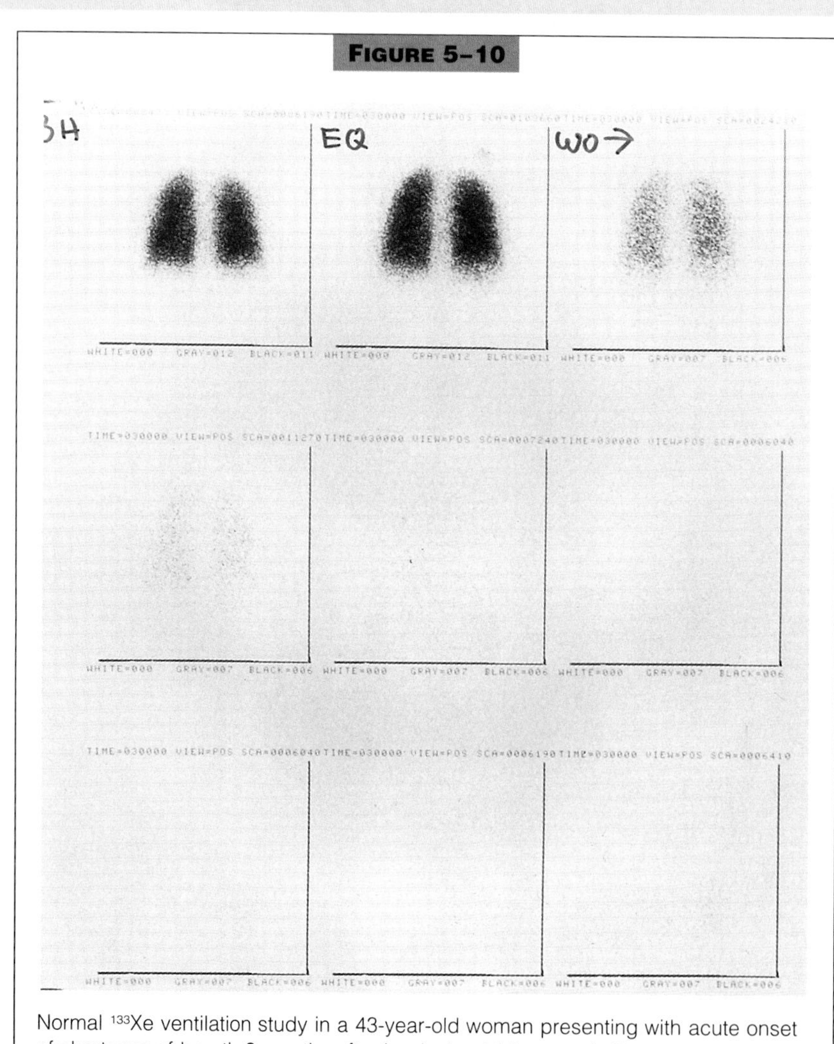

Normal ^{133}Xe ventilation study in a 43-year-old woman presenting with acute onset of shortness of breath 3 months after beginning birth control pills.

CLINICAL EXAMPLES

ACUTE PULMONARY EMBOLISM

FIGURE 5–11

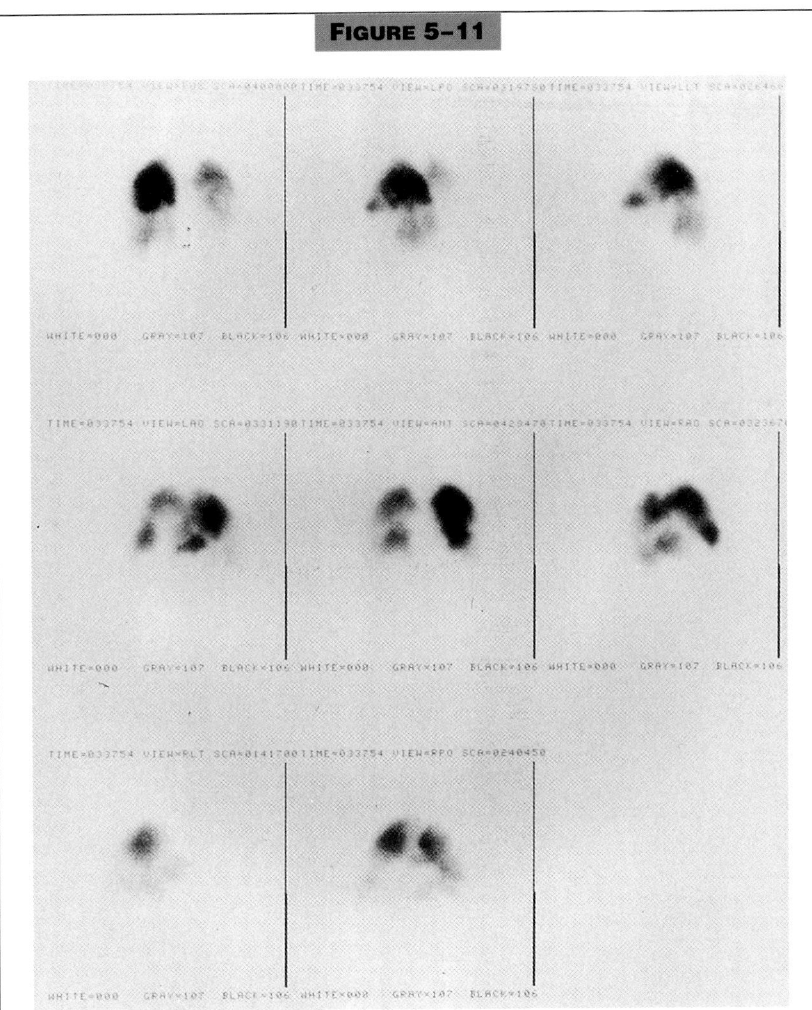

Perfusion scan (^{99m}Tc-MAA) demonstrating multiple bilateral major segmental and subsegmental perfusion defects bilaterally in the same patient as in FIGURE 5–10. In association with a normal chest x-ray and the normal ventilation study, this results in a high probability for acute pulmonary embolism.

CLINICAL EXAMPLES

ACUTE PULMONARY EMBOLISM

FIGURE 5-12

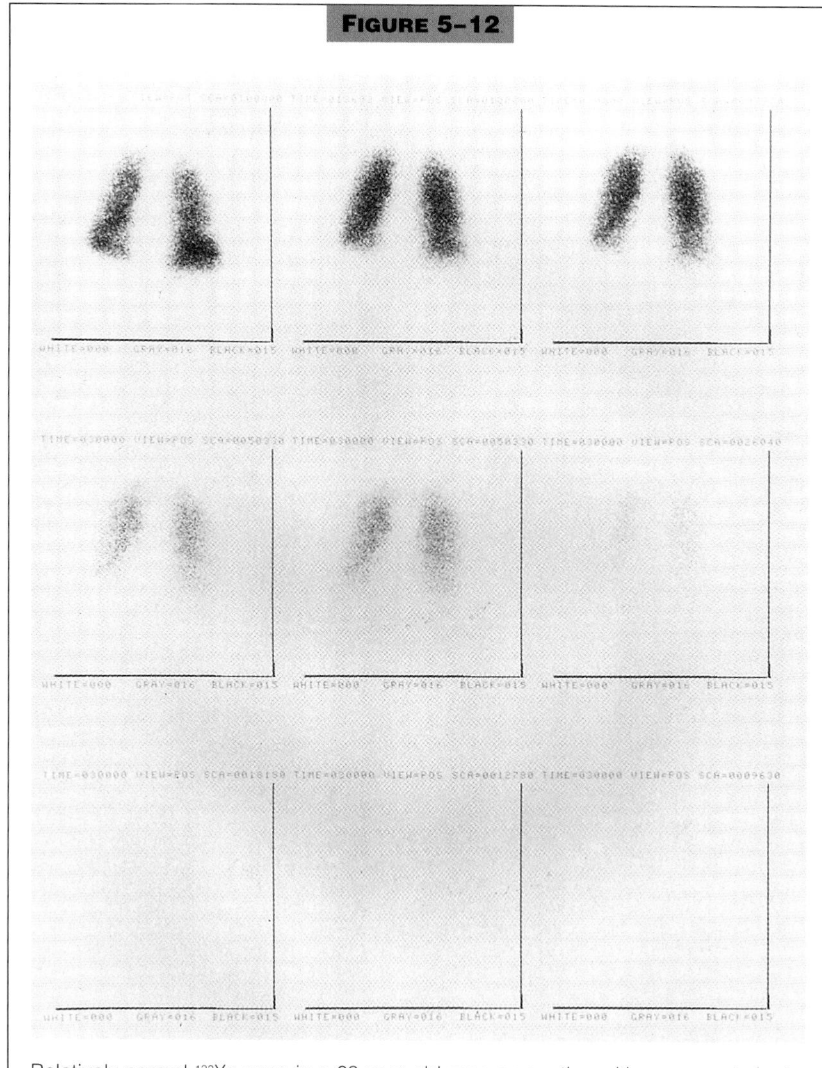

Relatively normal ^{133}Xe scan in a 69-year-old man presenting with new-onset shortness of breath.

CLINICAL EXAMPLES

ACUTE PULMONARY EMBOLISM

FIGURE 5–13

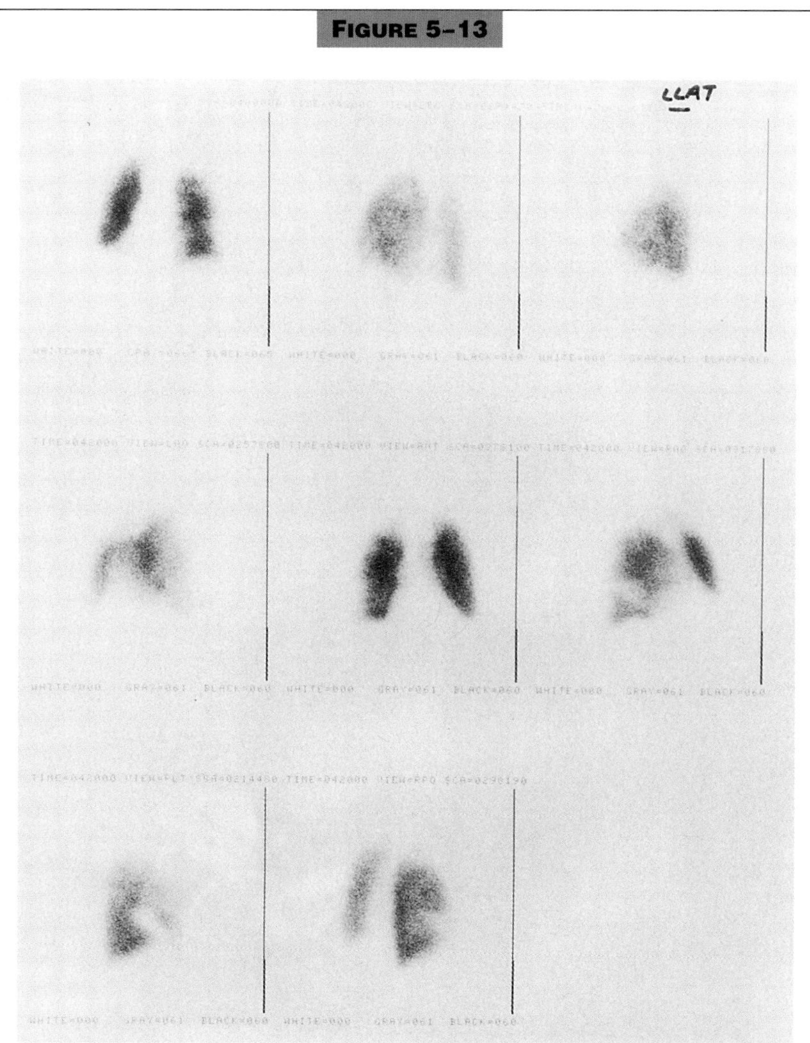

Perfusion scan (^{99m}Tc-MAA) in the same patient as in FIGURE 5–12, demonstrating a single segmental perfusion defect in the lateral segment of the right middle lobe. In conjunction with the patient's normal chest x-ray and ventilation scan, this would be associated with an intermediate probability of acute pulmonary embolism (33%, Biello criteria). The patient's pulmonary angiogram was positive.

CLINICAL EXAMPLES

ACUTE PULMONARY EMBOLISM

FIGURE 5–14

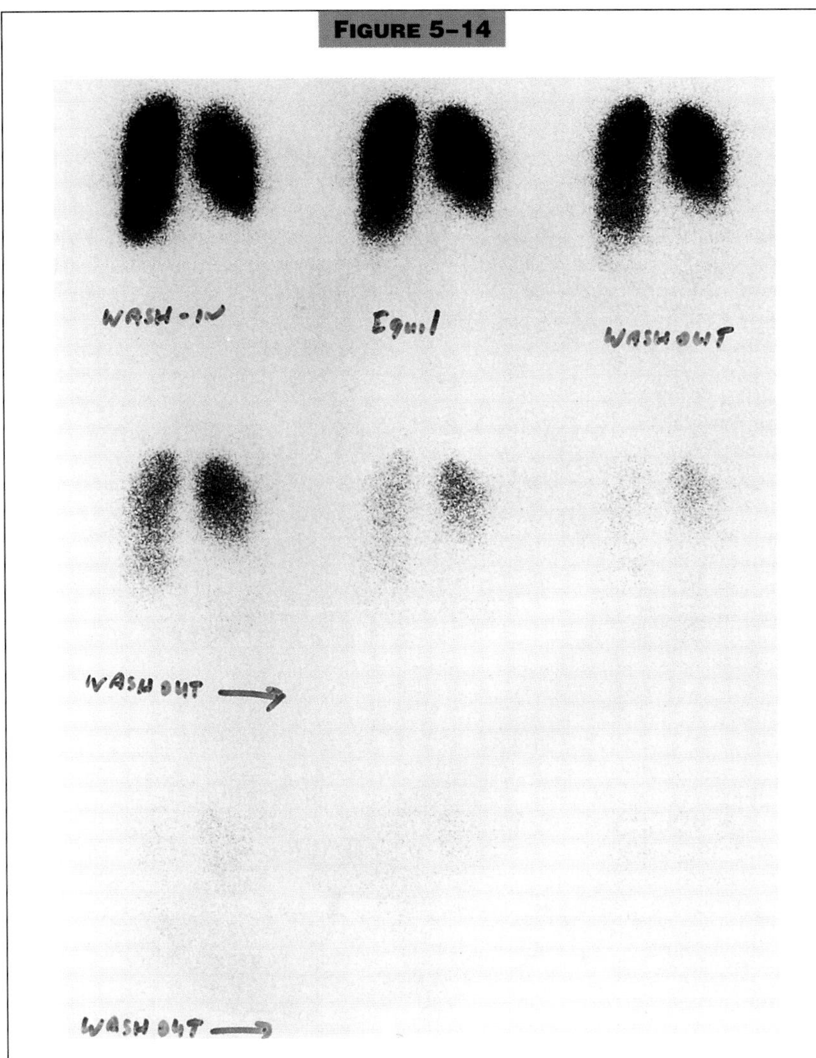

Ventilation scan (^{133}Xe) in a 50-year-old cardiac transplant patient with a 2-day history of shortness of breath and right pleuritic chest pain. The study demonstrates major loss of ventilation in the right lower lung.

CLINICAL EXAMPLES

ACUTE PULMONARY EMBOLISM

FIGURE 5–15

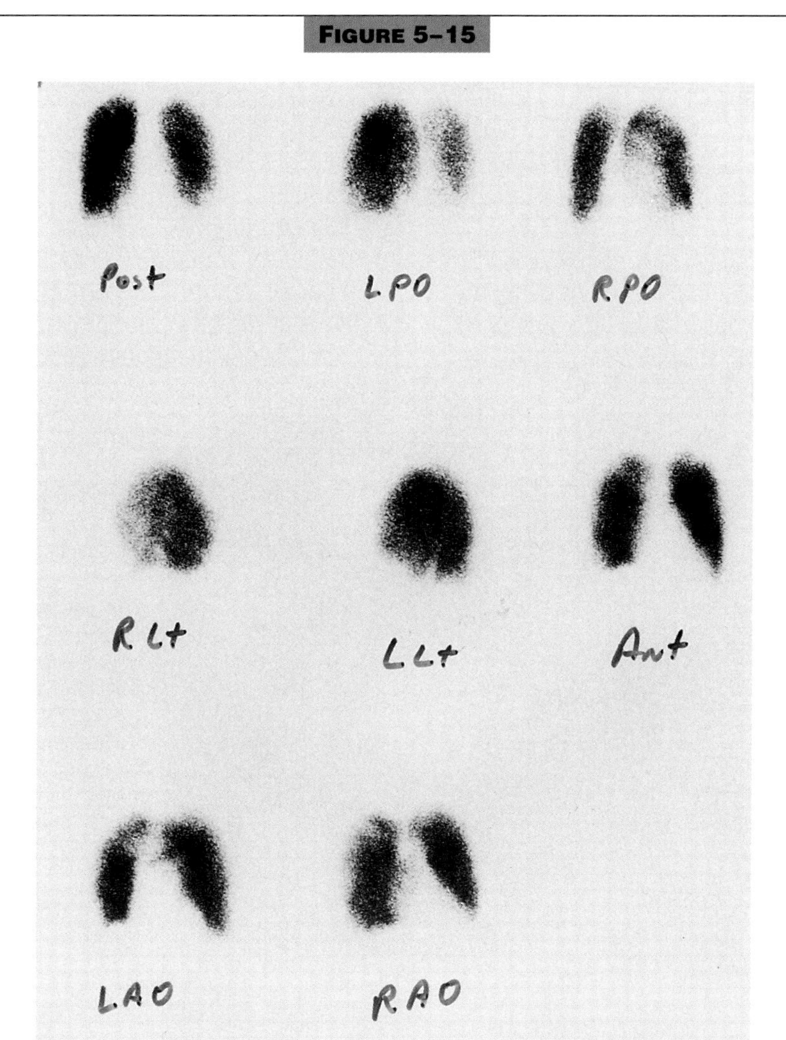

Perfusion scan (^{99m}Tc-MAA) in the same patient as in FIGURE 5–14. There is major perfusion loss to the right lower lobe, matching the ventilation defect, and a corresponding right lower lobe radiographic infiltrate. The probability of acute pulmonary embolism would be intermediate (triple match).

CLINICAL EXAMPLES

NONEMBOLIC PULMONARY DISEASE

Diseases with Airflow Obstruction

- Most nonembolic pulmonary parenchymal diseases (COPD, alpha$_1$-antitrypsin deficiency, bullous emphysema, etc.) are characterized by relatively equivalent effects on pulmonary vasculature and pulmonary airways.
- V/Q scans generally show matched ventilation/perfusion defects in the absence of comparable radiographic changes, resulting in a low probability for acute pulmonary embolism by both the Biello and PIOPED criteria.
- FIGURES 5–16 and 5–17 show matched ventilation/perfusion defects in a 29-year-old man with cystic fibrosis and severe chronic parenchymal disease under consideration for lung transplantation.
- These findings are relevant to the consideration of acute pulmonary embolism in such patients as well as to determine the extent of regional and global parenchymal disease prior to lung volume reduction surgery or lung transplantation.

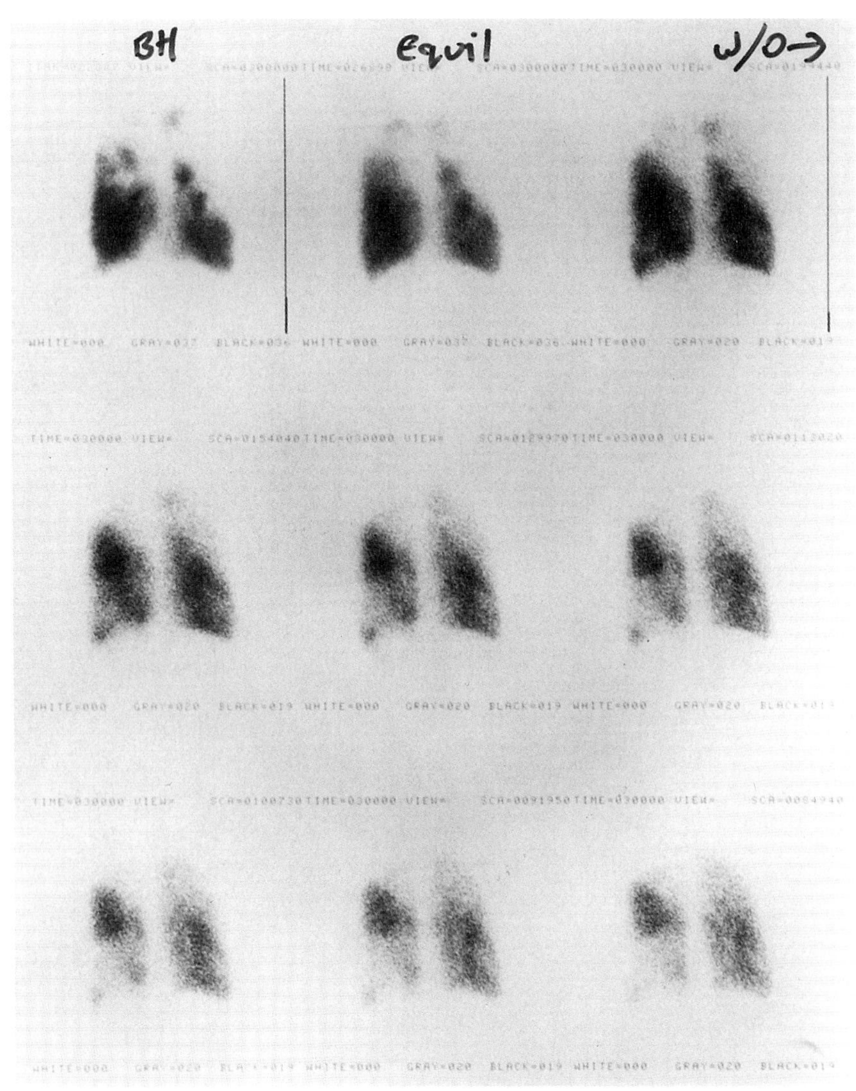

FIGURE 5–16

Ventilation scan (^{133}Xe) in a 29-year-old man with cystic fibrosis and severe pulmonary parenchymal disease leading to consideration of possible lung transplantation. Note that the best ventilation (single breath and equilibrium phase) is in the left middle lower lung and the right lower lung, also reflected in the complementary pattern of washout delay persisting at 3.5 minutes.

CLINICAL EXAMPLES

NONEMBOLIC PULMONARY DISEASE

Diseases with Airflow Obstruction

FIGURE 5–17

Perfusion scan (^{99m}Tc-MAA) in the same patient as FIGURE 5–16, demonstrating an exact match between the best areas of ventilation and of perfusion (left middle lower lung and right lower lung).

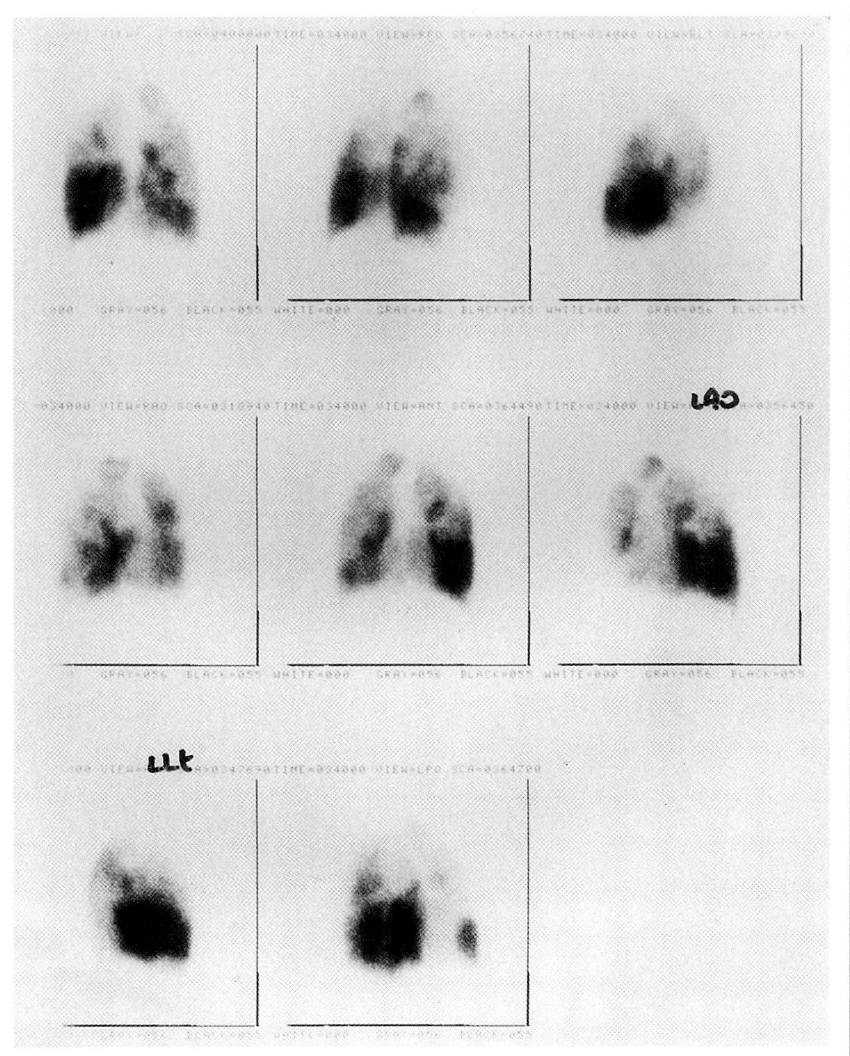

CLINICAL EXAMPLES

NONEMBOLIC PULMONARY DISEASE

Infection

See also Chapter 7, Laboratory Diagnosis of Respiratory Tract Infection

- Any one of several different nuclear imaging strategies can most effectively carry out assessment for pulmonary infection in a patient with fever of unknown origin and pulmonary radiographic abnormality.
- For many years the use of ^{111}In (indium)-labeled autologous white blood cells (In-WBC) has been associated with the highest sensitivity and specificity for acute infection.
- ^{67}Ga (gallium) has demonstrated greater effectiveness with chronic or indolent infections, in particular with regard to *Pneumocystis carinii* pneumonia (PCP).[15]
- FIGURE 5–18 illustrates the typical ^{67}Ga pulmonary image in an AIDS patient with grade IV PCP.
- FIGURE 5–19 shows an interesting contrast between ^{67}Ga (*left*) and ^{111}In-WBC (*right*) imaging in a patient with active tuberculosis, in whom the indolence of the tuberculous lesions clearly predisposes to much higher sensitivity with the gallium.
- FIGURE 5–20 illustrates an immunosuppressed patient with a fever of unknown origin and mild pulmonary symptoms but a clear x-ray who demonstrates intense diffuse pulmonary uptake due to cytomegaloviral pneumonia. Unrecognized clinically was an intense bacterial vaginitis, which had been overlooked because of the concern regarding the patient's pulmonary status.

FIGURE 5–18

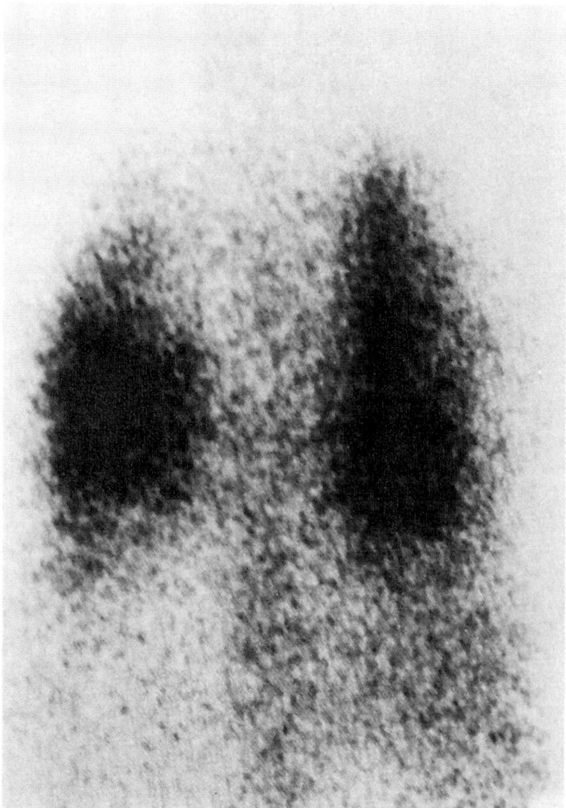

Intensely positive ^{67}Ga uptake diffusely throughout both lungs in a patient with AIDS, fever, cough, and a normal chest x-ray in spite of the presence of grade IV *Pneumocystis carinii* pneumonia, clearly confirmed by the gallium scan.

CLINICAL EXAMPLES

NONEMBOLIC PULMONARY DISEASE

Infection

FIGURE 5–19

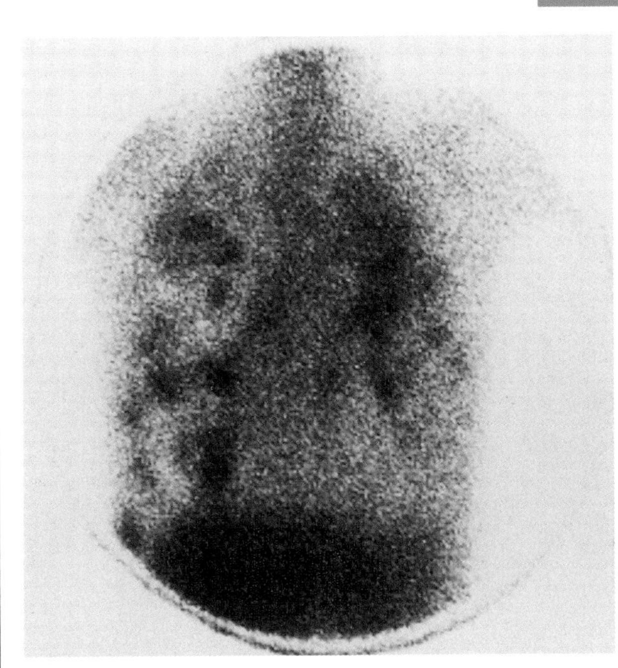

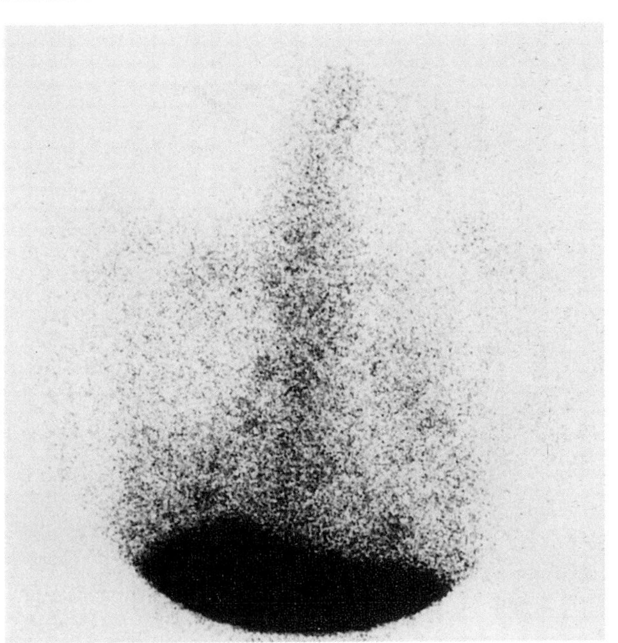

Positive ^{67}Ga (*left*) and ^{111}In-WBC (*right*) scans in a patient with active pulmonary tuberculosis. Note the much greater number and intensity of positive lesions with ^{67}Ga than with ^{111}In-WBC, presumably because of the relative chronicity and indolence of many of the lesions.

CLINICAL EXAMPLES

NONEMBOLIC PULMONARY DISEASE

Infection

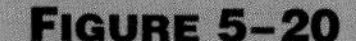

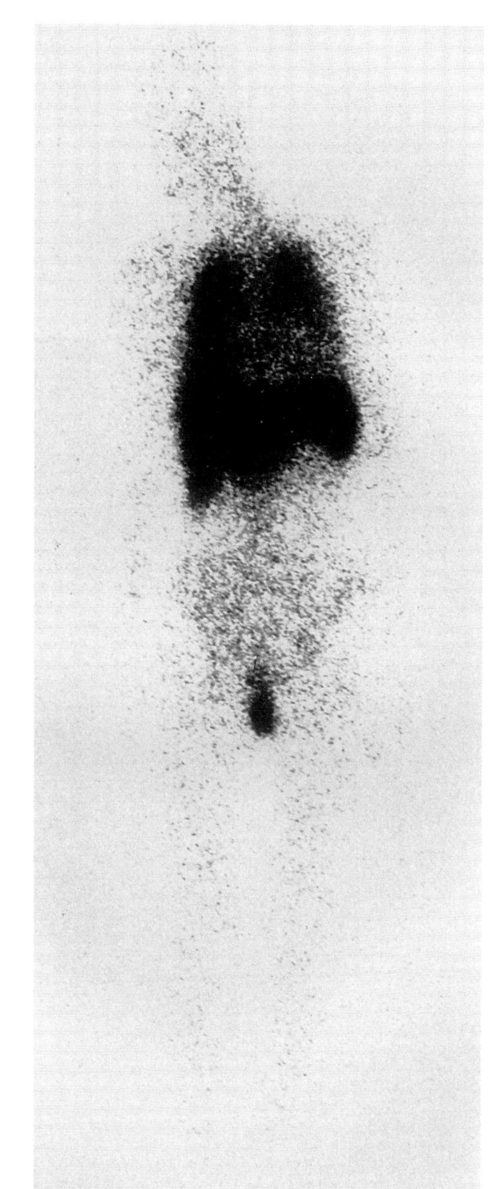

Intense diffuse pulmonary uptake of ^{111}In-WBC in an immunosuppressed renal transplant patient (right pelvis) with fever of unknown origin and cough who proved to have diffuse bilateral pneumonia due to cytomegalovirus. Unrecognized by her clinicians was the fact that she also suffered from an intense bacterial vaginitis, first identified on the indium-WBC scan.

CLINICAL EXAMPLES

NONEMBOLIC PULMONARY DISEASE

Sarcoidosis

- It has been recognized for many years that ^{67}Ga is highly sensitive and specific for the diagnosis and the staging of pulmonary sarcoidosis.[16] It is significantly more sensitive than ^{111}In-WBC.[17]

- FIGURE 5–21 illustrates the typical pulmonary and nonpulmonary findings on a ^{67}Ga scan of a 37-year-old woman with acute and extensive bihilar pulmonary sarcoidosis, as well as extensive salivary and lacrimal gland involvement.

FIGURE 5–21

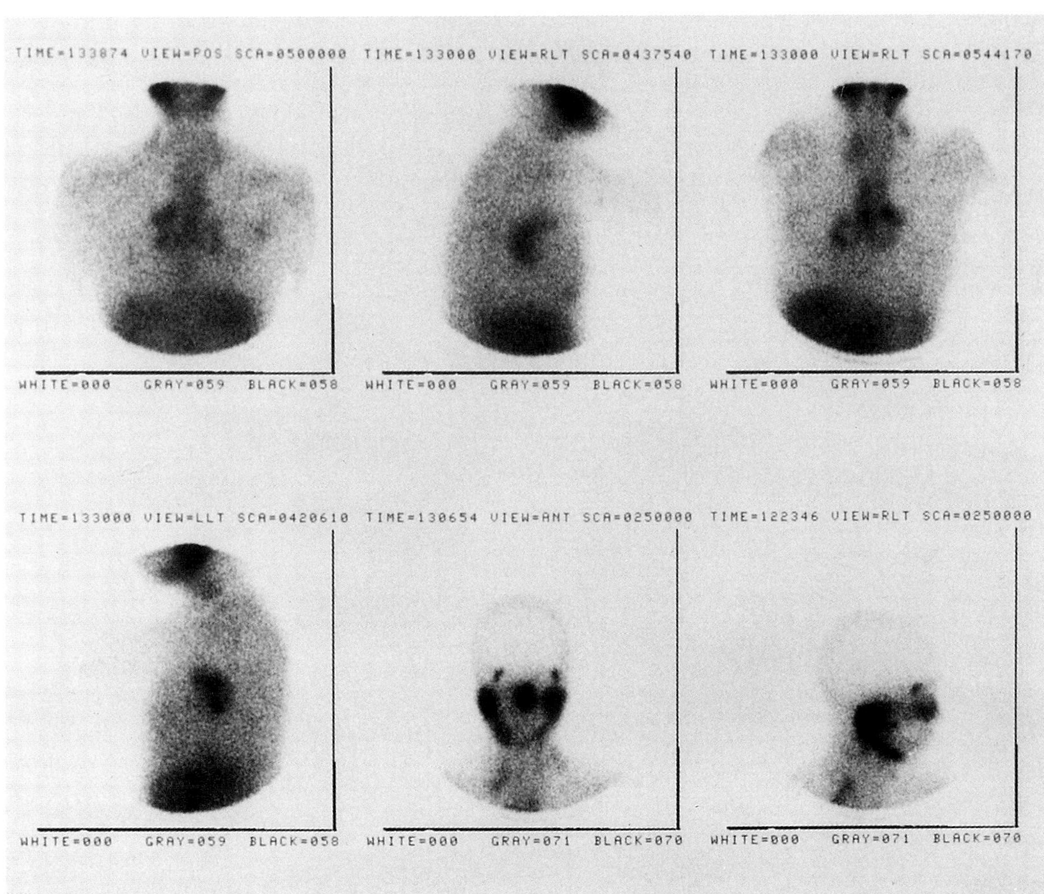

Characteristic 48-hour ^{67}Ga scan spot views of the head and thorax in a 35-year-old woman with known sarcoidosis, demonstrating positive bihilar pulmonary disease as well as intense salivary gland and lacrimal gland involvement (note "panda sign" of the anterior head).

CLINICAL EXAMPLES

NONEMBOLIC PULMONARY DISEASE

Congenital Cardiopulmonary Disease

- Quantitative pulmonary perfusion scintigraphy is a useful technique in the evaluation of children with a variety of cardiac and pulmonary vascular disorders predisposing to surgical or angioplastic intervention.
- Anterior and posterior ^{99m}Tc-MAA scintigraphy with calculation of the geometric mean right/left pulmonary perfusion ratio will help assess quantitatively the degree of benefit of angioplasty for pulmonary artery stenosis, or the effectiveness of unifocalization for severe pulmonary artery atresia or stenosis.*[17a, 17b]
- In FIGURE 5–22, the pulmonary perfusion ratio is 45% on the right and 55% on the left in an 8-month-old boy with a single ventricle, Glenn shunt, and subsequent Norwood procedure, also demonstrating considerable right-to-left shunting.
- FIGURES 5–23 and 5–24 show the ventilation and perfusion images in a 16-year-old girl with a cardiac shunt similar to that in FIGURE 5–22. These images demonstrate dextrocardia and spleen reversal, and such extensive right-to-left shunting (single ventricle) that the right anterior oblique view reveals a myocardial perfusion image analogous to a left anterior oblique view with intracoronary injection of ^{99m}Tc-MAA in a normal subject.

*Unifocalization is a surgical procedure designed to improve pulmonary blood flow in patients with pulmonary atresia or severe pulmonary artery stenosis. In a one-stage or two-stage procedure, bronchial arteries are gathered to form a right and left pulmonary artery replacement, which is connected to the right ventricular outflow tract.[17a,17b]

FIGURE 5–22

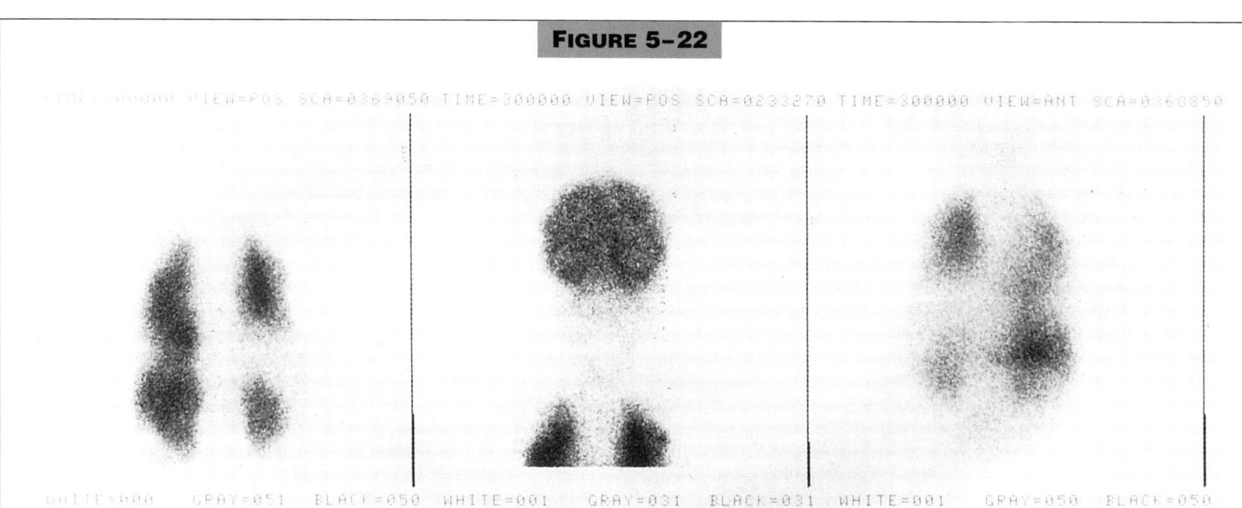

Quantitative pulmonary perfusion scan (^{99m}Tc-MAA) in an 8-month-old boy with multiple congenital cardiac defects, including single ventricle of the left ventricular type with transposition of the great vessels, and widespread regions of pulmonary vessel stenosis. Treatment has included end-to-side anastomosis of the proximal main pulmonary artery to the aortic arch, right-sided bidirectional Glenn shunt, and left-sided Blalock-Taussig, as well as repair of aortic coarctation. The ^{99m}Tc-MAA study demonstrates a pulmonary perfusion ratio of 45% to the right and 55% to the left, within the range of normal, and a major right-to-left shunt visible as intense cerebral labeling. (Left image = posterior torso; middle image = anterior head; right image = anterior torso.)

CLINICAL EXAMPLES

NONEMBOLIC PULMONARY DISEASE

Congenital Cardiopulmonary Disease

FIGURE 5–23

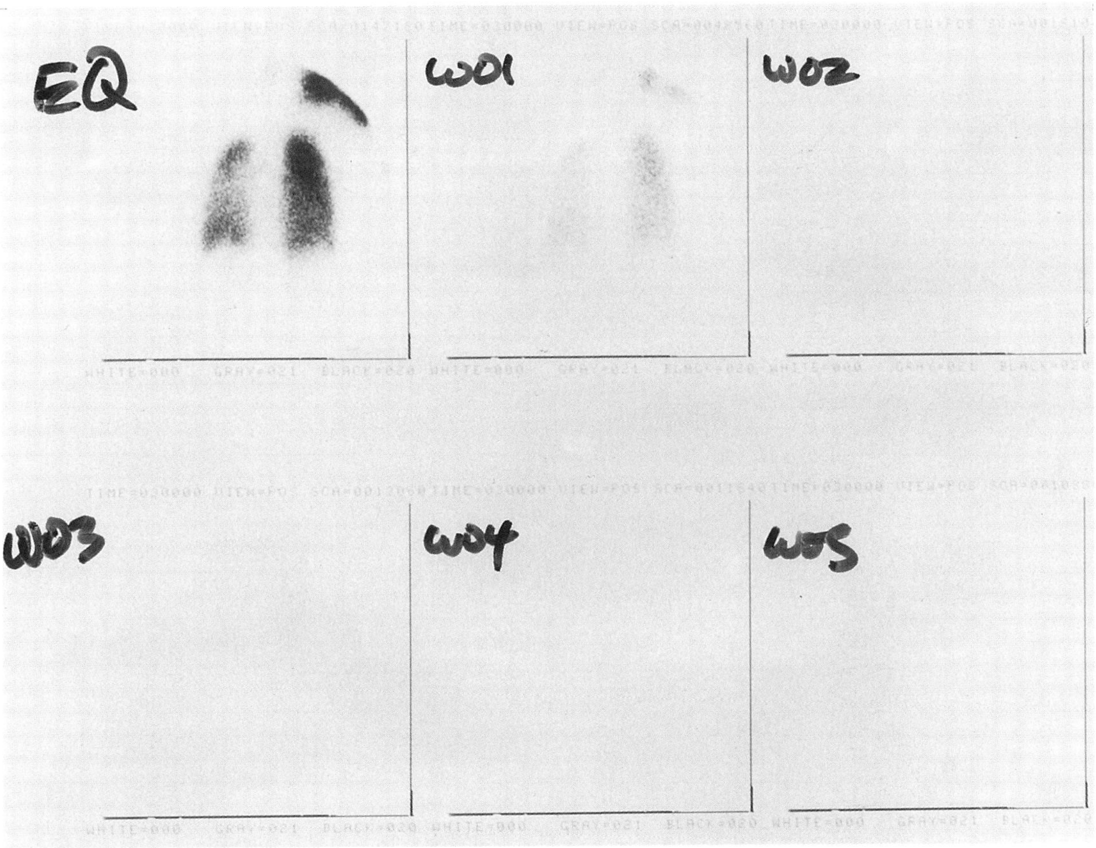

Pulmonary ventilation scan (^{133}Xe) in a 16-year-old girl with multiple congenital abnormalities including situs inversus totalis with transposition of the great vessels and multiple surgical interventions. Ventilation of the left lung is generally reduced compared to the right, but there are no regions of delayed washout on either side.

CLINICAL EXAMPLES

NONEMBOLIC PULMONARY DISEASE

Congenital Cardiopulmonary Disease

FIGURE 5-24

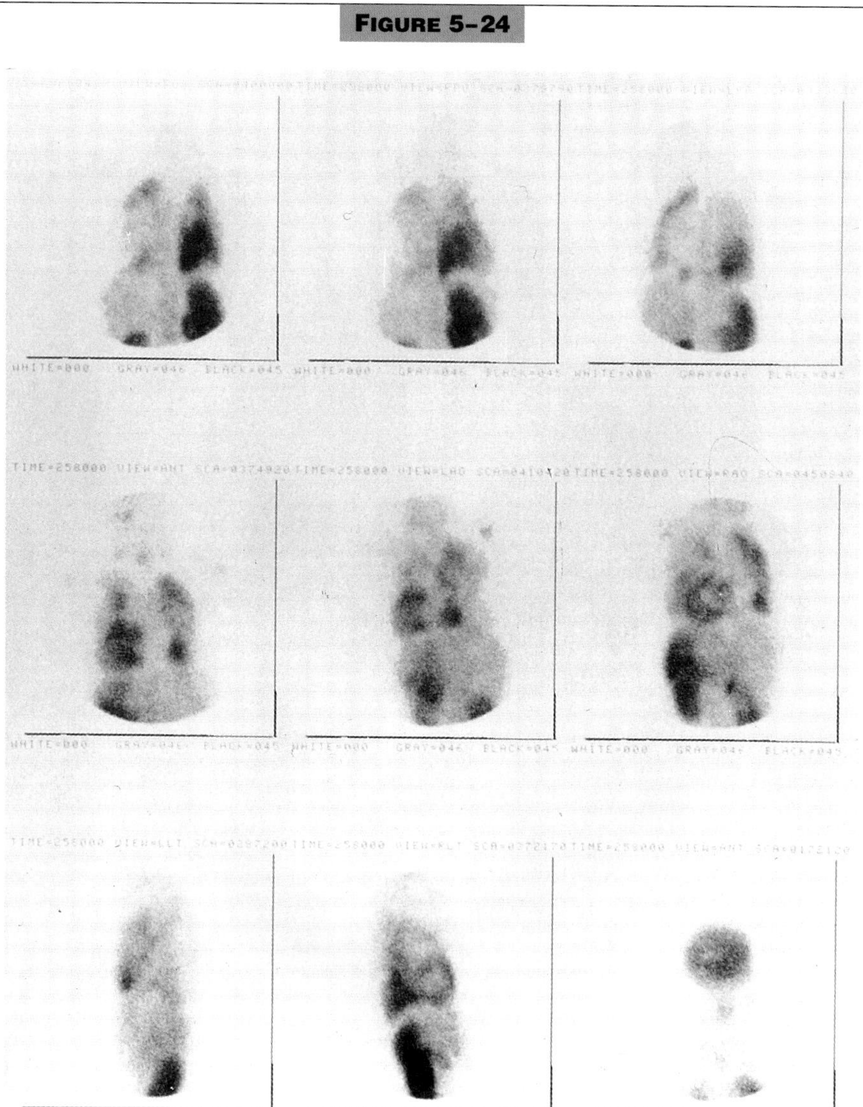

Pulmonary perfusion scan (^{99m}Tc-MAA) in the same patient as shown in FIGURE 5-23. Perfusion to the entire left lung and the right upper lung is reduced compared to the right lower lung in the upper three images in posterior, right posterior oblique, and left posterior oblique projections, as a result of bilateral Glenn shunting. Extensive right-to-left cardiac shunting through the single ventricle results in striking visualization of the various manifestations of situs inversus, including dextrosplenia (posterior views in the upper row), dextrocardia (circular myocardial outline in the right anterior oblique view, middle row right, and right lateral view, lower row center) and markedly positive brain visualization (lower row right).

CLINICAL EXAMPLES

NONEMBOLIC PULMONARY DISEASE

Carcinoma

- Within the last few years there has been a tremendous increase in interest in and use of PET imaging with ^{18}F fluorodeoxyglucose (FDG) for tumor diagnosis and staging in general.
- Commonly used applications of PET in pulmonary medicine include
  - Evaluation of the newly discovered pulmonary nodule
  - Staging of confirmed non–small cell lung cancer (identification of regional metastases in the absence of CT or MRI findings)
  - Possibly, to monitor response to therapy.[18]

Current usage patterns have identified significant cost savings in the investigation of lung cancer patients when PET is included as one of the primary diagnostic procedures.

- FIGURE 5–25 illustrates the whole-body volume-rendered image of a patient with a newly discovered large left hilar lung mass and a negative hilum/mediastinum on CT.
- FIGURE 5–26 represents the more detailed coronal images through the thorax, which clearly demonstrate one positive mediastinal lymph node, precluding cure by surgical resection of the primary site alone.
- The use of PET in oncologic diagnosis and management will continue to increase rapidly in the coming years as its considerable effectiveness is even better demonstrated by wide usage.

FIGURE 5–25

Whole-body volume-rendered ^{18}F-FDG PET scan in a 65-year-old woman with newly diagnosed carcinoma of the lung after biopsy of a left hilar mass. Normal biodistribution of the FDG is visible in the brain, liver, kidneys, urinary collecting system, bladder, and bowel. The heart is poorly visualized in this diabetic patient. The left hilar mass is clearly visible, but is the only positive finding in the volume-rendered image.

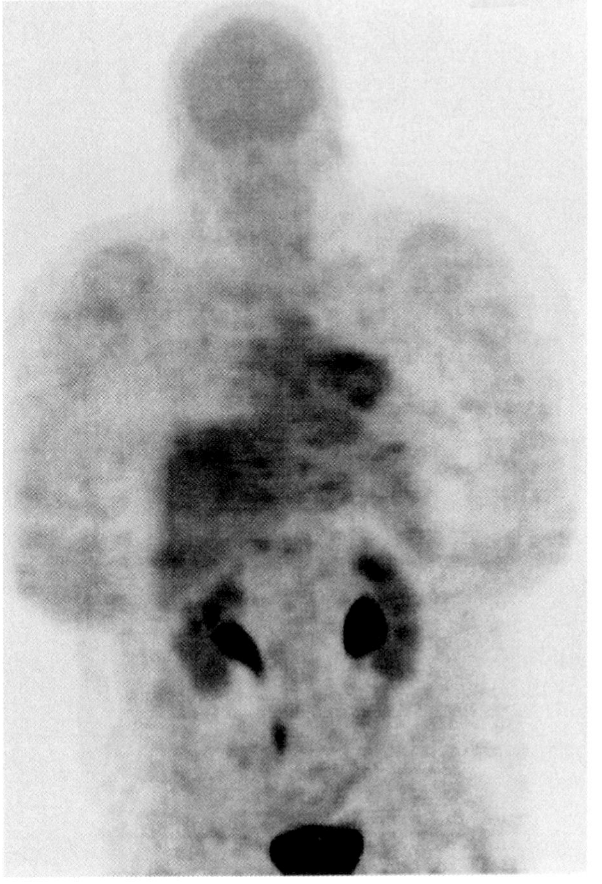

CLINICAL EXAMPLES

NONEMBOLIC PULMONARY DISEASE

Carcinoma

FIGURE 5-26

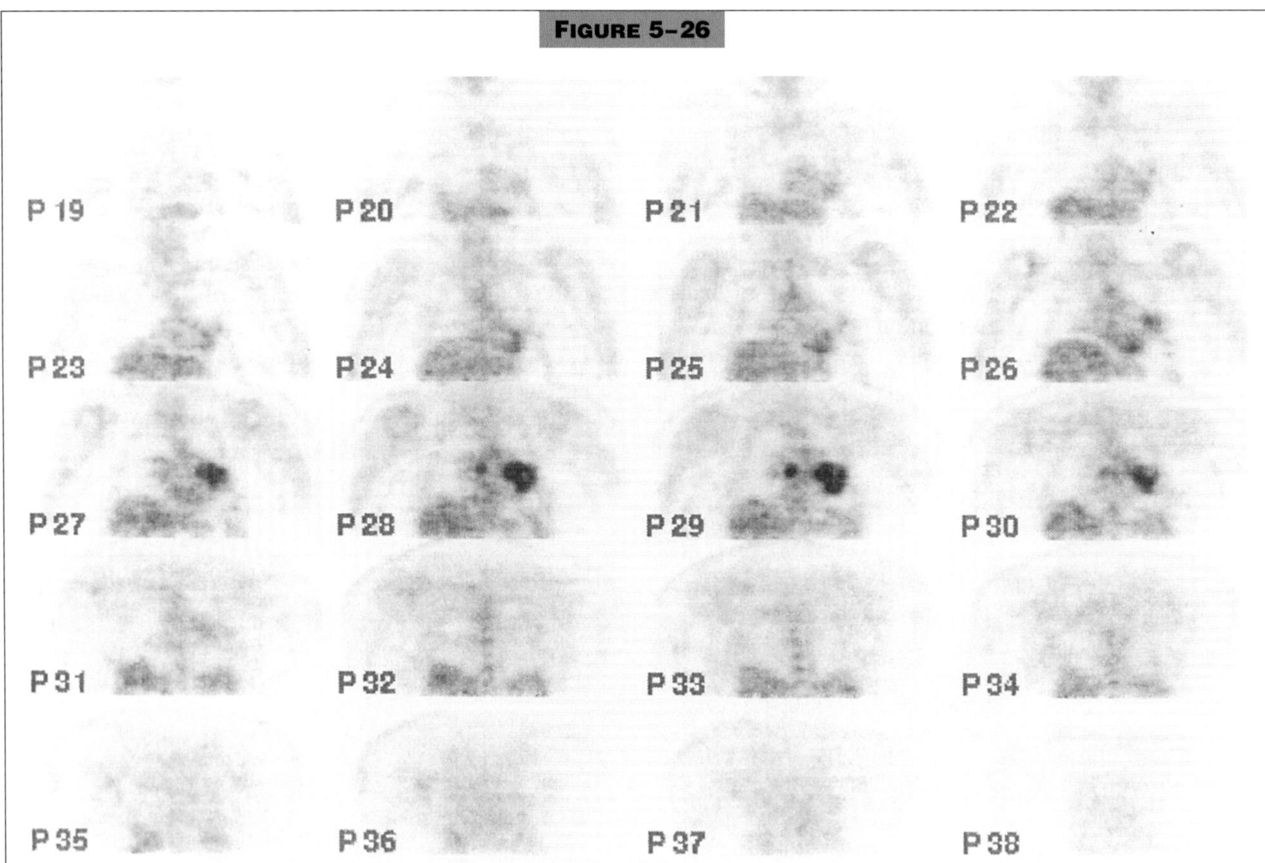

Detailed ^{18}F-FDG coronal images in the same patient shown in FIGURE 5–25 (anterior, P19, to posterior, P38). The intense uptake in the left hilar mass is much more definitive than in the volume-rendered image, and an additional positive right hilar node is now clearly detectable (images P27–P30).

CONCLUSION

Pulmonary nuclear medicine continues to thrive with the continuing use of long-term established procedures such as the V/Q scan, with newer techniques such as PET, and with potential future applications of such radiolabeled tracers as tumor antibodies and receptor-specific peptides (e.g., ^{111}In-octreotide). The combination of such procedures with the anatomic imaging modalities of CT and MRI creates powerful tools for the clinician with which may evaluate the pulmonary patient.

REFERENCES

1. Knipping H, Bolt W, Venrath H, et al: Eine neue Methode zur Pruefung der Herz- und Lungenfunktion; die regionale Funktionsanalyse in der Lungen- und Herzklinik mit Hilfe des radioaktiven Edelgases Xenon-133. Deutsch Med Wschr 80:1146–1147, 1955.

2. Dyson NA, Hugh-Jones P, Newbery GR, et al: Studies of regional lung function using radioactive oxygen. Br Med 1:213–238, 1960.

3. Ball W, Stewart P, Newsham LGS, Bates D: Regional pulmonary function studied with xenon-133. J Clin Invest 41:519–531, 1962.

4. Cassen B, Curtis L, Reed C, Libby R: Instrumentation of I^{131} used in medical studies. Nucleonics 9:46–50, 1951.

5. Anger H: Scintillation camera. Rev Sci Instr 29:27–33, 1958.

6. Taplin G, Johnson D, Dore E, Kaplan H: Lung photoscans with macroaggregates of human serum radioalbumin: Experimental basis and initial clinical trials. Health Phys 10:1219–1227, 1964.

7. Wagner H Jr, Sabiston D Jr, McAfee J, et al: Diagnosis of massive pulmonary embolism in man by radioisotope scanning. N Engl J Med 271:377–384, 1964.

8. McNeil B: A diagnostic strategy using ventilation-perfusion studies in patients suspected for pulmonary embolism. J Nucl Med 17:319–323, 1976.

9. Biello D, Mattar A, McKnight R, et al: Ventilation-perfusion studies in suspected pulmonary embolism. Am J Radiol 133:1033–1037, 1979.

10. PIOPED Investigators: Value of the ventilation-perfusion scan in acute pulmonary embolism. Results of the prospective investigation of pulmonary embolism diagnosis (PIOPED). JAMA 263:2753–2759, 1990.

11. Gottschalk A, Juni J, Sostman H, et al: Ventilation-perfusion scintigraphy in the PIOPED study. Part I. Data collection and tabulation. J Nucl Med 34:1109–1118, 1993.

12. Gottschalk A, Sostman H, Coleman R, et al: Ventilation-perfusion scintigraphy in the PIOPED study. Part II. Evaluation of the scintigraphic criteria and interpretations. J Nucl Med 34:1119–1126, 1993.

13. Morrell N, Roberts C, Jones B: The anatomy of radioisotope lung scanning. J Nucl Med 33:676–683, 1992.

14. Morrell N, Nijran K, Jones B, et al: The underestimation of segmental defect size in radionuclide lung scanning. J Nucl Med 34:370–374, 1993.

15. Fineman D, Palestro C, Kim C, et al: Detection of abnormalities in febrile AIDS patients with In-111–labeled leukocyte and Ga-67 scintigraphy. Radiol 170:677–680, 1989.

16. Israel H, Albertine K, Park C, Patrick H: Whole-body gallium 67 scans. Role in diagnosis of sarcoidosis. Am Rev Respir Dis 144:1182–1186, 1991.

17. Palestro C, Schultz B, Horowitz M, Swyer A: Indium-111–leukocyte and gallium-67 imaging in acute sarcoidosis: Report of two patients. J Nucl Med 33:2027–2029, 1992.

17a. Amin Z, McElhinney DB, Reddy VM, et al: Coronary to pulmonary artery collaterals in patients with pulmonary atresia and ventricular septal defect. Ann Thorac Surg 70: 119–123, 2000.

17b. Reddy VM, McElhinnery DB, Amin Z, et al: Early and intermediate outcomes after repair of pulmonary atresia with ventricular septal defect and major aortopulmonary collateral arteries: Experience with 85 patients. Circulation 101:1826–1832, 2000.

18. Al-Sugair A, Coleman R: Applications of PET in lung cancer. Semin Nucl Med 28:303–319, 1998.

CHAPTER

6

Bronchoscopy

Udaya B. S. Prakash, M.D.

and

Sergio Cavaliere, M.D.

INTRODUCTION

- The field of bronchoscopy has rapidly emerged as a major component of pulmonary and critical care medicine.
- Bronchoscopy is perhaps the most commonly employed minimally invasive diagnostic procedure in the field of pulmonary medicine.
- Currently, bronchoscopy is used not only for diagnostic purposes but also for therapy of various types of airway lesions.
- Of the two main types of bronchoscopes, the flexible (fiberoptic) bronchoscope is most commonly employed in clinical practice. The rigid bronchoscope, however, remains an important instrument in the diagnosis and treatment of many pulmonary disorders.
- The quality of instrumentation continues to improve, and newer applications have evolved.
- In addition to many diagnostic and therapeutic roles in clinical pulmonology, bronchoscopy has emerged as a major procedure in research protocols designed to study asthma, interstitial lung diseases, lung infections, and other respiratory disorders.
- This chapter discusses the fundamental aspects of bronchoscopy as they relate to clinical practice of pulmonary medicine.

FIGURE 6–1

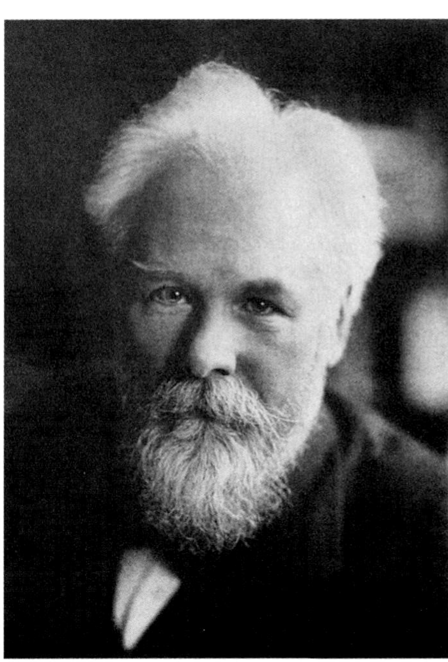

Gustav Killian is considered the father of bronchoscopy. The medical science of bronchoscopy had its origins in 1897 in the small town of Freiburg, Germany, where Killian, using a Kirstein laryngoscope, examined the trachea and main-stem bronchi of a hospital janitor. Later in the same year, Killian employed an esophagoscope to extract a bone from the right main-stem bronchus of a 63-year-old farmer.[1] One year later, Killian coined the word "directe bronkoskopie" to describe the extraction of tracheobronchial foreign bodies in three patients.[2] Thus was born the new field of bronchoscopy.[2] Chevalier Jackson, of Philadelphia, and others popularized bronchoscopy and modified the rigid bronchoscope.[2a] (Photograph courtesy of Heinrich D. Becker, M.D.)

FIGURE 6–2

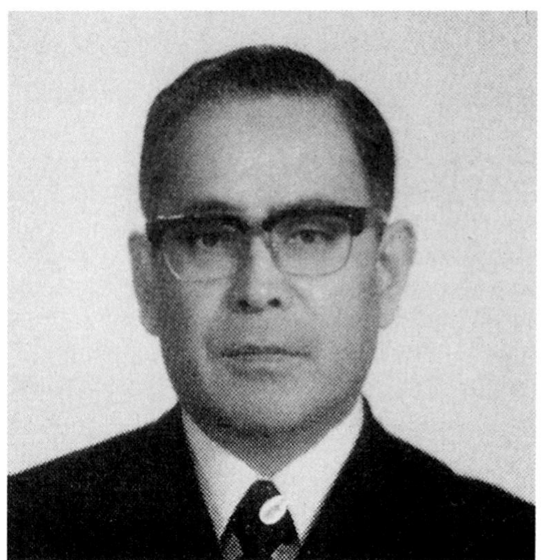

Shigeto Ikeda of Tokyo, Japan, was responsible for developing and introducing the flexible fiberoptic bronchoscope into clinical practice in the early 1970s.[3] The rapid application of flexible bronchoscopy into clinical practice revolutionized the practice of pulmonology. The flexible bronchoscope continues to undergo frequent modifications. Newer techniques have increased the indications for bronchoscopy.

INTRODUCTION

INDICATIONS FOR BRONCHOSCOPY

There are numerous indications for both diagnostic and therapeutic bronchoscopy (see TABLES 6–1 and 6–2). The list of indications continues to expand as newer techniques are introduced into practice.[4] Most of the indications listed in TABLES 6–1 and 6–2 are also applicable to pediatric patients. It is important to recognize that the diagnostic and therapeutic indications are not strictly isolated from one another. Frequently, both diagnostic and therapeutic procedures are indicated, and are therefore performed simultaneously.

TABLE 6–1

Indications for Diagnostic Bronchoscopy

- Cough
- Hemoptysis
- Wheeze and stridor
- Abnormal chest roentgenogram
- Diagnostic bronchoalveolar lavage
  - Pulmonary infections
  - Diffuse lung disease (noninfectious)
- Intrathoracic lymphadenopathy or mass
- Bronchogenic carcinoma
  - Positive or suspicious sputum cytologic findings
  - Staging of bronchogenic carcinoma
  - Follow-up of bronchogenic carcinoma
- Metastatic carcinoma
- Esophageal and mediastinal tumors
- Foreign body in the tracheobronchial tree
- Tracheobronchial strictures and stenoses
- Chemical and thermal burns of tracheobronchial tree
- Thoracic trauma
- Vocal cord paralysis and hoarseness
- Diaphragmatic paralysis
- Pleural effusion
- Persistent pneumothorax
- Miscellaneous
  - Suspected tracheoesophageal or bronchoesophageal fistula
  - Bronchopleural fistula
  - Bronchography
  - Assessment of endotracheal tube placement
  - Assessment of potential endotracheal tube related injury
  - Postoperative assessment of tracheal, tracheobronchial, or bronchial anastomosis

Adapted from Utz JP, Prakash UBS: Indications and contraindications to bronchoscopy. *In* Prakash UBS (ed): Bronchoscopy. New York, Raven Press, 1994, pp. 81–89.

TABLE 6–2

Indications for Therapeutic Bronchoscopy

- Retained secretions, mucous plugs, clots, and necrotic debris
- Foreign body in the tracheobronchial tree*
- Neoplasms of the tracheobronchial tree
  - Bronchoscopic removal*
  - Laser therapy*
  - Brachytherapy
  - Placement of tracheobronchial stent*
- Strictures and stenoses
  - Bronchoscopic dilatation*
  - Laser*
  - Balloon dilatation*
  - Stent placement*
- Lung abscess
- Mediastinal cysts
- Bronchogenic cysts
- Pneumothorax
- Bronchopleural fistula
- Miscellaneous
  - Intralesional injection
  - Endotracheal tube placement
  - Cystic fibrosis
  - Asthma
  - Thoracic trauma
  - Therapeutic lavage (pulmonary alveolar proteinosis)

* Rigid bronchoscopy may be required in these situations.

INTRODUCTION

CONTRAINDICATIONS

- Contraindications are important to consider before scheduling the procedure (TABLE 6–3).
- However, absolute contraindications to either diagnostic or therapeutic bronchoscopy are few.
- Bronchoscopy and diagnostic bronchoalveolar lavage (BAL) are safe, even in those requiring mechanical ventilation.[5–7]
- Severe thrombocytopenia and renal failure are not contraindications for diagnostic BAL.
- Hemorrhagic diatheses are contraindications to bronchoscopic biopsies of endobronchial lesions and bronchoscopic lung biopsy.
- A platelet count below 50,000 cells/dL and a serum creatinine level above 3.0 mg/dL are considered contraindications for biopsy procedures.
- On the other hand, bronchoscopic needle aspiration of subcarinal lymph nodes can be performed without great risk of bleeding in patients with coagulopathies.
- Studies in animal models have shown that an elevated international normalized ratio (INR) does not correlate with an increased risk of bleeding following bronchoscopic lung biopsy.[6]
- Most bronchoscopists prefer an INR below 1.6 if biopsies are contemplated. It should be stressed, however, that routine screening of all patients to detect underlying coagulopathy is not necessary.[4, 9]

TABLE 6–3

Contraindications to Bronchoscopy

- Lack of patient cooperation*
- Lack of skilled personnel*
- Lack of appropriate facilities*
- Unstable angina*
- Uncontrolled arrhythmias*
- Refractory hypoxia unresponsive to oxygen*
- Severe hypercarbia
- Severe bullous emphysema
- Severe asthma
- Severe coagulopathy
- Significant tracheal obstruction
- High positive end-expiratory pressure
- Severe systemic illness

* Absolute contraindications to either diagnostic or therapeutic bronchoscopy.

FIGURE 6–3

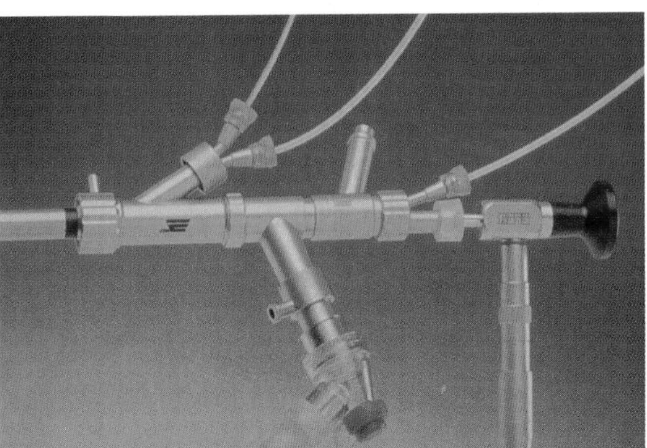

The rigid bronchoscope remains an indispensable instrument. The superiority of the rigid bronchoscope for the management of massive hemoptysis, laser procedures, removal of tracheobronchial foreign bodies, dilatation of tracheobronchial strictures, and placement of airway prostheses (stents) is well established.[9, 10] The rigid bronchoscope has undergone many modifications. The newer rigid bronchoscope, shown in this figure, permits introduction of a laser fiber, suction catheter, and at the same time allows excellent airway management and ventilation of the patient. (Photograph courtesy of Jean-François Dumon, M.D.)

FIGURE 6–4

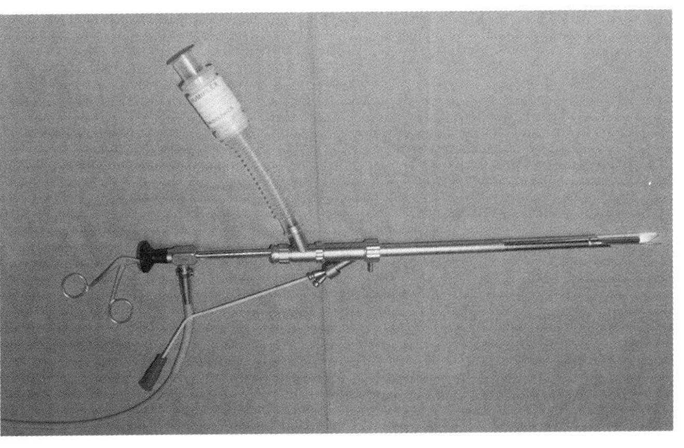

With the rigid bronchoscope and its ancillary equipment it is possible to obtain large biopsy specimens and manipulate various types of instruments within the airways. The optical telescopes employed for visualization provide superb imaging of airways. This photograph shows the optical telescope attached to a biopsy forceps. At the top is the tubing for delivery of anesthetic gases and oxygen. (Photograph courtesy of J. Pablo-Diaz Jimenez, M.D.)

INTRODUCTION

FIGURE 6–5

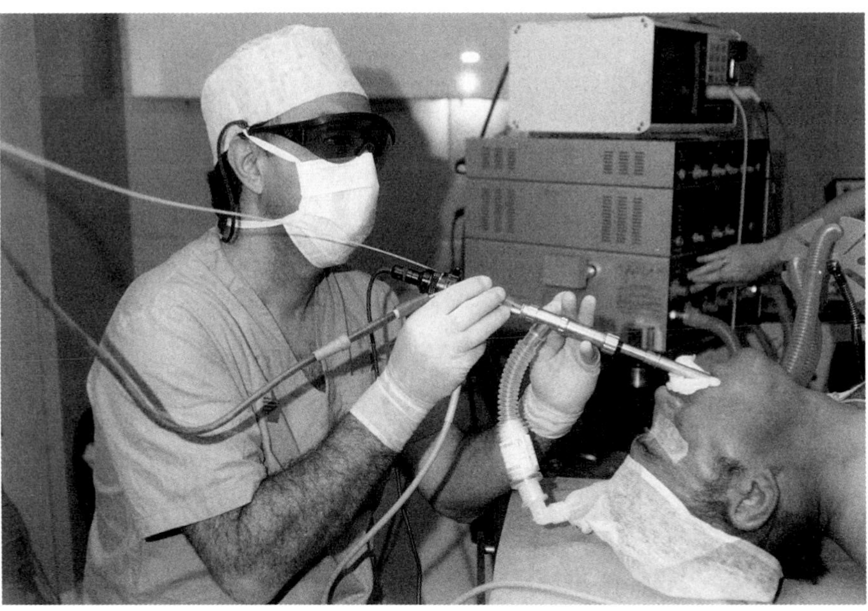

Rigid bronchoscopy under general anesthesia. The bronchoscopist is able to visualize the bronchoscopic findings on a video monitor by attaching a camera to the proximal end of the optical telescope. Oxygen and anesthetic gases are delivered through the side vent attachment (shown proximal to the operator's left hand). (Courtesy of J. Pablo-Diaz Jimenez, M.D.)

FIGURE 6–6

Rigid bronchoscopy is more difficult to learn and perform. As this diagram shows, it requires hyperextension of the patient's neck to permit passage of the instrument into the airways. To prevent discomfort, intravenous sedation or general anesthesia is required in most patients. Contraindications to rigid bronchoscopy include an unstable neck, severe arthritis or ankylosis of the cervical spine, severe kyphoscoliosis, microstomia, restricted motion of temporomandibular joints, and certain dental abnormalities.[11] Complications of rigid bronchoscopy include damage to teeth and transient aches in the throat and neck. (From Zavala DC: Flexible Fiberoptic Bronchoscopy: A Training Handbook. University of Iowa Press, Iowa City, IA, 1978.)

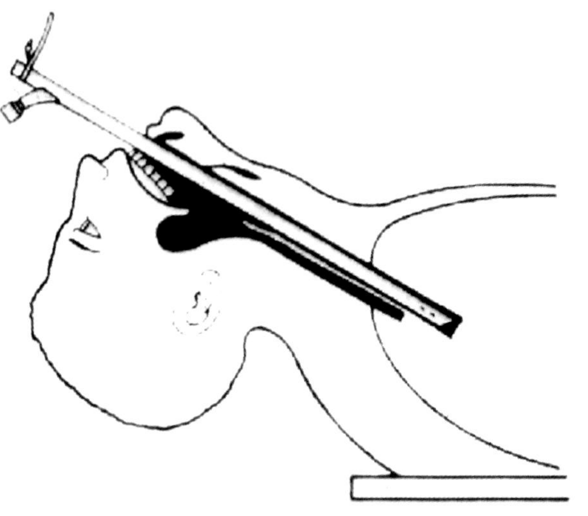

INTRODUCTION

FIGURE 6–7

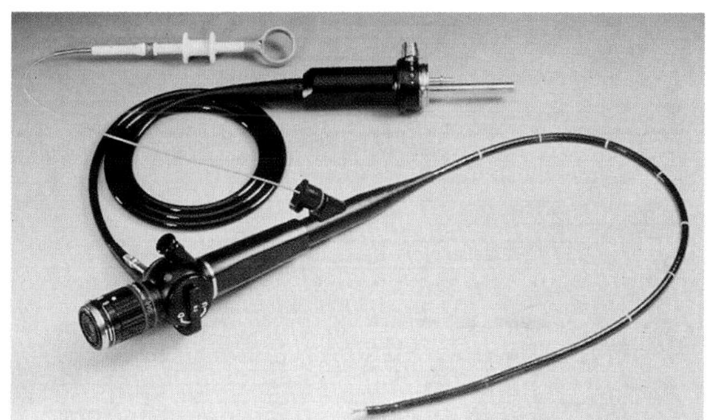

The flexible bronchoscope is used in more than 90% of all bronchoscopy procedures. Recent modifications in the optics and the development of video bronchoscopes have enabled better visualization of the airways. The working channel permits passage of various ancillary instruments to obtain specimens from the airways and the lung. In this figure, the biopsy forceps has been inserted into the working channel. The working channel also allows suction of mucous secretions and blood from the tracheobronchial tree. (Courtesy of Olympus Corp.)

FIGURE 6–8

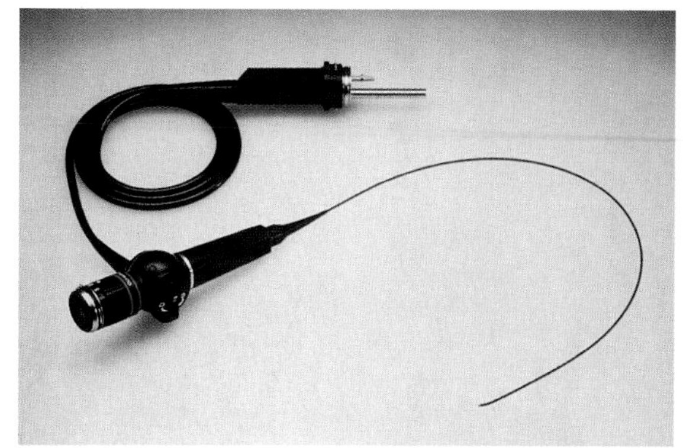

The ultrathin flexible bronchoscope is used in infants and small children whose air passages do not permit insertion of a standard flexible bronchoscope. The ultrathin bronchoscopes are available in diameters as small as 2.5 mm. The lack of a suction channel in the most narrow ultrathin bronchoscopes is a distinct disadvantage. The availability of the ultrathin flexible bronchoscope has obviated the need to use rigid bronchoscopies in pediatric patients in many cases.

FIGURE 6–9

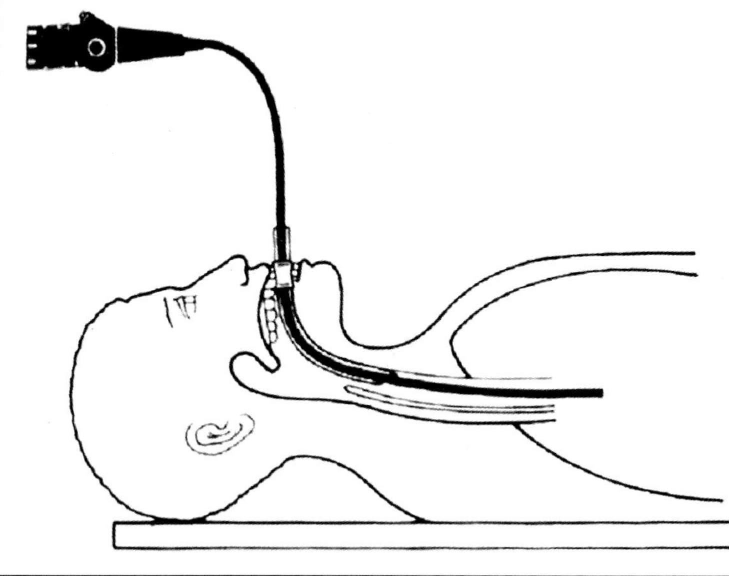

Flexible bronchoscopy performed via oral insertion. Comparison with Figure 6–6 readily demonstrates the differences in the rigid and flexible bronchoscopes. The patient is situated comfortably without the need for hyperextension of the neck. Most flexible bronchoscopy procedures can be performed with topical anesthesia applied to airways. Most bronchoscopists also use mild intravenous sedation to facilitate the procedure. When oral insertion is used, it is important to protect the delicate bronchoscope from damage from patient's teeth. A "bite-block" as shown here provides protection of the instrument. (From Zavala DC: Flexible Fiberoptic Brochoscopy: A Training Handbook. University of Iowa Press, Iowa City, IA, 1978.)

INTRODUCTION

FIGURE 6–10

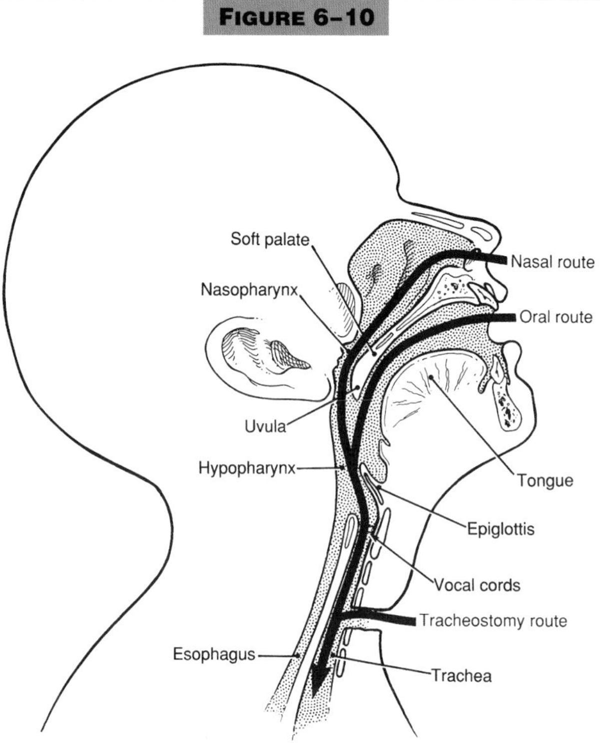

Bronchoscopy can be performed via nasal passages, mouth, or the stoma of the tracheostomy site. Each mode of insertion has its advantages and disadvantages.[12] Advantages of the nasal insertion include diminished gagging during preparation and insertion of the instrument, better control of the bronchoscope during its advancement into the upper airway, improved visualization of the nasopharynx, and the greatly reduced risk of trauma (induced by patients' teeth or gums) to the delicate structure of the flexible bronchoscope.[13] The disadvantages include the risk of trauma to the nasal passages, epistaxis, relative inability to repeatedly remove the instrument to clean it, particularly if the suction channel of the instrument gets plugged by thick mucous plugs or blood clots, greater difficulty controlling massive hemorrhage following bronchoscopic procedures, and difficulty in inserting a large enough nasotracheal tube that would facilitate passage of the standard flexible bronchoscope. The oral route, on the other hand, carries with it the advantage of being able to insert a large enough orotracheal tube through which the flexible bronchoscope can be easily removed and reinserted at will. Another major advantage of the oral route, when used with an orotracheal tube, is the great control over the airway and ventilation. This control is an important consideration because some patients who receive intravenous sedation tend to develop respiratory suppression and hypoventilate. In case of significant hemorrhage in the airways, an indwelling orotracheal tube will facilitate rapid suction of blood.[14] Disadvantages include the risk of damage to the instrument by patients' teeth or gums and increased gagging. (Figure modified from Prakash UBS: Bronchoscopy. New York, Raven Press, 1994, copyright © Mayo Foundation.)

INTRODUCTION

FIGURE 6–11

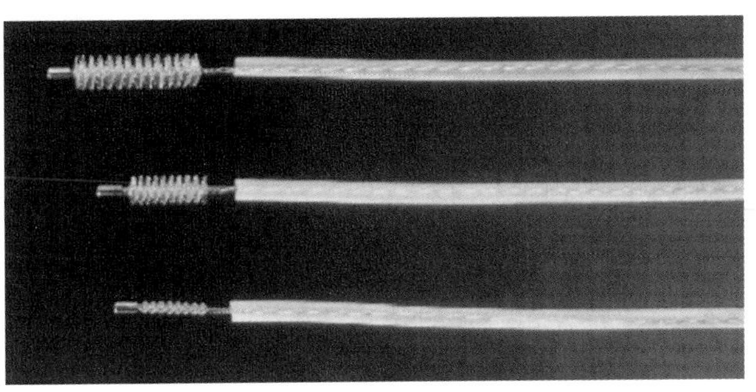

Cytologic specimen brushes for use through the bronchoscope are available in different bristle sizes and diameters. The brush is inserted through the working channel of the flexible bronchoscope to obtain material for cytologic examination. The brush can be used to sample either an endobronchial lesion or peripheral nodule or mass. Most bronchoscopists withdraw the brush completely from the bronchoscope, after brushing the lesion, before the cytoprep is made. This decreases the cellularity of the specimen obtained. Withdrawing the bronchoscope with the brush still protruding at the distal end and preparing the cytologic specimen provides better cytologic samples, even though the diagnostic accuracy is not affected.[15] (Courtesy of Olympus Corp.)

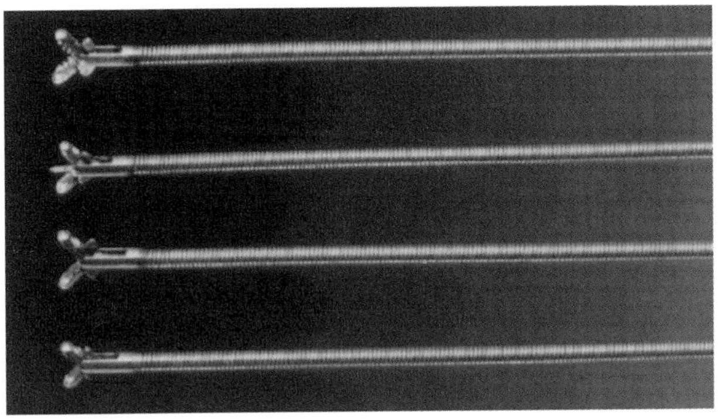

FIGURE 6–12

Biopsy forceps for insertion through the working channel of the flexible bronchoscope are available in different sizes and types. Serrated or toothed forceps (*top*) are better suited for grasping slippery tumor samples and foreign bodies, and the forceps with a needle in the middle (*second from top*) helps prevent slippage during biopsy of lesions on the walls of the trachea or the major bronchi. The two lower forceps are non-serrated and are used in obtaining lung biopsies. Although there are no special biopsy forceps designed solely for the purpose of bronchoscopic lung biopsy, larger flexible biopsy forceps obtain significantly more lung tissue than small biopsy forceps without increasing the risk of postbiopsy bleeding.[16] (Courtesy of Olympus Corp.)

FIGURE 6–13

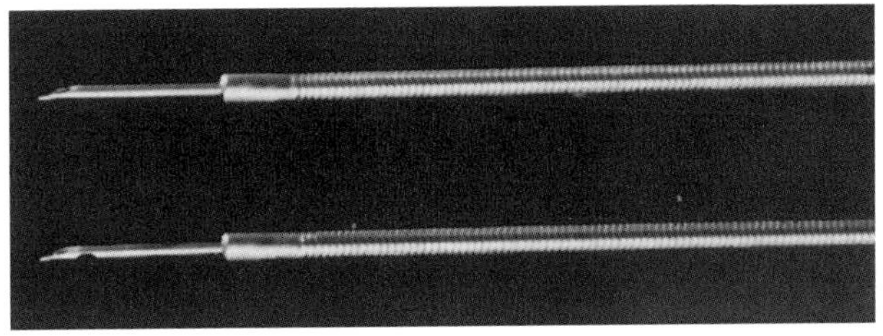

These needles are used to obtain bronchoscopic needle aspiration and biopsy from extrabronchial lymph nodes and masses. The needles are retractable, and some are equipped with a notched fenestration to secure a piece or core of tissue. Appropriate use of a needle is essential to prevent damage to the inner lining of the flexible bronchoscope.[17] Bronchoscopic needle aspiration has been used to improve diagnostic yield from endobronchial lesions presenting as either an exophytic mass lesions or submucosal and peribronchial disease.[18] (Courtesy of Olympus Corp.)

INTRODUCTION

FIGURE 6–14

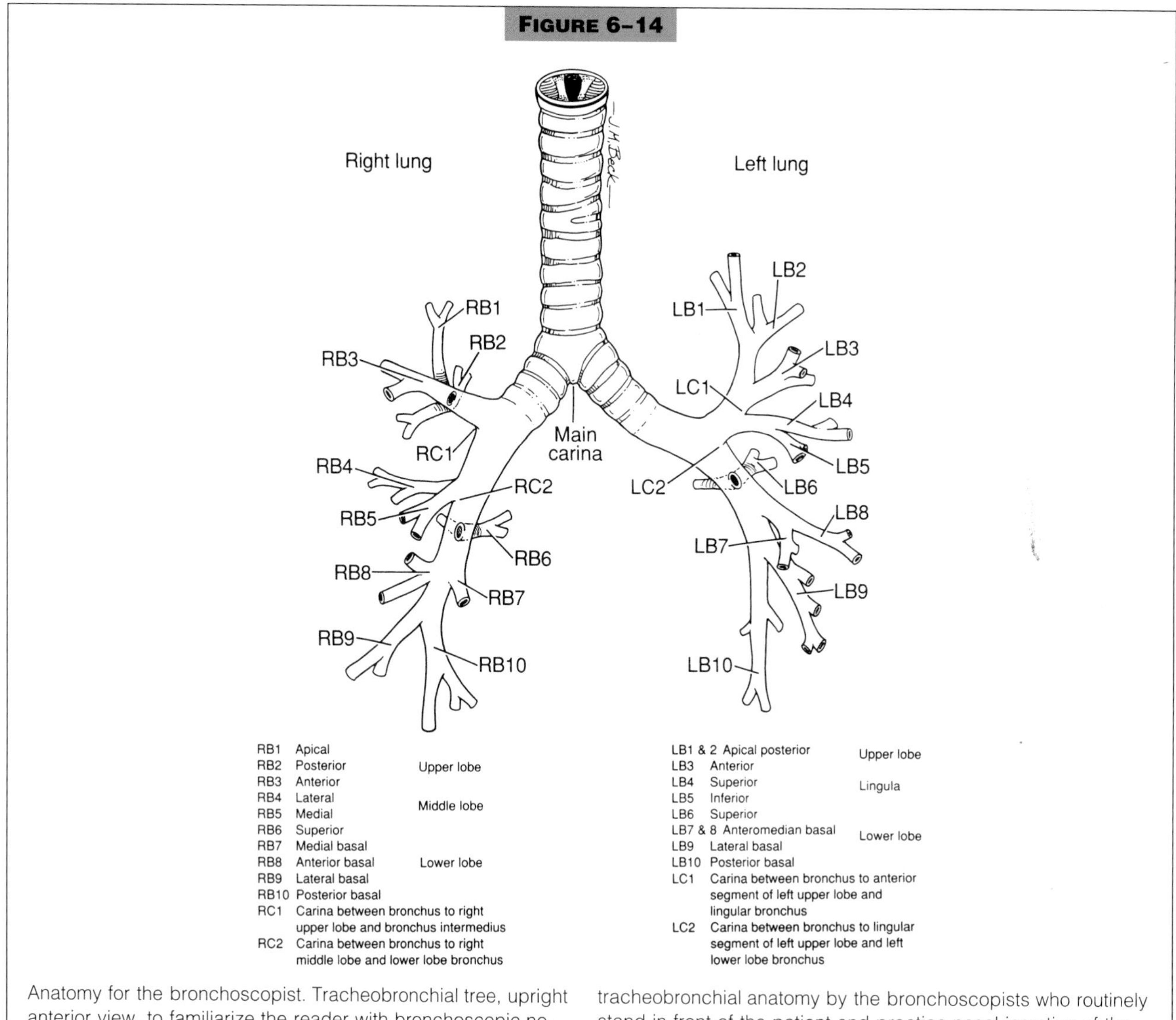

Anatomy for the bronchoscopist. Tracheobronchial tree, upright anterior view, to familiarize the reader with bronchoscopic nomenclature of bronchial branching. This orientation of the tracheobronchial tree is used for mental conceptualization of tracheobronchial anatomy by the bronchoscopists who routinely stand in front of the patient and practice nasal insertion of the bronchoscope. (From Prakash UBS: Bronchoscopy. New York Raven Press, 1994, copyright © Mayo Foundation.)

INTRODUCTION

FIGURE 6–15

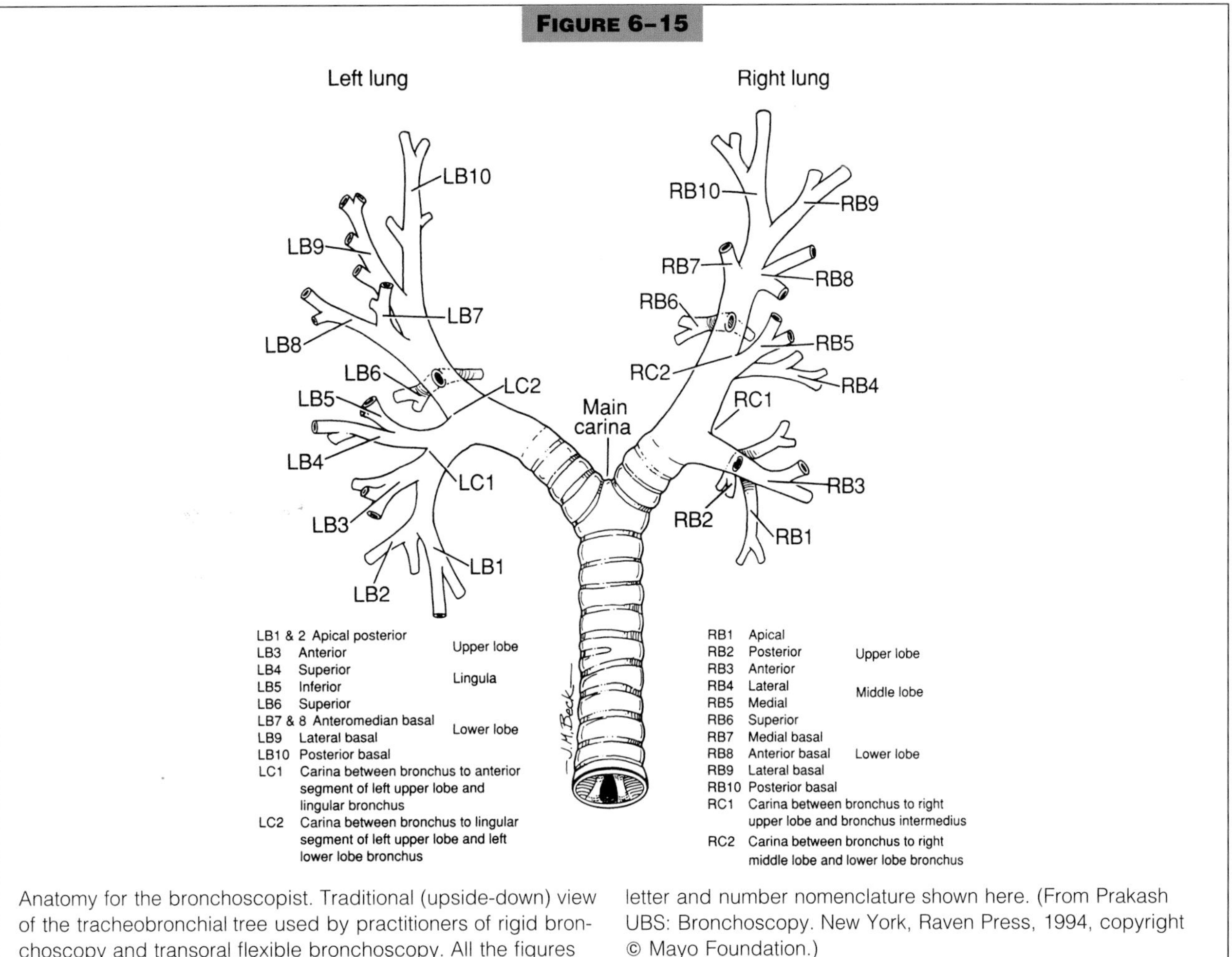

Anatomy for the bronchoscopist. Traditional (upside-down) view of the tracheobronchial tree used by practitioners of rigid bronchoscopy and transoral flexible bronchoscopy. All the figures that demonstrate bronchoscopic findings in this chapter use the letter and number nomenclature shown here. (From Prakash UBS: Bronchoscopy. New York, Raven Press, 1994, copyright © Mayo Foundation.)

PREPARATION FOR BRONCHOSCOPY

Reviewing a prebronchoscopy checklist (TABLE 6–4) is important before proceeding with any bronchoscopic procedure.[19] Many of the time-consuming procedures such as laser therapy, stent placement, and pediatric procedures will require deep intravenous sedation or general anesthesia. Extensive blood tests, pulmonary function tests, and blood gas analysis on a routine basis before all bronchoscopies are not necessary.[4] Chest roentgenography and computed tomography of the chest will help guide the brush biopsy equipment to the appropriate area. Not all patients with heart murmurs or artificial heart valves require prophylactic antibiotics before bronchoscopy.[20]

TABLE 6–4

Prebronchoscopy Checklist

- ☐ Is there an appropriate indication for bronchoscopy?
- ☐ Has there been a previous bronchoscopy?
- ☐ If the answer to the above question is yes, were there any problems or complications?
- ☐ Does the patient [or legal guardian(s), if patient is unable to communicate] fully understand the goal, risks, and potential complications of bronchoscopy?
- ☐ Does the patient's past medical history (allergy to medication or topical anesthesia) and present clinical condition pose special problems or predispose to complications?
- ☐ Are all the appropriate tests completed and are the results available?
- ☐ Are the premedications appropriate and the dosages correct?
- ☐ Does the patient require special consideration before bronchoscopy (e.g., corticosteroids for asthma, insulin for diabetes mellitus, or prophylaxis against bacterial endocarditis) or during bronchoscopy (e.g., supplemental oxygen, extra sedation, or general anesthesia)?
- ☐ Is the plan for postbronchoscopy care appropriate?
- ☐ Are all the appropriate instruments and personnel available to assist during bronchoscopy and to handle the potential complication?

Adapted from Prakash UBS, Cortese DA, Stubbs SE: Technical solutions to common problems in bronchoscopy. *In* Prakash UBS (ed): Bronchoscopy. New York, Raven Press, 1994, pp. 111–133.

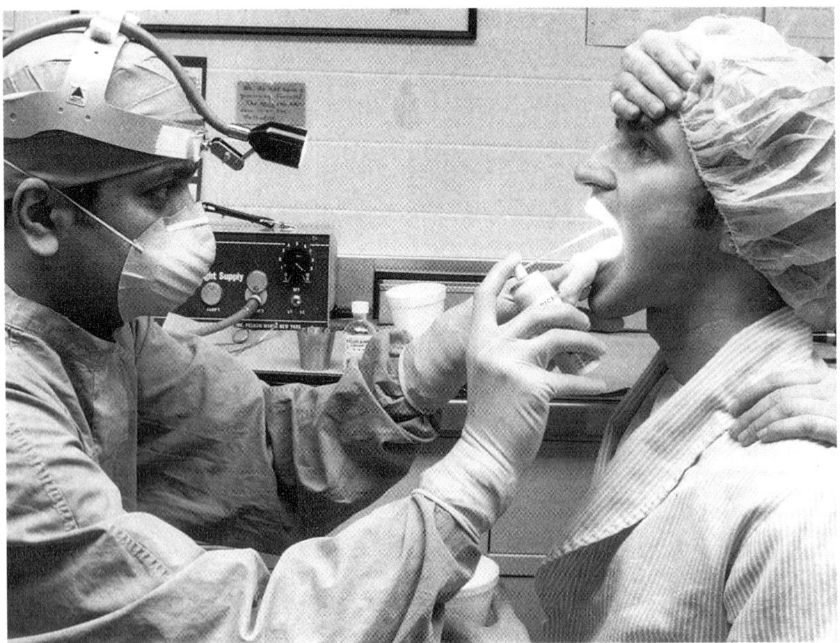

FIGURE 6–16

Preparation of the patient for bronchoscopy requires application of topical anesthetic to the upper airways. After the initial anesthetization of the upper supraglottic areas and larynx by hand spraying, as shown, further application of topical anesthetic can be accomplished via the working channel of the bronchoscope. Normally, a 2% solution of lidocaine is used. It is important to limit the total dose of lidocaine to less than the permitted maximum so that complications of lidocaine-related toxicity can be prevented.[21] Intravenous sedation is used commonly by most bronchoscopists.[21a] Use of antisialogogues (atropine or glycopyrrholate) is not helpful when sedatives are employed.[21b] (From Prakash UBS, Stubbs SE: Bronchoscopy: Indications and techniques. Semin Respir Med 3:17–24, 1981.)

PREPARATION FOR BRONCHOSCOPY

FIGURE 6–17

Superior laryngeal nerve block provides excellent anesthesia of the airway from the epiglottis to the vocal cords. Transtracheal block, through the cricothyroid membrane, results in excellent anesthetization of the vocal cords and trachea.[22] Currently, however, most bronchoscopists use the spray method as described in Figure 6–16. (From Prakash UBS: Bronchoscopy. New York, Raven Press, 1994, copyright © Mayo Foundation.)

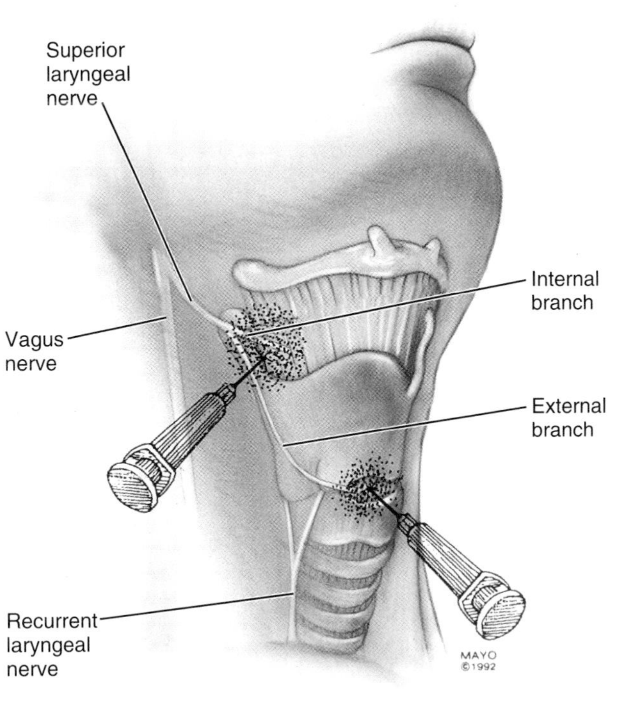

FIGURE 6–18

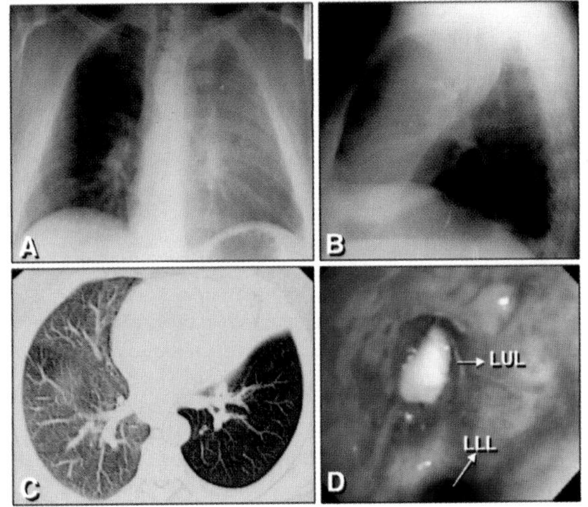

Roentgenographic images often lead to diagnostic bronchoscopy. Posteroanterior **(A)** and lateral **(B)** chest roentgenograms show atelectasis of the left upper lobe. Computed tomography of the chest **(C)** shows significantly reduced vascular supply to the left upper lobe. This excellent example of reflex vasoconstriction was caused by a squamous cell carcinoma that completely obstructed the left upper lobe (LUL) bronchus **(D)**. LLL = left lower lobe bronchus.

FIGURE 6–19

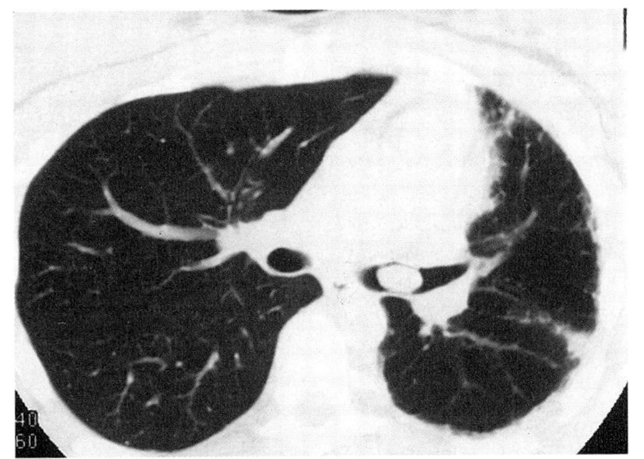

Special roentgenographic imaging prior to bronchoscopy provides valuable information in guiding the bronchoscopist to the appropriate area. A computed tomography shows an obstructing lesion in the left main-stem bronchus in a patient with chronic wheezing. Bronchoscopy showed a large carcinoid tumor. In patients with normal chest roentgenogram, both computed tomography and bronchoscopy detect airway neoplasms in only 5%.[23] In patients with hemoptysis caused by bronchiectasis, CT helps detect bronchiectasis.

PREPARATION FOR BRONCHOSCOPY

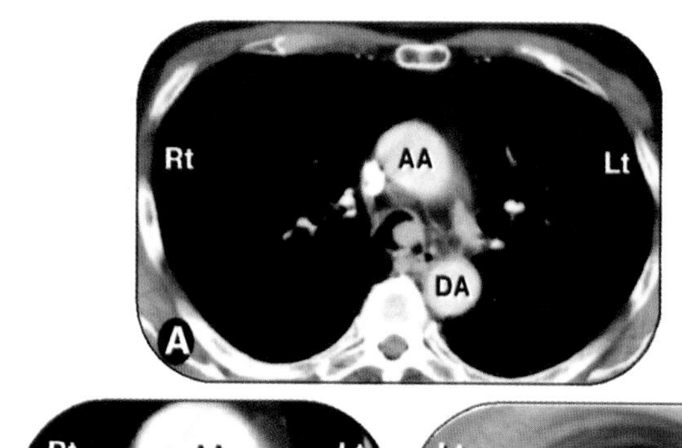

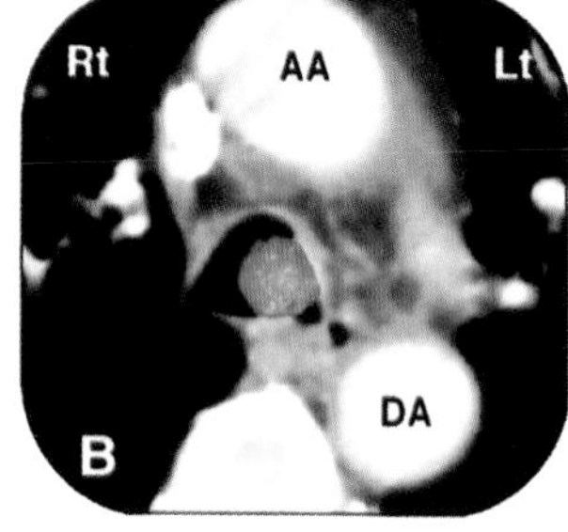

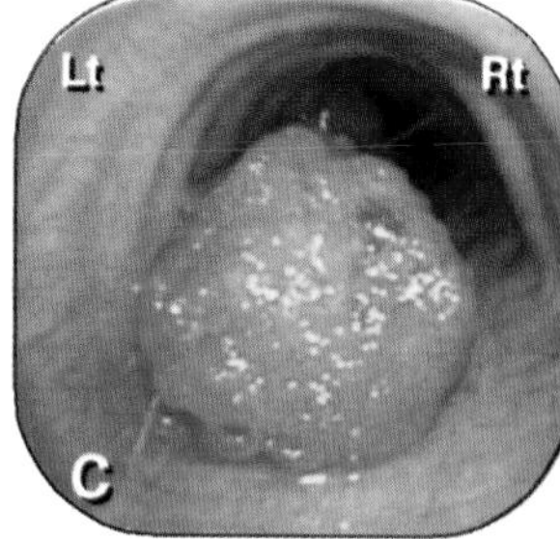

FIGURE 6–20

Computed tomography of the lower trachea showing a partially obstructing mass **(A)** is compared with the bronchoscopic image superimposed on the CT image **(B)** and the bronchoscopic appearance of the tracheal lesion **(C)**. Even though the bronchoscopic examination showed two identical lesions in the distal trachea, the CT study could not discern the more distal tracheal lesion. The distal lesion can be seen in **C,** just beyond the obvious tumor. Biopsy of both lesions revealed metastatic squamous cell carcinoma. Both lesions were successfully ablated with Nd:YAG laser via rigid bronchoscopy. DA = descending aorta; AA = ascending aorta.

FIGURE 6–21

Tracheal tomography before bronchoscopy (the latter to assess tracheobronchial stenosis) is helpful in assessing the airway lumen distal to the narrowed area. If laser or other types of therapeutic procedures are planned, tomography may provide the necessary information to plan appropriate therapy. **A,** Tracheal tomography shows a mild upper tracheal stricture caused by tracheopathia osteoplastica. Bronchoscopy here is most likely to establish the diagnosis. **B,** In this patient with metastatic chondrosarcoma of the upper trachea, the tomographic evidence indicates that the trachea distal to the neoplasm has a normal lumen, and therefore, bronchoscopic laser therapy is most likely to benefit this patient. (See Chapter 8, Pulmonary Function Testing, for examples of physiologic consequences of tracheal stenosis.)

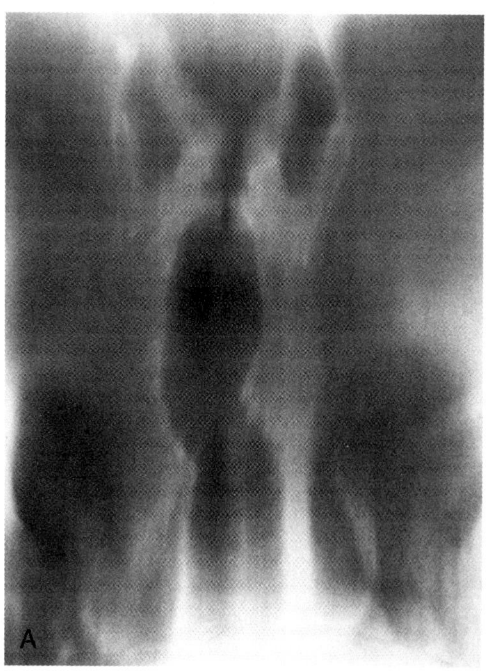

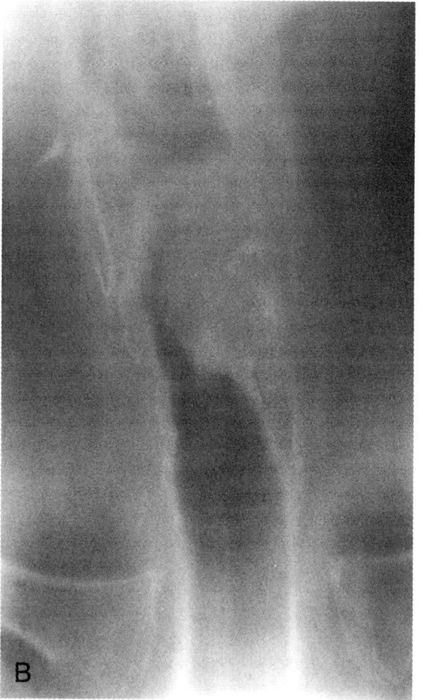

DIAGNOSTIC BRONCHOSCOPY

(See also Chapter 7, Laboratory Diagnosis of Respiratory Tract Infections.)

BRONCHOSCOPIC TECHNIQUES IN PULMONARY INFECTIONS

TABLE 6–5

Bronchoscopic Techniques and Applications in Respiratory Infections

Bronchoscopic Technique	Clinical Application
Bronchoscopy (visualization)	• Assess mucosal, intraluminal, and extraluminal pathology • Evaluate endobronchial tuberculosis, mycoses, viral vesicles (AIDS) • Evaluate invasive tracheobronchial aspergillosis, candidiasis, and others • Follow-up of endobronchial disease (tuberculosis, etc.)
Bronchial washings	• Culture of mycobacteria, fungi, *Pneumocystis carinii,* and viruses
Bronchoalveolar lavage	• Culture of all organisms, especially for identification of *Pneumocystis carinii,* mycobacteria, fungi, cytomegalovirus, and other viruses
Protected specimen brushing	• Culture of aerobic and anaerobic bacteria
Nonprotected bronchial brushing	• Stains and culture for mycobacteria, fungi, *Pneumocystis carinii,* and viruses • Mucosal lesions caused by mycobacteria, fungi, protozoa, etc.
Endobronchial biopsy	• Removal of obstructing lesions responsible for infection (tumor, foreign body, etc.) • Drainage of lung abscess, piecemeal removal of mycetomas (aspergilloma and other types of fungus ball)
Bronchoscopic needle aspiration	• Stains and culture of extrabronchial lymph nodes for identification of mycobacteria and fungi • Drainage of bronchogenic cyst and instillation of sclerosing agent
Bronchoscopic lung biopsy	• Stains and culture of all organisms, especially for identification of *Pneumocystis carinii,* mycobacteria, and fungi; also detection of parasitic lung infections
Rigid or flexible bronchoscope	• Insertion of tracheobronchial prosthesis (stent) to overcome airway obstruction caused by intrinsic stenosis (post-tuberculous or fungal), extrinsic compression caused by mediastinal fibrosis due to histoplasmosis

DIAGNOSTIC BRONCHOSCOPY FOR RESPIRATORY INFECTIONS (TABLE 6–6)

- Bronchoalveolar lavage (BAL) is more commonly used than protected brush catheter to identify bacterial pneumonia; counts above 10^4 colony-forming units (cfu)/mL are indicative of active infection.
- BAL is safe even in patients with severe coagulation problems.
- Cultures obtained by protected brush catheter (PBC) indicate active infection when bacterial count exceeds 10^3 cfu/mL.[24]
- In patients with ventilator-associated pneumonia, when more than 10^3 cfu/mL organisms are identified by PBC, over 75% of patients are likely to have pneumonia caused by isolated organisms.[25]

TABLE 6–6

Diagnostic Bronchoscopy in Respiratory Infections

Type of Infection	Diagnostic Yield (% range, average)
Bacterial pneumonia	30–75, 65 (BAL, PBC)
Ventilator-associated bacterial pneumonia	50–80, 75 (BAL, PBC)
Mycobacteriosis	58–98, 75 (BAL, BLB)
Mycosis	30–80, 55 (BAL, BLB)
HIV	>90 (BAL), >95 (BAL + BLB)

HIV = human immunodeficiency virus; BAL = bronchoalveolar lavage; PBC = protected brush catheter; BLB = bronchoscopic lung biopsy.

DIAGNOSTIC BRONCHOSCOPY

DIAGNOSTIC BRONCHOSCOPY FOR RESPIRATORY INFECTIONS

FIGURE 6–22

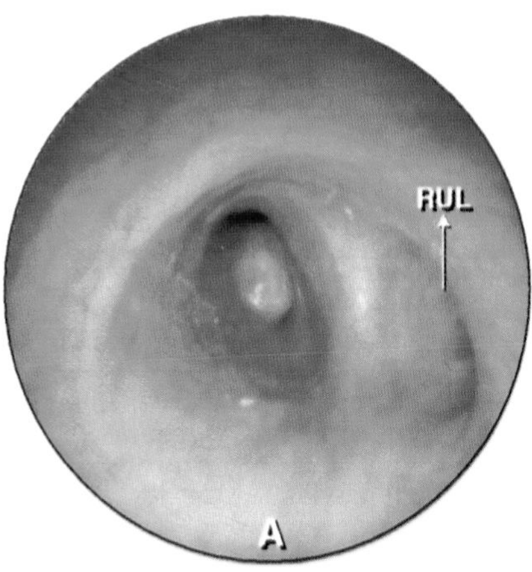

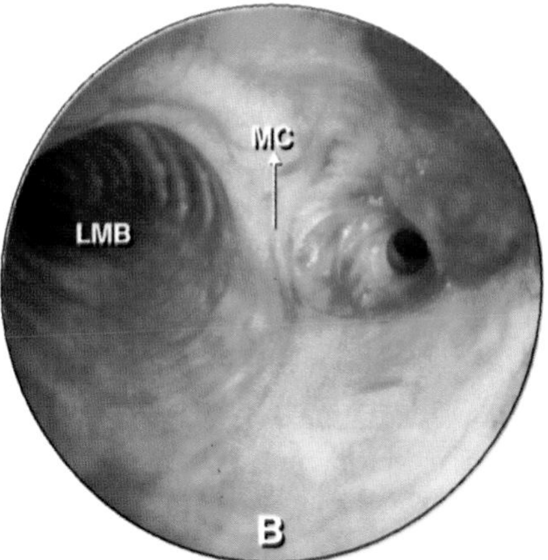

A, Endobronchial tuberculosis with endobronchial granuloma distal to right upper lobe bronchus (RUL). **B,** Tuberculous stricture of right main-stem bronchus. Main carina (MC) and left main-stem bronchus (LMB) are normal. Postinfectious strictures usually follow endobronchial tuberculosis.[26–28] Tuberculosis can lead to mucosal and submucosal granulomas, mucosal ulcerations, endobronchial polyps, and bronchial stenosis. Erosion into a bronchus by a mediastinal lymph node may mimic a neoplasm. The diagnostic rate from bronchoscopy in tuberculosis is about 72%,[29] and bronchoscopy is the only procedure to provide the diagnosis in 20% to 45% of patients with active tuberculosis.[30] However, routine culture of bronchoscopic specimens has a diagnostic yield of only 6%. In miliary tuberculosis, bronchoscopic brushings, washings, and bronchoscopic lung biopsy (BLB) are diagnostic in up to 80% of patients.[31]

FIGURE 6–23

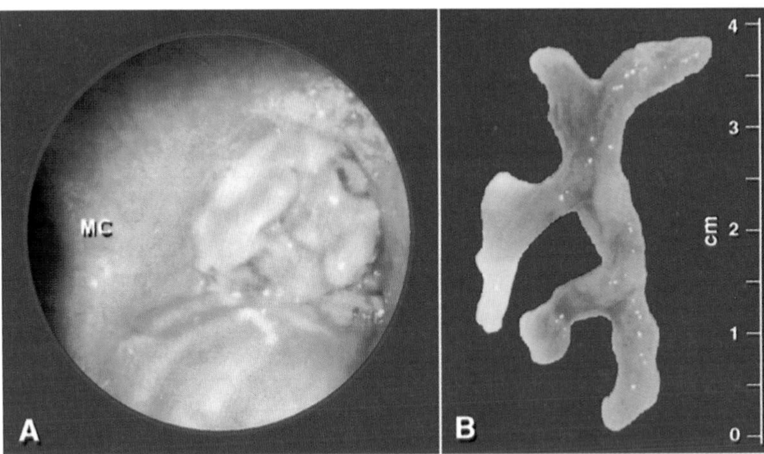

A, Endobronchial aspergillosis obstructing the right main-stem bronchus. **B,** Extracted bronchial cast cultured *Aspergillus fumigatus*. Bronchoscopic identification of fungal organisms responsible for histoplasmosis, coccidioidomycois, blastomycosis, cryptococcosis, and mucormycosis is highly indicative of respiratory infection. However, growth of *Aspergillus* and *Candida* species from bronchoscopic washings does not establish the diagnosis of respiratory aspergillosis or candidiasis because these organisms frequently colonize the respiratory tract. In invasive aspergillosis, bronchoscopic specimens are positive for *Aspergillus* species in only 23% of patients.[32] In pulmonary histoplasmosis, bronchoscopy helps in documenting the diagnosis in patients with cavitated lesions, localized infiltrates, and miliary disease caused by histoplasmosis. In 11% of patients with histoplasmosis, bronchoscopy is the only test to document the diagnosis.[33]

DIAGNOSTIC BRONCHOSCOPY

BRONCHOSCOPY IN HEMOPTYSIS

FIGURE 6–24

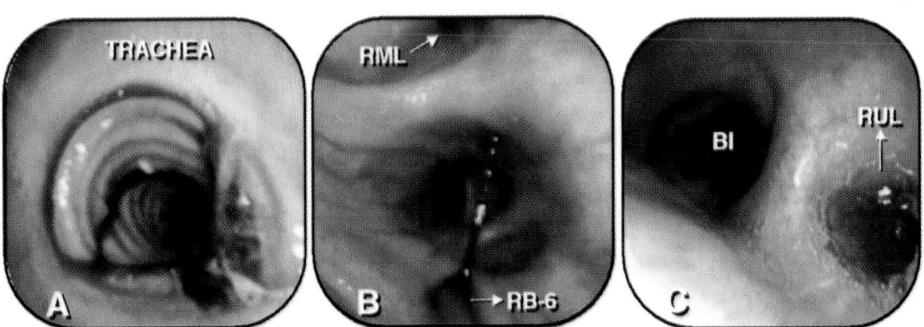

Hemoptysis is a common indication for bronchoscopy. In this patient with an aspergilloma in the right upper lobe, bronchoscopy revealed dark blood streak in the trachea **(A)** and distal bronchus intermedius (BI) **(B),** and eventually, fresh blood was identified in the right upper lobe (RUL) bronchus **(C).** When blood is seen in the tracheobronchial tree, it is essential to trace its origin before suctioning and clearing the airways. The most common causes of significant hemoptysis worldwide are tuberculosis, bronchiectasis, necrotizing pneumonia, and bronchogenic carcinoma. Aspergilloma, cystic fibrosis, mitral stenosis, and metastatic carcinomas also lead to significant hemoptysis. Even though the majority of patients with hemoptysis should undergo bronchoscopy, the examination is nondiagnostic in 25% of patients.[34] RML = right middle lobe; RB-6 = superior segment of right lower lobe (see Fig. 6–15).

FIGURE 6–25

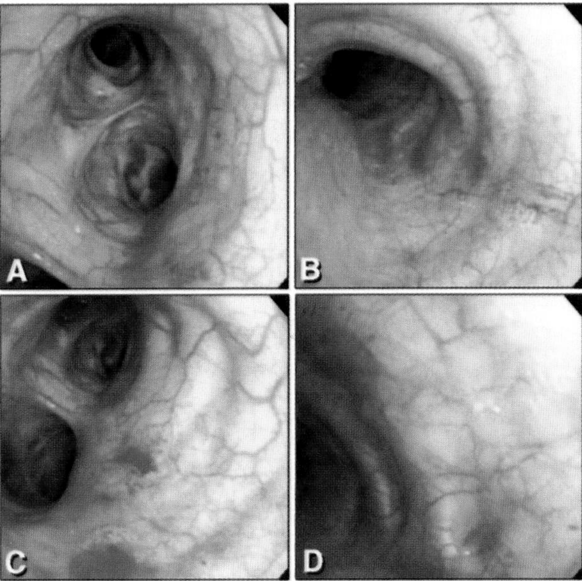

Chronic bronchitis is responsible for nearly 25% of all cases of nonmassive hemoptysis.[34] Bronchoscopy in this figure shows significantly hypertrophied and prominent submucosal capillaries in many lobar and segmental bronchi in a patient with chronic bronchitis and frequent streaky hemoptysis. The capillaries tend to bleed on hard coughing and instrumentation with the bronchoscope. The capillaries are branches of the bronchial arterial system. Similar prominent mucosal capillary hypertrophy can be seen in bronchiectasis, mitral stenosis, and severe congestive cardiac failure. Early (within 48 hours of onset) bronchoscopy is more likely to provide the diagnosis than when it is delayed.[35]

DIAGNOSTIC BRONCHOSCOPY

EVALUATION OF THE LARYNX

FIGURE 6–26

Laryngeal examination, before the bronchoscope is introduced into the trachea and distal bronchial tree, is an essential aspect of bronchoscopy. Unexpected findings may provide diagnostic clues to the underlying respiratory symptoms. This figure depicts an unexpected finding of a benign epiglottic cyst in **(A).** A close-up view of the cyst **(B).** The patient had no symptoms referable to the cyst. Large or symptomatic epiglottic cysts can be drained or removed by direct laryngoscopy.[35]

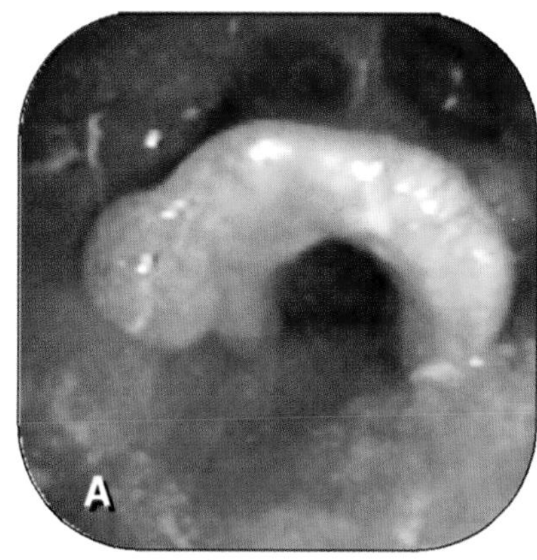

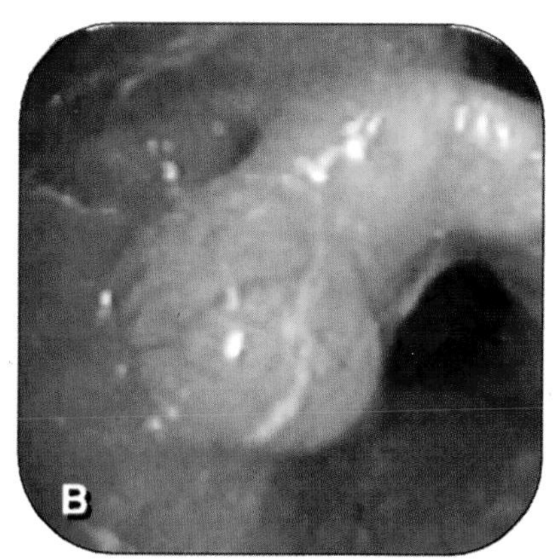

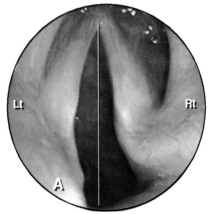

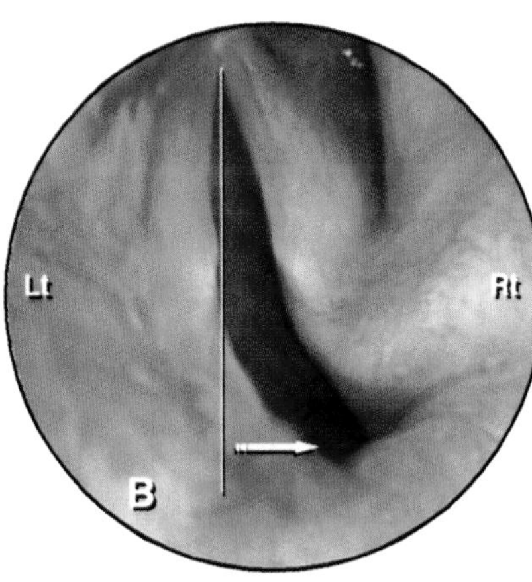

FIGURE 6–27

Right vocal cord paralysis. During quiet breathing **(A),** the paralyzed right vocal cord remains in abducted position. During phonation **(B),** when the patient is asked to say "eee" or "hee," there is no movement of the paralyzed side, but the normal left vocal cord is trying to compensate by hyperadducting (*arrow*) to the right by crossing the midline (*white line*). Proximal stationing of the bronchoscope and instructing the patient to engage in different forms of phonation may reveal clinically inapparent vocal cord paralysis, laryngeal abnormalities, or disorders of the epiglottis or hypopharyngeal structures.

FIGURE 6–28

Laryngeal papillomatosis involving the posterior aspect of the larynx and subglottic trachea in an adult. **A,** Distal view. **B,** Close-up view. The causative agent of the disease is the human papillomavirus (HPV), and HPV types 6 and 11 are the most common genotypes associated with recurrent respiratory papillomatosis.[37] Visual diagnosis is usually obtained with laryngoscopy or bronchoscopy and the appearance is pathognomonic, being "grape-bunch," "cauliflower-like," or "mulberry nodules" that are translucent, whitish, warty growths projecting into the airway lumen.[38, 39] Complications of the disease include webbing, stenosis, obstruction of upper airway, bleeding, respiratory arrest, respiratory infections, tracheoesophageal fistula, and pneumothorax.[39] Squamous cell carcinoma develops in 2% to 10% of patients.[39] A study reported the occurrence of squamous cell carcinoma in 16 of 102 patients with respiratory papillomatosis; the mean time between onset of papilloma and diagnosis of carcinoma was 24 years.[40] In addition to other treatments, bronchoscopic removal, laser therapy, and bronchoscopic photodynamic therapy have been attempted to treat papillomatosis.[41, 42]

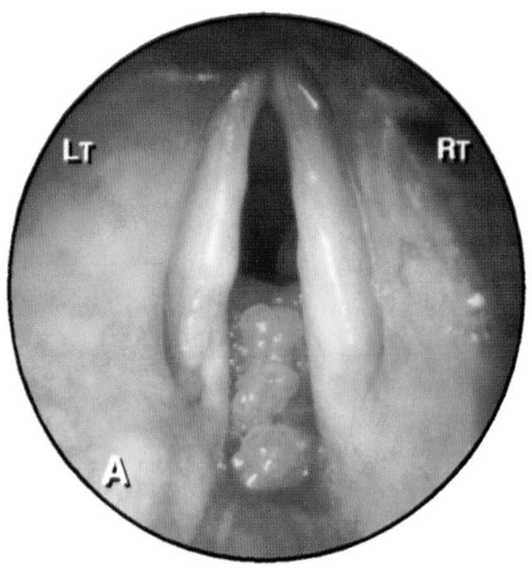

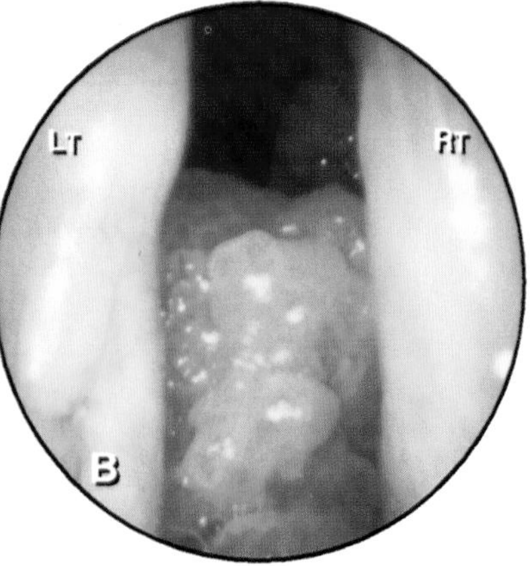

DIAGNOSTIC BRONCHOSCOPY

EVALUATION OF THE LARYNX

FIGURE 6–29

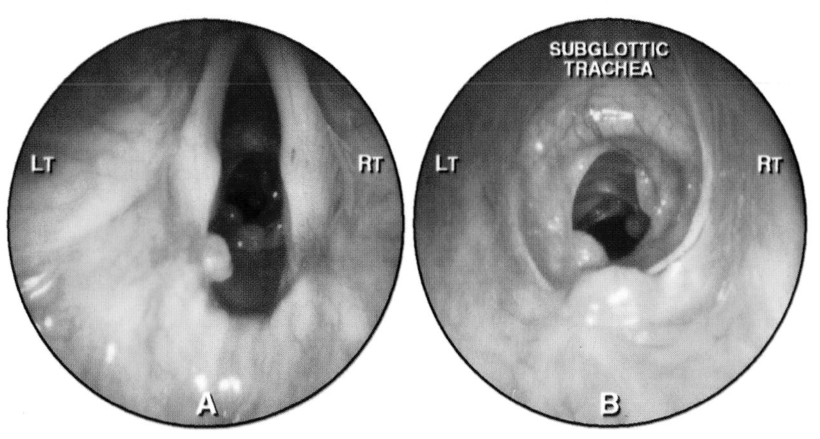

Laryngeal granulomatosis resulting from prolonged endotracheal intubation. **A,** Vocal cords with a granuloma at the posterior aspect of the right vocal cord and involvement of the subglottic trachea. **B,** A close-up view of the subglottic trachea shows significant tracheal narrowing. The degree of postintubation stenosis and resultsymptoms vary from patient to patient. Significant posttracheostomy tracheal stenosis occurs in 8% of patients.[43] Bronchoscopy is important in the evaluation of postintubation stenosis.

FIGURE 6–30

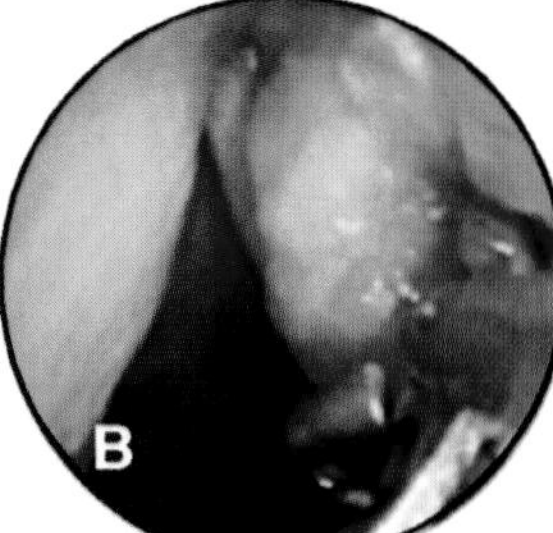

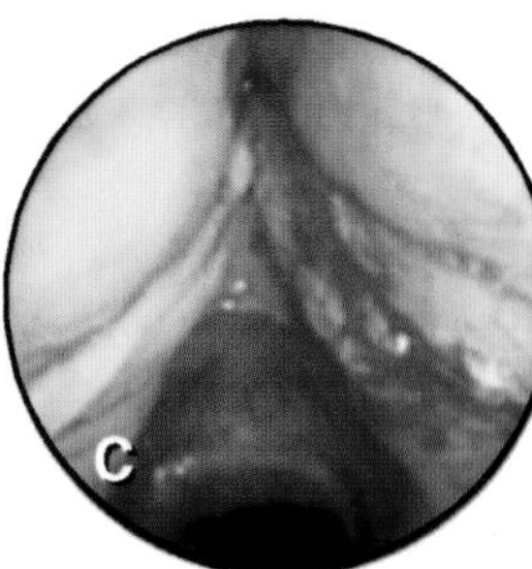

Leukoplakia of right vocal cord detected during bronchoscopy for evaluation of cough. The use of cytologic brush **(A)** and biopsy forceps **(B)** to obtain specimens for diagnosis and postbiopsy appearance of vocal cords **(C)** is shown.

BRONCHOSCOPIC EVALUATION OF RESPIRATORY NEOPLASMS

FIGURE 6–31

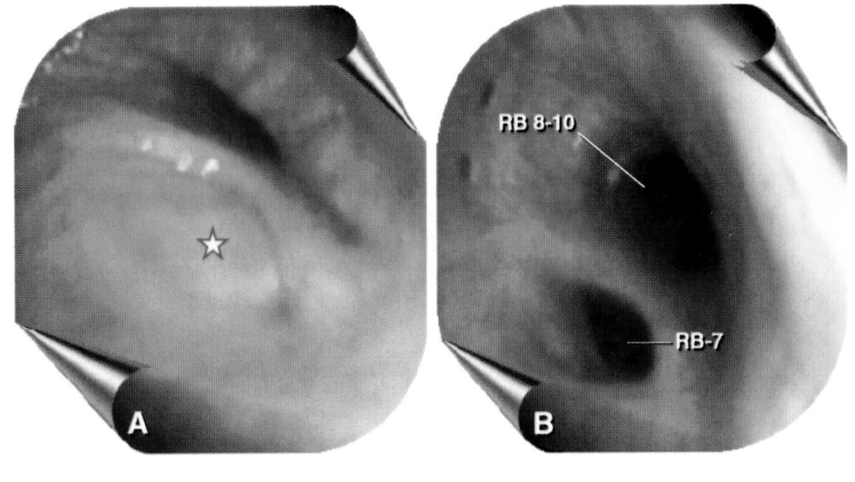

Bronchoscopy in this patient who was referred for evaluation of an obstructing tumor in the RB-7 (medial basal segment of right lower lobe; see Figure 6–15) segmental bronchus showed that during the end-expiratory phase of breathing, the invagination of bronchial mucosa causes a tumor-like protrusion (*star*) into the lumen **(A),** but during full inspiration, the bronchus opens normally **(B).** There was no evidence of a tumor. Various maneuvers by the patient, such as forced expiratory breathing, deep inspiration, coughing, phonation, and flexion and extension of neck during bronchoscopy will help in identifying unusual airway complications.[19]
(RB 8–10-anterior basal, lateral basal, and posterior basal segments, respectively, of the right lower lobe.)

DIAGNOSTIC BRONCHOSCOPY

BRONCHOSCOPIC EVALUATION OF RESPIRATORY NEOPLASMS

FIGURE 6-32

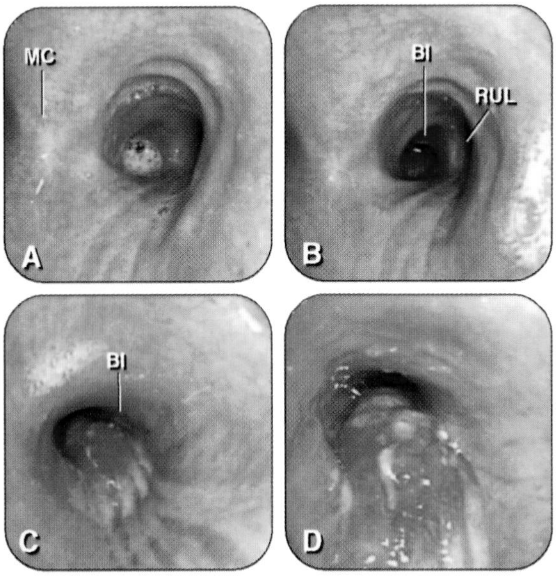

Bronchogenic carcinoma. Bronchoscopy is commonly used to diagnose respiratory neoplasms. **A,** View from the distal trachea reveals collection of mucus in the right bronchus intermedius (BI). **B,** Following suctioning of the mucus, an obstructing lesion can be seen in the BI. **C,** Close-up reveals partial obstruction of BI. **D,** Further close-up indicates distal extension of the tumor. It is important to clear the mucus and necrotic tissue before attempting brush or biopsy. Biopsy in this patient revealed squamous cell carcinoma. MC = main carina.

FIGURE 6-33

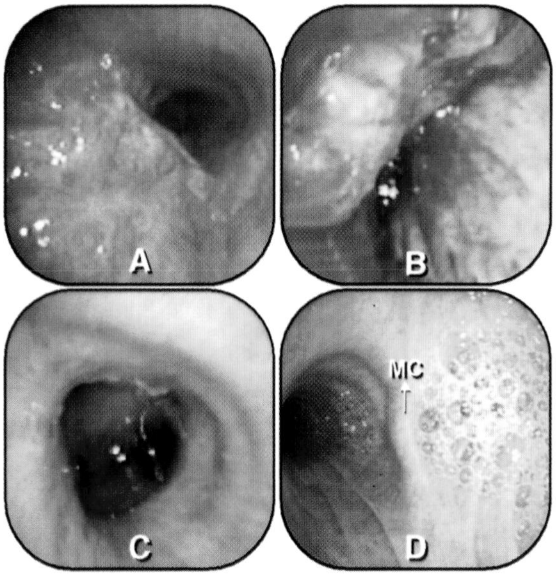

Bronchogenic carcinoma; bronchoscopic views of the four main histologic types are shown. **A,** Squamous cell carcinoma involving proximal bronchus intermedius. **B,** Small cell carcinoma of left main-stem bronchus. **C,** Adenocarcinoma protruding from right upper lobe bronchus. **D,** Bronchorrhea in a patient with diffuse bronchoalveolar cell carcinoma involving the right lung. Bronchorrhea is defined as expectoration of more than 100 mL of thin mucous secretion in 24 hours. Bronchorrhea is encountered in about 20% of patients with diffuse alveolar cell carcinoma. MC = main carina. (See Chapter 3, Pathology.)

FIGURE 6-34

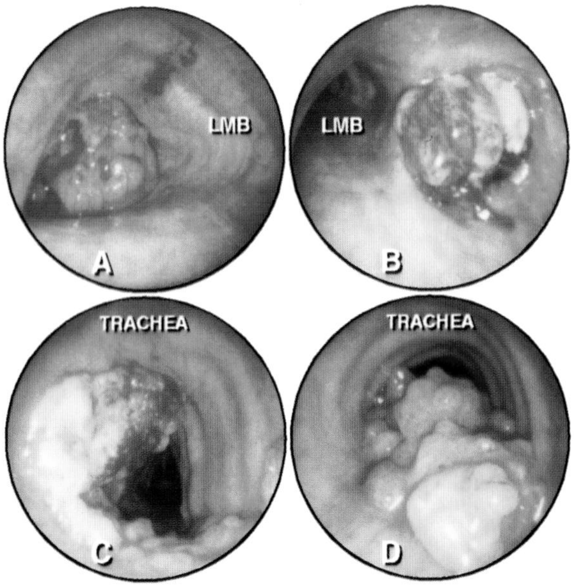

Bronchogenic carcinoma. Further examples of common types of primary bronchogenic cancers. **A,** Squamous cell carcinoma of left main-stem bronchus (LMB). **B,** Squamous cell carcinoma of proximal right main bronchus. **C,** Squamous cell carcinoma of the upper trachea, as a complication of tracheal papillomatosis (see Fig. 6–28). **D,** Squamous cell carcinoma of the midtrachea. Squamous cell carcinoma of the trachea is among the common tumors of the trachea. One study of 198 primary tracheal tumors found the following histologic types: squamous (36%), cylindroma (40%), and carcinoid (5%).[44] A mail survey of British physicians over a 10-year period recorded 321 tracheal tumors, consisting of squamous cell cancer (174), adenoid cystic carcinoma (34), large cell carcinoma (19), small cell carcinoma (16), adenocarcinoma (13), and other neoplasms.[45]

DIAGNOSTIC BRONCHOSCOPY

BRONCHOSCOPIC EVALUATION OF RESPIRATORY NEOPLASMS

FIGURE 6–35

Small cell carcinoma involving right bronchial tree. The typical submucosal spread of this type of lung cancer is shown in this figure. Thickening of mucosa over RC-1 **(A)** and distal right bronchial tree **(B)** indicates an underlying pathologic process. Deep submucosal biopsies are essential to document small cell lung cancer. Bronchoscopic needle aspiration of the submucosal process may increase the diagnostic yield in such lesions.[18] (RC-1 = carina between bronchus to right upper lobe and bronchus intermedius; RUL = right upper lobe; RML = right middle lobe; RC-2 = carina between bronchus to right upper lobe and lower lobe bronchus; RB7-10 = medial basal, anterior basal, lateral basal, and posterior basal segments, respectively, of the right lower lobe; RB6 = superior segment of the right lower lobe.) (See Figure 6–15.)

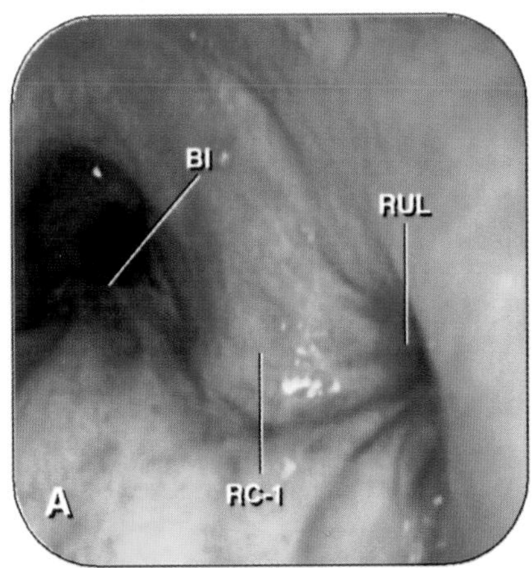

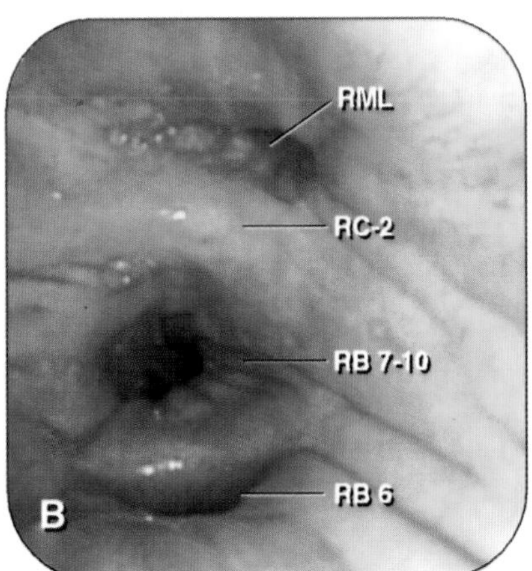

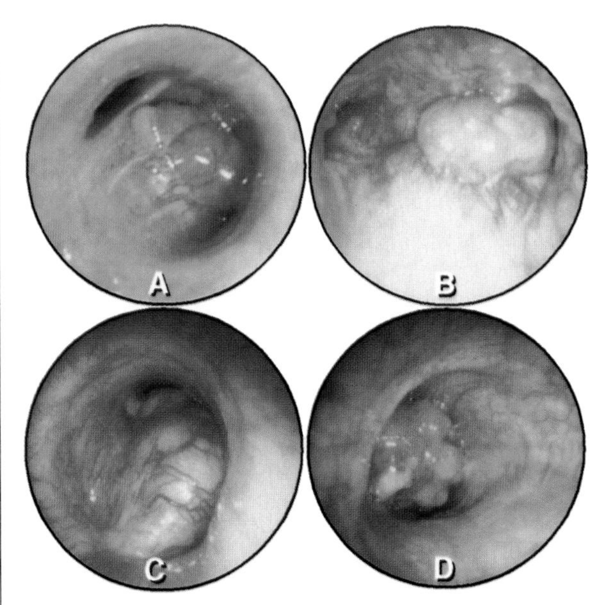

FIGURE 6–36

Uncommon tumors of the airway. **A,** Typical bronchial carcinoid. **B,** Atypical carcinoid tumor involving the trachea and both main-stem bronchi. Atypical carcinoid tumors exhibit clinical and histologic features suggestive of an aggressive behavior. Atypical carcinoids constitute less than 10% of all pulmonary carcinoids. **C,** Cylindroma (adenoid cystic carcinoma) of distal trachea. Cylindroma is a neoplasm of the tracheobronchial mucous glands. Nearly 80% of the tumors occur in the trachea and main-stem bronchi, and the rest arise from lobar bronchi. In the trachea, most tumors arise in the upper or lower third and along the junction of cartilaginous and membranous portions of the airway. Cylindroma is locally invasive. Symptoms include cough, hemoptysis, dyspnea, wheezing, and recurrent pneumonitis. **D,** Mucoepidermoid carcinoma of right main-stem bronchus. This rare neoplasm constitutes less than 0.5% of all pulmonary carcinomas. The tumors are located in the main-stem or lobar bronchi. Tracheal involvement is unusual and occurs in the region of the main carina. Bronchoscopic appearance is similar to that in cylindroma.

DIAGNOSTIC BRONCHOSCOPY

BRONCHOSCOPIC EVALUATION OF RESPIRATORY NEOPLASMS

FIGURE 6-37

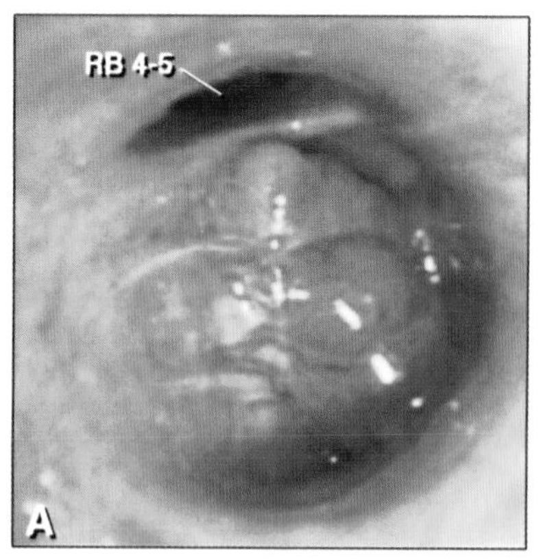

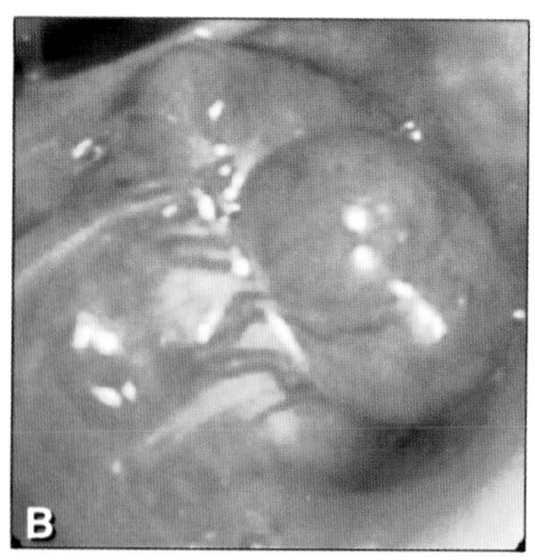

Typical bronchial carcinoid tumor obstructing right lower lobe bronchus **(A).** A close-up view reveals that the tumor is vascular and smooth **(B),** which is typical of carcinoid. This appearance is not exclusive to carcinoid. Pulmonary carcinoid is separate and different from gastrointestinal carcinoid. Carcinoids constitute less than 3% of all pulmonary neoplasms. The tumor is slightly more common in females, and the mean age at diagnosis is about 45 years. Central carcinoids make up 80% of pulmonary carcinoids and originate in lobar or segmental bronchi, and present earlier with cough, hemoptysis, and localized or posture-dependent wheezing (particularly if the tumor is pedunculated). The average tumor is 3 cm in diameter, and most tumors extend extraluminally (iceberg tumors). Hemoptysis is present in at least 50% of patients.[45, 47] In a study of 126 bronchial carcinoid tumors, bronchoscopy suggested carcinoid in 81%, bronchoscopic brushing and washing were positive in 50%, and bronchoscopic biopsy was diagnostic in 40%.[48] The bronchoscopic suspicion of carcinoid is not a contraindication to bronchoscopic biopsy. Significant or uncontrollable postbiopsy bleeding is rarely a problem.[49] (RB4-5 = lateral and medial segments of the right middle lobe.)

FIGURE 6-38

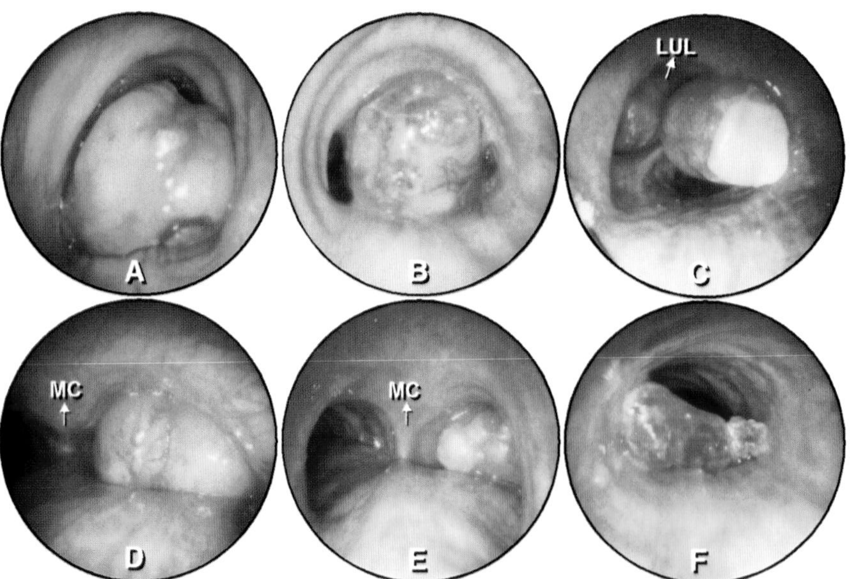

Rare neoplasms of the airways. **A,** Plasmacytoma of trachea. Extramedullary plasmacytoma can present as a solitary tracheal lesion.[50] Rarely, an unusual plasma cell proliferative disorder of the upper aerodigestive tract typically produces a cobblestone or warty appearance of the upper airways, including the larynx and trachea.[51] **B,** Schwannoma (neurilemoma) of trachea. Schwannoma of airways can grow in size and lead to obstruction of airways.[52] **C,** Lipoma at distal end of left main-stem bronchus, just before the take-off of left upper lobe (LUL) bronchus. Lipoma of tracheobronchial tree usually arises from the membranous portion of the airway.[53] They can be large and cause airway obstruction. **D,** Hamartoma of trachea and right main-stem bronchus. Among 128 benign tumors of the tracheobronchial tree, 38 (30%) were hamartomas.[54] **E,** Chondroma involving right main-stem bronchus. One study of 250 cartilaginous tumors of the larynx observed that 72% were benign chondromas; only eight were tracheal in location.[55] **F,** Fibrohistiocytoma of distal trachea. The tumors shown here are indistinguishable from other types of tracheal tumors; bronchoscopic biopsy for histologic analysis is essential to identify their histologic type.[56] MC = main carina.

DIAGNOSTIC BRONCHOSCOPY

BRONCHOSCOPIC EVALUATION OF RESPIRATORY NEOPLASMS

FIGURE 6-39

Metastatic neoplasms of airways. **A,** Metastatic breast cancer involving the left main-stem bronchus. In a study of 42 patients with endobronchial metastases from primary carcinoma of breast, the clinical features included cough (71%), hemoptysis (25%), and segmental atelectasis (57%).[57] **B,** Hodgkin's lymphoma involving the main carina (MC) and both main-stem bronchi. Hodgkin's lymphoma can cause lobar atelectasis and tracheal compression. Mucosal involvement by lymphoma is also common and may lead to bronchial stenosis.[58] Multiple endobronchial tumors and lobar collapse caused by non-Hodgkin's lymphoma have been described.[59] **C,** Metastatic colon cancer protruding from left lower lobe bronchus. **D,** Metastatic renal cell carcinoma obstructing right bronchus intermedius. Airway metastasis is common in patients with nonpulmonary malignancies. Renal, breast, thyroid, and colon cancers are the most common malignancies associated with tracheobronchial metastases.[60] In one study of patients with nonpulmonary malignancies and pulmonary metastases, bronchoscopy was most diagnostic in patients with primary colorectal cancer (79%) and breast cancer (57%), and least helpful (33%) in genitourinary tract cancer (33%).[61] (LB4-5 = superior and inferior segments of the lingula, left upper lobe.)

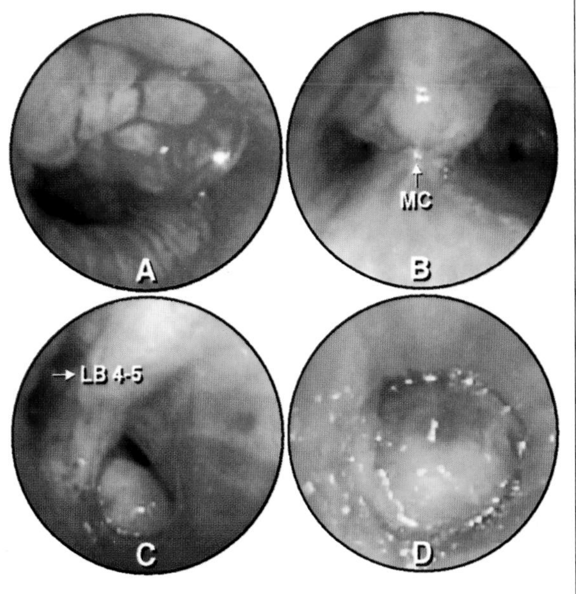

FIGURE 6-40

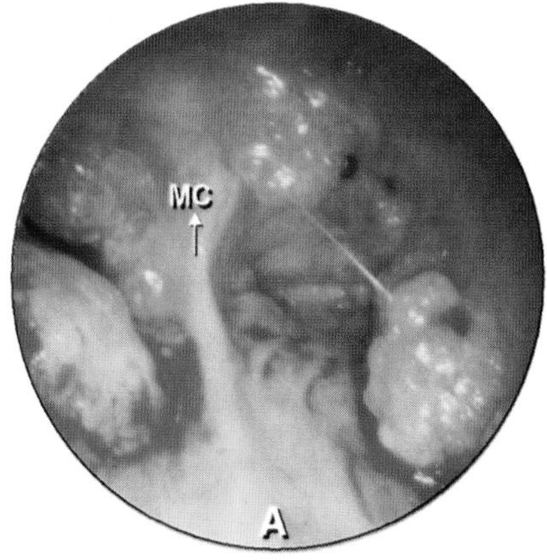

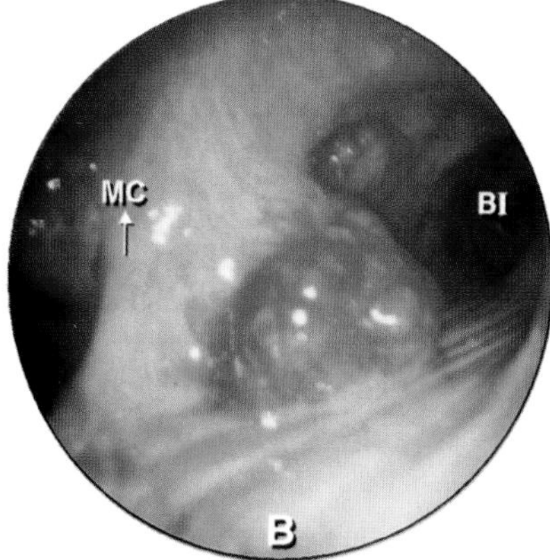

Tracheobronchial metastasis from recurrent squamous cell carcinoma of lung after bilobectomy on the right **(A).** Endobronchial metastases from renal cell carcinoma involving right main-stem bronchus **(B).** These tumors tend to be vascular, grow rapidly, and cause hemoptysis.[62-64] Occasionally, patients with endobronchial metastasis from renal cell carcinoma expectorate necrotic tumor fragments. (MC = main carina; BI = right bronchus intermedius.)

DIAGNOSTIC BRONCHOSCOPY

BRONCHIECTASIS, FISTULAS, AND UNUSAL LESIONS

FIGURE 6–41

Bronchiectasis, with purulent secretions coming out of left main-stem bronchus. Bronchoscopy is helpful in obtaining respiratory secretions for cultures, and in identifying the site of bleeding in patients who develop this complication. Occasionally, bronchoscopy can aid in performing bronchography.

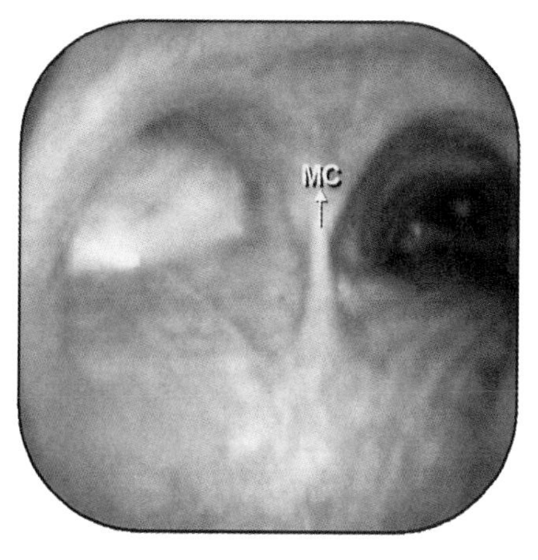

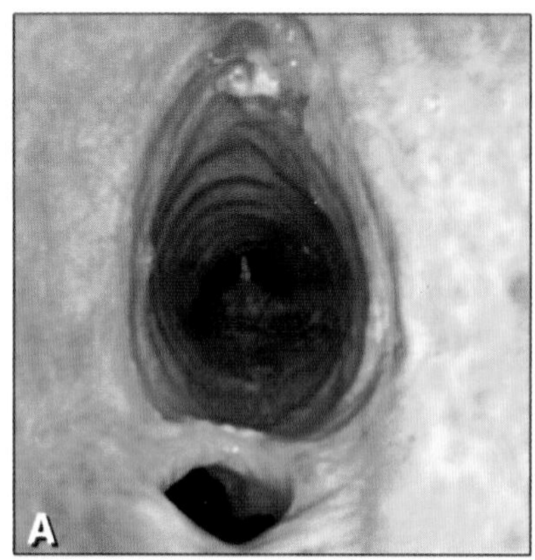

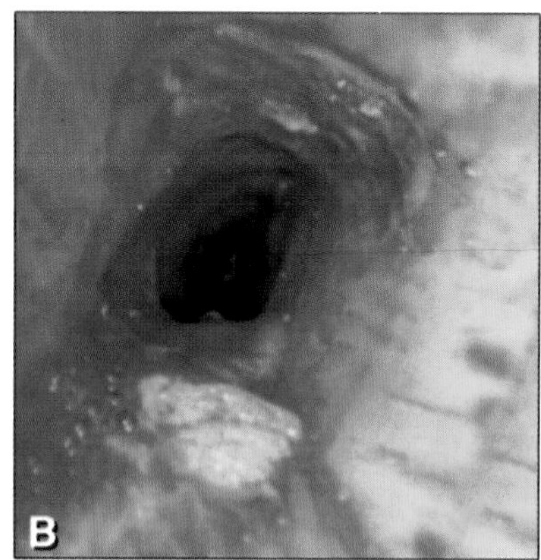

FIGURE 6–42

Tracheoesophageal fistula, benign, at the level of cricoid cartilage **(A).** Bronchoscopy immediately after thoracotomy and surgical closure of fistula with muscle flap; portion of the muscle flap interposed between trachea and esophagus is seen along the posterior wall of the trachea **(B).**

FIGURE 6–43

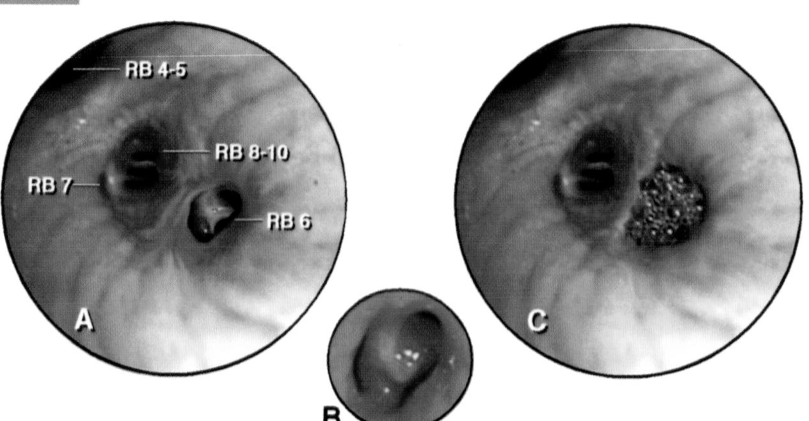

Bronchoesophageal fistula, benign. Normal appearing right bronchial tree **(A).** Superior segment bronchus (RB-6) appears inflamed, but there is no evidence of fistula **(B).** Instillation of several drops of methylene blue into the proximal esophagus through nasogastric tube reveals that the site of communication with esophagus is through RB-6 bronchus **(C).**[64a] The fistula was the result of previous esophageal surgery. Such abnormal communications can exist as tracheoesophageal, bronchoesophageal, bronchopleural, bronchovascular, or bronchoperitoneal fistulas. Bronchoscopic laser coagulation, fibrin glue application, and stent placements have been used to treat tracheoesophageal, bronchoesophageal, and bronchopleural fistulas.[65-68] The results from such bronchoscopic therapies have been disappointing. (RB6 = superior segment of right lower lobe; RB4-5 = lateral and medial segment of right middle lobe; RB7 = medial basal segment of the right lower lobe; RB8-10 = anterior basal, lateral basal, and posterior basal segments of the right lower lobe.) (See Fig. 6–15.)

DIAGNOSTIC BRONCHOSCOPY

BRONCHIECTASIS, FISTULAS, AND UNUSAL LESIONS

FIGURE 6–44

Tracheoesophageal fistula caused by esophageal cancer. Gastric secretions are seen coming out of the fistula **(A).** The size of the fistula can be assessed after suctioning the secretions **(B).** Tracheoesophageal fistula following radiation therapy in a different patient **(C).**[64a] Fistula complicating right upper lobe sleeve resection **(D).** (MC = main carina)

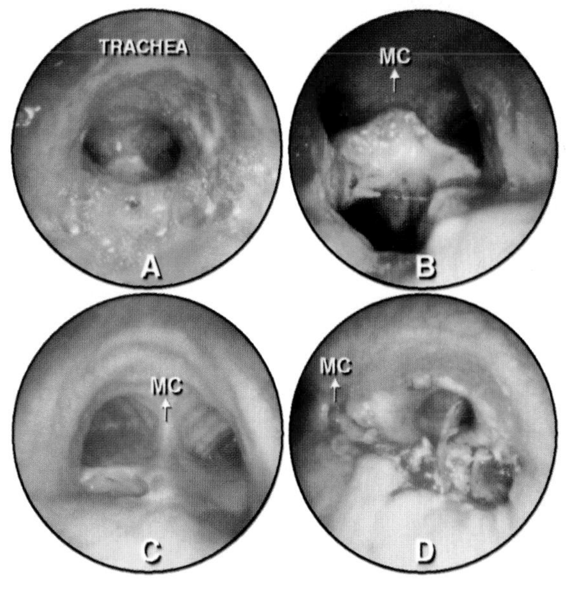

FIGURE 6–45

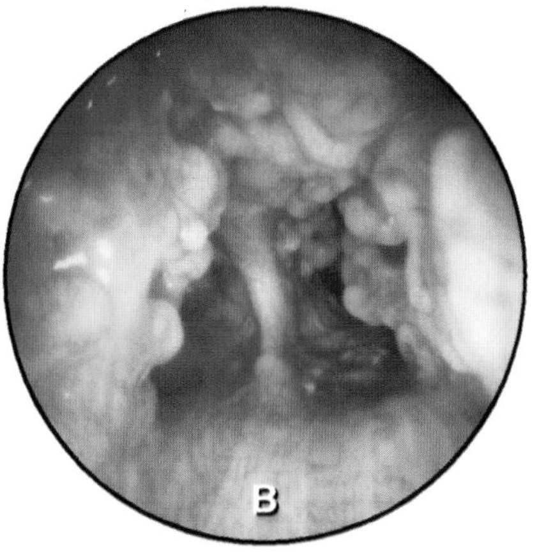

Tracheobronchopathia osteoplastica. **A,** Midtrachea. **B,** Distal trachea. This rare disease of obscure etiology is characterized by cartilaginous or bony outgrowths into the lumen of the tracheobronchial tree. The nodular excrescences represent exostoses or enchondroses from the cartilaginous trachea that often ossifies. The posterior membranous trachea is always spared from the development of bony/cartilaginous enchondroses. Clinical manifestations include cough, wheeze, and occasional hemoptysis. Bronchoscopy is diagnostic.[69, 70]

FIGURE 6–46

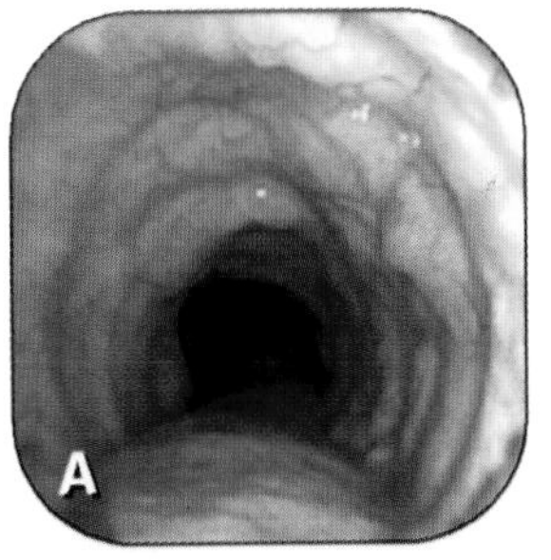

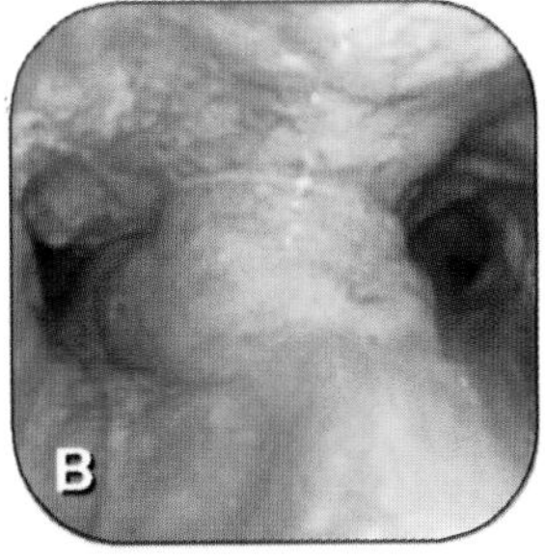

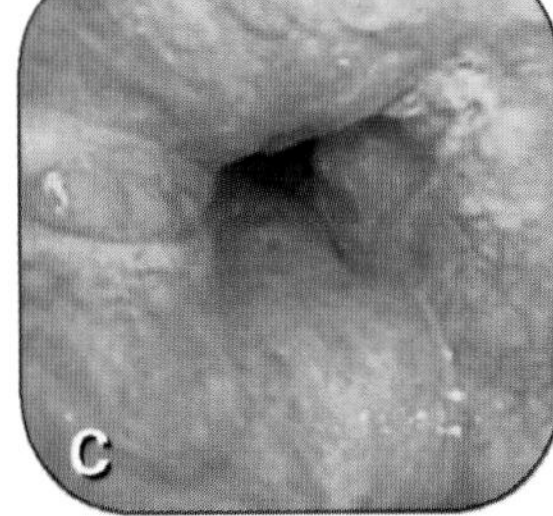

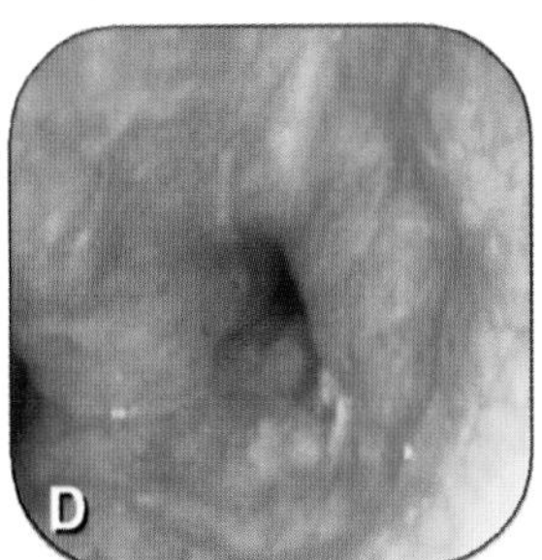

Amyloidosis of the tracheobronchial tree shows that the trachea **(A),** main carina **(B),** left main-stem bronchus **(C),** and right upper lobe bronchus **(D)** are all involved by the pathologic process. Submucosal depositions of amyloid produce gradual narrowing of the major airways and lead to respiratory distress.[71] Deep biopsy of mucosal and submucosal lesions usually provides diagnosis. Laser therapy has been described in the treatment of tracheobronchial amyloidosis.[72, 73]

DIAGNOSTIC BRONCHOSCOPY

BRONCHIECTASIS, FISTULAS, AND UNUSAL LESIONS

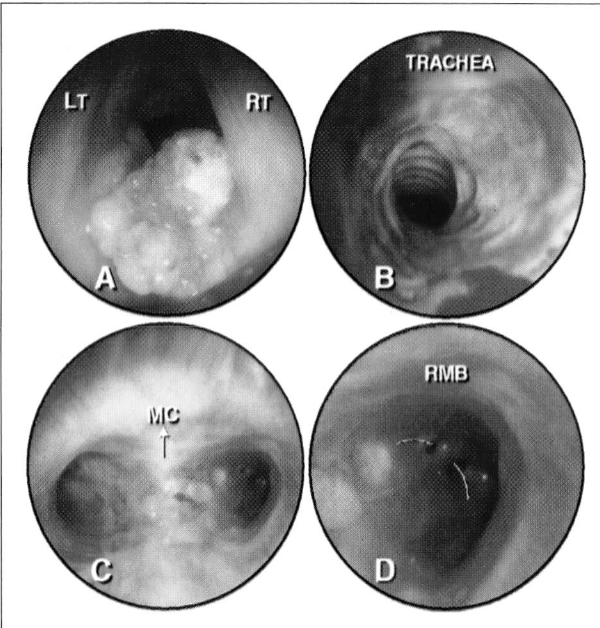

FIGURE 6-47

Wegener's granulomatosis involving the tracheobronchial tree. **A,** Subglottic pseudotumoral mass. **B,** Midtracheal stenosis in chronic Wegener's granulomatosis. **C,** Main carinal involvement. **D,** Submucosal communication with tunnel formation; the interruption in the middle of the white line identifies the tunnel. Tracheobronchial mucosal ulcerations and stenoses are common in this disorder.[74-76] Lobar atelectasis caused by endobronchial Wegener's granulomatosis has been described.[74] Repeated bronchoscopic dilatations have been used to dilate chronic stenotic lesions.[75] In a study of 51 patients with biopsy-proven Wegener's granulomatosis, 30 (59%) exhibited endobronchial abnormalities. The bronchoscopic findings consisted of subglottic stenosis in 5 (17%), ulcerating tracheobronchitis with or without inflammatory pseudotumors in 18 (60%), cicatricial tracheal or bronchial stenosis without inflammation in 4 (13%), and hemorrhage without identifiable source in 2 (4%).[77]

FIGURE 6-48

Tracheobronchomegaly (Mounier-Kuhn syndrome) demonstrates a large tracheal lumen **(A),** a patulous trachea **(B),** and collapsibility during expiration **(C).** Tracheal diverticulum is also noted in **C.** Pathologic states associated with tracheobronchomegaly include Mounier-Kuhn syndrome, Ehlers-Danlos syndrome, cutis laxa, and acromegaly. However, many cases of asymptomatic tracheobronchomegaly are idiopathic in nature.[78, 79]

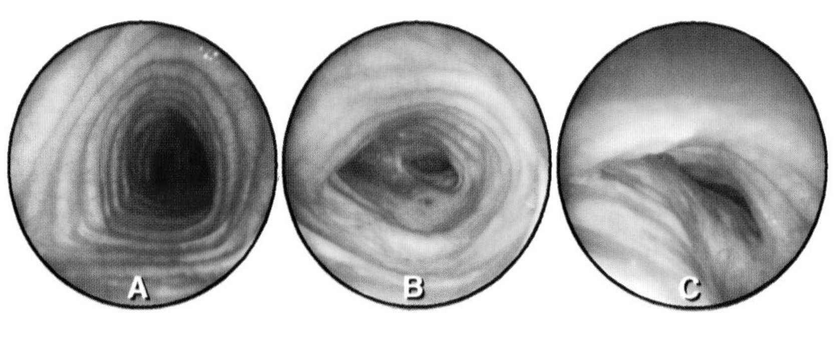

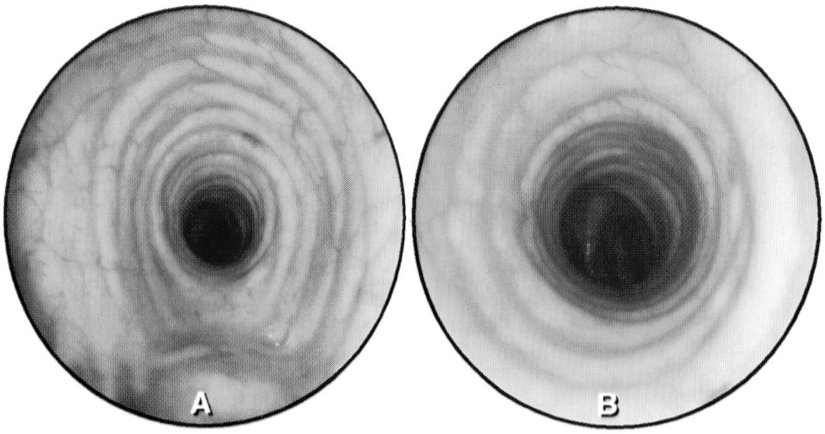

FIGURE 6-49

Congenital tracheal anomaly shows complete tracheal rings in proximal trachea **(A)** and distal trachea **(B).** Such anomalies are usually incidental findings during bronchoscopy.

DIAGNOSTIC BRONCHOSCOPY

BRONCHOALVEOLAR LAVAGE, BIOPSIES, ULTRASOUND, AND OTHER NEWER TECHNIQUES

FIGURE 6–50

Bronchoalveolar lavage (BAL) in Langerhans cell granuloma of lung. Finding more than 5% CD1a (OKT6) cells (brightly stained cells) in the BAL effluent establishes the diagnosis. BAL is diagnostic of lung disorders such as Langerhans cell granuloma, lymphangitic carcinoma, and lipoid pneumonia.[80] BAL is also diagnostic in chronic eosinophilic pneumonia, fat embolism syndrome, alveolar phospholipoproteinosis, alveolar hemorrhage, and pulmonary endometriosis. BAL findings in other interstitial lung diseases are supportive of the diagnoses provided the clinical features are compatible with the diagnosis. Tables 6–5 and 6–6 provide further information on the role of BAL in lung infections. (See Chapter 7, Laboratory Diagnosis of Respiratory Tract Infections.)

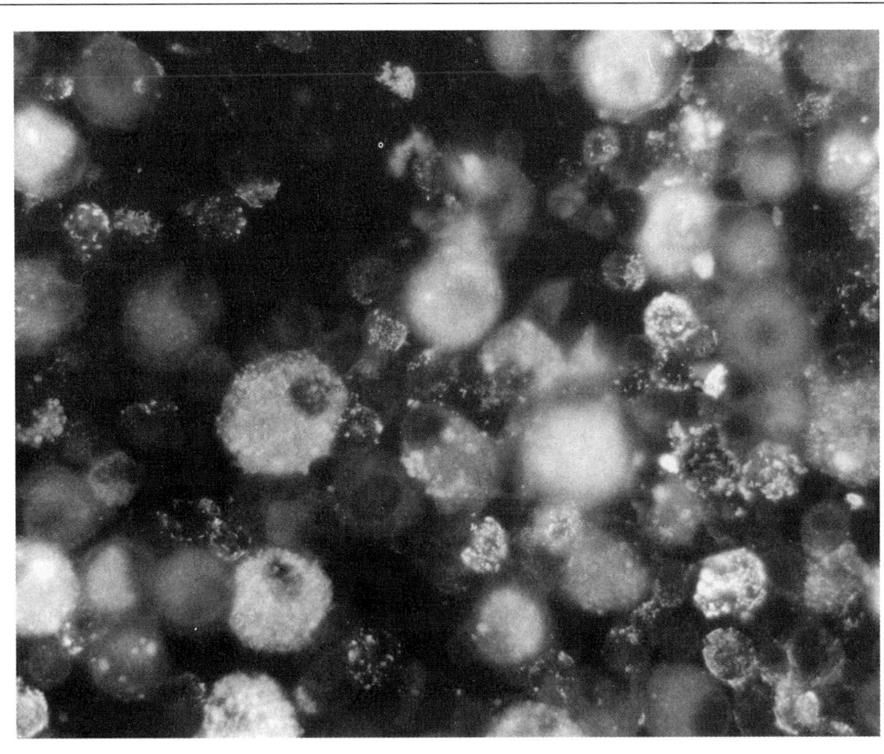

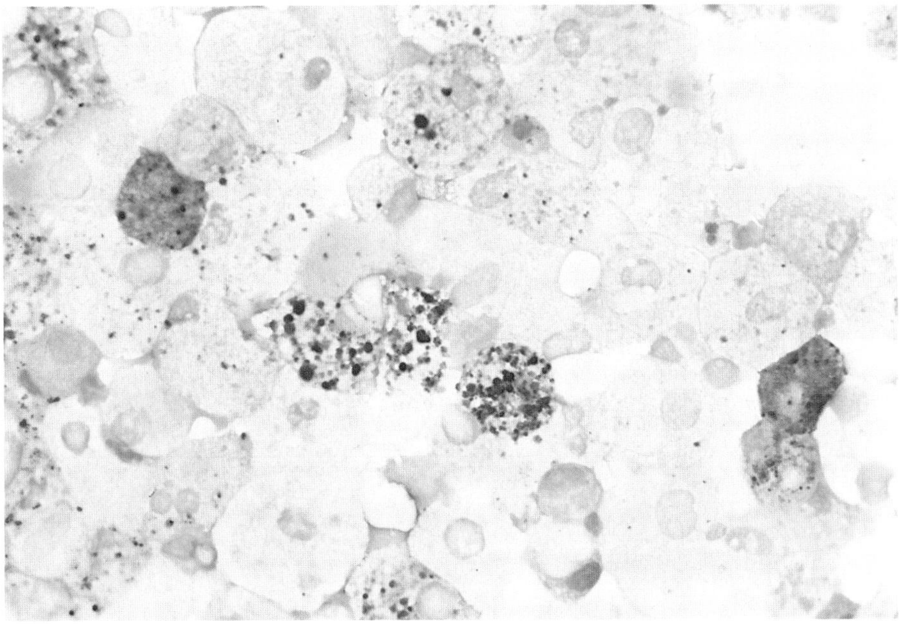

FIGURE 6–51

Alveolar hemorrhage diagnosed by BAL. Special iron stain of the BAL effluent shows hemosiderin-laden macrophages, estimated at 44% of total cells. Finding more than 20% hemosiderin-laden macrophages is an indicator of alveolar hemorrhage.[81]

DIAGNOSTIC BRONCHOSCOPY

BRONCHOALVEOLAR LAVAGE, BIOPSIES, ULTRASOUND, AND OTHER NEWER TECHNIQUES

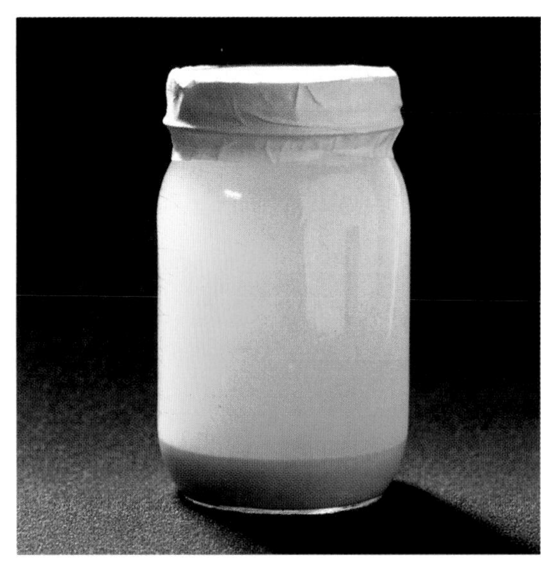

FIGURE 6-52

Pulmonary alveolar phospholipoproteinosis diagnosed by BAL. The characteristic appearance of the BAL effluent, with thick sediment at the bottom and lipoid layer at the top, is diagnostic. A lung biopsy can be waived when the BAL effluent has the typical appearance (From Prakash UBS: Bronchoscopy. New York, Raven Press, 1994, copyright Mayo Foundation).

FIGURE 6-53

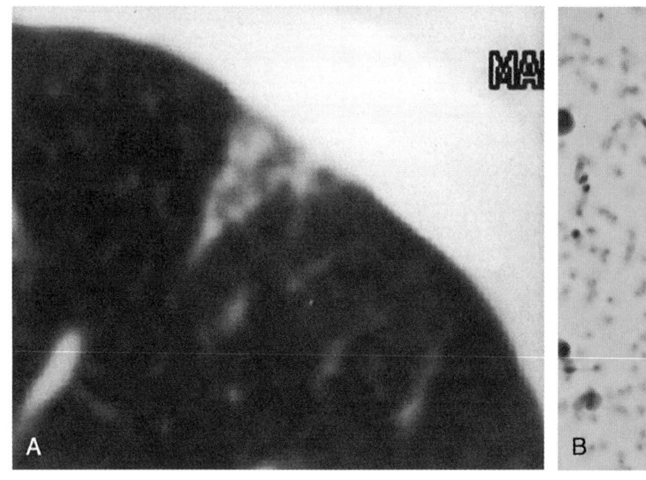

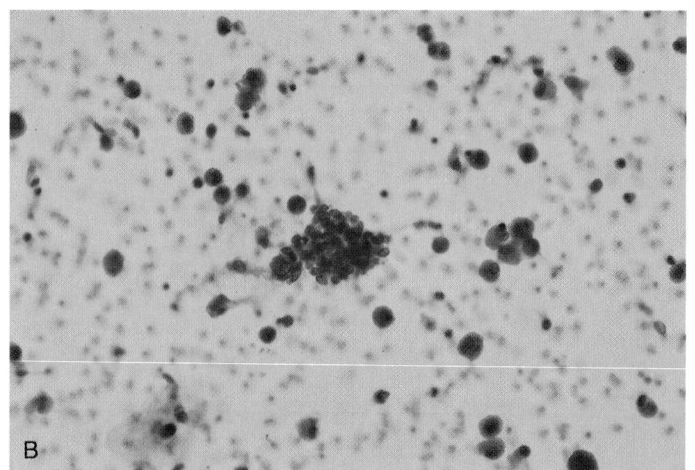

Pulmonary endometriosis diagnosed by BAL. Computed tomography in this patient with hemoptysis at the time of menstrual period shows a wedge-shaped peripheral infiltrate in the left upper lung **(A).** A diagnostic BAL showed endometrial cells in the BAL effluent **(B).**[82]

DIAGNOSTIC BRONCHOSCOPY

BRONCHOALVEOLAR LAVAGE, BIOPSIES, ULTRASOUND, AND OTHER NEWER TECHNIQUES

FIGURE 6-54

Bronchial biopsy using biopsy forceps through the flexible bronchoscope. **A,** The forceps is opened and pushed firmly against the abnormal mucosa. **B,** The forceps cups are closed; the forceps is withdrawn after the cups firmly close around the biopsied tissue. Various types of biopsy forceps, shown in Figure 6-12, can be used to obtain specimens from the endobronchial lesions.

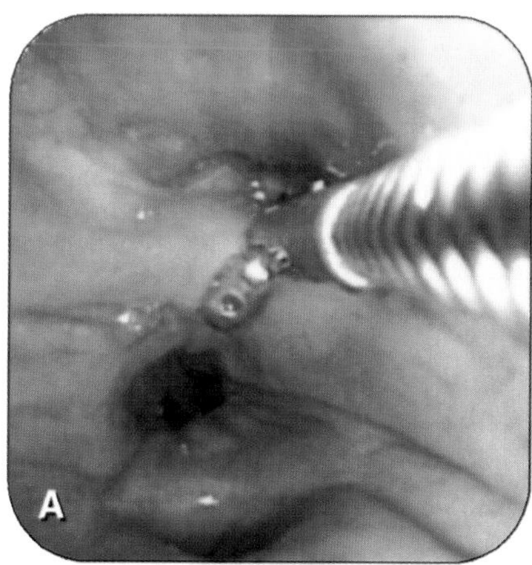

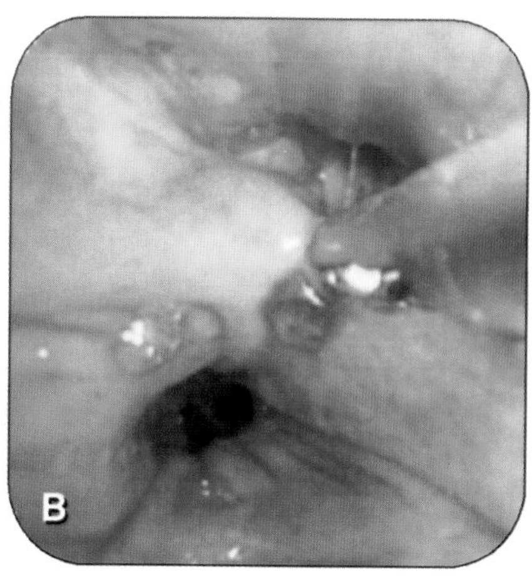

TABLE 6-7

Pulmonary Diseases in Which Bronchoscopic Lung Biopsy Provides High Diagnostic Yield (>70%)*

- Sarcoidosis
- Hypersensitivity pneumonitis
- Eosinophilic granuloma (histiocytosis X)
- Alveolar proteinosis
- Lymphangitic metastasis
- Diffuse pulmonary lymphoma
- Diffuse alveolar cell carcinoma
- *Pneumocystis carinii* pneumonia
- Mycobacterioses
- Mycoses
- Cytomegalovirus
- Pneumoconioses
- Rejection process in lung transplant recipients

* Addition of bronchoalveolar lavage may increase diagnostic yield in most of these conditions.

FIGURE 6-55

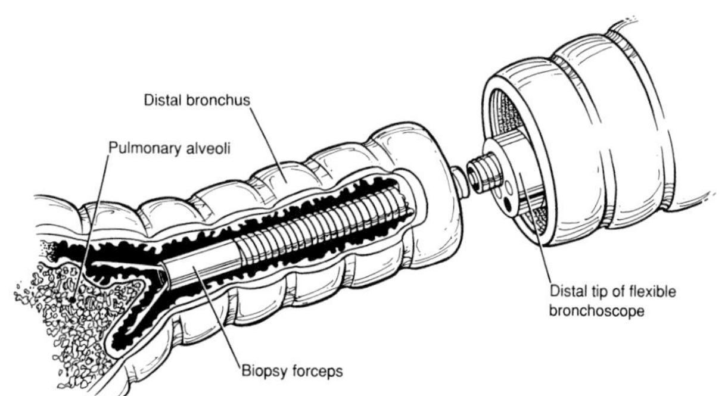

Bronchoscopic lung biopsy technique shown here assumes that the forceps pinches off the lung tissue in between two terminal bronchioles. Larger forceps obtain better specimens.[16] (From Prakash UBS: Bronchoscopy. New York, Raven Press, 1994, copyright © Mayo Foundation.)

DIAGNOSTIC BRONCHOSCOPY

BRONCHOALVEOLAR LAVAGE, BIOPSIES, ULTRASOUND, AND OTHER NEWER TECHNIQUES

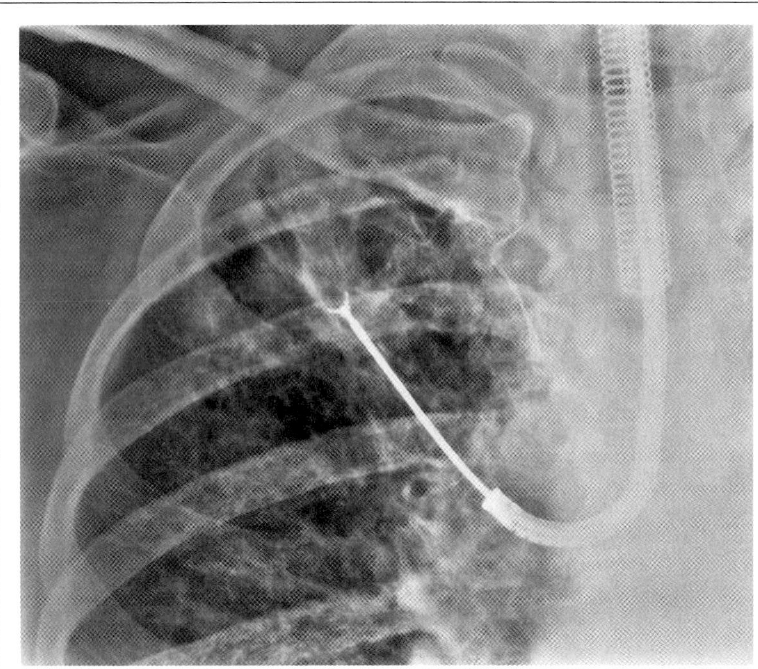

FIGURE 6–56

Bronchoscopic lung biopsy of right upper lobe nodular lesion under fluoroscopic guidance. Localized lesions are best approached with biplane fluoroscopic guidance to ensure that the specimen obtained is representative of the abnormality being investigated. Diffuse processes can be biopsied without fluoroscopy. A mail survey of 231 bronchoscopists reported that the incidence of pneumothorax associated following bronchoscopic lung biopsy was 1.8% when fluoroscopy was used, and the incidence significantly increased to 2.9% when fluoroscopy was not used.[83]

FIGURE 6–57

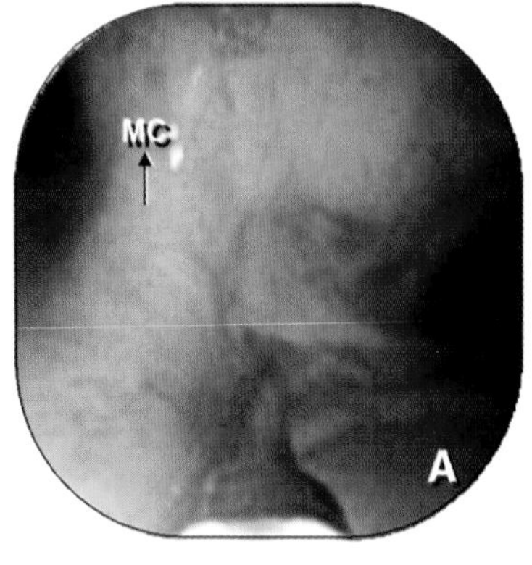

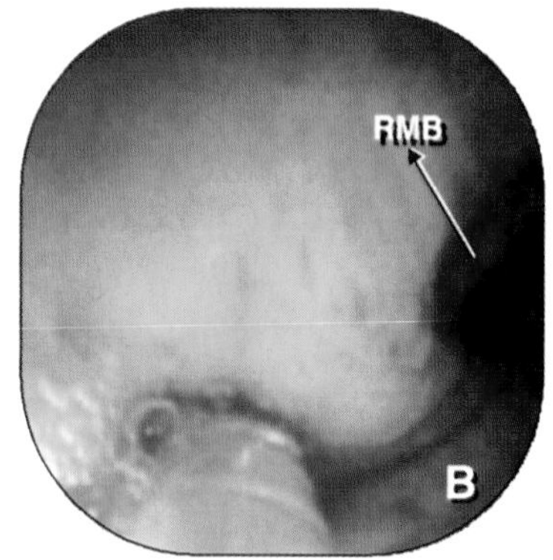

Bronchoscopic needle aspiration of subcarinal lymph node. **A,** The needle is about to be inserted into the mucosa just to the right of the main carina (MC). **B,** The needle has been inserted fully into the subcarinal lymph node, and only the catheter sheath is seen. The diagnostic rate of this technique in malignant disease ranges from 38% to 71% when a main carinal abnormality is present on bronchoscopic examination and 17% to 100% when mediastinal lymphadenopathy is present on imaging studies.[84] RMB = right main-stem bronchus.

DIAGNOSTIC BRONCHOSCOPY

BRONCHOALVEOLAR LAVAGE, BIOPSIES, ULTRASOUND, AND OTHER NEWER TECHNIQUES

FIGURE 6–58

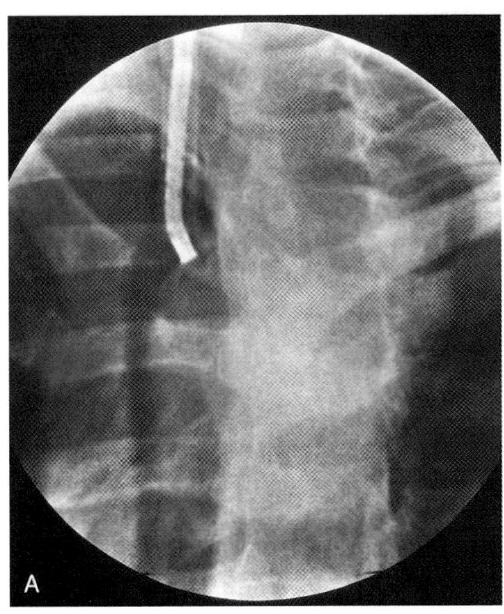

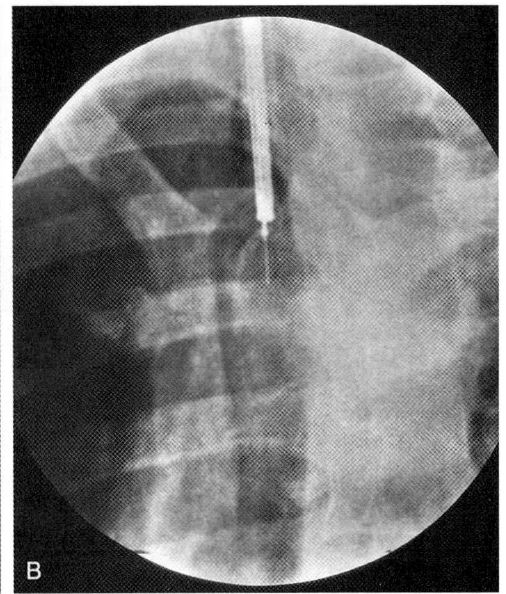

Bronchoscopic needle aspiration of upper paratracheal lymph node as visualized by fluoroscopy. **A,** The tip of the flexible bronchoscope is seen. **B,** The needle has been inserted fully into the paratracheal lymph node. The diagnostic rates are somewhat lower in sampling the paratracheal lymph nodes compared with subcarinal lymph node aspiration. Fluoroscopy is not always necessary in this technique. However, improved diagnostic rate with the use of simultaneous computed tomographic guidance has been reported.[85, 86]

FIGURE 6–59

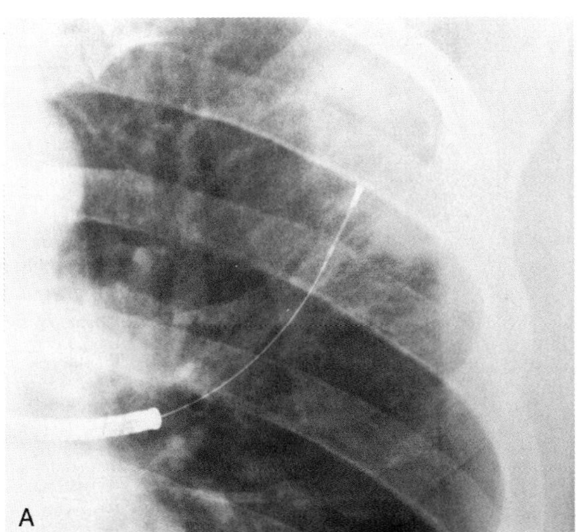

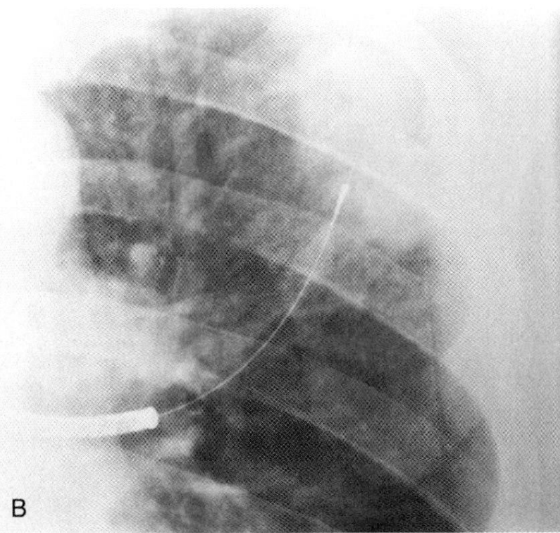

Bronchoscopic needle aspiration of a peripheral mass in the left upper lobe. **A,** The tip of the catheter containing the retracted needle has been inserted into the mass. **B,** The needle has been advanced beyond the tip of the sheath to obtain specimen from the mass. Needle aspirations in this patient yielded *Blastomyces dermatitidis* on staining and culture. The use of bronchoscopic needle aspiration in peripheral nodules and masses yields diagnosis in 36% to 69% of cases.[84] Bronchoscopic needle aspiration is best suited for nodules and masses with diameters exceeding 3 cm.[87]

DIAGNOSTIC BRONCHOSCOPY

BRONCHOALVEOLAR LAVAGE, BIOPSIES, ULTRASOUND, AND OTHER NEWER TECHNIQUES

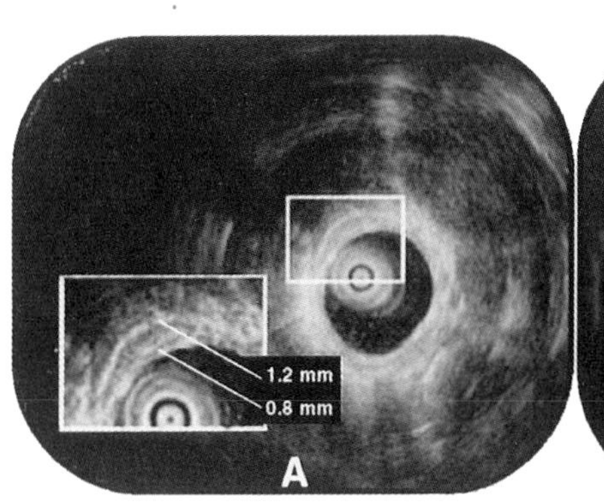

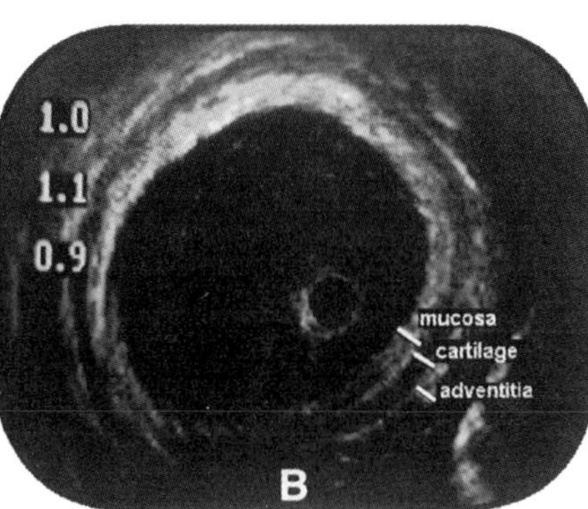

FIGURE 6-60

Bronchoscopic ultrasound is a newer technique that is undergoing clinical evaluations.[88,89] A flexible bronchoscope with an ultrasound probe enables the bronchoscopist to map the airways and surrounding structures. **A,** Ultrasound examination of the tracheobronchial wall in vitro. **B,** The various layers of the tracheal wall and their thickness (in mm) seen in vivo. The distinct layers of the wall of the trachea can only be recognized in higher magnification. (Courtesy of Heinrich D. Becker, M.D.)

FIGURE 6-61

Bronchoscopic ultrasound of the right main-stem bronchus (RMB). The following structures are identified: aorta (AO), superior vena cava (SVC), azygos vein (AZ), right pulmonary artery (RPA), and esophagus (ES). The posterior wall of the bronchus is thickened due to neoplastic infiltration and its structure is destroyed by tumor infiltration (TU). (Courtesy of Heinrich D. Becker, M.D.)

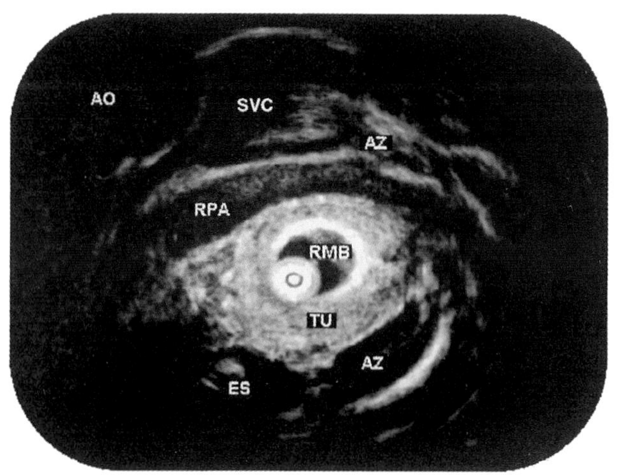

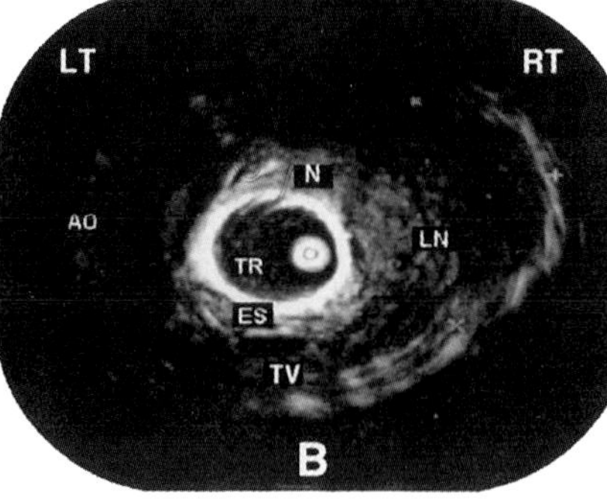

FIGURE 6-62

Bronchoscopic ultrasound in clinical practice. **A,** Computed tomography shows the tumor in the right upper lobe (TU) and enlarged right paratracheal lymph nodes (LN); trachea (TR) and aortic arch (AO) are also identified. **B,** Bronchoscopic ultrasound images at the level of the aortic arch (AO) show the enlarged right paratracheal lymph nodes (LN), which can be separated clearly from the tracheal wall. A smaller lymph node is seen anterior to the trachea (N), and the esophagus is seen posterior to the trachea (ES). Thoracic vertebral column (TV) is also seen. (Courtesy of Heinrich D. Becker, M.D.)

DIAGNOSTIC BRONCHOSCOPY

BRONCHOALVEOLAR LAVAGE, BIOPSIES, ULTRASOUND, AND OTHER NEWER TECHNIQUES

FIGURE 6–63

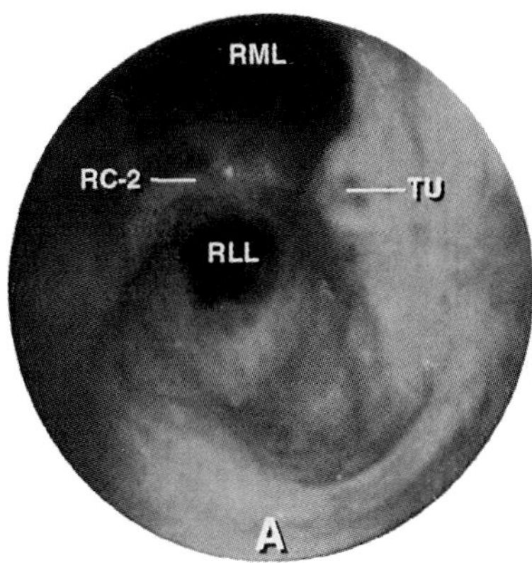

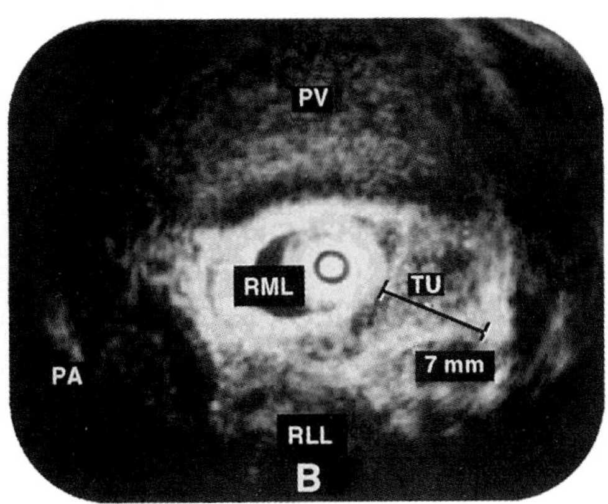

Bronchoscopic ultrasound imaging compared with bronchoscopic findings. **A,** Flexible bronchoscopic image shows a small tumor (TU) protruding into the lumen between the origins of the right middle lobe (RML) and the right lower lobe (RLL) bronchi. The tumor was not visible on plain chest roentgenograph or computed tomography. **B,** Bronchoscopic ultrasound image at the level of the right middle lobe bronchus reveals a lesion with a diameter of 7 mm (TU) and confined to the bronchial wall. The pulmonary artery (PA) and vein (PV) are intact. RC-2 = carina between bronchus to right middle lobe and lower bronchus (see Figure 6–15). (Courtesy of Heinrich D. Becker, M.D.)

FIGURE 6–64

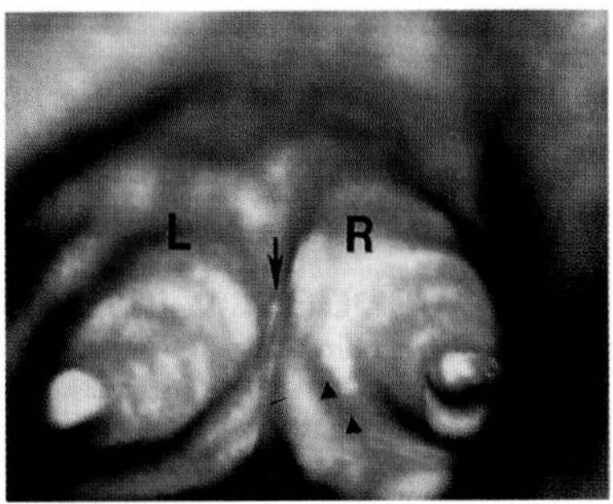

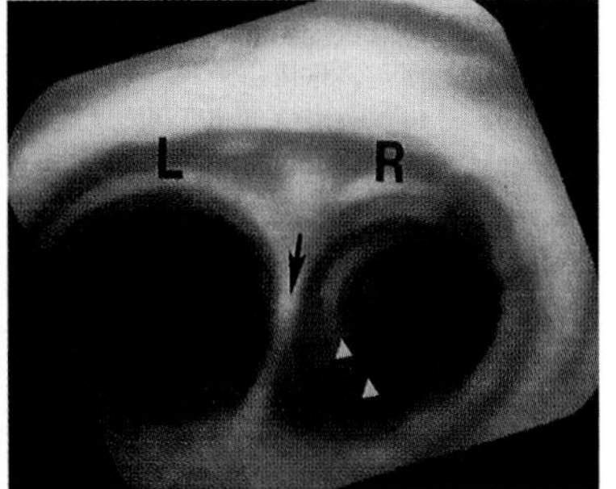

Virtual bronchoscopy does not utilize bronchoscopy to obtain bronchoscopic images. Instead, data obtained with computed tomographic technique are used to create images of the airways. **Left,** Virtual bronchoscopic image of the main carina and main bronchi. **Right,** The corresponding image obtained with a standard flexible bronchoscope.[90] The major advantage of virtual bronchoscopy is the ability to obtain images of the airways without actually performing bronchoscopy. Another advantage is the capacity to visualize the structures adjacent to the airways and the external aspect of major airways. However, if biopsy specimens or other samples are to be obtained from the respiratory tract, standard bronchoscopy is required. Currently, virtual bronchoscopy has a minimal clinical role and continues to undergo clinical trials. (From McAdams HP, Goodman PC, Kussin P: Virtual bronchoscopy for directing transbronchial needle aspiration of hilar and mediastinal lymph nodes: A pilot study. Am J Roentgenol 170:1361–1364, 1998.)

DIAGNOSTIC BRONCHOSCOPY

BRONCHOALVEOLAR LAVAGE, BIOPSIES, ULTRASOUND, AND OTHER NEWER TECHNIQUES

FIGURE 6–65

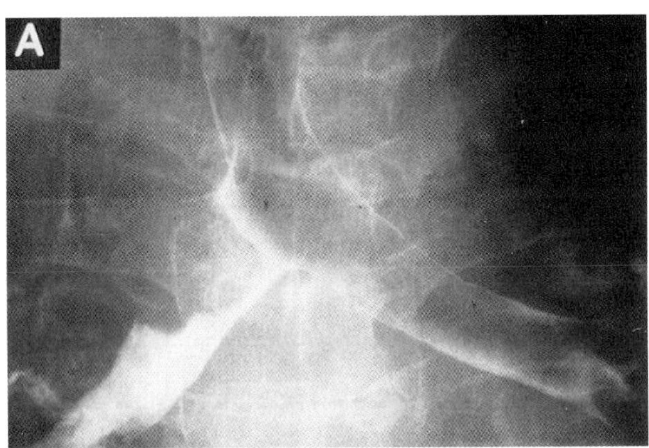

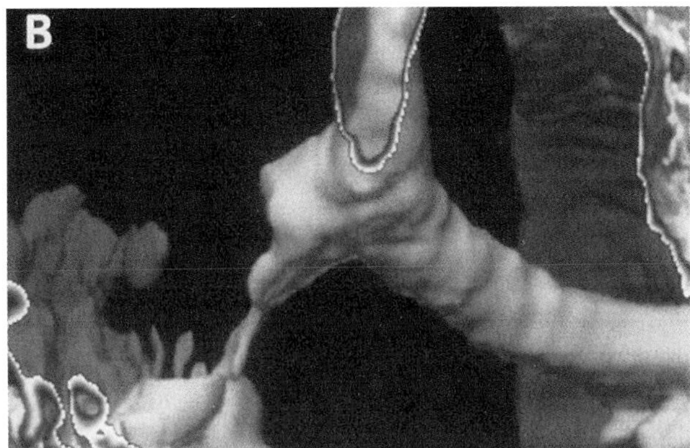

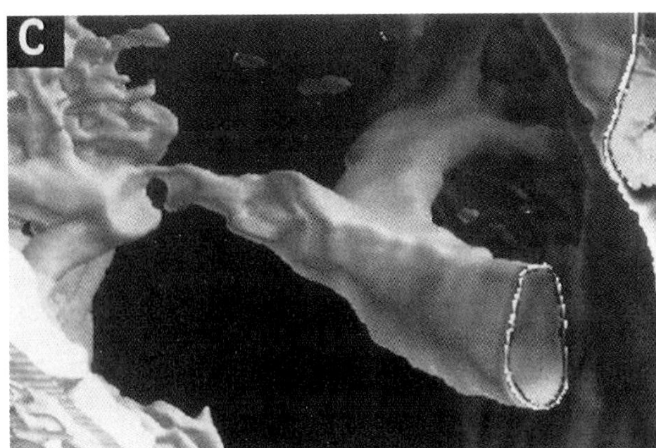

Virtual bronchoscopy with three-dimensional reconstruction of airways is accomplished by obtaining special helical images from computed tomography.[91] **A,** Conventional bronchography using contrast material shows significant constriction of the right main-stem bronchus. **B** and **C,** Three-dimensional images of the affected bronchus provide excellent external views of the stenotic segment. The 3D reconstruction has been used to assess the degree of airway stenosis prior to placement of tracheobronchial stents.[92] (From Doi M, Miyazawa T, Mineshita M, et al: Three-dimensional bronchial imaging by spiral computed tomography as applied to tracheobronchial stent placement. J Bronchol 6:155–158, 1999.)

FIGURE 6–66

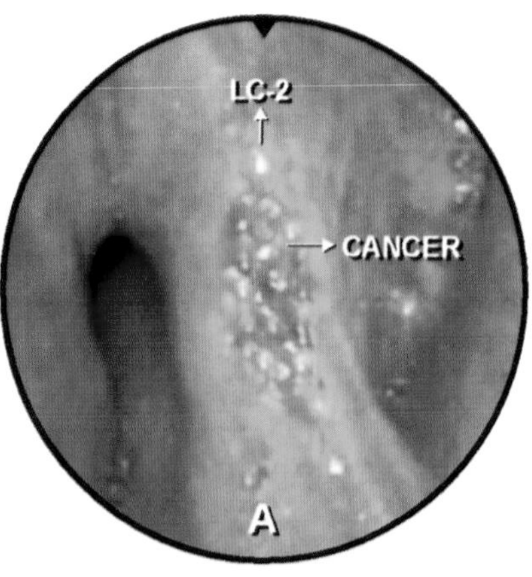

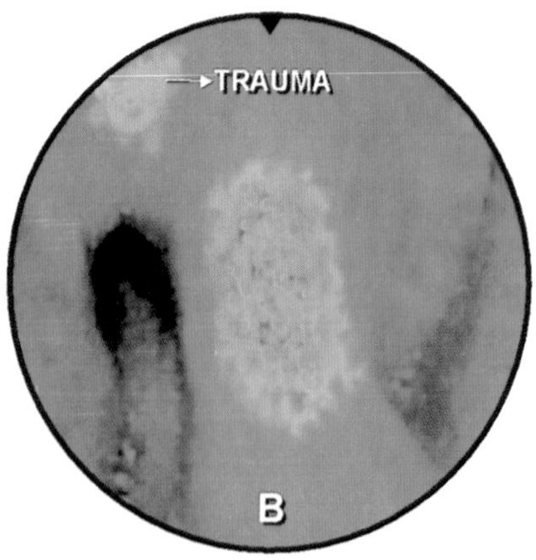

Autofluorescence bronchoscopy is based on the premise that nonmalignant and malignant cells differ in their light reflectance. A standard bronchoscopic image using the normally used white light (WL) shows obvious cancerous lesion **(A).** The same lesion is visualized by special autofluorescence system has a different color (brownish orange) compared to uniformly green color reflected by the normal mucosa **(B).** Even minor trauma to the mucosa or mucosal bleeding can produce abnormal reflectance. Autofluorescence bronchoscopy, when used as an adjunct to standard WL bronchoscopy, appears to increase the bronchoscopist's ability to localize small neoplastic lesions, particularly precancerous intraepithelial lesions.[93] Analysis of bronchial biopsies obtained by fluorescence bronchoscopy may help study the natural history of preinvasive bronchial lesions and the outcome of interventions, such as with chemopreventive treatment. This figure has been computer-enhanced.

THERAPEUTIC BRONCHOSCOPY

FIGURE 6–67

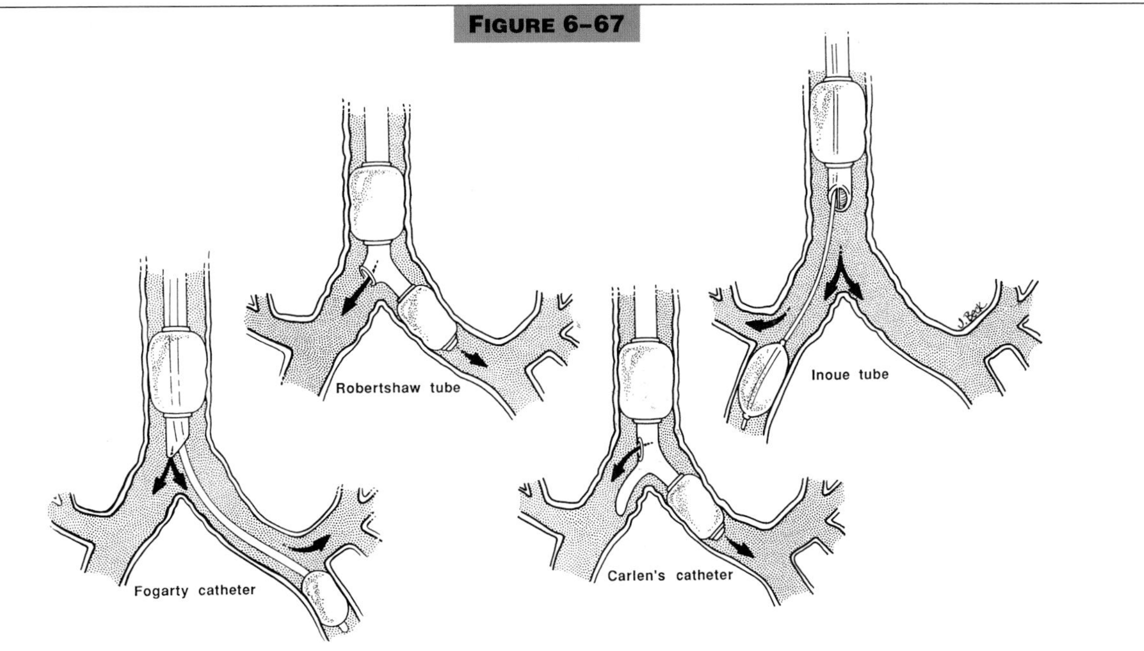

Therapeutic bronchoscopy in massive hemoptysis may require the use of special types of endotracheal tubes to simultaneously control the bleeding and provide adequate ventilation. The types of endotracheal tubes available are shown. It is important for the bronchoscopist to recognize that the standard flexible bronchoscope cannot be inserted through the Robertshaw tube or Carlen's catheter.[49] Bronchoscopy plays a major role in the diagnosis and treatment of massive hemoptysis, as shown in Table 6–8.[49, 94] (From Prakash UBS: Bronchoscopy. New York, Raven Press, 1994, copyright © Mayo Foundation.)

TABLE 6–8

Bronchoscopic Management of Massive Hemoptysis

- Repeated bronchoscopic suctioning
- Iced saline irrigation
- Topical application of vasoactive drugs
- Bronchoscopic tamponade*
- Balloon tamponade
- Tamponade with gauze or Gelfoam
- Fibrin glue tamponade
- Laser coagulation
- Electrocautery†
- Isolation of bronchial tree (see Fig. 6–67)
- Bronchoscopic brachytherapy

* Either flexible or rigid bronchoscope can be used.

† May help in slow bleeding endobronchial neoplasms.

FIGURE 6–68

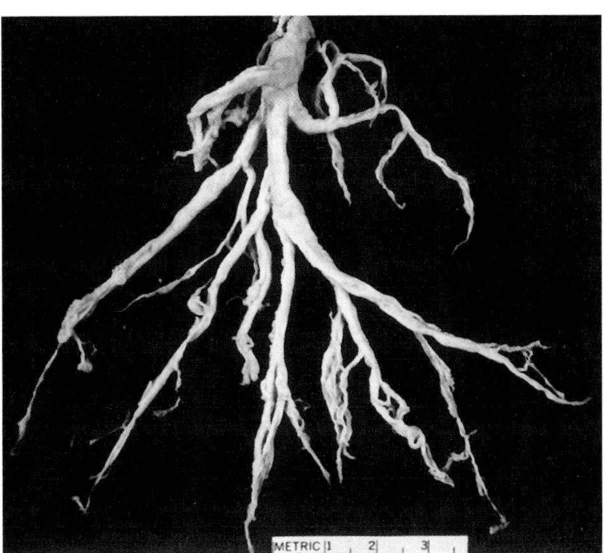

Therapeutic bronchoscopy to aspirate mucoid secretions and plugs. This figure shows a bronchial cast removed with a flexible bronchoscope in a patient with asthma. This condition has been called plastic bronchitis and can be seen in patients with asthma, allergic bronchopulmonary aspergillosis, bronchiectasis, and cystic fibrosis.[95–97] (Courtesy of James R. Jett, M.D.)

THERAPEUTIC BRONCHOSCOPY

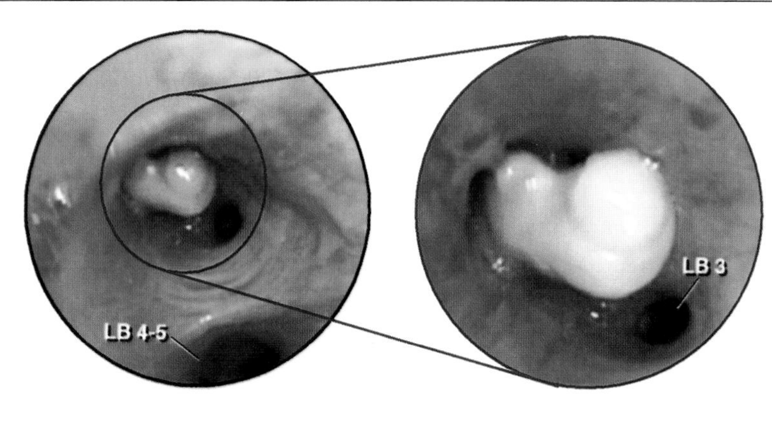

FIGURE 6-69

Therapeutic bronchoscopy to remove an inspissated mucous plug from the left upper lobe bronchus of a patient with asthma. Repeated suctioning or biopsy forceps may be needed to extract tightly stuck mucous plugs and blood clots. Among all indications for bronchoscopy, therapeutic reasons constitute more than half. A large survey of bronchoscopists in North America observed that 56% of therapeutic bronchoscopy procedures were performed to treat lobar and segmental atelectasis, and therapeutic bronchoscopy was one of the five most common indications for bronchoscopy. LB4-5 = superior/inferior segment bronchus of the lingula; LB-3 = anterior segment of left upper lobe.

TABLE 6–9 lists various types of bronchoscopic therapeutic procedures for airway lesions and the expected results and potential complications.

The gamut of therapeutic bronchoscopy ranges from simple bronchoscopic aspiration of retained airway mucus to complicated procedures such as laser bronchoscopy, dilation of tracheobronchial strictures and stenosis, airway stenting, brachytherapy, cryotherapy, electrocautery, and extraction of airway foreign bodies.[97a] Not infrequently, a diagnostic bronchoscopy may dictate that an immediate therapeutic bronchoscopic procedure be undertaken. For instance, a diagnostic bronchoscopy for significant hemoptysis may disclose a bleeding tumor in the tracheobronchial lumen and an urgent therapeutic bronchoscopy may be indicated to control the bleeding. Or, a diagnostic bronchoscopy for evaluation of wheezing may reveal an airway foreign body, and a bronchoscopy to extract the foreign body makes it a therapeutic procedure. Because the diagnostic and therapeutic bronchoscopy are combined into a single procedure in many instances, the bronchoscopist should be prepared to proceed with both procedures. The following examples demonstrate several of the therapeutic bronchoscopic procedures listed above and in TABLE 6–9.

TABLE 6-9

Bronchoscopic Therapies

Type of Therapy	Type of Lesion	Type of Bronchoscope	Rapidity of Positive Result	Repeatability of Therapy	Complications
Mechanical débridement	E/Sm	R/F1	++++	+++	Hmg
Laser	E	R/F1	++++	++++	Hmg, Fis
Brachytherapy	E/Sm	F	+	+	Hmg, Fis
Cryotherapy	E	R/F	++	+++	Minimal
Balloon dilatation	E/Sm/Ext	R/F1	++++	++++	Minimal
Photodynamic therapy	E	F	++	+++	Skin, PM
Electrocautery	E	R/F	+++	++++	Hmg
Stent	E/W/Ex	R/F2	++++	+++	Mig, Muc, Inf, Gran

R = rigid bronchoscope; F = flexible bronchoscope; E = endoluminal lesion; Sm = submucosal lesion; Ex = extraluminal compression; 1 = rigid bronchoscope preferable; 2 = Dumon stent requires rigid bronchoscope; ++++ = most rapid or repeatable; Hmg = hemorrhage; Fis = fistula; Skin = photosensitivity reaction; PM = pseudomembrane formation; Mig = migration of stent; Muc = inspissated mucus in the stent; Inf = infection of airways; Gran = granulation tissue growth. Wall stents and Gianturco stents require fluoroscopy.

Adapted from Ramser ER, Beamis JF Jr: Laser bronchoscopy. Clin Chest Med 16:415–26, 1995.

THERAPEUTIC BRONCHOSCOPY

FIGURE 6–70

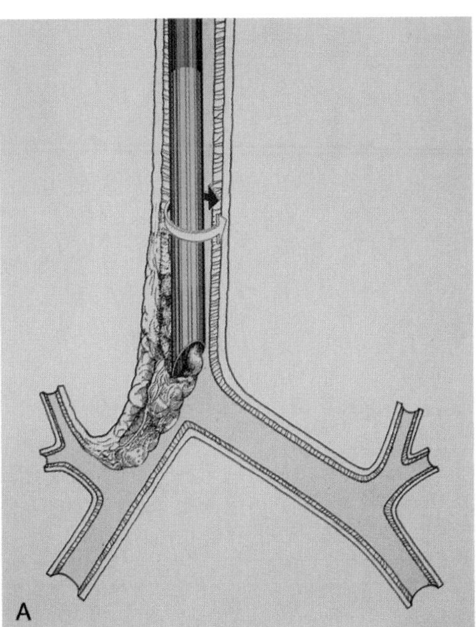

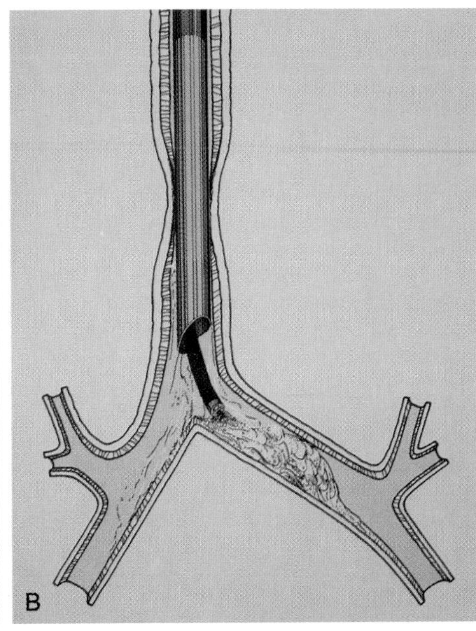

Therapeutic bronchoscopy to relieve airway obstruction from neoplastic process. Either flexible or rigid bronchoscopy can be employed for this purpose. The advantage of the rigid bronchoscope is that the instrument itself can be used to "core out" the tumor **(A).** Another advantage is that a flexible bronchoscope can be passed through the rigid bronchoscope to treat distal lesions or lesions that cannot be reached with the rigid bronchoscope **(B).** Thus, the two instruments complement each other.[4] (From Prakash UBS: Bronchoscopy. New York, Raven Press, 1994, copyright © Mayo Foundation.)

FIGURE 6–71

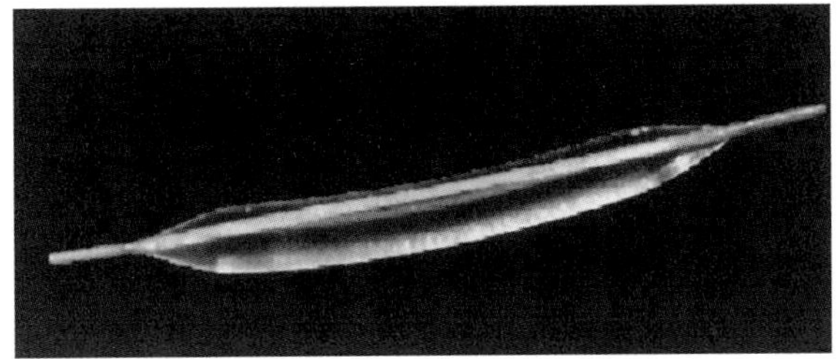

Therapeutic bronchoscopy using balloon dilatation to treat tracheobronchial strictures and stenoses. The balloon shown here is an esophageal balloon used for dilatation of esophageal strictures. This and other balloons can be used either through the flexible or rigid bronchoscope or adjacent (external) to the instrument to dilate the strictures. If the balloon cannot be passed through the bronchoscope, a guidewire can be passed and the bronchoscope withdrawn; then the balloon is passed over the guidewire to dilate the stenosis under bronchoscopic vision.[99]

FIGURE 6–72

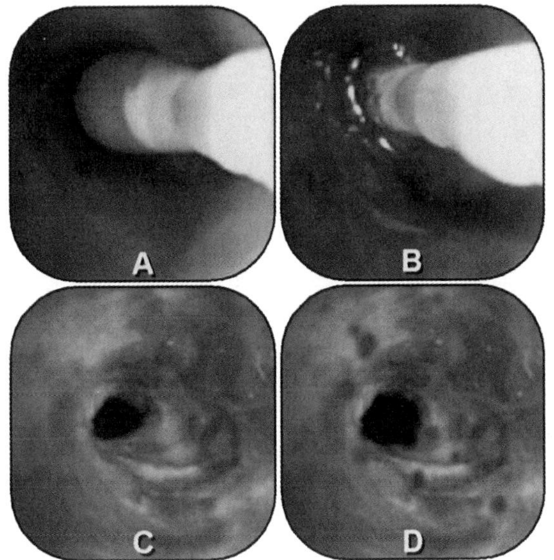

Therapeutic balloon bronchoplasty to dilate right bronchus intermedius. **A,** Balloon catheter being inserted into the stenotic segment of the bronchus. **B,** The balloon is being inflated. **C,** Stenotic area before dilatation. **D,** Postdilatation appearance of the stenosis. Balloon bronchoplasty alone can provide only short-term relief.[100] Most patients will require other types of treatments. Balloon bronchoplasty helps prepare the airway for stent placement and brachytherapy.

THERAPEUTIC BRONCHOSCOPY

FIGURE 6–73

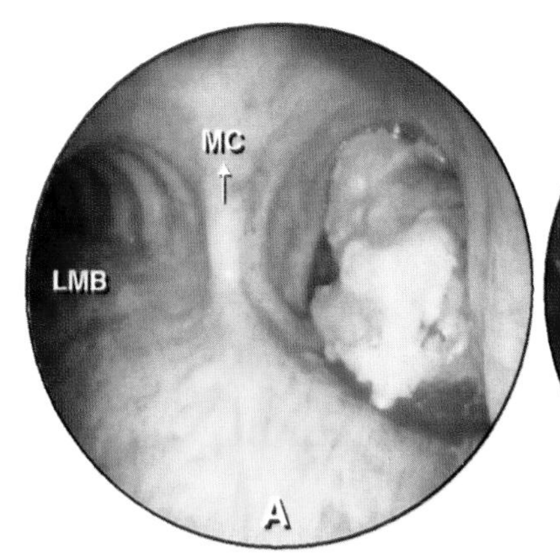

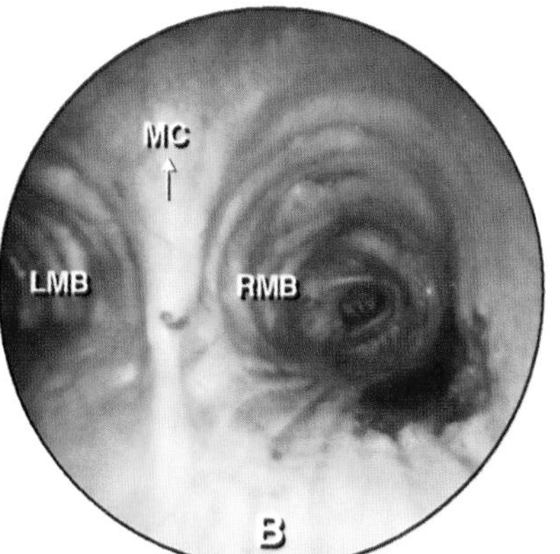

Bronchoscopic laser therapy using Nd:YAG laser to treat unresectable malignant tumor obstructing the proximal right main-stem bronchus **(A).** After laser therapy the image shows normal luminal diameter of the right main-stem bronchus and normal distal bronchial tree **(B).** Laser therapy provides immediate relief of symptoms caused by obstructing tumors in over 90% of patients. Among 1585 patients who underwent 2253 Nd:YAG laser therapeutic procedures, 78% had non–small cell lung cancer, 6% had small cell lung cancer, 7% had metastatic tumors, and 5% had unclassifiable tumors; almost all procedures were performed under general anesthesia utilizing rigid bronchoscopy. More than 93% showed immediate good results. Complications included 18 instances of hemorrhage, 6 pneumothoraces, and 10 deaths.[101] LMB = left main bronchus; MC = main carina; RMB = right main bronchus.

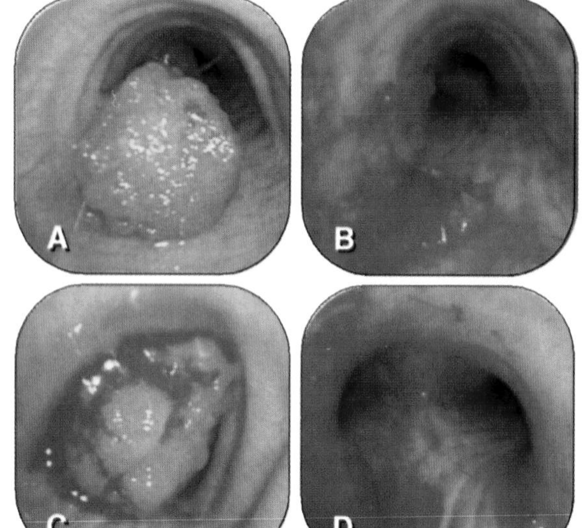

FIGURE 6–74

Bronchoscopic laser therapy using Nd:YAG laser to treat a malignant tumor obstructing the distal trachea. **A** A large tracheal lesion is seen in the distal trachea, but another lesion is also present slightly more distal to it. **B,** The appearance immediately after the more proximal lesion is resected. The more distal tracheal lesion is now obvious **(C).** Normal-appearing main carina is visualized after both tracheal lesions are resected by Nd:YAG laser **(D).** Patients who are on mechanical ventilators because of progressive or acute respiratory failure resulting from large airway lesions can be successfully weaned off the ventilator following rigid bronchoscopic laser therapy.[102]

FIGURE 6–75

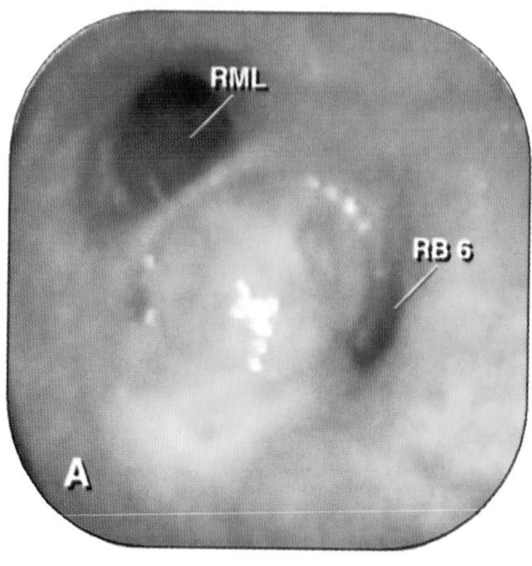

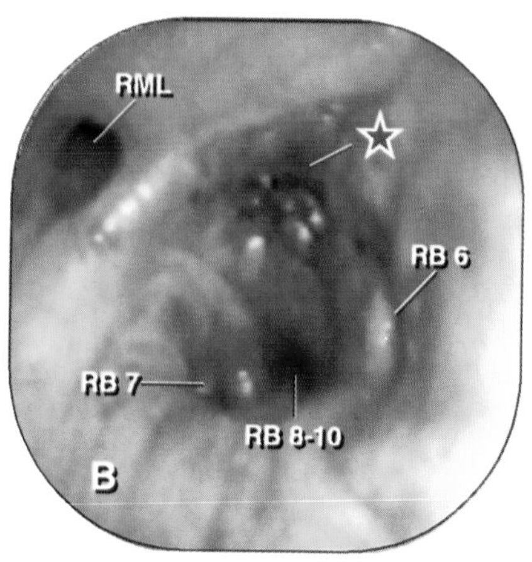

Bronchoscopic laser therapy using Nd:YAG laser to treat a benign pedunculated fibroma obstructing the right lower lobe bronchus **(A).** After laser therapy, examination shows previously obscured distal bronchi and the star indicates laser burn marks **(B).** Laser therapy has been used to cure benign airway tumors.[103] RML = right middle lobe; RB-6 = superior segment of right lower lobe; RB-7 = medial basal segment of right lower lobe; RB8-10 = anterior, lateral, and posterior basal segments of right lower lobe.

THERAPEUTIC BRONCHOSCOPY

FIGURE 6–76

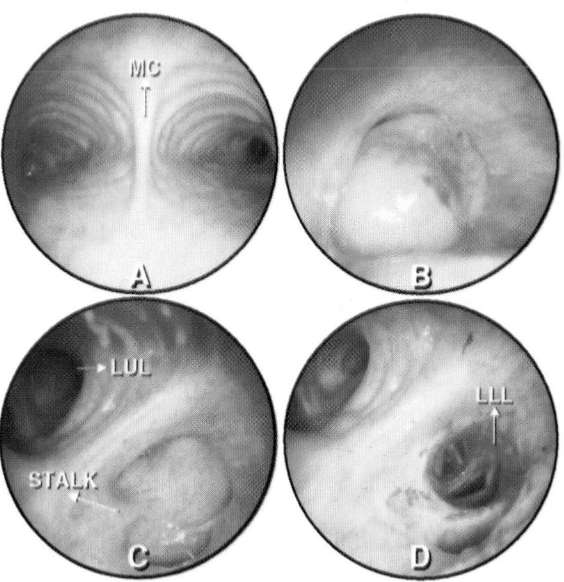

Bronchoscopic laser therapy using Nd:YAG laser to treat a benign pedunculated leiomyoma obstructing the left lower lobe bronchus proximally **(A).** A close-up of the lesion shows the smooth surface of tumor **(B).** After the lesion is pushed down distally, the stalk is apparent **(C).** After laser therapy, examination shows that the tumor along with the stalk has been completely obliterated **(D).** Left lower lobe (LLL) bronchi are now visible. (MC = main carina; LUL = left upper lobe.)

FIGURE 6–77

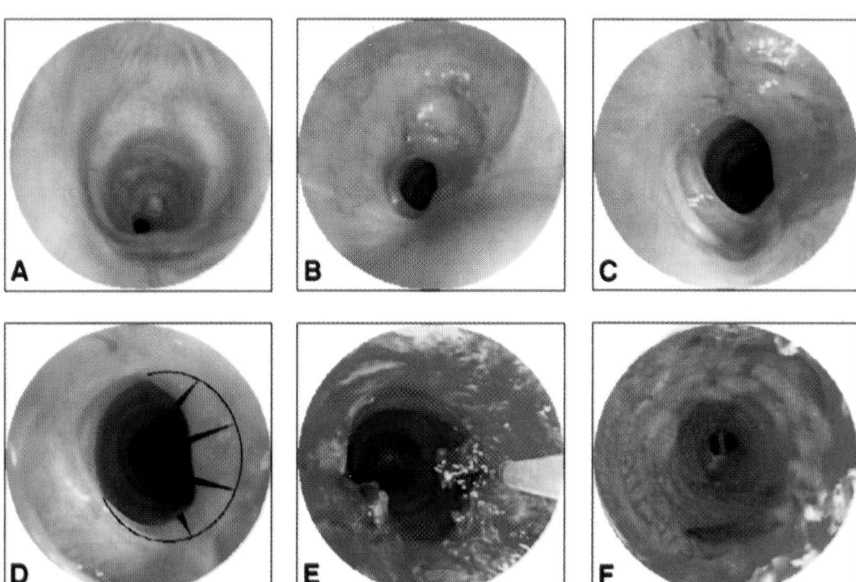

Bronchoscopic laser therapy using Nd:YAG laser to treat a benign tracheal stricture located below the cricoid **(A).** Closer views of the stricture reveal that it involves a short segment of the trachea **(B** and **C).** Conceptualization of radial laser cuts to be made using a laser fiber **(D).** Appearance of stricture after several laser cuts have been made; laser fiber is seen on the right **(E).** Examination after laser treatment shows normal caliber of trachea, and the main carina is seen distally **(F).** Different types of lasers including CO_2 laser and Nd:YAG laser have been used to treat benign tracheal strictures.[104]

THERAPEUTIC BRONCHOSCOPY

FIGURE 6-78

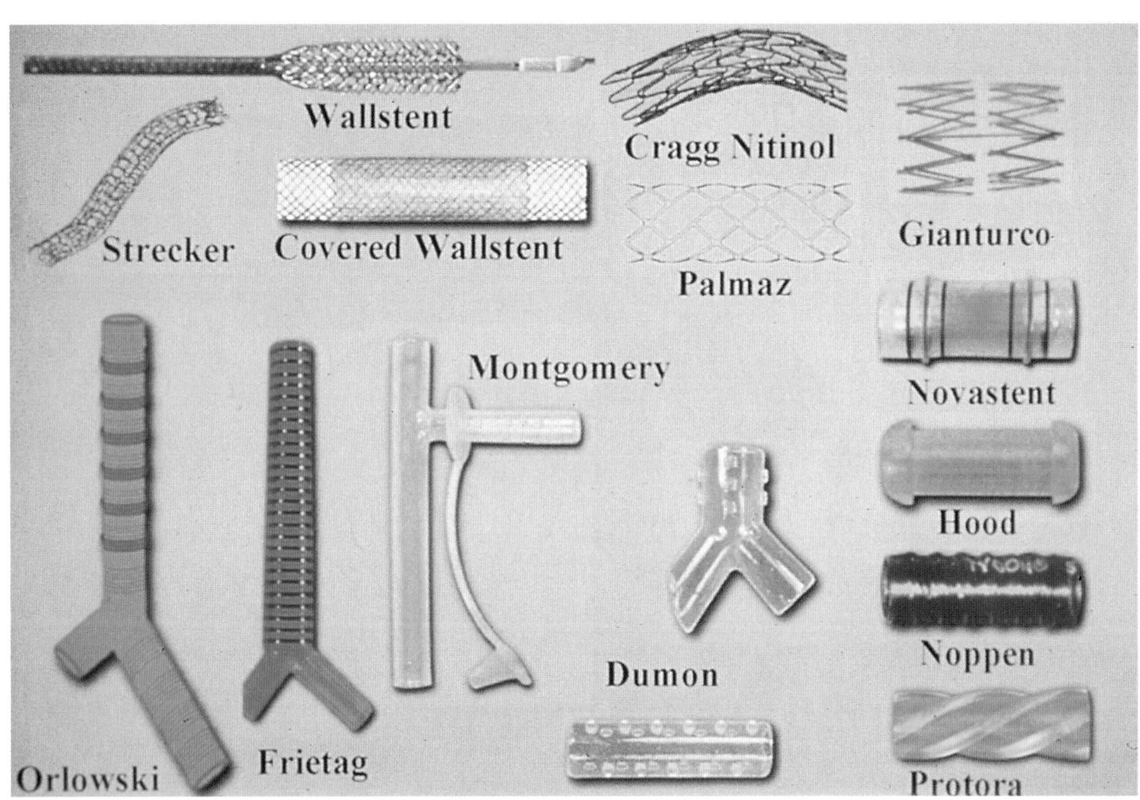

Tracheobronchial prostheses (stents) for treatment of airway stenoses and strictures employ various types of stents, some of which are shown here. There is no ideal stent. Generally, silicone or nonmetallic stents are advisable for benign strictures. Stents work best in the trachea and main-stem bronchi but are not well suited for lobar and distal bronchial stenoses. (Courtesy of Jean-Francois Dumon, M.D.)

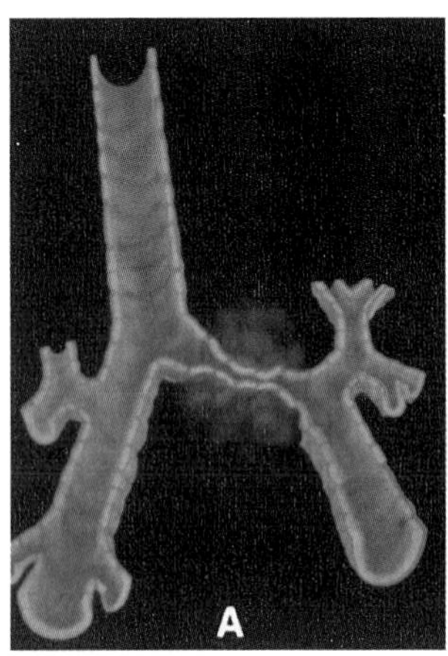

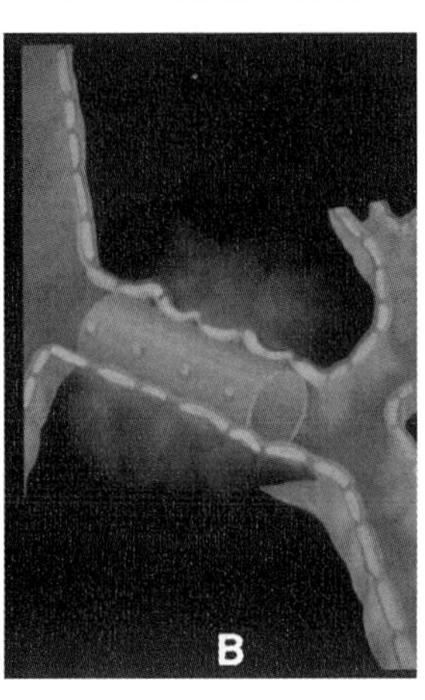

FIGURE 6-79

Bronchial prosthesis (stent) therapy for extrinsic compression of left main-stem bronchus, as envisioned by the artist **(A).** Placement of a silicone stent has resulted in the proper ventilation of distal airways in the left lung **(B).** Silicone stents require rigid bronchoscopy and sedation or general anesthesia. In a multicenter study of 1574 stents in 1058 patients with high-grade stenoses, the stents were placed in the trachea in 54%, in the left main-stem bronchus in 21%, in the right main-stem bronchus in 18%, and in miscellaneous areas in 8%. The indications were malignancy in 677 patients (926 stents), benign stenoses in 263 patients (419 stents), and other causes in the remaining patients. The main complications included migration (9.5%), obstruction by secretions (3.6%), and granulation tissue formation (8%).[105] (Courtesy of Jean-Francois Dumon, M.D.)

THERAPEUTIC BRONCHOSCOPY

FIGURE 6–80

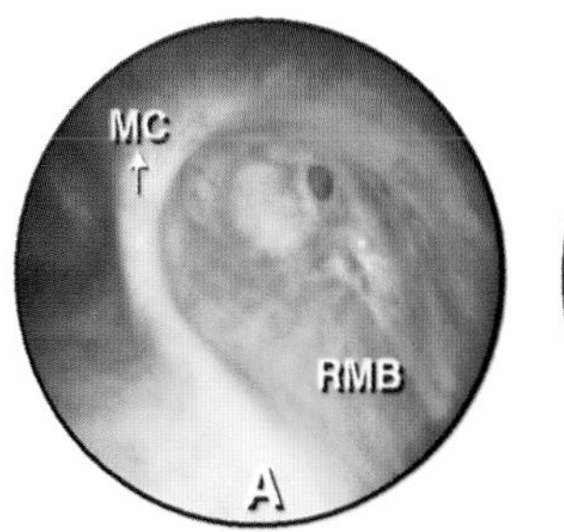

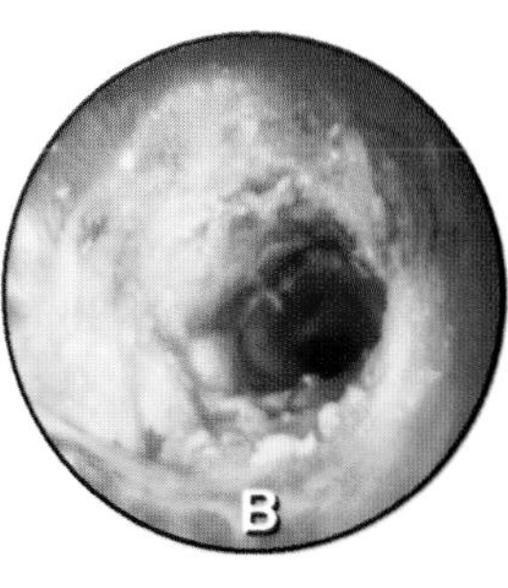

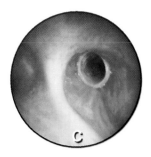

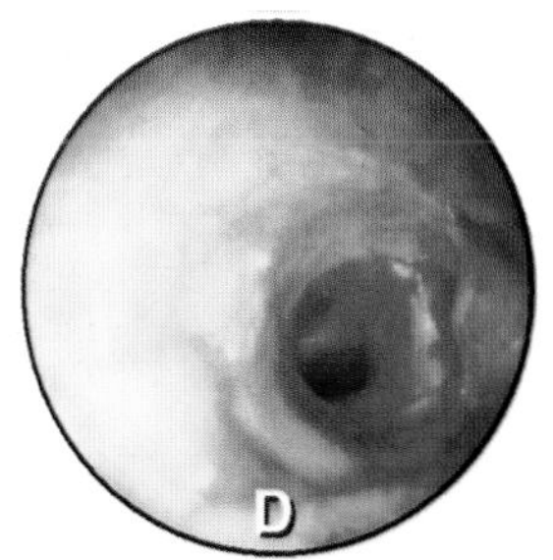

Bronchial prosthesis (stent) therapy for treatment of benign stricture of right main-stem bronchus **(A).** Laser therapy has enlarged the airway lumen **(B).** The proximal end of the stent is seen in the right main-stem bronchus **(C).** Distal end of the stent is seen in distal bronchus intermedius **(D).** Preparation of the airway by rigid bronchoscopic dilatation, balloon bronchoplasty, or laser resection is necessary if the stenosis is tight. MC = main carina; RMB = right main bronchus.

FIGURE 6–81

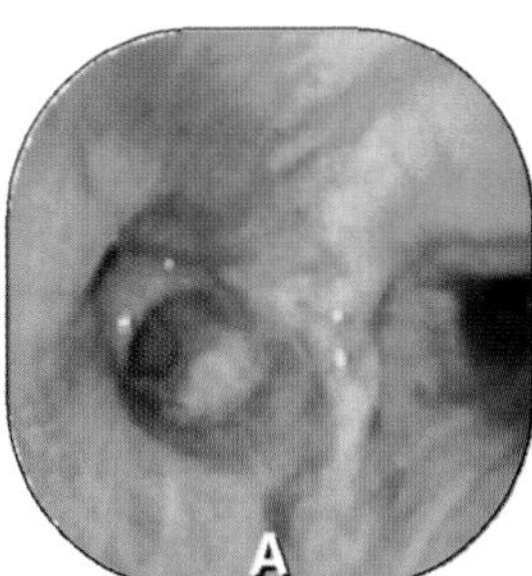

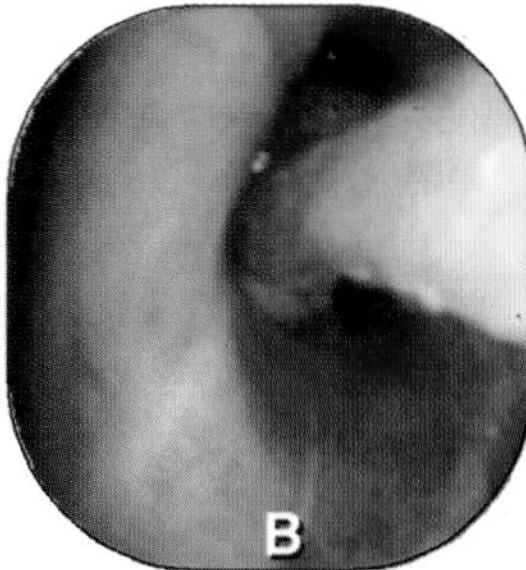

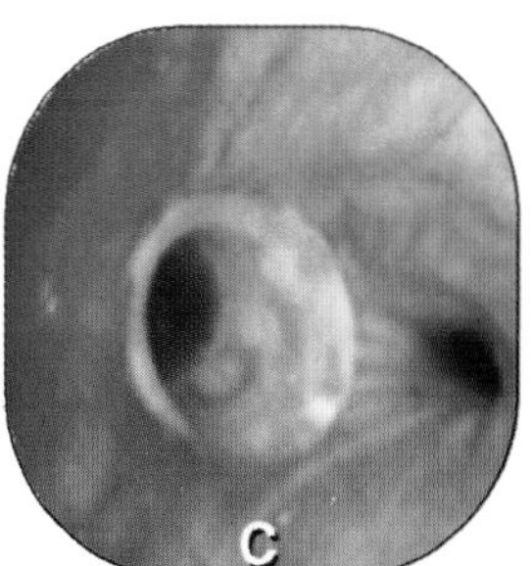

Bronchial prosthesis (stent) therapy for treatment of benign stricture of left main-stem bronchus **(A).** The small diameter of the silicone stent caused complete obstruction by thick inspissated mucus, being suctioned here **(B).** Removal of the smaller stent and placement of a silicone stent with a larger diameter prevented recurrence of mucous obstruction **(C).** Up to 5% of patients with silicone stents develop significant problems with retention of secretions and mucous plugs. Regular inhalation of aerosolized saline keeps the secretions thin and helps keep open the stent lumen. (MC = main carina; RMB = right main bronchus.)

FIGURE 6–82

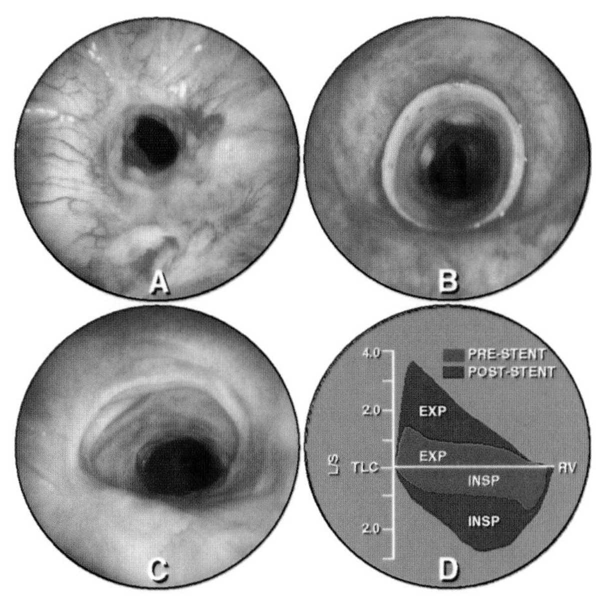

Tracheal prosthesis (stent) therapy for treatment of benign stricture of midtrachea **(A).** Silicone stent is properly placed in the trachea **(B). C,** Appearance of trachea after 1 year of stent therapy. Flow-volume studies in a similar patient, showing significant improvement in flow rates after prolonged stent therapy **(D).**

THERAPEUTIC BRONCHOSCOPY

FIGURE 6-83

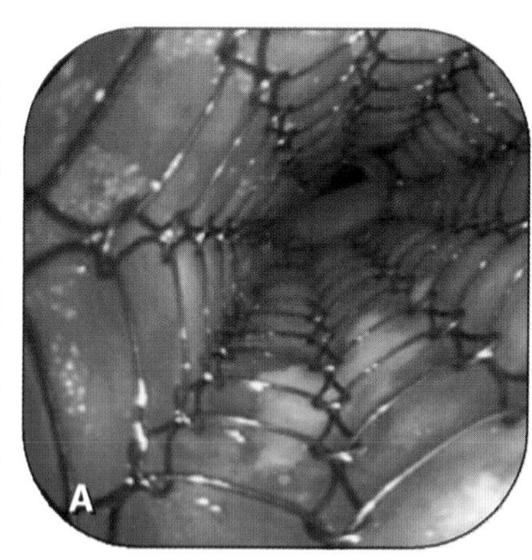

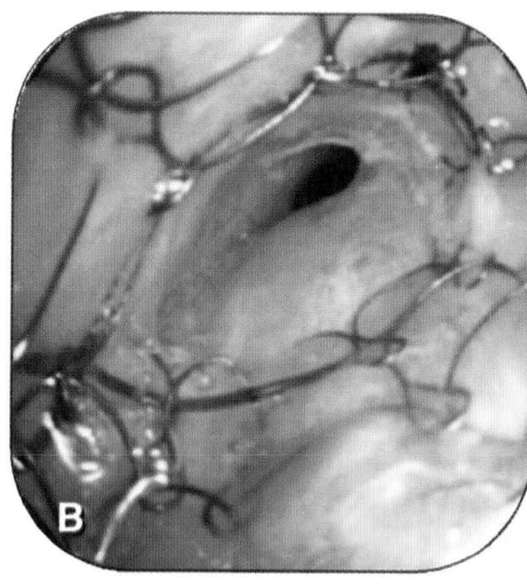

Bronchial prosthesis (stent) therapy for treatment of benign stricture of right main-stem bronchus. A newly placed nitinol stent in the airway lumen **(A)** and the distal end of the stent **(B).** (From Prakash UBS: Chest 116:1403–1408, 1999.)

FIGURE 6-84

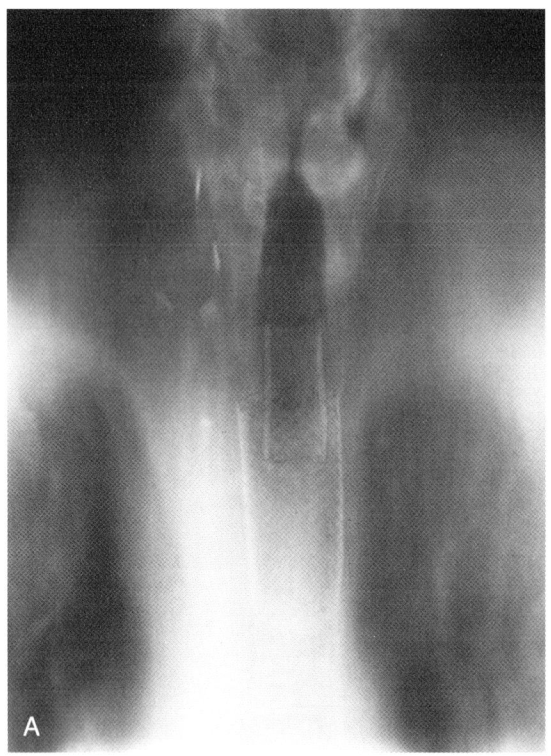

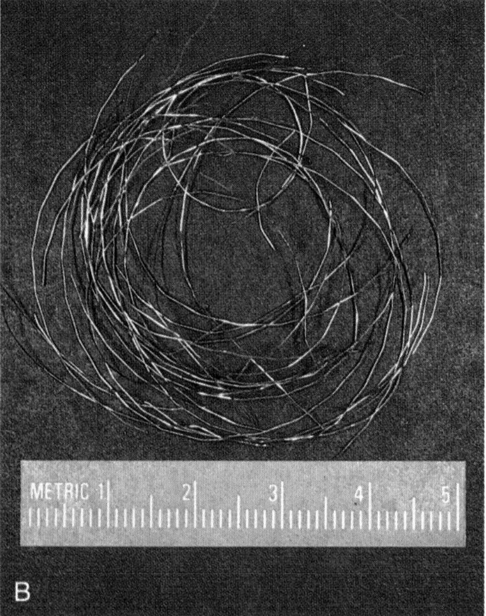

Stent within a stent shown by tracheal tomography of a patient who was treated with a Wall stent for a benign stricture of the upper trachea. The stent slipped distally without providing relief of symptoms caused by the stricture. Because of significant epithelialization and growth of granulation tissue of the metallic stent, the metallic stent was left in place, and a silicone stent (upper stent in the figure) was placed to treat the stricture **(A).** This stent provided relief for several months, but continued growth of granulation tissue in the distal aspect of the Wall stent necessitated removal of both stents and placement of a Montgomery tube. **B,** Individual wires of the Wall stent after the stent was removed with a rigid bronchoscope.

FIGURE 6–85

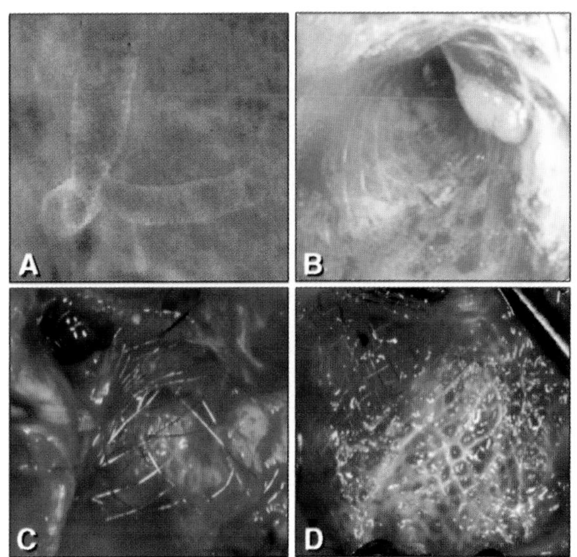

Three Wall stents in the right bronchial tree **(A)** in this patient who developed upper lobectomy stenosis of the bronchus intermedius. The stents caused growth of significant granulation tissue in the distal bronchus intermedius **(B)** and resultant postobstructive pneumonias. The patient required thoracotomy for complete pneumonectomy. Resected specimen showed extensive formation of granulation tissue **(C)** and complete epithelialization of one of the three stents **(D).** A major complication of the metallic stents is the exuberant growth of granulation tissue.

FIGURE 6–86

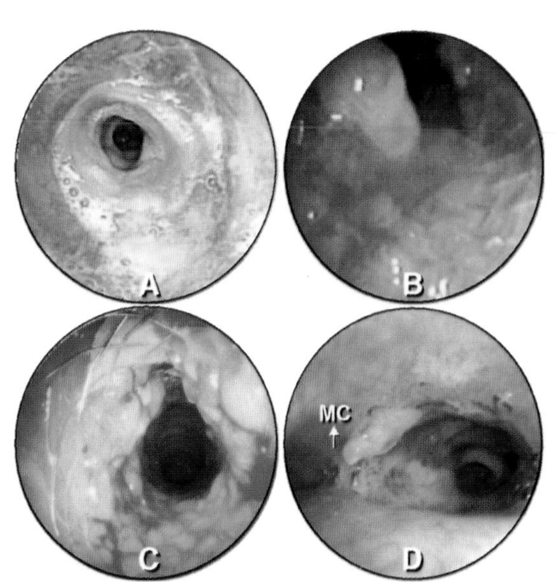

Complications of tracheobronchial stents include retention of mucous secretions within and around the silicone stent **(A),** epithelialization of metallic mesh and growth of significant granulation tissue through the mesh in Wall stent **(B),** tissue necrosis caused by Wall stent **(C),** and gram-negative (*Pseudomonas aeruginosa*) tracheobronchial bacterial infection in a patient who had a nitinol stent placed for bronchomalacia of right bronchial tree **(D).**

FIGURE 6–87

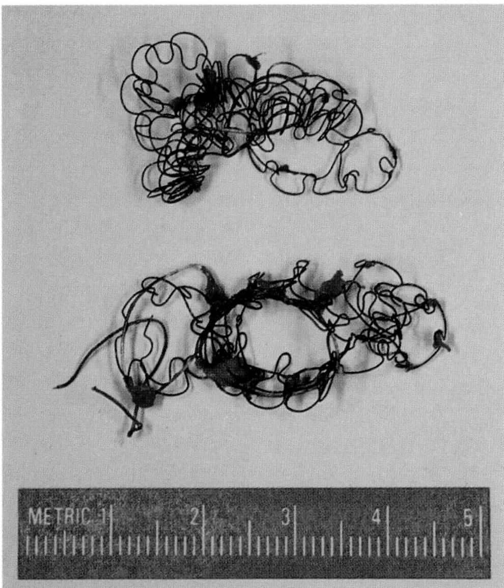

Nitinol stents after both were extracted from the patient described in Figure 6–86*D*.

THERAPEUTIC BRONCHOSCOPY

FIGURE 6-88

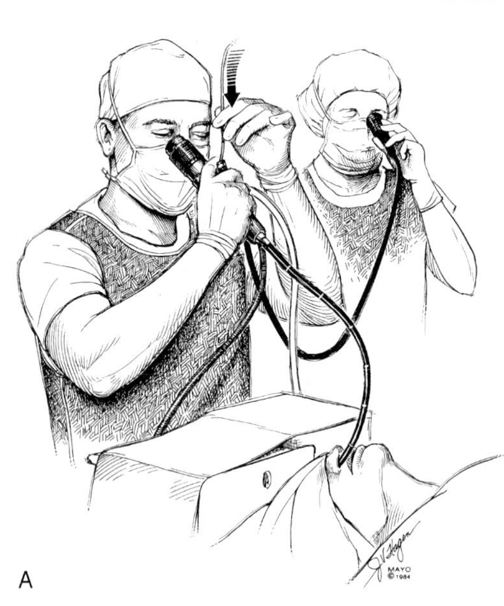

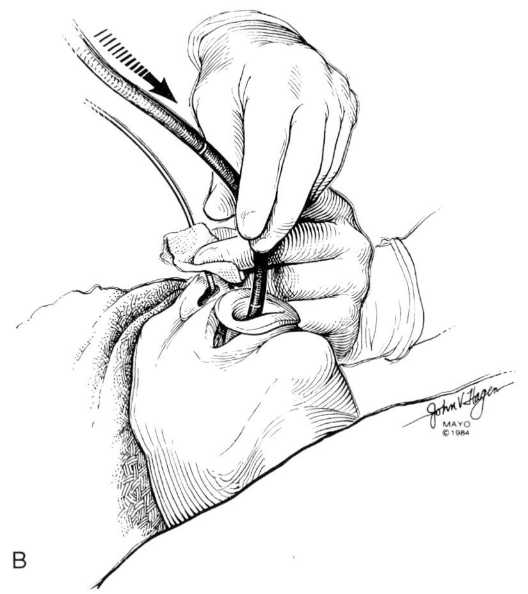

Brachytherapy is used as an adjunct in the therapy of unresectable bronchogenic cancer that has already received maximal external beam radiation. Brachytherapy catheter placement under bronchoscopic visualization, with nasal insertion of the bronchoscope **(A).** After the brachytherapy catheter placement is secured, bronchoscopy is repeated to ensure that the catheter is stationed in the proper location **(B).** A wire containing radioactive seeds is then placed through the catheter to begin radiation treatment from within the airways. (From Prakash UBS: Bronchoscopy. New York, Raven Press, 1994, copyright © Mayo Foundation.)

FIGURE 6-89

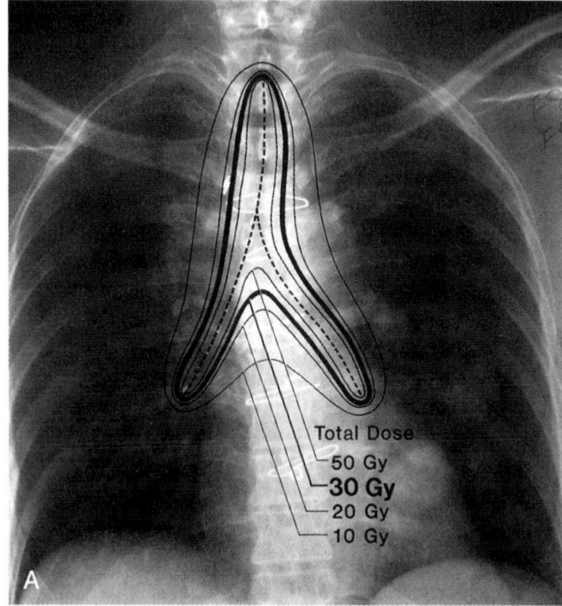

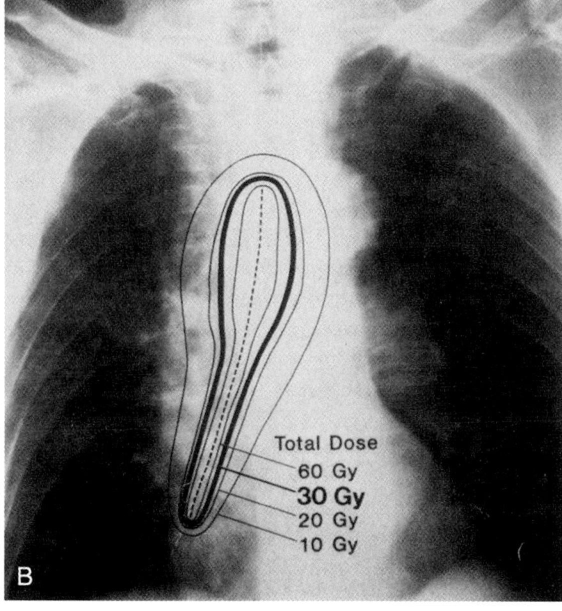

A, Brachytherapy dosage is shown in the chest roentgenographic depiction of location of brachytherapy source within the tracheobronchial tree. Dose distribution is superimposed over a chest roentgenograph from a combined tracheal and bilateral main-stem bronchial placement delivering 30 Gy to a 0.5- to 1.0-cm radius from the ^{192}Ir wire. **B,** Dose distribution superimposed over a chest roentgenograph from a tracheal and right main-stem bronchial placement delivering 30 Gy to a 0.5- to 1.0-cm radius from the ^{192}Ir wire. (From Prakash UBS: Bronchoscopy. New York, Raven Press, 1994, copyright © Mayo Foundation.)

THERAPEUTIC BRONCHOSCOPY

FIGURE 6–90

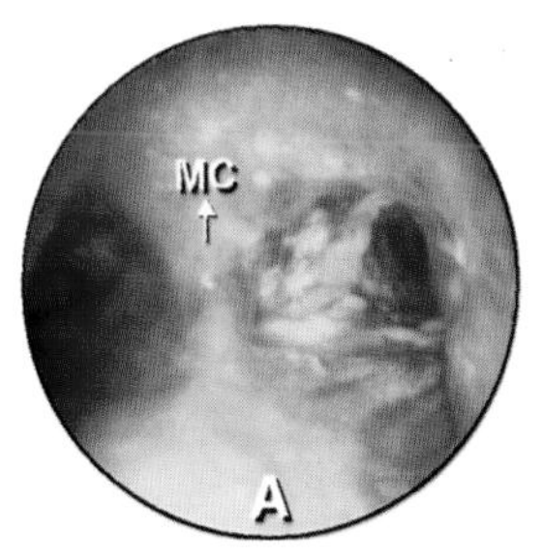

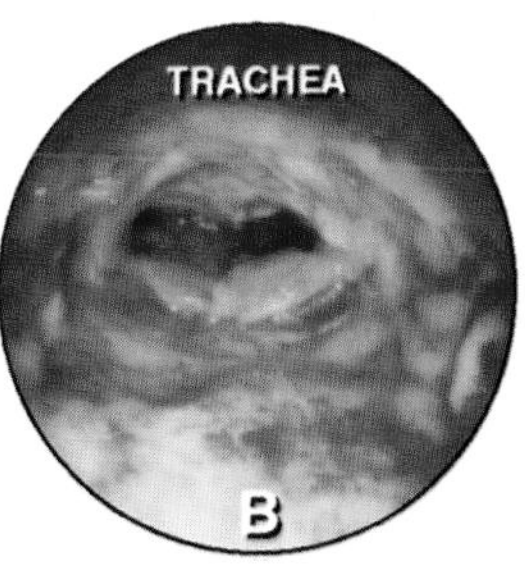

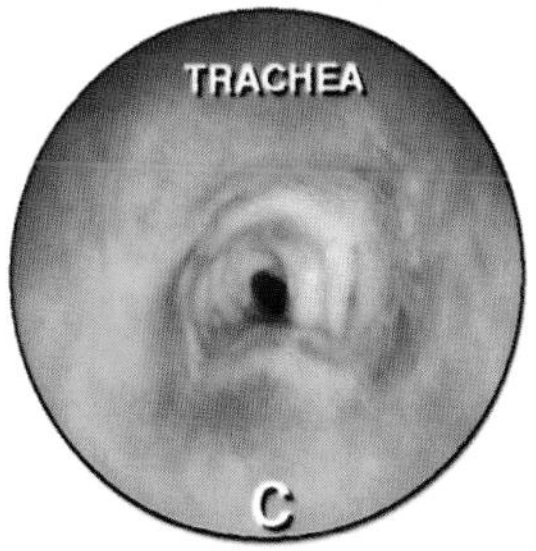

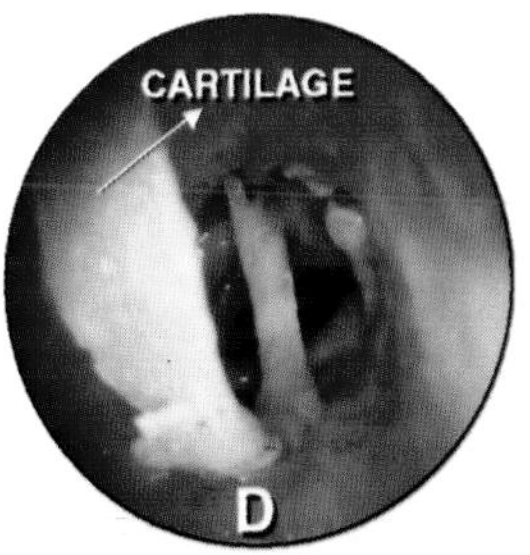

Radiation-induced injury to tracheobronchial tree. Both external beam radiation therapy and brachytherapy can cause significant damage to the airways. Necrotic tissue is seen in the right main-stem bronchus following intense brachytherapy **(A).** Significant necrosis of the distal trachea and main carina **(B).** Purulent-appearing midtrachea following radiotherapy **(C).** Radiation therapy has resulted in necrosis and loosening of tracheal cartilages into airway lumen **(D).** *Arrow* indicates main carina, MC.

FIGURE 6–91

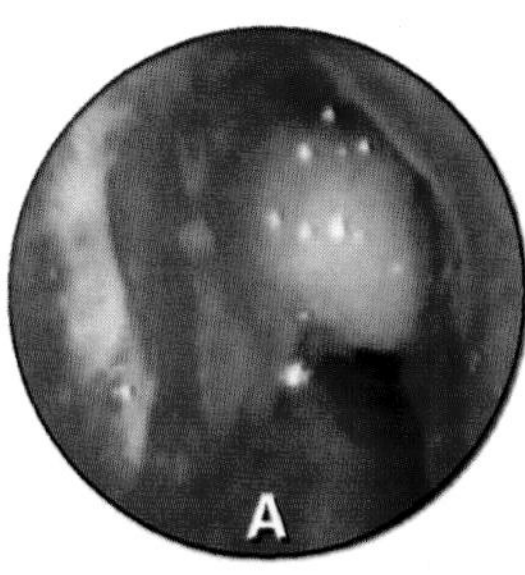

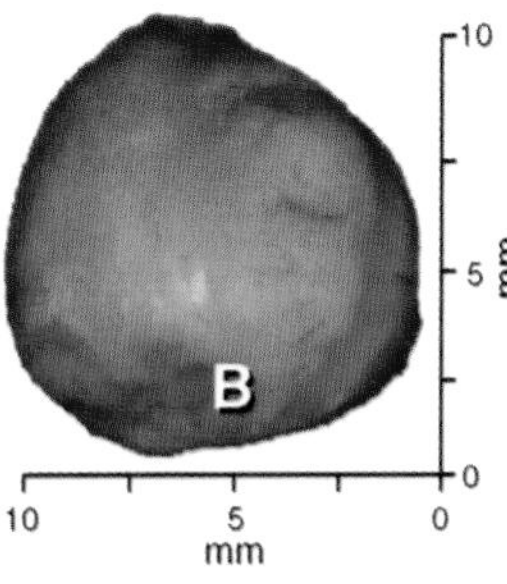

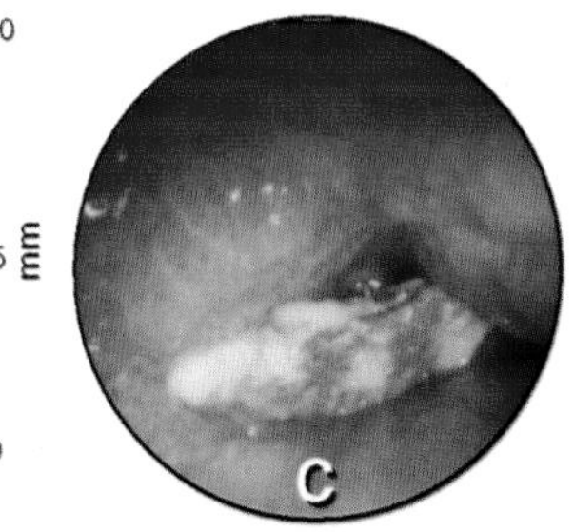

Foreign body impacted in the trachea of an adult was successfully removed with a rigid bronchoscope because of the respiratory distress **(A).** The foreign body was a macadamia nut **(B).** In another patient a chicken bone was extracted without difficulty using a rigid bronchoscope **(C).** Tracheobronchial foreign bodies can also be removed with flexible bronchoscope. However, a study of 60 adults with tracheobronchial foreign bodies noted that the rigid bronchoscope was successful in 90% of removals, and the flexible instrument was able to extract the foreign bodies in 60% of patients.[106]

FIGURE 6–92

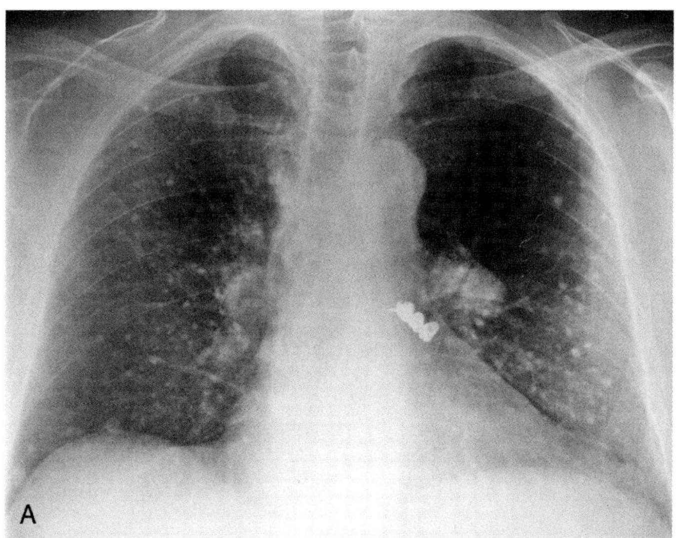

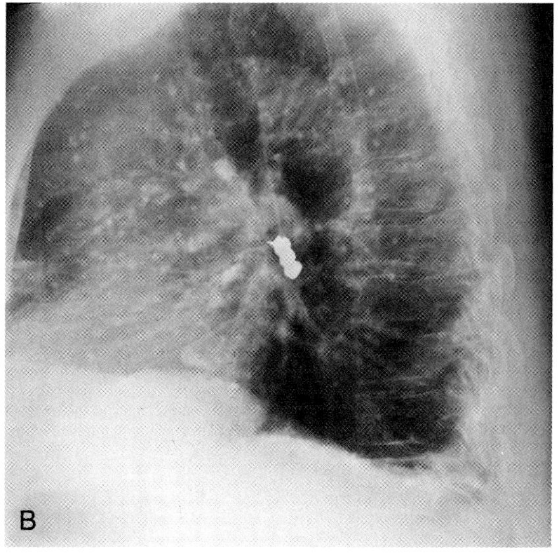

Foreign body in the left main-stem bronchus is radiopaque (partial dental bridge). The posteroanterior **(A)** and lateral **(B)** views are helpful to identify the location of the foreign body. The foreign body was extracted using flexible bronchoscope and a ureteral basket. Calcified granulomas in both lungs indicate old histoplasmosis.

THERAPEUTIC BRONCHOSCOPY

FIGURE 6–93

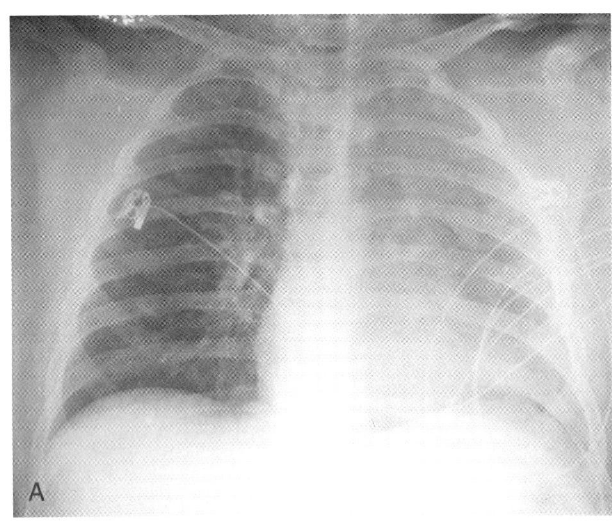

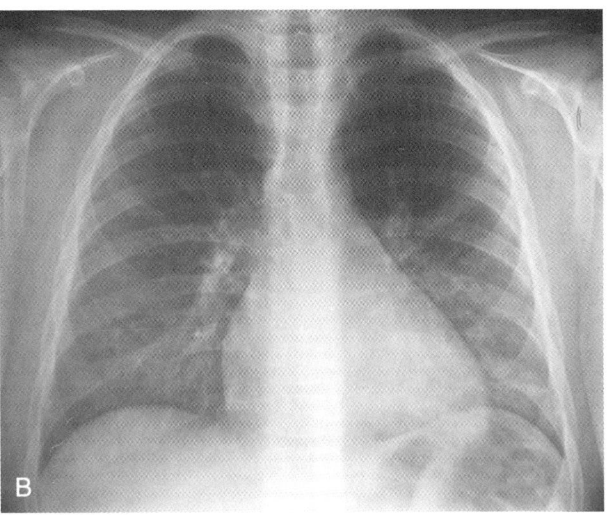

Foreign body in the left main-stem bronchus causes atelectasis of the left lung **(A).** Chest roentgenograph after the extraction of foreign body shows full expansion of left lung **(B).** The plastic object aspirated into the left main-stem bronchus was radiolucent and therefore cannot be seen on the roentgenograph. Clinical suspicion is important in the diagnosis of airway foreign bodies.

FIGURE 6–94

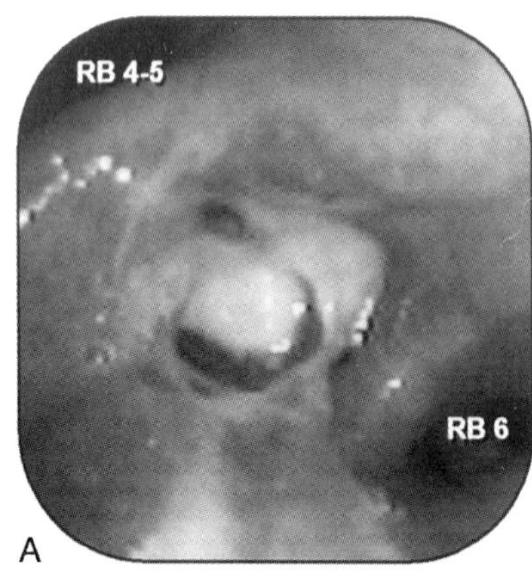

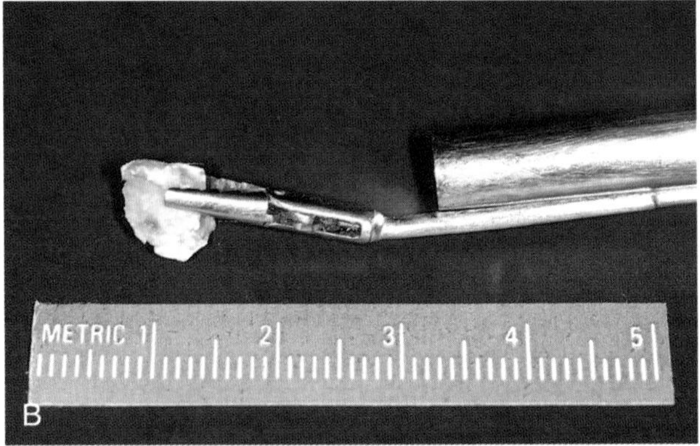

Foreign body in the right lower lobe bronchus **(A)** was extracted with a rigid bronchoscope **(B)** in a child who had aspirated this small pebble. Rigid bronchoscopy remains the instrument of choice for removal of airway foreign bodies in children. RB 4-5 = lateral and medial segment of right middle lobe; RB-6 = superior segment of right middle lobe (see Fig. 6–15).

FIGURE 6–95

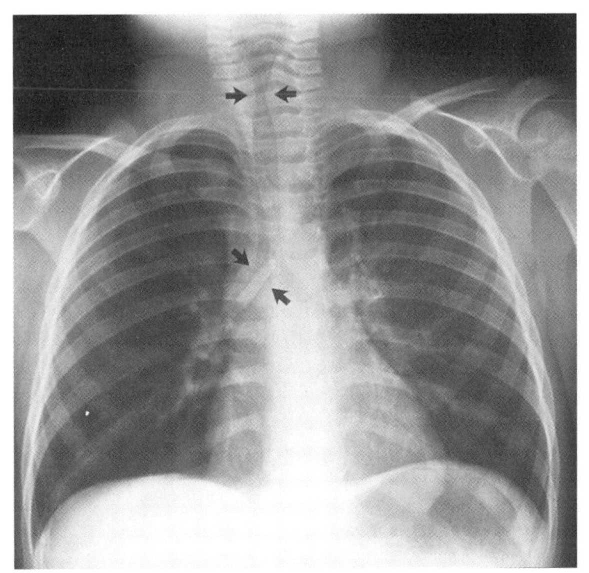

A foreign body impacted in the right main-stem bronchus (*slanting arrows*) of a child is shown in this chest roentgenograph. The subglottic area (*horizontal arrows*) in children is smaller in diameter compared with the rest of trachea, and the foreign body may be sheared off by this area during bronchoscopic attempt to remove the foreign body.

FIGURE 6–96

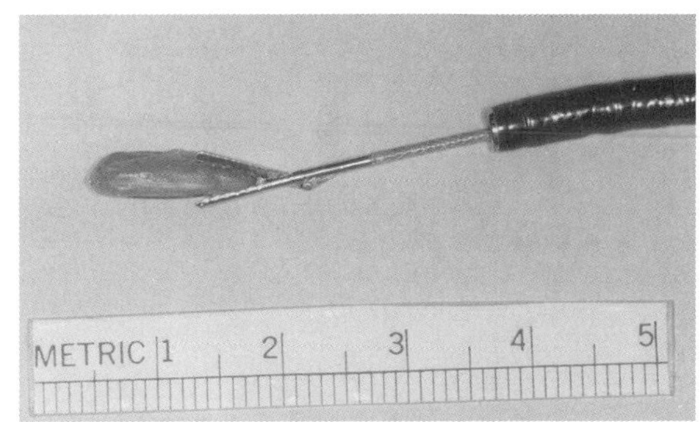

Foreign bodies in children can be removed with pediatric flexible bronchoscope (external diameter 3.2 mm), provided the bronchoscopist is prepared to proceed immediately with rigid bronchoscopy if the flexible bronchoscope fails. A foreign body (sunflower seed) is shown being grasped by a flexible ureteral stone forceps that has traversed the working channel of a pediatric flexible bronchoscope. The suction channel of the pediatric flexible bronchoscope has a diameter of 1.0 mm.

FIGURE 6–97

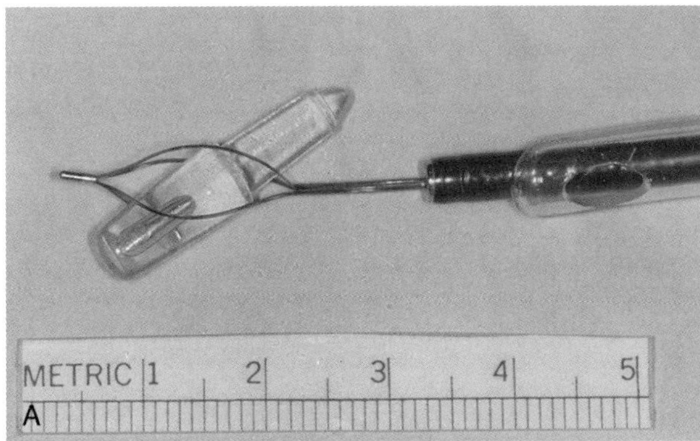

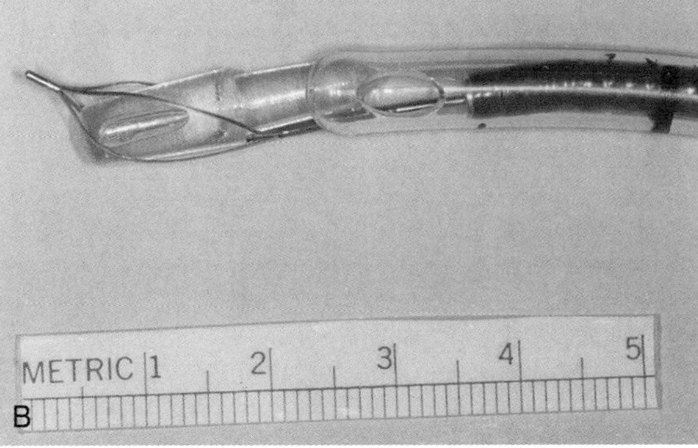

Foreign body impacted in the right main-stem bronchus (see Fig. 6–95) was removed using pediatric flexible bronchoscope. The in vitro demonstration shows the methods used. The pediatric flexible bronchoscope with an external diameter of 3.2 mm is passed through a 4.5-mm endotracheal tube. A ureteral stone basket is used to grasp the foreign body **(A).** The basket with the captured foreign body is gradually pulled proximally until the tip of the foreign body is inside the tip of the endotracheal tube and the entire unit (endotracheal tube, bronchoscope, and the foreign body) is removed en masse **(B).** Many types of airway foreign bodies have been extracted using the pediatric flexible bronchoscope.[107]

THERAPEUTIC BRONCHOSCOPY

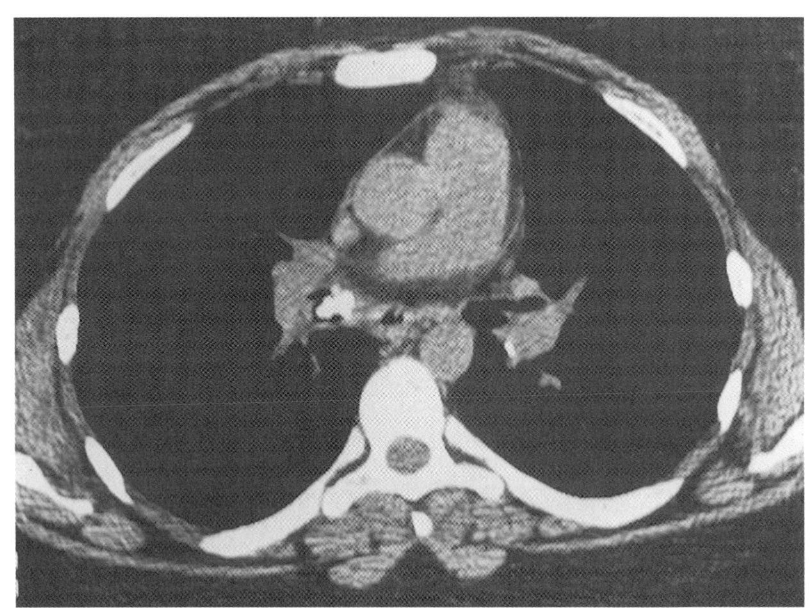

FIGURE 6-98

Broncholithiasis is an uncommon disorder and is usually caused by calcified lymph nodes that erode into the tracheobronchial tree. Symptoms include cough, hemoptysis, and lithoptysis. An imaging study such as computed tomography of the chest may indicate the possibility of broncholithiasis. Here the computed tomography scan of the chest shows a large calcified mass in the right hilar region, partially obstructing the bronchus intermedius. The most important diagnostic test, however, is bronchoscopic visualization of the broncholith.

FIGURE 6-99

Broncholithiasis involving left main-stem bronchus was successfully removed with bronchoscope **(A)**. **B,** Fragments of broncholiths in another patient who underwent bronchoscopic removal, which is described in Figure 6-100. Broncholiths are usually made up of calcium phosphate. The most common etiologies of broncholithiasis include infections by *Histoplasma capsulatum, Coccidioides immitis,* and *Mycobacterium tuberculosis.* Symptoms include cough, hemoptysis (in 50%), and localized wheezing.

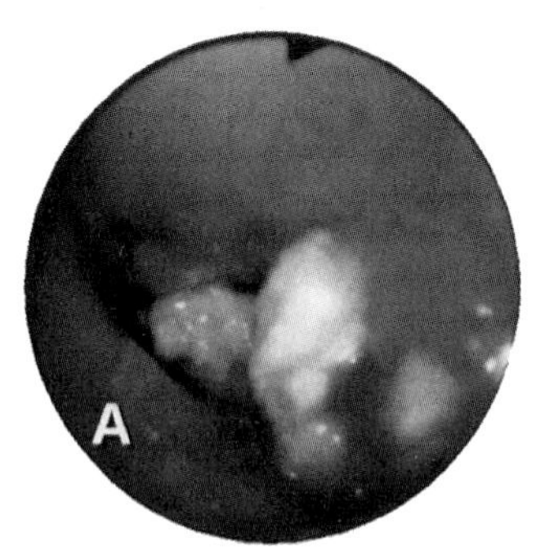

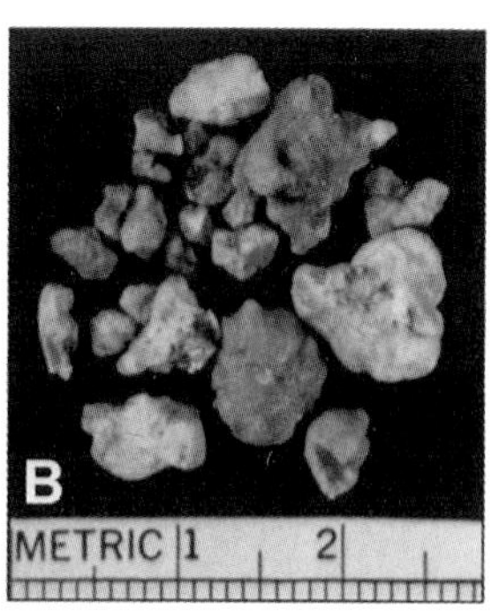

Rigid bronchoscope
Rt
Lt
Flexible bronchoscope
Normal saline
Electrohydraulic lithotriptor or Pulsed-dye laser probe
Broncholith
Fogarty balloon (air inflated)

FIGURE 6-100

Broncholithotripsy to extract the broncholiths shown in Figure 6-99*B*. The diagram shows immersion of the broncholith and the lithotriptor tip in normal saline. This step is essential for the optimal discharge and transmission of energy by electrohydraulic and pulsed dye laser lithotriptors.[108] (From Aust MR, Prakash UBS, McDougall JC, et al: Bronchoscopic broncholithotripsy. J Bronchol 1:37–41, 1994.)

THERAPEUTIC BRONCHOSCOPY

FIGURE 6–101

Broncholithiasis of left upper lobe bronchus (LB 4–5) with mild bleeding upon manipulation **(A).** Flexible bronchoscopic extraction of the broncholith **(B).** Bronchoscopic removal of broncholiths has been successful in 19% to 67% of patients.[109, 110] If the broncholiths are loose within the airway lumen, either a flexible or rigid bronchoscope can be used to remove them.[111]

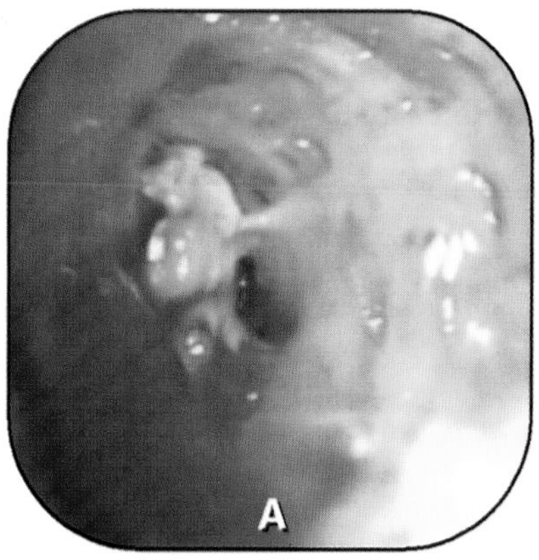

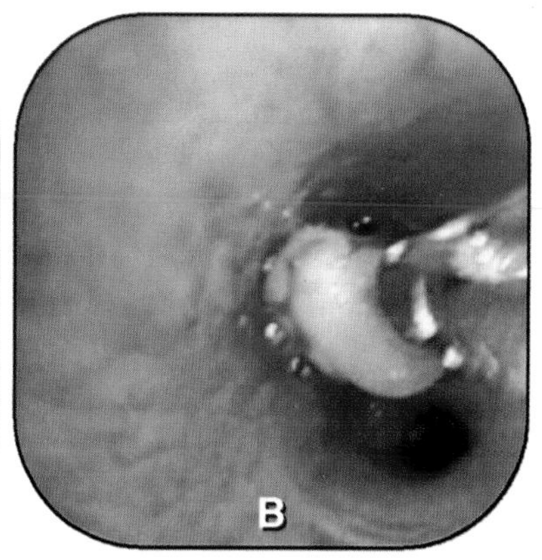

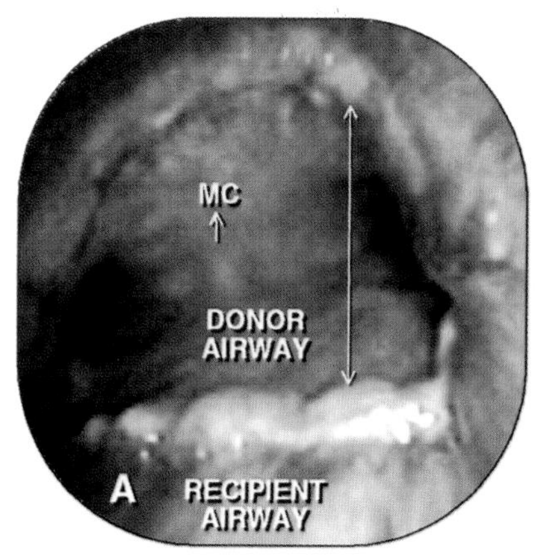

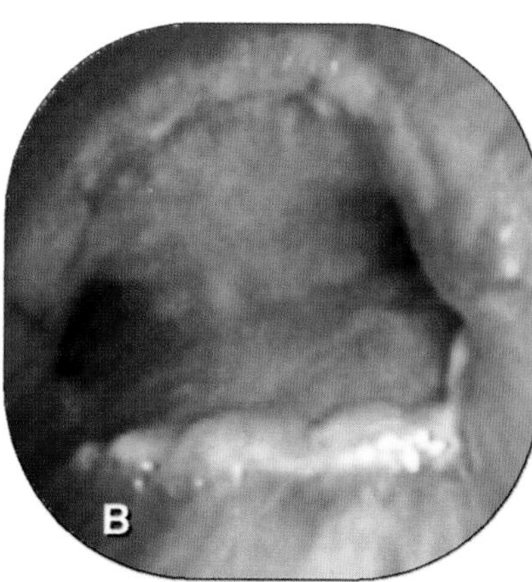

FIGURE 6–102

Lung transplant recipients require bronchoscopy to diagnose opportunistic infections and transplant rejection, and to diagnose and treat anastomotic strictures.[112] This figure shows the appearance of airways of the donor and the recipient. The anastomotic site appears healthy, and there is no evidence of tracheal stricture. Flexible bronchoscopic balloon dilatation and bronchial stent therapy have been utilized to treat bronchial strictures that follow lung transplantation.[113, 114] Surveillance bronchoscopy denotes regular periodic bronchoscopy with lung biopsy to identify opportunistic infections as well as lung rejection process.[115] MC = main carina.

FIGURE 6–103

Lung transplant recipient with dehiscence of an anastomotic site in the right main-stem bronchus (RMB) **(A).** **B,** Close-up view shows loose sutures and purulent material surrounding it. Occasionally, loose sutures inside the airway lumen lead to cough. Bronchoscopic removal of sutures resolves the cough. MC = main carina; RUL = right upper lobe.

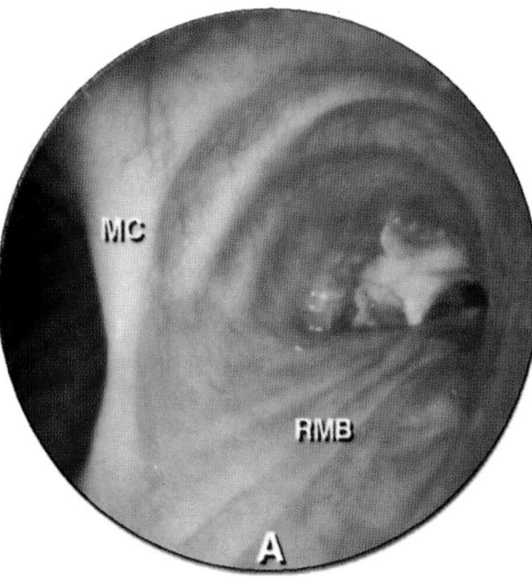

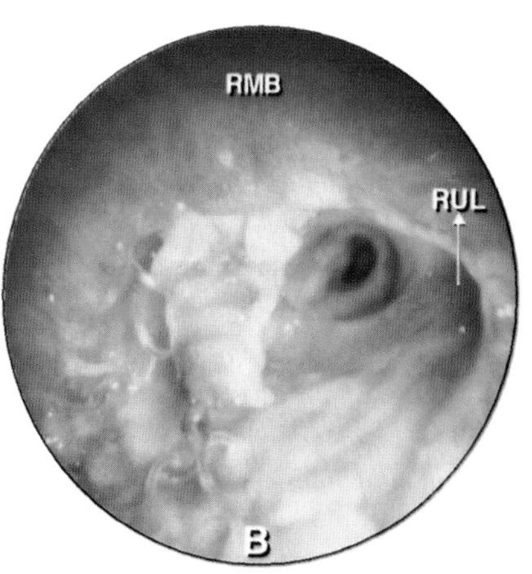

REFERENCES

1. Killian G: Removal of a bone splinter from the right bronchus with help of direct laryngoscopy. Münch Med Wochenschr 24:86, 1897.

2. Killian G: Ueber directe Bronkoskopie. Münch Med Wochenschr 27:844–847, 1898.

2a. Jackson C: Bronchoscopy: Past, present, and future. N Engl J Med 199:758–763, 1928.

3. Ikeda S, Yanai N, Ishikawa S: Flexible bronchofiberscope. Keio J Med 17:1–10, 1968.

4. Prakash UBS, Stubbs SE: The bronchoscopy survey: Some reflections. Chest 100:1660–1667, 1991.

5. Prakash UBS: Bronchoscopy in the critically ill patient. Semin Respir Med 18:583–591, 1997.

6. Olapade CS, Prakash UBS: Bronchoscopy in the critical care unit. Mayo Clin Proc 64:1255–1263, 1989.

7. Stover DE, Zaman MB, Hajdu SI, et al: Bronchoalveolar lavage in the diagnosis of diffuse pulmonary infiltrates in the immunocompromised host. Ann Intern Med 101:107, 1984.

8. Brickey DA, Lawlor DP: Transbronchial biopsy in the presence of profound elevation of the international normalized ratio. Chest 115:1667–1671, 1999.

9. Prakash UBS: Optimal bronchoscopy. J Bronchol 1: 44–62, 1994.

10. Prakash UBS, Diaz-Jimenez JP: The rigid bronchoscope. *In* Prakash UBS (ed): Bronchoscopy. New York, Raven Press, 1994, pp. 53–69.

11. Zavala DC: Flexible fiberoptic bronchoscopy: A training handbook. Iowa City, IA, University of Iowa Press, 1978, p. 123.

12. Mehta AC, Dweik RA: Nasal versus oral insertion of the flexible bronchoscope. Pro-nasal insertion. J Bronchol 3:224–228, 1996.

13. Guntupalli KK, Siddiqi AJ: Nasal versus oral insertion of the flexible bronchoscope. Pro-oral insertion. J Bronchol 3:229–233, 1996.

14. Prakash UBS: Nasal versus oral insertion of the bronchoscope: Advantages and disadvantages. J Bronchol 3:173–176, 1996.

15. Elkus RL, Miller MB, Kini SR, et al: Comparison of withdrawn and nonwithdrawn brushes in the diagnosis of lung cancer. J Bronchol 1:269–275, 1994.

16. Loube DI, Johnson JE, Wiener D, et al: The effect of forceps size on the adequacy of specimens obtained by transbronchial biopsy. Am Rev Respir Dis 148:1411–1413, 1993.

17. Mehta AC, Curtis PS, Scalzitti M, Meeker DP: The high price of bronchoscopy: Maintenance and repair of the flexible fiberoptic bronchoscope. Chest 98:448–454, 1990.

18. Dasgupta A, Jain P, Minai OA, et al: Utility of transbronchial needle aspiration in the diagnosis of endobronchial lesions. Chest 115:1237–1241, 1999.

19. Prakash UBS, Cortese DA, Stubbs SE: Technical solutions to common problems in bronchoscopy. *In* Prakash UBS (ed): Bronchoscopy. New York, Raven Press, 1994, pp. 111–133.

20. Prakash UBS: Prophylactic antibacterial therapy for bronchoscopy: Indications. J Bronchol 4:281–285, 1997.

21. Wu FL, Razzaghi A, Souney PF: Seizure after lidocaine for bronchoscopy: Case report and review of the use of lidocaine in airway anesthesia. Pharmacotherapy 13:72–78, 1993.

21a. Cowl CT, Prakash UBS, Kruger BR: The role of anticholinergic drugs in bronchoscopy: A randomized clinical trial. Chest 118:188–192, 2000.

21b. Colt HG, Prakash UBS, Offord, KP: Bronchoscopy in North America: Survey by the American Association for Bronchology, 1999. J Bronchol 7:8–25, 2000.

22. Reed AP: Preparation of the patient for awake fiberoptic bronchoscopy. Chest 101:244–253, 1992.

23. Set PAK, Flower CDR, Smith IE, et al: Hemoptysis: Comparative study of the role of CT and fiberoptic bronchoscopy. Radiology 189:677–680, 1993.

24. Gerbeaux P, Ledoray V, Boussuges A, et al: Diagnosis of nosocomial pneumonia in mechanically ventilated patients: Repeatability of the bronchoalveolar lavage. Am J Respir Crit Care Med 157:76–80, 1998.

25. Fagon JY, Chastre J, Hance AJ, et al: Detection of nosocomial lung infection in ventilated patients: Use of a protected specimen brush and quantitative culture techniques in 147 patients. Am Rev Respir Dis 138:110–116, 1988.

26. Kurasawa T, Kuze F, Kawai M, et al: Diagnosis and management of endobronchial tuberculosis. Intern Med 31:593–598, 1992.

27. Nakamura K, Terada N, Ohi M, et al: Tuberculous bronchial stenosis: Treatment with balloon bronchoplasty. Am J Roentgenol 157:1187–1188, 1991.

28. Van-den-Brande P, Lambrechts M, Tack J, Demedts M: Endobronchial tuberculosis mimicking lung cancer in elderly patients. Respir Med 85:107–109, 1991.

29. Danek SJ, Bower JS: Diagnosis of pulmonary tuberculosis by flexible fiberoptic bronchoscopy. Am Rev Respir Dis 119:677–679, 1979.

30. Russell MD, Torrington KG, Tenholder MF: A ten year experience with fiberoptic bronchoscopy for mycobacterial isolation: Impact on the Bactec system. Am Rev Respir Dis 133:1069–1071, 1986.

31. Willcox PA, Potgieter PD, Bateman ED, et al: Rapid diagnosis of sputum negative miliary tuberculosis using the flexible fiberoptic bronchoscope. Thorax 41:681–684, 1986.

32. Kahn FW, Jones JM, England DM: The role of bronchoalveolar lavage in the diagnosis of invasive pulmonary aspergillosis. Am J Clin Pathol 86:518–523, 1986.

REFERENCES

33. Prechter GC, Prakash UBS: Bronchoscopy in the diagnosis of pulmonary histoplasmosis. Chest 95:1033–1036, 1989.

34. Thompson AB, Teschler H, Rennard SI: Pathogenesis, evaluation, and therapy for massive hemoptysis. Clin Chest Med 13:69–82, 1992.

35. Gong H Jr, Salvatierra C: Clinical efficacy of early and delayed fiberoptic bronchoscopy in patients with hemoptysis. Am Rev Respir Dis 124:221–225, 1981.

36. Kawaida M, Kohno N, Kawasaki Y, Fukuda H: Surgical treatment of large epiglottic cysts with a side-opened direct laryngoscope and snare. Auris Nasus Larynx 19:45–49, 1992.

37. Dickens P, Srivastava G, Loke SL, Larkin S: Human papillomavirus 6, 11, and 16 in laryngeal papillomas. J Pathol 165:243–246, 1991.

38. Prakash UBS, Cavaliere S: Atlas of bronchoscopy. *In* Prakash UBS (ed): Bronchoscopy. New York, Raven Press, 1994, Chap. 32, pp. 443–532.

39. Adlakha A, Prakash UBS: Tracheobronchial papillomatosis. J Bronchol 6:42–45, 1999.

40. Lie ES, Engh V, Boysen M, et al: Squamous cell carcinoma of the respiratory tract following laryngeal papillomatosis. Acta Otolaryngol (Stockh) 114:209–212, 1994.

41. Saleh EM: Complications of treatment of recurrent laryngeal papillomatosis with the carbon dioxide laser in children. J Laryngol Otol 106:715–718, 1992.

42. Abrammson AL, Shikowitz MH, Mullooly VM, et al: Clinical effects of photodynamic therapy on recurrent laryngeal papillomas. Arch Otolaryngol Head Neck Surg 118:25–29, 1992.

43. Wood DE, Mathisen DJ: Late complications of tracheotomy. Clin Chest Med 12:597–609, 1991.

44. Grillo HC, Mathisen DJ: Primary tracheal tumors: Treatment and results. Ann Thorac Surg 49:69–77, 1990.

45. Gelder CM, Hetzel MR: Primary tracheal tumours: A national survey. Thorax 48:688–692, 1993.

46. Davila DG, Dunn WF, Tazelaar HD, et al: Bronchial carcinoid tumors. Mayo Clin Proc 68:795–803, 1993.

47. Warren WH, Faber LP, Gould VE: Neuroendocrine neoplasms of the lung: A clinicopathologic update. J Thorac Cardiovasc Surg 98:321–332, 1989.

48. Harpole DH Jr, Feldman JM, Buchanan S, et al: Bronchial carcinoid tumors: A retrospective analysis of 126 patients. Ann Thorac Surg 54:50–55, 1992.

49. Prakash UBS, Freitag L: Hemoptysis and bronchoscopy-induced hemorrhage. *In* Prakash UBS (ed): Bronchoscopy. New York, Raven Press, 1994, pp. 227–251.

50. Jerray M, Benzarti M, Hayouni A, et al: Extramedullary solitary plasmacytoma of the trachea. Eur J Med 1: 249–250, 1992.

51. Ferreiro JA, Egorshin EV, Olsen KD, et al: Mucous membrane plasmacytosis of the upper aerodigestive tract. A clinicopathologic study. Am J Surg Pathol 18:1048–1053, 1994.

52. Robin J, Wilson AC: Polypoid neurilemmoma of the trachea: An unusual cause of major airway obstruction. Aust N Z J Surg 58:912, 1988.

53. Chen TF, Braidley PC, Shneerson JM, Wells FC: Obstructing tracheal lipoma: Management of a rare tumor. Ann Thorac Surg 49:137–139, 1990.

54. Hurt R: Benign tumours of the bronchus and trachea, 1951–1981. Ann R Coll Surg Engl 66:22, 1984.

55. Neis PR, McMahon MF, Norris CW: Cartilaginous tumors of the trachea and larynx. Ann Otol Rhinol Laryngol 98:31, 1989.

56. Miller DL, Allen MS: Rare pulmonary neoplasms. Mayo Clin Proc 68:492–498, 1993.

57. Ettensohn DB, Bennett JM, Hyde RW: Endobronchial metastases from carcinoma of the breast. Med Pediatr Oncol 13:9, 1985.

58. Cordier JF, Chailleux E, Lauque D, et al: Primary pulmonary lymphomas. A clinical study of 70 cases in nonimmunocompromised patients. Chest 103:201–208, 1993.

59. Ieki R, Goto H, Kouzai Y, et al: Endobronchial non-Hodgkin's lymphoma. Respir Med 83:87–89, 1989.

60. Shapshay SM, Strong MS: Tracheobronchial obstruction from metastatic distant malignancies. Ann Otol Rhinol Laryngol 91:648, 1982.

61. Poe RH, Ortiz C, Israel RH, et al: Sensitivity, specificity, and predictive values of bronchoscopy in neoplasm metastatic to lung. Chest 88:84, 1985.

62. Rovirosa-Casino A, Bellmunt J, Salud A, et al: Endobronchial metastases in colorectal adenocarcinoma. Tumori 78:270–273, 1992.

63. Merine D, Fishman EK: Mediastinal adenopathy and endobronchial involvement in metastatic renal cell carcinoma. J Comput Tomogr 12:216, 1988.

64. Noy S, Michowitz M, Lazebnik N, Baratz M: Endobronchial metastasis of renal cell carcinoma. J Surg Oncol 31:268, 1986.

64a. Prakash UBS: Role of methylene blue in bronchoscopy. J Bronchol 7:54–57, 2000.

65. Schmittenbecher PP, Mantel K, Hofmann U, Berlien HP: Treatment of congenital tracheoesophageal fistula by endoscopic laser coagulation: Preliminary report of three cases. J Pediatr Surg 27:26–28, 1992.

66. Antonelli M, Cicconetti F, Vivino G, Gasparetto A: Closure of a tracheoesophageal fistula by bronchoscopic application of fibrin glue and decontamination of the oral cavity. Chest 100:578–579, 1991.

67. York EL, Lewall DB, Hirji M, et al: Endoscopic diagnosis and treatment of postoperative bronchopleural fistula. Chest 97:1390–1392, 1990.

REFERENCES

68. Sippel JM, Chestnutt MS: Bronchoscopic therapy for bronchopleural fistulas. J Bronchol 5:61–69, 1998.

69. Prakash UBS, McCullough AE, Edell ES, Nienhuis DM: Tracheopathia osteoplastica: Familial occurrence. Mayo Clin Proc 64:1091–1096, 1989.

70. Nienhuis DM, Prakash UBS, Edell ES: Tracheobronchopathia osteochondroplastica. Ann Otol Rhinol Laryngol 99:689–694, 1990.

71. Chen KT: Amyloidosis presenting in the respiratory tract. Pathol Annu 73:253–273, 1989.

71a. Capizzi SA, Betancourt EM, Prakash UBS: Tracheobronchial amyloidosis. Mayo Clin Proc 75:1148–1152, 2000.

72. Russchen GH, Wouters B, Meinesz AF, et al: Amyloid tumour resected by laser therapy. Eur Respir J 3:932–933, 1990.

73. Fukumura M, Mieno T, Suzuki T, Murata Y: Primary diffuse tracheobronchial amyloidosis treated by bronchoscopic Nd:YAG laser irradiation. Jpn J Med 29:620–622, 1990.

74. Amin R: Endobronchial involvement in Wegener's granulomatosis. Postgrad Med J 59:452, 1983.

75. Eagleton LE, Rosher RB, Hawe A, Bilinsky RT: Radiation therapy and mechanical dilation of endobronchial obstruction secondary to Wegener's granulomatosis. Chest 76:609, 1979.

76. Lebovics RS, Hoffman GS, Leavitt RY, et al: The management of subglottic stenosis in patients with Wegener's granulomatosis. Laryngoscope 102:1341, 1992.

77. Daum TE, Spechs U, Colby TV, et al: Tracheobronchial involvement in Wegener's granulomatosis. Am J Respir Crit Care Med 151:522–526, 1995.

78. Van-Schoor J, Joos G, Pauwels R: Tracheobronchomegaly—The Mounier-Kuhn syndrome: Report of two cases and review of the literature. Eur Respir J 14:1303–1306, 1991.

79. Woodring JH, Barrett PA, Rehm SR, Nurenberg P: Acquired tracheomegaly in adults as a complication of diffuse pulmonary fibrosis. Am J Roentgenol 152:743–747, 1989.

80. Baughman RP: Is bronchoalveolar lavage clinically useful for everyday practice in interstitial lung disease? J Bronchol 6:211–216, 1999.

81. De Lassence A, Fleury Feith J, Escudier E, et al: Alveolar hemorrhage. Diagnostic criteria and results in 194 immunocompromised hosts. Am J Respir Crit Care Med 151:157–163, 1995.

82. Di Boscio, Prakash UBS: Diagnosis of pulmonary endometriosis by bronchoalveolar lavage. J Bronchol 4:231–234, 1997.

83. Simpson FG, Arnold AG, Purvis A, et al: Postal survey of bronchoscopic practice by physicians in the United Kingdom. Thorax 41:311–317, 1986.

84. Dasgupta A, Mehta AC: Transbronchial needle aspiration. An underused diagnostic technique. Clin Chest Med 20:39–51, 1999.

85. Solomon SB, White P Jr, Acker DE, et al: Real-time bronchoscope tip localization enables three-dimensional CT image guidance for transbronchial needle aspiration in swine. Chest 114:1405–1410, 1998.

86. Rong F, Cui B: CT scan directed transbronchial needle aspiration biopsy for mediastinal nodes. Chest 114:36–39, 1998.

87. Shankar S, Gulati M, Gupta D, et al: CT-guided transthoracic fine-needle aspiration versus transbronchial fluoroscopy-guided needle aspiration in pulmonary nodules. Acta Radiol 39:395–399, 1998.

88. Steiner RM, Liu JB, Goldberg BB, Cohn JR: The value of ultrasound-guided fiberoptic bronchoscopy. Clin Chest Med 16:519–534, 1995.

89. Summers RM, Selbie WS, Malley JD, et al: Polypoid lesions of airways: Early experience with computer-assisted detection by using virtual bronchoscopy and surface curvature. Radiology 208:331–337, 1998.

90. McAdams HP, Goodman PC, Kussin P: Virtual bronchoscopy for directing transbronchial needle aspiration of hilar and mediastinal lymph nodes: A pilot study. Am J Roentgenol 170:1361–1364, 1998.

91. Ferretti GR, Knoplioch J, Bricault I, et al: Central airway stenoses: Preliminary results of spiral-CT-generated virtual bronchoscopy simulations in 29 patients. Eur Radiol 7:854–859, 1997.

92. Doi M, Miyazawa T, Mineshita M, et al: Three-dimensional bronchial imaging by spiral computed tomography as applied to tracheobronchial stent placement. J Bronchol 6:155–158, 1999.

93. Lam S, Kennedy T, Unger M, et al: Localization of bronchial intraepithelial neoplastic lesions by fluorescence bronchoscopy. Chest 113:696–702, 1998.

94. Dweik RA, Stoller JK: Role of bronchoscopy in massive hemoptysis. Clin Chest Med 20:89–105, 1999.

95. Cairns-Bazarian AM, Conway EE Jr, Yankelowitz S: Plastic bronchitis: An unusual cause of respiratory distress in children. Pediatr Emerg Care 8:335–337, 1992.

96. Jett JR, Tazelaar HD, Keim LW, Ingrassia TS 3d: Plastic bronchitis: An old disease revisited. Mayo Clin Proc 66:305–311, 1991.

97. Muller W, von-der-Hardt H, Rieger CH: Idiopathic and symptomatic plastic bronchitis in childhood. A report of three cases and review of the literature. Respiration 52:214–218, 1987.

97a. Prakash UBS: Advances in bronchoscopic techniques. Chest 116:1403–1408, 1999.

98. Prakash UBS, Offord KP, Stubbs SE: Bronchoscopy in North America: The ACCP Survey. Chest 100:1668–1675, 1991.

REFERENCES

99. Sheski FD, Mathur PN: Balloon bronchoplasty using the flexible bronchoscope. J Bronchol 5:242–246, 1998.

100. Sheski FD, Mathur PN: Long-term results of fiberoptic bronchoscopic balloon dilation in the management of benign tracheobronchial stenosis. Chest 114:796–800, 1998.

101. Cavaliere S, Foccoli P, Toninelli C, Feijo S: Nd:YAG laser therapy in lung cancer: An 11-year experience with 2,253 applications in 1,585 patients. J Bronchol 1:105–111, 1994.

102. Colt HG, Harrell JH: Therapeutic rigid bronchoscopy allows level of care changes in patients with acute respiratory failure from central airways obstruction. Chest 112:202–206, 1997.

103. Shah H, Garbe L, Nussbaum E, et al: Benign tumors of the tracheobronchial tree. Endoscopic characteristics and role of laser resection. Chest 107:1744–1751, 1995.

104. Vansteenkiste JF, Lacquet LM: Possibilities and indications for Nd-YAG laser and dilation therapy in the management of tracheal stenosis. Acta Otorhinolaryngol Belg 49:359–365, 1995.

105. Dumon JF, Cavaliere S, Diaz-Jimenez JP, et al: Seven-year experience with the Dumon prosthesis. J Bronchol 3:6–11, 1996.

106. Limper AH, Prakash UBS: Tracheobronchial foreign bodies in adults. Ann Intern Med 112:604–609, 1990.

107. Castro M, Midthun DE, Edell ES et al: Flexible bronchoscopic removal of foreign bodies from pediatric airways. J Bronchol 1:92–98, 1994.

108. Aust MR, Prakash UBS, McDougall JC, et al: Bronchoscopic broncholithotripsy. J Bronchol 1:37–41, 1994.

109. Trastek VF, Pairolero PC, Ceithaml EL, et al: Surgical management of broncholithiasis. J Thorac Cardiovasc Surg 90:842–849, 1985.

110. Cole FH, Cole FH Jr, Khandekar A, Watson DC: Management of broncholithiasis: Is thoracotomy necessary? Ann Thorac Surg 42:255–259, 1986.

111. Olson ES, Utz JP, Prakash UBS: Therapeutic bronchoscopy in broncholithiasis. Am J Respir Crit Care Med 160:776–770, 1999.

112. Ward C, Snell GI, Zheng L, et al: Endobronchial biopsy and bronchoalveolar lavage in stable lung transplant recipients and chronic rejection. Am J Respir Crit Care Med 158:84–91, 1998.

113. Keller C, Frost A: Fiberoptic bronchoplasty. Description of a simple adjunct technique for the management of bronchial stenosis following lung transplantation. Chest 102:995–998, 1992.

114. Colt HG, Janssen JP, Dumon JF, Noirclerc MJ: Endoscopic management of bronchial stenosis after double lung transplantation. Chest 102:10–16, 1992.

115. Kukafka DS, O'Brien GM, Furukawa S, Criner GJ: Surveillance bronchoscopy in lung transplant recipients. Chest 111:377–381, 1997.

Microbiology Laboratory Diagnosis of Respiratory Tract Infections

W. Keith Hadley, M.D., Ph.D.

INTRODUCTION

COLONIZING MICROBIAL POPULATIONS IN THE HOST

- The presence of a large and diverse microbial population in the secretions at the entrance to the lower respiratory tract, sinuses, and middle ears complicates diagnosis of respiratory tract infections.
- Saliva contains 10^8 to 10^9 anaerobic bacteria per milliliter and 10^7 to 10^8 aerobic bacteria per milliliter (FIGURE 7–1).
- Increased colonization by gram-negative bacilli occurs during hospitalization and is associated with the appearance of nosocomial respiratory infections.
- Antimicrobial therapy or prophylaxis selects for a population of intrinsically resistant or adapting resistant microorganisms.[1–3]

FIGURE 7–1

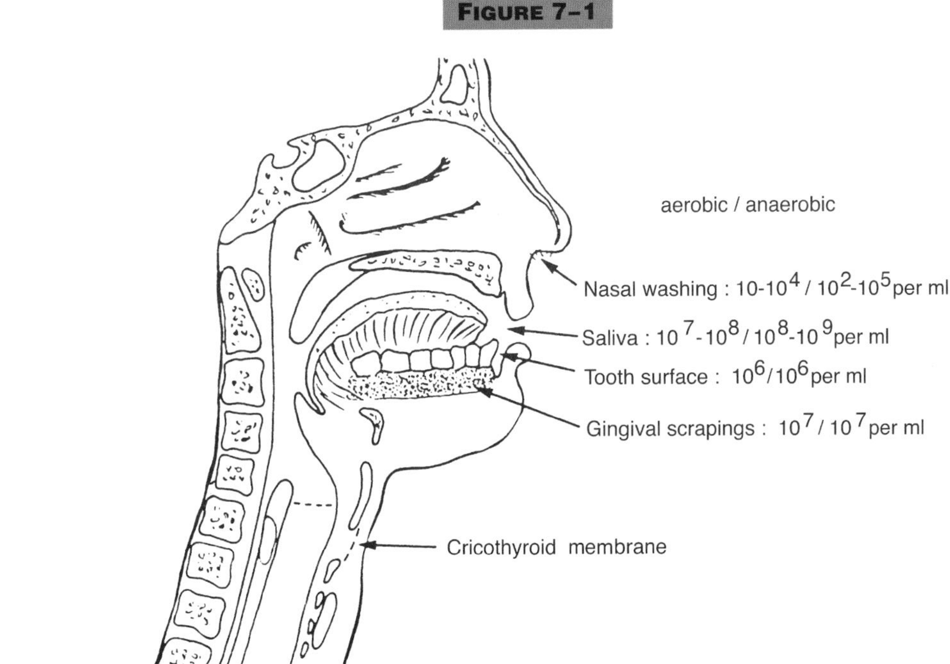

Counts of indigenous microflora at sites in the upper respiratory tract. The dotted horizontal line indicates the level below which the tracheobronchial tree normally is sterile. (From Hoeprich PD: Etiologic diagnosis of lower respiratory tract infections. Calif Med 112:1, 1970.)

RELATIONSHIP BETWEEN HOST AND COLONIZING ORGANISMS

- There is a complicated relationship between the colonizing microorganisms and the host.
- Some agents are nearly always commensals, which live upon the host without producing disease.
- Other agents are usually pathogens.
- Production of disease is dependent upon the virulence and dose of the agent and the resistance of the host (TABLE 7–1).[4]

INTRODUCTION

RELATIONSHIP BETWEEN HOST AND COLONIZING ORGANISMS

TABLE 7–1

Commensal and Pathogenic Agents in the Respiratory Tract

Commensal Agents

Aerobic bacteria
- *Corynebacterium*
- *Enterobacteriaceae*
- *Haemophilus*
- *Lactobacillus*
- *Micrococcus*
- *Moraxella*
- *Mycoplasma*
- *Neisseria*
- *Staphylococcus aureus*
- *Staphylococcus* (coagulase-negative)
- *Streptococcus pneumoniae*
- *Streptococcus pyogenes* (group A)
- *Streptococcus* sp.

Anaerobic bacteria
- *Actinomyces*
- *Bacteroides*
- *Bifidobacterium*
- *Eubacterium*
- *Fusobacterium*
- *Peptostreptococcus*
- *Porphyromonas*
- *Prevotella*
- *Propionibacterium*

Fungi
- *Candida* sp.
- Environmental molds and yeasts

Parasites
- *Entamoeba gingivalis*
- *Trichomonas tenax*

Pathogenic Agents

UPPER RESPIRATORY TRACT

Aerobic bacteria
- *Arcanobacterium (Corynebacterium) haemolyticum*
- *Chlamydia pneumoniae*
- *Corynebacterium diphtheriae*
- *Mycoplasma pneumoniae*
- *Neisseria gonorrhoeae*
- *Streptococcus pyogenes* (group A)

Fungi
- *Candida sp.*

Viruses
- Adenovirus
- Coronavirus
- Coxsackievirus A
- Epstein-Barr virus
- Herpes simplex viruses
- Influenzavirus, A and B
- Parainfluenza viruses
- Rhinovirus

LOWER RESPIRATORY TRACT

Aerobic bacteria
- *Bordetella pertussis*
- *Chlamydia pneumoniae*
- *Chlamydia psittaci*
- *Chlamydia trachomatis*
- *Enterobacteriaceae (Escherichia coli, Klebsiella,* others*)*
- *Haemophilus influenzae*
- *Branhamella (Moraxella) catarrhalis*
- *Mycobacterium tuberculosis* (others)
- *Mycoplasma pneumoniae*
- *Staphylococcus aureus*
- *Streptococcus pyogenes* (group A)

Anaerobic bacteria
- *Mixed anaerobic bacteria*

Fungi
- *Aspergillus* sp.
- *Blastomyces dermatitidis*
- *Coccidioides immitis*
- *Cryptococcus neoformans*
- *Histoplasma capsulatum*
- *Pneumocystis carinii*

Viruses
- Adenovirus
- Coronavirus
- Coxsackievirus A
- Hantavirus
- Influenzavirus, A and B
- Parainfluenza viruses
- Respiratory syncytial virus
- Rhinovirus

CLINICAL HISTORY

- The clinical history is necessary to interpret the significance of microbiologic laboratory data. This information is especially important when microorganisms, which may be either commensals or pathogens, are present.
- The laboratory finding of large numbers of bacteria resembling *Streptococcus pneumoniae* in sputum smear and culture may indicate pneumonia. However, the diagnosis of pneumonia must be supported by the clinical history, symptoms, signs, and radiographic evidence.
- In some cases it will be necessary to use more invasive and expensive procedures to bypass the indigenous microorganisms in order to make a specific diagnosis.
- Some of the commensal and pathogenic agents are listed in TABLE 7–1.
- Even with pathogenic agents, clinical signs of disease should be sought. Intermittent, convalescent, or asymptomatic carriage can occur with these agents.

COLLECTION, PRESERVATION, AND TRANSPORT OF RESPIRATORY TRACT SPECIMENS

GENERAL PRINCIPLES[5-7]

- Microbiologic diagnostic procedures are complicated and expensive.
- Every effort should be made to obtain the best possible initial specimen and to preserve the specimen properly before the procedure is started.
- Collect samples as directly as possible from the infected site, considering the need and cost of an invasive procedure.
- Avoid contamination by indigenous flora of the patient, e.g., mouth, nose, throat, or skin, when possible.
- Avoid contaminating patients' specimens with the flora from examiner's hands or respiratory droplets or environmental microorganisms from surfaces or dust.
- Use sterile instruments to collect specimens and sterile containers for specimens.

VOLUME OF SPECIMEN

- Obtain a sufficient volume of the specimen so that microorganisms can be recovered even when small numbers are present.
- Always send as much pleural fluid or bronchoalveolar lavage (BAL) sample as can be safely obtained for smear and culture.
- Chronic infections (e.g., mycobacterial or fungal infections) may have few microorganisms/volume so that greater volume or several specimens may be necessary.

COLLECTION ENVIRONMENT

- The specimen must be kept in an environment that maintains viability of the organisms initially present. *Note:* Drying rapidly inactivates many microorganisms and viruses.
- Appropriate bacterial, chlamydial, or viral transport media are used to contain the specimen, prevent overgrowth by microorganisms, and control pH.
- Viral transport media contain Eagle's MEM (minimum essential medium) or Hank's balanced salt solution along with a protein such as fetal bovine serum or bovine serum albumin.
- Antibiotics are added to prevent overgrowth of bacteria without killing the agent.
- Sucrose phosphate 2SP is a suitable transport medium for all three agents.
- Time between collection and inoculation into media for culture should be minimized.
- In general, swabs with wood sticks or certain lots of calcium alginate swabs may be toxic. Dacron or rayon swabs are usually preferable, but some lots may contain toxic materials.
- Use appropriate transport media for nucleic acid amplification tests.
- Refrigerate the specimen at 4°C when it must be held for culture. This temperature prevents overgrowth by microorganisms in a specimen and will keep most infectious agents alive for subsequent culture.
  - Specimens for anaerobic cultivation should be held at room temperature.
  - If specimen must be frozen, use −70°C, not −20°C.
- Fastidious bacteria, such as *Neisseria gonorrhoeae, N. meningitidis, Haemophilus influenzae,* and *Bordetella pertussis,* grow best when the specimen is inoculated onto media directly and incubated as soon as possible.
- Growth is enhanced when inoculated plates are put into a candle jar and sent to the laboratory for incubation. The candle jar provides an atmosphere of reduced oxygen, 5 to 7% CO_2, and increased humidity, all of which increase growth of these fastidious bacteria.

COLLECTION, PRESERVATION AND TRANSPORT OF RESPIRATORY TRACT SPECIMENS

AEROBIC TRANSPORT SYSTEMS[5-7]

- Amies and Stuart's transport media are designed to provide water, prevent acid accumulation, and may contain charcoal to absorb toxic substances.
- Hold at room temperature for respiratory cultures.
- Use a protected brush or catheter through a bronchoscope to avoid contamination by anaerobes.

ANAEROBIC COLLECTION AND SYSTEMS[8]

- Do not use swabs with holding medium for specimens that should be cultured anaerobically, e.g., from wounds or abscesses.
- Collect specimens by needle and syringe aspiration, eject air bubbles, and then inject into a special anaerobe collection tube that has a rubber diaphragm and contains oxygen-free CO_2. This tube serves to collect anaerobes and aerobes.
- An ordinary sterile tube that contains greater than 2 mL of pus, fluid, or tissue is satisfactory for anaerobic cultivation if it is not shaken.
- Sputum and swabs from mucosal or skin surfaces are not cultured anaerobically because they contain a large mixed anaerobic flora.[8]

TRANSPORTATION[5-7]

- Specimens must be transported and processed as rapidly as possible, generally within 2 hours of collection.
- Some agents need more rapid processing.

ANTIBACTERIAL AGENTS

- The "caine" local anesthetics, such as lidocaine (Xylocaine), are antibacterial.
- Some anticoagulants such as SPS (sodium polyanethol sulfonate), which is present in blood culture media, and heparin may have specific or mild antibacterial action against certain microorganisms.
  - They may interfere with culture when used.[9]
  - Use as necessary for culture collection, but understand the potential problems.
- Multiple-use vials of saline, lidocaine, heparin, etc., contain antibacterial preservatives (benzoate, methyl- or propylparabens) to prevent growth of bacteria in these vials, which are used more than once.
- Use IV bottle saline for specimen collection, when possible.[10]

TYPES OF SPECIMENS[7, 11-13]

- A swab is used to collect samples from mucosal or skin surfaces.
- Collections for culture or nucleic acid amplification of viruses, chlamydiae, or other intracellular parasites require moderate abrasion so that cells are obtained.
- For transport, put swabs in appropriate holding medium to prevent drying.
- For group A *Streptococcus* antigen detection, use the swab and tube from the antigen test kit.
- Use thorough swabbing in order to obtain sufficient antigen for analysis.

COLLECTION, PRESERVATION, AND TRANSPORT OF RESPIRATORY TRACT SPECIMENS

TYPES OF SPECIMENS

Anterior Nares

- Moisten a swab with saline or broth and swab the anterior 1 to 2 cm of the nose.
- *Staphylococcus aureus* and various *Staphylococcus* sp. (coagulase-negative), *Corynebacterium* spp., and *Streptococcus pyogenes* may colonize the nose.
- This specimen is used to find an infecting agent in the nose or to find carriage of a strain responsible for a nosocomial infection.

Pharyngeal Swab

- Rub vigorously and rotate a pair of moistened Dacron or rayon swabs on the posterior pharynx, tonsils, and inflamed regions.
- Using two swabs held together obtains maximum antigen or specimen for culture.
- In the presence of epiglottitis, airway obstruction can occur during pharyngeal swabbing. In these circumstances, a physician in a facility where intubation can be done in an emergency should be responsible for the pharyngeal swabbing.
- Vigorous swabbing obtains host cells, which may contain intracellular or adherent infecting agents.

Transtracheal Aspirate[12, 13]

- This procedure is rarely done because there are few physicians trained and experienced with the procedure.
- Bleeding, infection, subcutaneous emphysema, and vasovagal reactions have occurred when this procedure has been performed.
- The technique in experienced hands can detect bacterial infections in the lower airway, particularly due to anaerobic bacteria, and can bypass the upper airway commensals.

Nasopharynx

- Nasopharyngeal aspirate is obtained by introducing 1 to 2 mL of saline into the nose followed by rapid aspiration with a catheter into a respiratory culture trap or rubber bulb.
- This method provides the best recovery of respiratory syncytial virus, influenza viruses, or other respiratory viruses.
- A calcium alginate swab ("calgiswab") on flexible wire introduced deep into the nasopharynx through the nose and rotated 5 seconds is more acceptable to some patients.

Sinus Aspirate

- Swabbings or superficial aspirations usually are heavily contaminated by nasopharyngeal microorganisms.
- A needle and syringe aspiration obtained operatively by a physician from the affected sinus yields the best specimen.
- This specimen may be cultured for aerobic or anaerobic bacteria, fungi, and viruses.

Tracheal or Bronchial Aspirates

- This specimen is similar to expectorated sputum or the aspirate through the central channel of the fiberoptic bronchoscope.

Catheter, Drain, or Stoma Sites

- If exudate comes in contact with the air and the environment, it may become colonized by *Pseudomonas* and other gram-negative bacteria from the patient or the environment.
- Specimens collected through these sites will contain these bacteria and may be falsely interpreted as evidence of deep-seated infection, e.g., *Pseudomonas* pneumonia.

COLLECTION, PRESERVATION, AND TRANSPORT OF RESPIRATORY TRACT SPECIMENS

TYPES OF SPECIMENS

Expectorated Sputum[11, 13–16]

- Rinse the mouth and throat with water to remove free, colonizing microorganisms.
- Brushing of tongue and gingiva, sometimes recommended, releases squamous epithelial cells with attached colonizing bacteria that are not removed by one rinse.
- Instruct the patient that what is needed is thick material brought up from the chest by a deep cough.
- When possible have an experienced person supervise the collection and explain to the patient that you do not want material snuffed from the nasopharynx.
- The first morning coughs yield the most concentrated sputum.
- Obtain 3 to 5 mL of sputum for sample. However, do not emphasize volume because a deficiency often is made up with saliva.
- Do not use 24- or 48-hour collections because they permit growth of rapid-growing microorganisms which overgrow mycobacteria or other slow-growing organisms.
- Children are usually unable to expectorate sputum, so more invasive procedures may be necessary.
- Sputum specimens should be screened by microscopic examination of a gram-stained smear.
- Specimens with more than 10 squamous epithelial cells per 100×, or low-power field, should be rejected because this represents saliva, not sputum.
- Some laboratories give weight to presence of alveolar macrophages or polymorphonuclear leukocytes (PMN).
  - PMN may come from gingiva, nasopharynx, or sinuses as well as the lower respiratory tract.
  - Some laboratories culture specimens with up to 25 squamous epithelial cells per 100×, or low-power field.[16]
- Screening is ordinarily not done for mycobacterial specimens, which are decontaminated during processing.
- Screening of sputum for fungal culture has not been studied but it is known that *Candida* sp. and rapid-growing bacteria, which colonize the mouth, overgrow and inhibit culture of pulmonary pathogenic fungi such as *Cryptococcus* and *Histoplasma.*
- It is not appropriate to screen respiratory specimens used for diagnosis of *Pneumocystis carinii* pneumonia (PCP).
  - *Pneumocystis* is detected morphologically, not by culture.[19]
  - The usual PCP specimen does not contain purulent sputum.
- Specimens for *Legionella* culture should not be screened for rejection. There is not a relationship between host cell content of specimens and presence of *Legionella* sp.[17]
- A first-morning-sputum sample (obtained on 3 successive days) is recommended for diagnosis of mycobacterial or fungal respiratory infection.

COLLECTION, PRESERVATION, AND TRANSPORT OF RESPIRATORY TRACT SPECIMENS

TYPES OF SPECIMENS

Host Cells Seen in Gram-Stained Sputum Smears[18, 24]

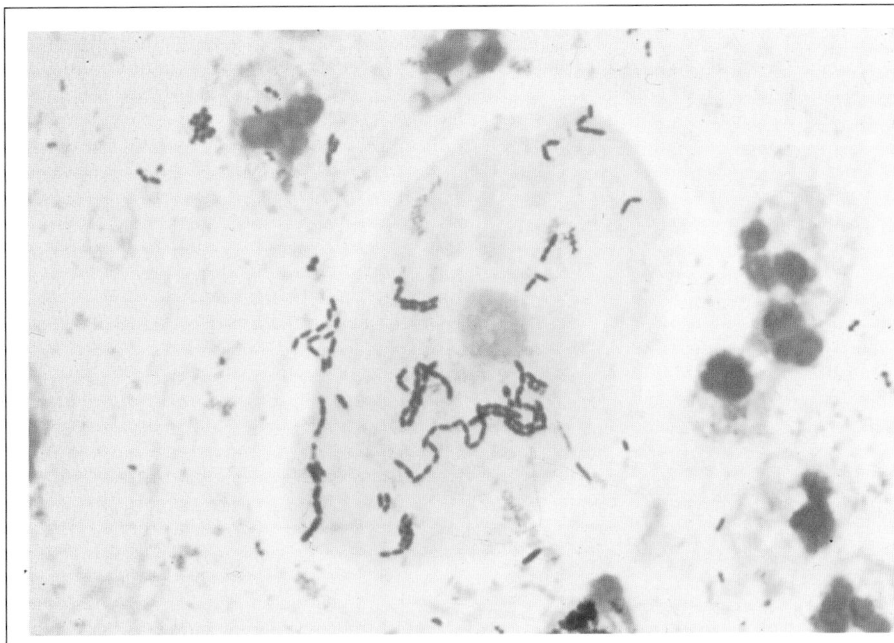

FIGURE 7–2

Gram-stained smear of a specimen submitted as expectorated sputum. This specimen was rejected because it contained more than 10 squamous epithelial cells per low-power microscopic field. Note the squamous epithelial cells with adherent commensal bacteria.

FIGURE 7–3

Multilobulated polymorphonuclear leukocytes 10 to 15 μm in diameter. In sputum smears these cells are often necrotic. Strands of safranin-staining, viscous nucleoprotein are pulled out across the field from nuclei.

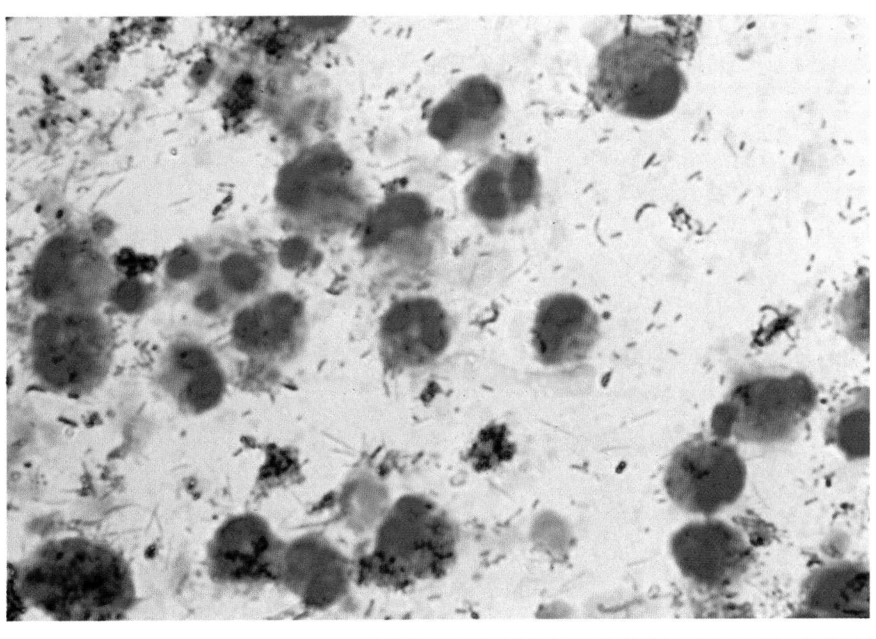

COLLECTION, PRESERVATION, AND TRANSPORT OF RESPIRATORY TRACT SPECIMENS

TYPES OF SPECIMENS

Host Cells Seen in Gram-Stained Sputum Smears

FIGURE 7-4

Macrophages, 10 to 40 μm in diameter, have an elliptical, sometimes eccentric, nucleus. They contain black dust particles, golden hemosiderin, or other particulates.

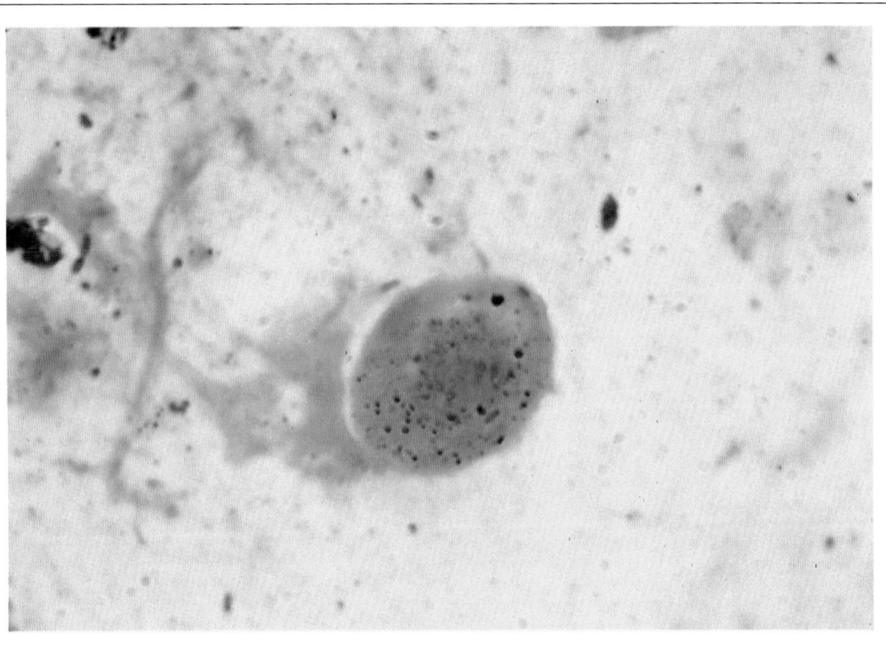

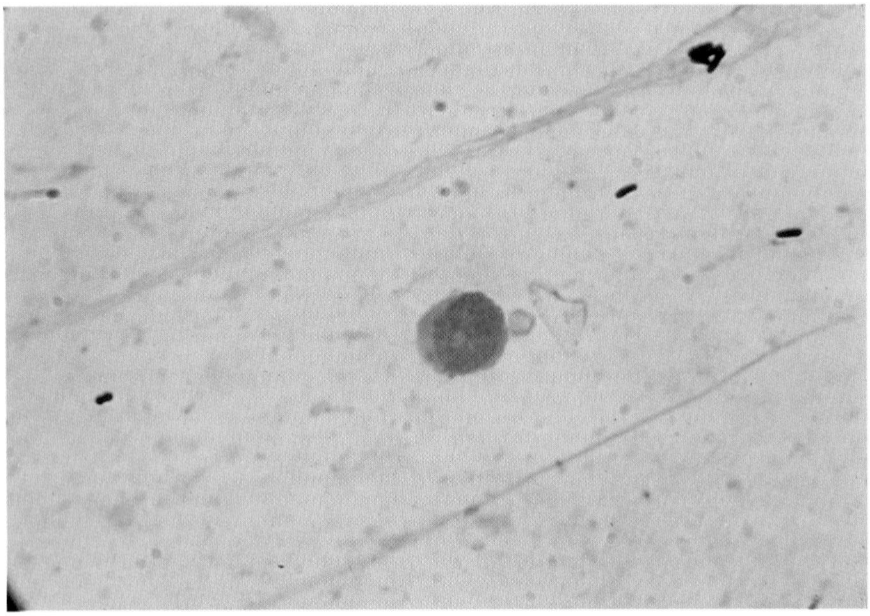

FIGURE 7-5

Lymphocytes, 7 to 10 μm in diameter, are usually present in sputum in small numbers.

COLLECTION, PRESERVATION, AND TRANSPORT OF RESPIRATORY TRACT SPECIMENS

TYPES OF SPECIMENS

Host Cells Seen in Gram-Stained Sputum Smears

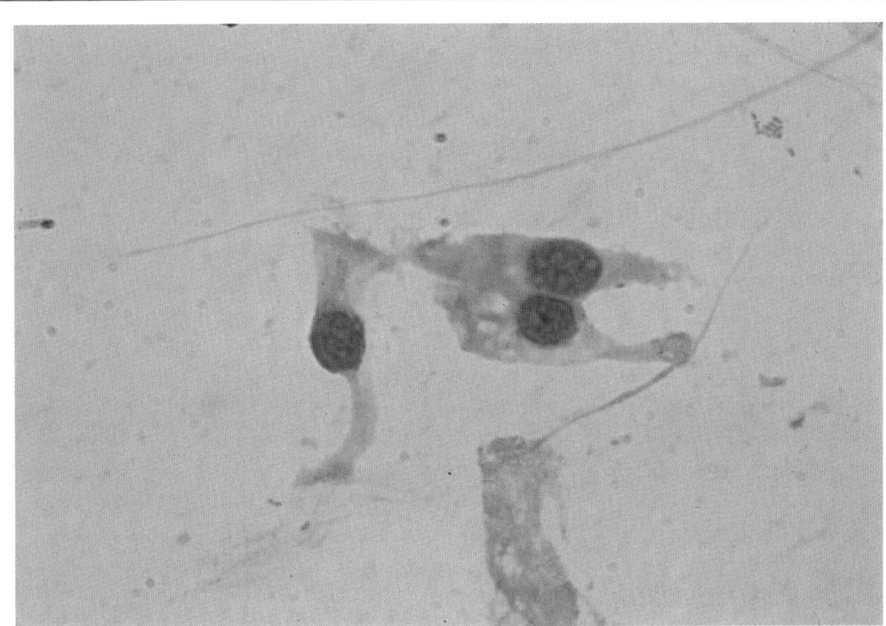

FIGURE 7–6

Exfoliated columnar bronchial epithelial cells with intact cilia appear in sputum cells post-bronchoscopy.

FIGURE 7–7

Curschmann's spirals contain mucinous material spirally twisted around a central thread. They are probably casts of smaller bronchial airways.

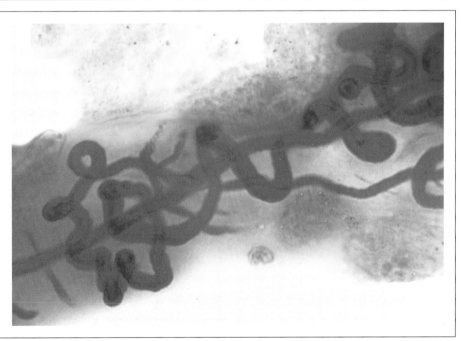

COLLECTION, PRESERVATION, AND TRANSPORT OF RESPIRATORY TRACT SPECIMENS

TYPES OF SPECIMENS

Induced Sputum[19, 20]

- Patients who do not expectorate sputum or who do not have diseases characterized by purulent sputum may produce a diagnostically useful specimen after inhalation of a 3% to 5% saline aerosol generated with an ultrasonic nebulizer.
  - Room temperature saline aerosol is produced at 3 to 7 mL/minute for a period of 20 minutes.
  - 5% saline produces more irritation and a more violent cough response. 10% saline may not be tolerated by many patients.
  - Sputum induction yields a specimen containing many squamous epithelial cells.
- Sputum induction is most useful for specimens that will be detected morphologically, such as *Pneumocystis,* or decontaminated prior to culture, such as *Mycobacterium.*
- The diagnosis of *Pneumocystis carinii* pneumonia (PCP) by means of induced sputum examination was studied in a population of HIV-1 infected patients (WK. Hadley, unpublished observations, 1998), and the following conclusions were drawn:
  - Patients who had sufficient respiratory reserve to cooperate with sputum induction were studied.
  - A sensitivity of 74% to 77% was obtained using induced sputum as compared to the composite final diagnosis made by induced sputum, bronchoalveolar lavage, and response to treatment.
  - Mycobacteria, usually *M. avium* complex, were found in 6% of the induced sputum specimens.
  - The induced sputum specimens were not useful for diagnosis of *Cryptococcus* or *Histoplasma* infection because of the overgrowth of culture medium by *Candida* sp., present in abundance in the induced sputum specimen.
  - Sputum induction provides an outpatient diagnostic method that avoids the discomfort and expense of bronchoscopy.

Transthoracic Needle Aspiration[12, 13]

- Transthoracic needle aspiration (TTNA) may be performed with a thin-walled needle (20 to 25 gauge) inserted during suspended respiration and slowly withdrawn during negative pressure.
- TTNA is most useful for diagnosis of small nodules, mediastinal masses, or airspace consolidation.
- TTNA is used for adults who are immunocompromised and in whom other procedures are not feasible.

Thoracentesis

- Empyema, an accumulation of pus in the pleural space, is much less common in the era of antibiotic therapy and is defined as a pleural effusion with greater than 25,000 leukocytes/mL.
- The predominant cell in the effusion is the polymorphonuclear leukocyte.
- The pleural fluid pH is usually less than 7.1.
- Microorganisms may be present in small numbers in the pleural fluid of patients with mycobacterial or fungal disease, and the cellular response may be principally mononuclear.
- As much fluid as possible should be collected and centrifuged at $3000 \times g$ in a refrigerated centrifuge.
- The sediment should be smeared, stained, and cultured.
- Most laboratories provide sterile containers for 50 to 250 mL of fluid to be centrifuged.

COLLECTION, PRESERVATION, AND TRANSPORT OF RESPIRATORY TRACT SPECIMENS

TYPES OF SPECIMENS

Bronchoscopy[12, 13, 19, 20, 97] (See Chapter 6, Bronchoscopy)

- The fiberoptic bronchoscope carries upper airway commensal and colonizing microorganisms when it is inserted into a bronchus.
- Unless a protected catheter or brush is used in the bronchoscope, the inner channel yields a specimen no better than expectorated sputum.
- The bronchoscope is especially effective at recovering microorganisms, which do not colonize the upper airway, but infect the lower airways, i.e., *M. tuberculosis, Legionella, Pneumocystis carinii,* other pathogenic fungi, and certain viruses.
- Bronchoalveolar lavage (BAL) done with successive 20-mL saline washes and aspirations can yield a 50-mL to 100-mL specimen of washings from distal airspaces.
- Packed aggregates of *Pneumocystis* cysts and trophic forms are washed out as plugs, which can be identified easily in concentrated, stained smears in 95% of *Pneumocystis* infections in AIDS patients.
- Bronchial brushings are useful for obtaining respiratory cells for detection of intracellular organisms such as *Chlamydia* and viruses but are not as efficient for recovery of *Pneumocystis* as the BAL.[12, 13, 19, 20]

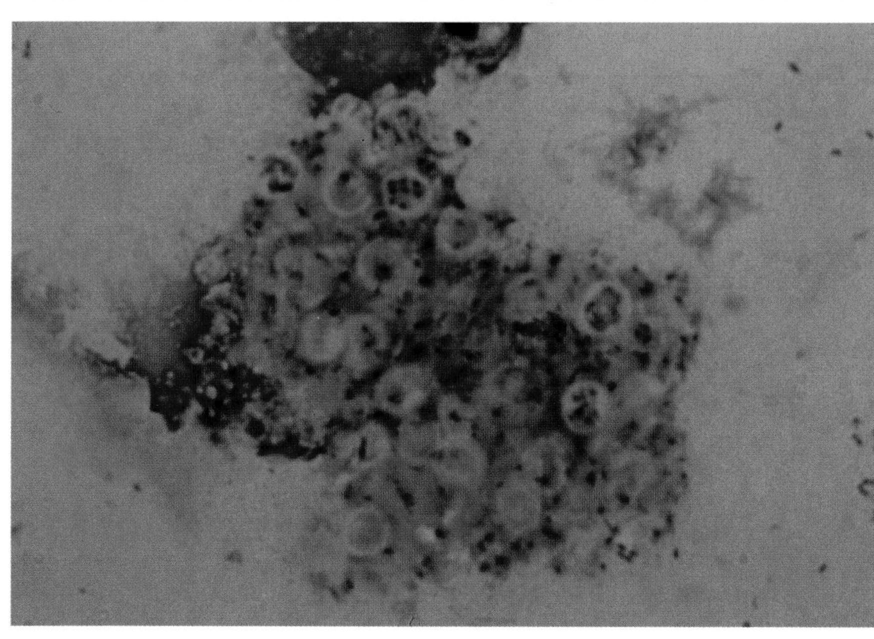

FIGURE 7–8

Packed aggregate of *Pneumocystis carinii* cysts and trophic forms stained by Diff-Quik® (Dade, Behring Inc.). Specimen has been obtained from bronchoalveolar lavage.

COLLECTION, PRESERVATION, AND TRANSPORT OF RESPIRATORY TRACT SPECIMENS

TYPES OF SPECIMENS

Tissue Biopsy[12, 13, 23]

- Tissue biopsies provide useful specimens for microbiologic diagnosis.
- Unfortunately tissue samples are often ruined because of the confusion between needs for histopathology and the microbiology laboratory.
- The microbiology laboratory should be informed when a biopsy will be obtained so that a plan can be developed for handling and processing the specimen.
- Handle the biopsy specimen aseptically.
- Collect the biopsy specimen on sterile Telfa that has been barely moistened with preservative-free saline, fold to prevent drying, and transport in a sterile container to the microbiology laboratory as rapidly as possible.
- Avoid drying, contact with fixatives (for pathologic examination), soaking in saline, and exposure to preservatives that are present in some saline solutions.
- The biopsy tissue may be examined by wet mount, touch-preparations (see below), stained by special stains, and will be ground in a glass tissue grinder for culture as appropriate.

METHODS FOR DIAGNOSIS

GENERAL

- Diagnosis of infections in the laboratory has depended upon direct observation of the infectious agent and culture in vitro or in cell culture or animal infection. Microbiology laboratories have the resources to accommodate these time-consuming procedures when necessary.
- When these procedures fail, serologic diagnostic methods have been adapted, as in detection of *Treponema pallidum* infection (syphilis). Serologic diagnostic tests are characterized as follows:
  - Antibody response is slow to develop and variable in result, depending upon the immune status of the patient.
  - Antigen detection and nucleic acid probe methods as well as nucleic acid amplification methods have high initial reagent and equipment cost.
  - Despite high initial costs, when these new diagnostic tests have been adapted to the laboratory, significant savings in microbiologic diagnostic time can be appreciated.
  - Savings also occur in more rapid diagnosis and therapy, reduced costs for hospitalization, and protection of family or community members against infection by communicable agents, e.g., tuberculosis.
  - These changes in diagnostic testing are useful but will require changes in funding for diagnostic testing and medical care.

DIRECT EXAMINATION

- Simple methods can give a rapid microbiologic diagnosis when supported by clinical information.
- The eukaryotic microorganisms such as the fungi and parasites have sufficient complexity so that a specific diagnosis can be made in a few moments of direct examination of a wet mount or a stained touch-preparation or smear.

METHODS FOR DIAGNOSIS

DIRECT EXAMINATION

Wet Mount[11, 19, 22, 24]

- A cover-slipped drop of a fluid or mucolysed specimen can be examined easily with a microscope.
- Nomarski or phase optics increase the contrast between the microorganism and the surrounding fluid.
- Alternately closing down the iris diaphragm of a bright-field condenser will increase contrast.
- The dark-field condenser is useful for observing motile microorganisms. A dark-field condenser designed for use with a 50× magnification objective lens avoids the cumbersome use of oil between the objective lens, cover-slipped slide, and condenser.
- These microscope optics are also useful for examining preparations from cultures.[20]
- A drop of saline serves to clear a field of dense purulent exudate so that a microorganism can be seen.
- Mucolysis with *N*-acetyl-L-cysteine or dithiothreitol permits centrifugation of viscous specimens.[19]
    - Mucolysed expectorated or induced sputum, sediment from centrifuged bronchoalveolar lavage, or purulent exudate can be useful for examination.
- Some observers prefer to use a 10% KOH wet mount.
    - Such preparations lyse the host leukocytes and other cellular material, but leave intact the dense walls that enclose fungi and certain stages of parasites.
    - The KOH preparation may obscure the relationship between microorganism and host leukocytes.
    - Stages of a parasite that lack a wall will be lysed.

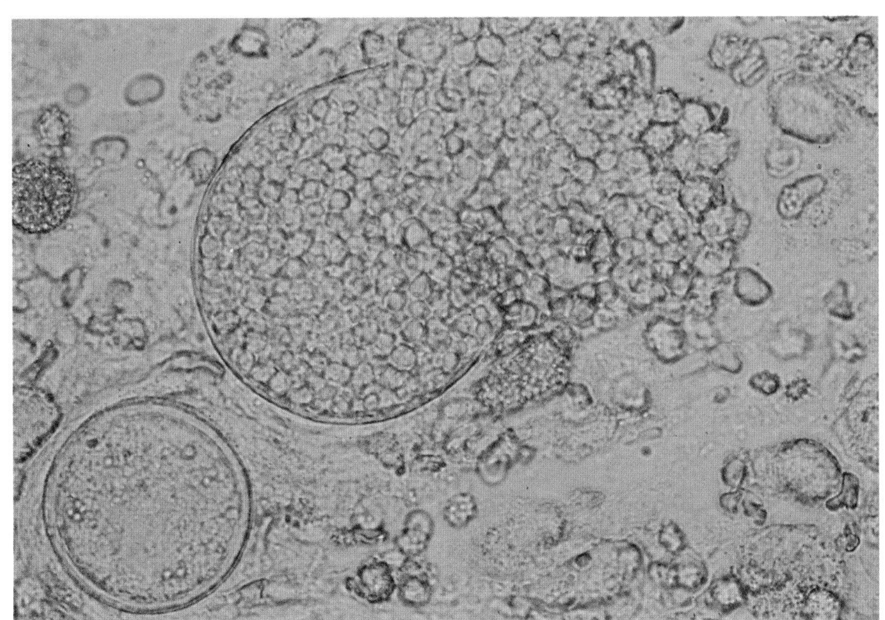

FIGURE 7–9

A wet mount preparation of centrifuged bronchoalveolar lavage sediment demonstrates a large ruptured *Coccidioides immitis* spherule spilling endospores. Smaller intact spherules are also present. This patient has disseminated disease. Culture to produce enough mycelial growth for cell lysis and performance of DNA probe test (Gen-Probe) would take 4 to 5 days.[101]

METHODS FOR DIAGNOSIS

DIRECT EXAMINATION

Wet Mount

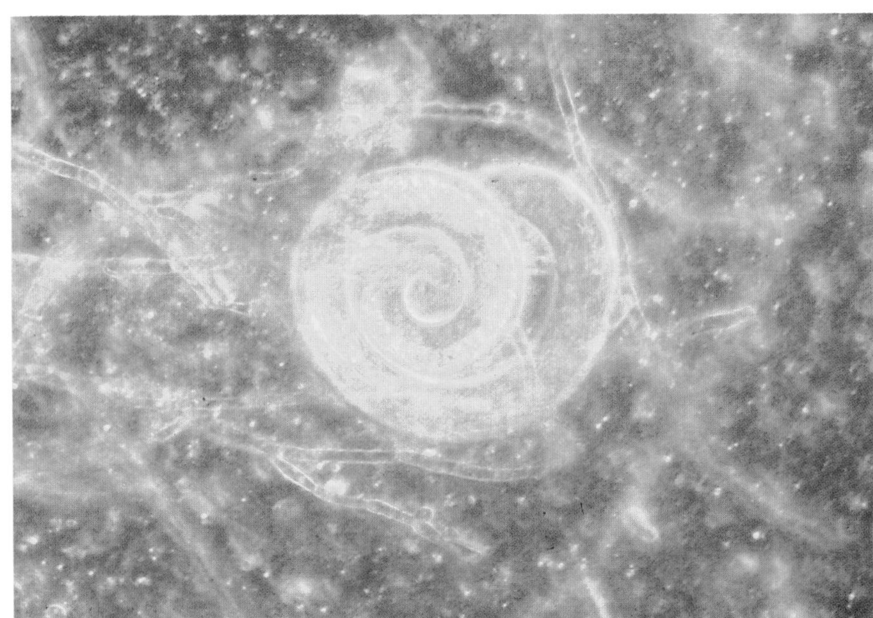

FIGURE 7–10

A wet mount of tracheal aspirate from a patient with *Strongyloides stercoralis* hyperinfection syndrome as a consequence of an overdose of corticosteroid. A *S. stercoralis* larva surrounded by *Candida albicans* pseudohyphae is visible by phase contrast microscopy with green filter.[111–115]

Touch-Preparations and Thin Smears[23, 24]

- A touch-preparation or thin smear provides tissue, exudate cells, and microorganisms spread out in a single-cell thickness so that they can be easily stained and examined.
- In order to prevent contamination of a biopsy sample, which will also be used for culture, cleaned slides are retained in a Coplin jar containing absolute methanol.
  - The slides are removed, air-dried, and used for the touch-preparation.
  - The biopsy material is handled aseptically.
- Biopsy specimens must not be allowed to dry and must be protected from tissue fixatives and from soaking in saline.
  - Saline removes tissue adhesins, which cause cell attachment to the slides.
  - The biopsy can be prevented from drying by placing it on Telfa that has been barely moistened with preservative-free saline.
  - The folded Telfa should be transported to the laboratory in a sterile cup.
  - Fresh-cut surfaces should be blotted to remove excess blood and pressed firmly several times to each slide.
- While moist, the slides with touch-preparations are fixed in absolute methanol for at least 5 minutes, then air-dried and stained.
- Giemsa, immunofluorescent stains, Gram, acid-fast, calcofluor white, silver, and other stains can be performed on these touch-preparations.

METHODS FOR DIAGNOSIS

DIRECT EXAMINATION

Touch-Preparations and Thin Smears

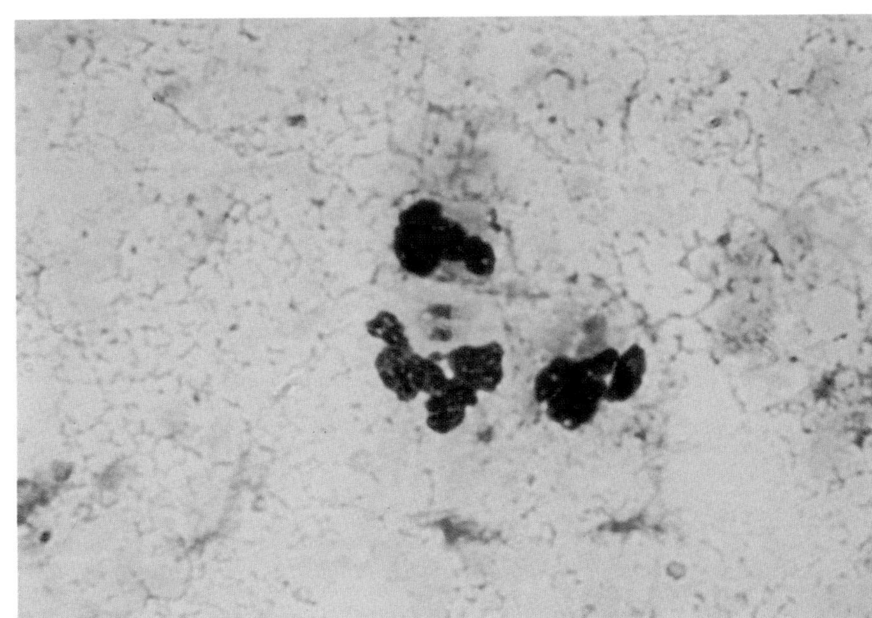

FIGURE 7–11

A touch-preparation of a transbronchial biopsy shows two *Toxoplasma gondii* tachyzoites surrounded by polymorphonuclear leukocytes. This preparation was stained with a rapid (3-minute) stain related to the Giemsa stain.[130, 131]

FIGURE 7–12

A touch-preparation of a transbronchial biopsy shows a *Pneumocystis carinii* cyst with intracystic bodies attached to a host cell. The preparation is stained by buffered Giemsa.[97]

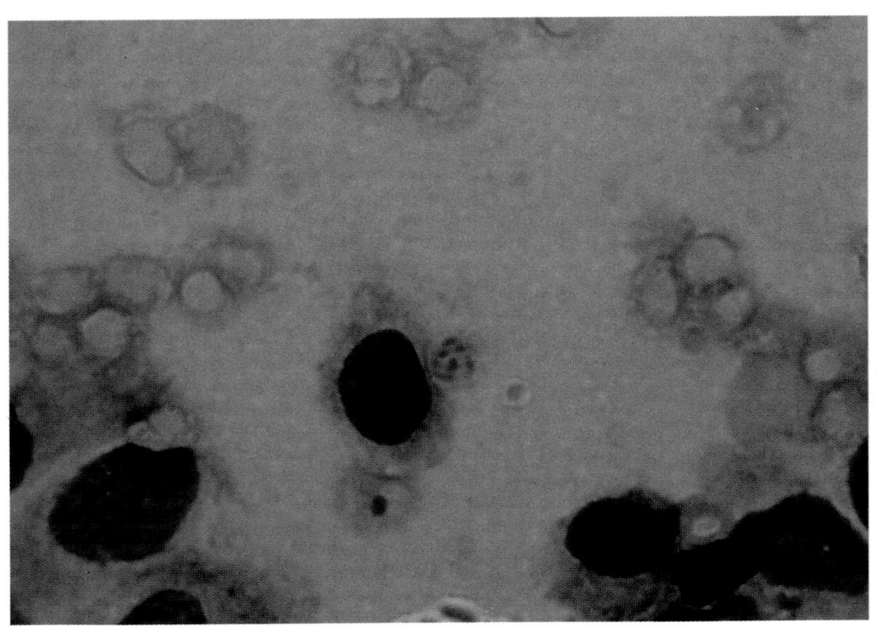

METHODS FOR DIAGNOSIS

DIRECT EXAMINATION

Touch-Preparations and Thin Smears

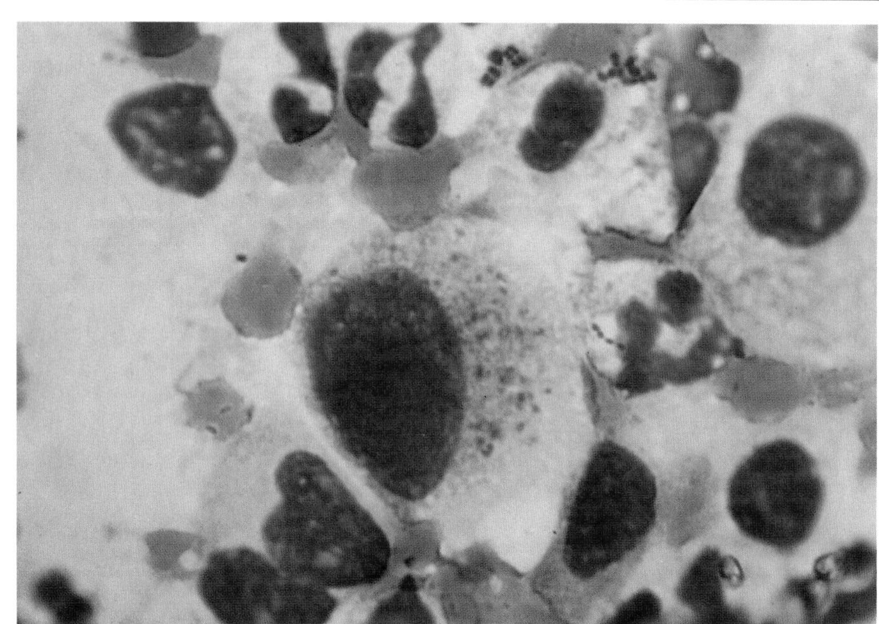

FIGURE 7–13

This touch-preparation was prepared from a transbronchial biopsy. It contains an enlarged macrophage with intranuclear and fine cytoplasmic inclusions of cytomegalovirus. The preparation was stained by buffered Giemsa.[138, 139, 141, 142]

METHODS FOR DIAGNOSIS

DIRECT EXAMINATION

Stains

- The Gram stain[24] distinguishes bacteria by their cell wall.
- Gram-positive bacteria have a thick interlinked peptidoglycan layer.
- Gram-negative bacteria have a thin peptidoglycan layer with an outer trilaminar membrane.
- The peptidoglycan layer is responsible for the rigidity and the shape of bacteria.
- Certain processes, which alter the peptidoglycan layer, may change the Gram reaction or the shape of a bacterium.
- The Gram reaction may be defective in old cultures, after the action of lysozyme produced by leukocytes and other host cells, and after the action of beta-lactam antibiotics (the penicillins and cephalosporins), which block the cross-linking of peptidoglycan chains.
- Defective shaped and gram-negative or granular *Streptococcus pneumoniae* are seen after the action of penicillin.
- Gram-negative bacteria, after the action of certain beta-lactam antibiotics, may appear swollen, vacuolated, and filamentous with no similarity in appearance to untreated bacteria.

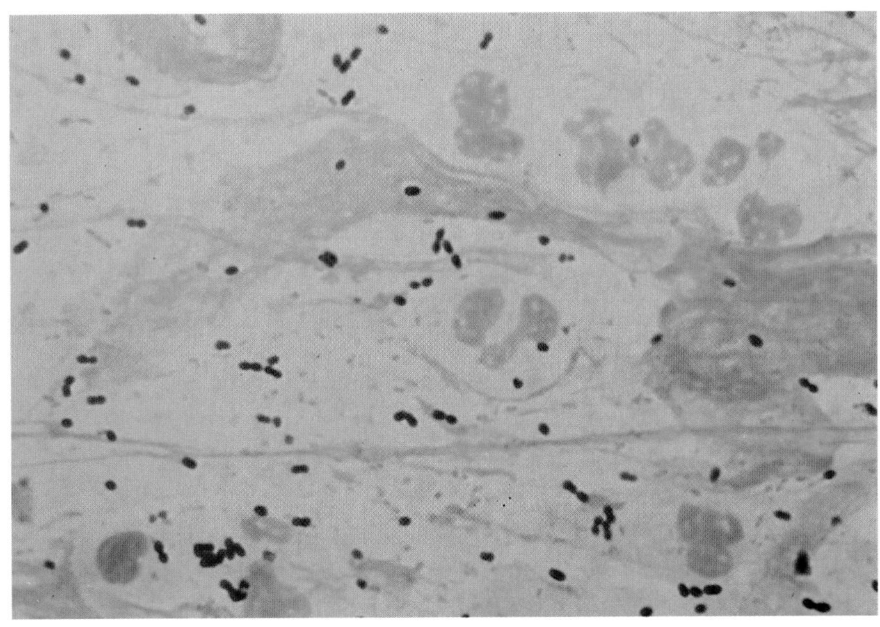

FIGURE 7-14

Streptococcus pneumoniae, Gram stain.[42] Gram-positive (purple) diplococci are present among polymorphonuclear leukocytes in this smear.

METHODS FOR DIAGNOSIS

DIRECT EXAMINATION

Stains

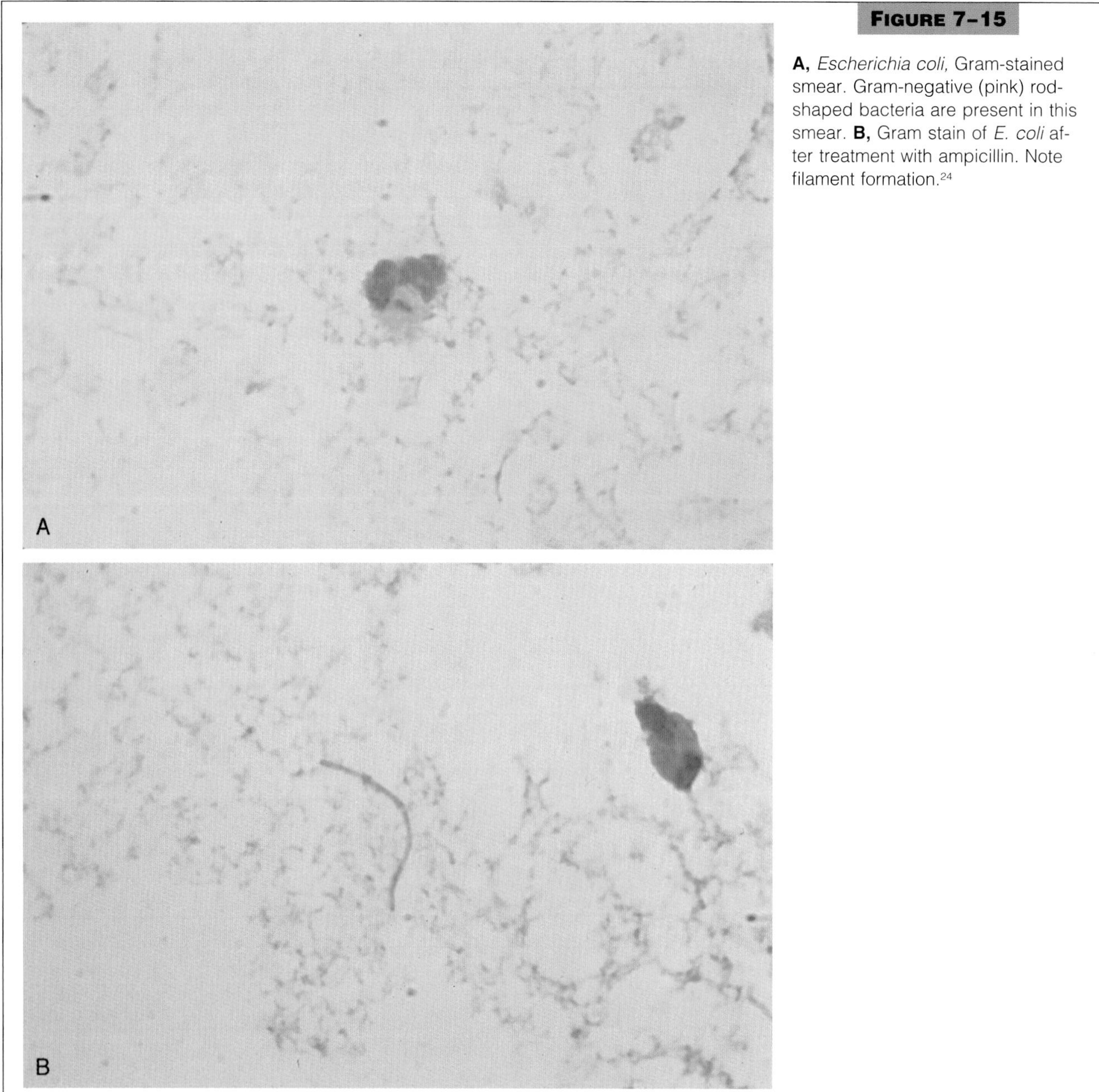

FIGURE 7–15

A, *Escherichia coli,* Gram-stained smear. Gram-negative (pink) rod-shaped bacteria are present in this smear. **B,** Gram stain of *E. coli* after treatment with ampicillin. Note filament formation.[24]

METHODS FOR DIAGNOSIS

DIRECT EXAMINATION

Stains

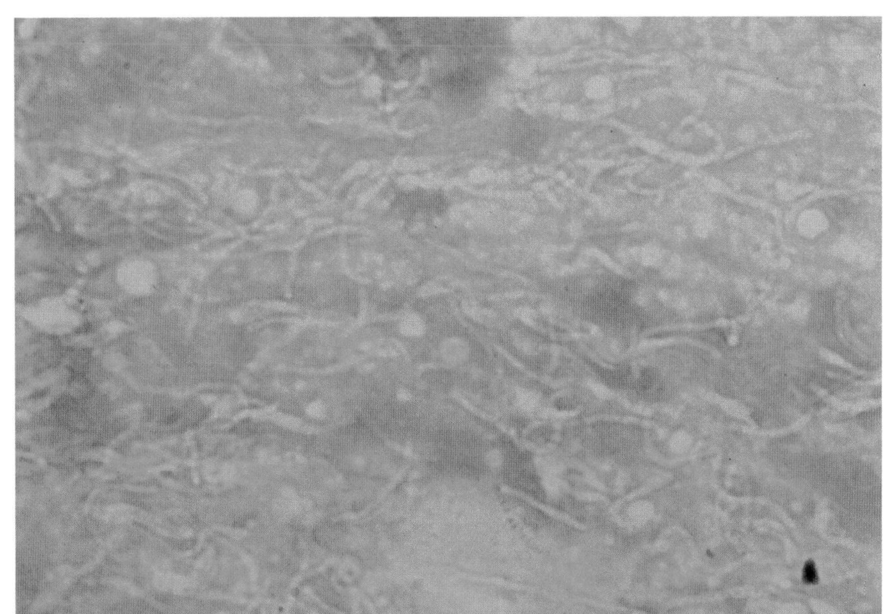

FIGURE 7-16

Gram-stained smear of *Mycobacterium kansasii* with unstained "ghost" cells and a granular gram-positive stain. Acid-fast bacteria such as the mycobacteria have a complex wall with long-chain fatty acids, the mycolic acids, outside the peptidoglycan layer that inhibits penetration by the Gram stain.[91]

FIGURE 7-17

Kinyon acid-fast stain[24, 87] of *M. tuberculosis*. In the Ziehl-Neelsen acid-fast stain use of phenol and heating to steaming enhances the entry of basic fuchsin into the acid-fast bacterium. Once stained, the dye is not easily removed by acid or alcohol. The Kinyon acid-fast stain does not require heating and uses a higher concentration of phenol and saturated basic fuchsin to increase penetration of the dye. The Ziehl-Neelsen stain is more laborious than the Kinyon stain.

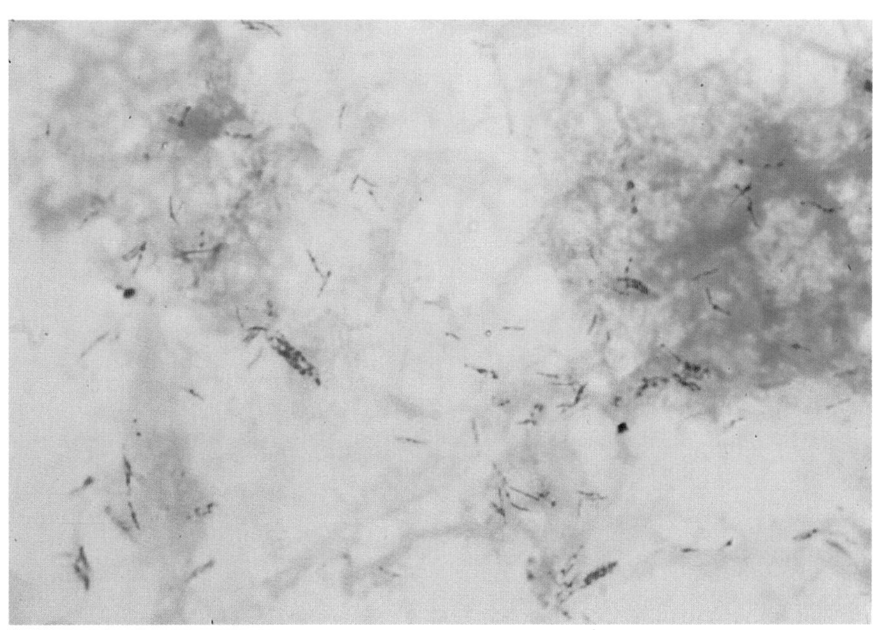

METHODS FOR DIAGNOSIS

DIRECT EXAMINATION

Stains

FIGURE 7–18

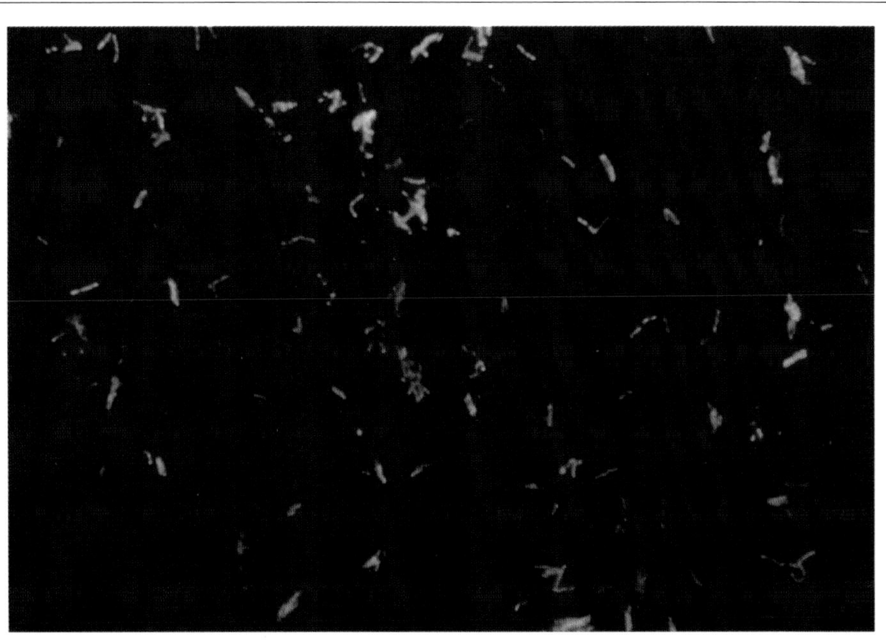

Auramine-orhodamine acid-fast stain of *M. tuberculosis.* Auramine-o and rhodamine are fluorochromes, which fluoresce upon ultraviolet radiation. Auramine-o binds to mycolic acid and resists acid alcohol destaining. Rhodamine, which fluoresces a dark red, covers autofluorescence often present in exudate smears. The acid-fast bacteria fluoresce orange-yellow against a black background when a potassium permanganate counterstain is used. Because of the contrast, preparations can be screened rapidly at magnifications of 125 to 400× using an epifluorescent microscope. Most laboratories that perform a large volume of acid-fast stains use this stain.

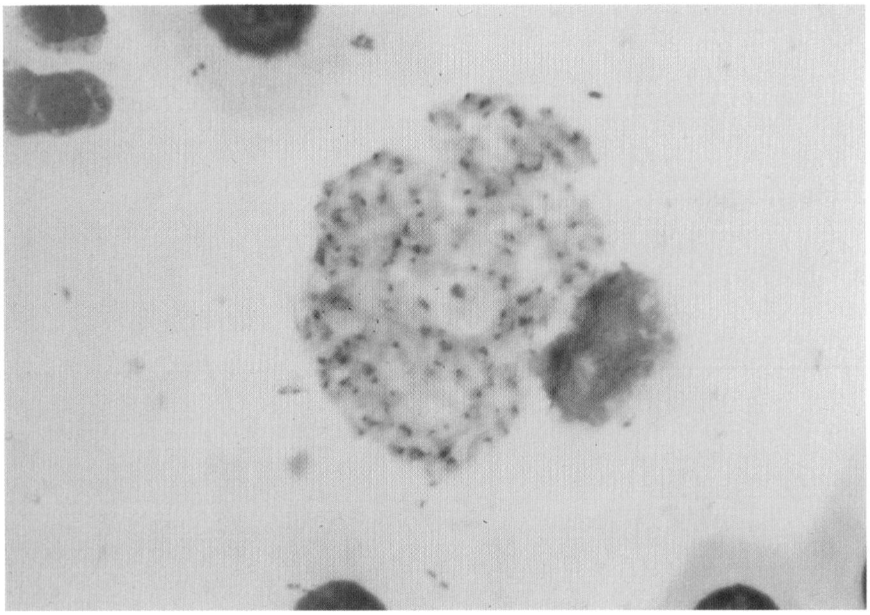

FIGURE 7–19

Giemsa-stained *Pneumocystis.*[22] The Giemsa stain is a Romanowski type stain[24, 97] in which the stain is a salt of a basic and acidic dye, e.g., azure II eosinate. Changing the pH of the buffer solution in which the dye is dissolved will emphasize the acidic or basic elements. Moist smears or touch-preparations are fixed with absolute methanol or acetone, air-dried, and stained.

METHODS FOR DIAGNOSIS

DIRECT EXAMINATION

Stains

- Wright stain combines methanol fixation and staining into one less time-consuming step.
- Nucleoprotein is stained purple. Cytoplasm is often blue.
- Acridine orange intercalates into DNA, producing orange fluorescence in bacterial and fungal cells and green fluorescence in mammalian DNA upon ultraviolet irradiation.
- Giemsa and acridine orange, a fluorescent stain, stain nucleoprotein structures in host inflammatory cells, bacteria, fungi, protozoa, and other organisms.
- This stain serves as an alternative to Gram stain for bacteria that are losing their cell walls or that stain faintly gram-negative and is preferred for certain fungi and protozoa.
- The periodic acid–Schiff (PAS) and Gomori methenamine silver (GMS) stains[24, 97, 101] use a strong acid to hydrolyze the polysaccharide coat of fungi, including *Pneumocystis.* The reducing sugars, which result, react to form the red color of the Schiff reagent and the black color of reduced silver.

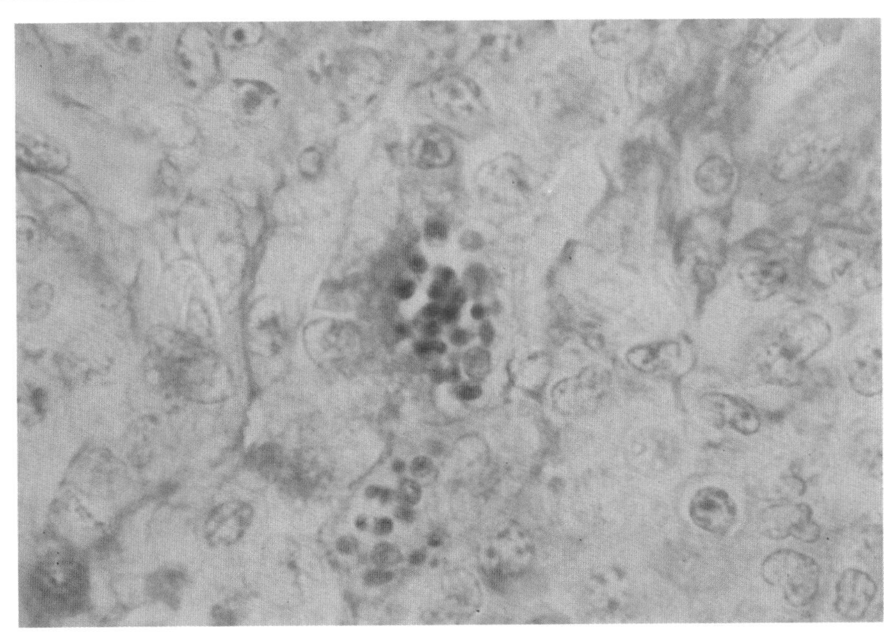

FIGURE 7–20

Periodic acid–Schiff stained *Histoplasma* yeasts appear red.

METHODS FOR DIAGNOSIS

DIRECT EXAMINATION

FIGURE 7-21

Gomori methenamine silver stained *Histoplasma* yeasts are black and 2.0 to 3.0 μm in diameter.

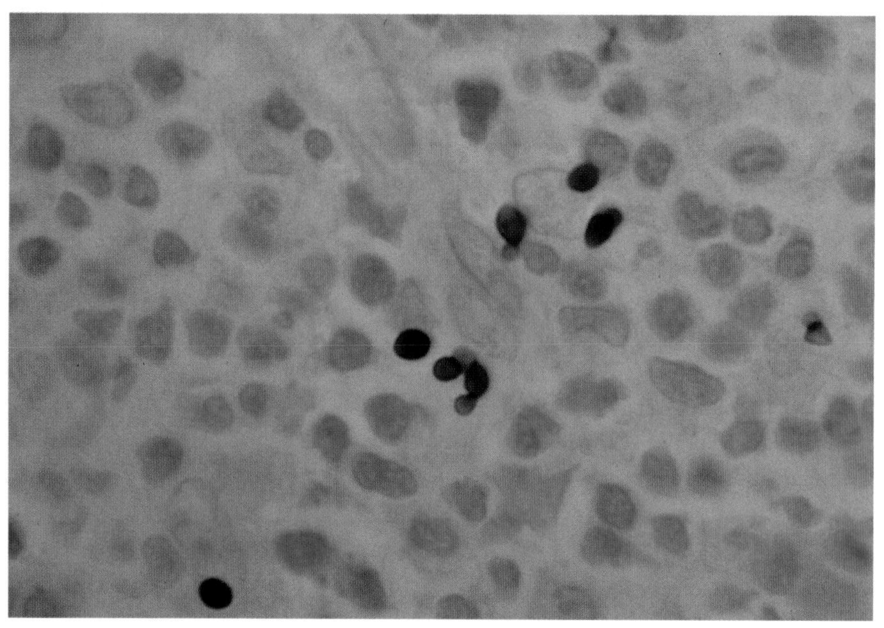

Culture[25–29]

- Media for microbial growth provide water, a balanced salt mixture, carbon and nitrogen sources, and an energy source.
- Dehydrated digested crude proteins, e.g., casein and soy (peptones), and infusions or extracts of animal tissue are used as inexpensive sources of nutrients.
- Certain organisms require specific growth factors; for example, *H. influenzae* requires factor X (hemin) and factor V (NAD).
- Media are either broth (liquid) or agar (solid) based:
- Broth media accommodate large volumes of inoculum, support growth of small numbers of some bacteria and other infectious agents, and can be easily diluted for inoculum.
- Agar media achieve separation of colony forming units (CFU) and permit estimation of microorganisms in the initial inoculum by counting CFU/volume inoculum.
- Media are sterilized by autoclaving at 121°C (15 lb pressure) for 15 to 30 minutes depending upon volume.
- Agar liquefies at 84°C and does not solidify until 38 to 40°C.

METHODS FOR DIAGNOSIS

DIRECT EXAMINATION

Culture Media

- *Transport media* provide water, balanced salt, and pH buffering, but lack an energy source. Microorganisms are kept alive but do not overgrow each other in this mixture.
- Different media are used in microbiology laboratories to grow and distinguish different microorganisms:
  - *General purpose media* provide the materials needed to grow and hold a wide variety of microorganisms.
- *Differential media* contain indicators, which distinguish different microorganisms; for example, chromogenic substrates that indicate presence of a specific enzyme, pH, or reduction/oxidation indicators.
- *Selective media* permit the growth of some bacteria and inhibit the growth of others.

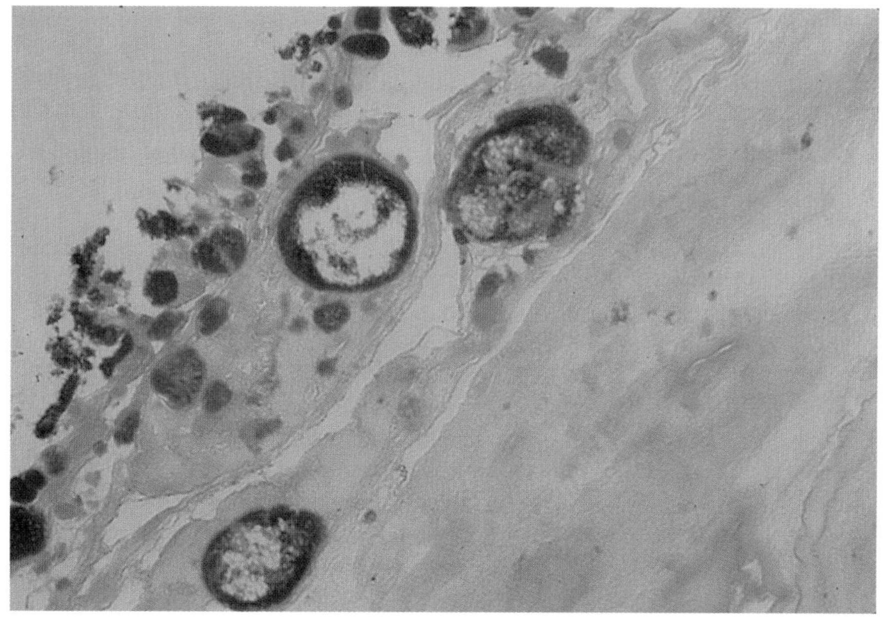

FIGURE 7-22

Diphtheritic pseudomembrane from pharynx. *Corynebacterium diphtheriae* (gram-positive stain) are present in the membrane.

FIGURE 7-23

Culture from base of pseudomembrane. Black colonies of *Corynebacterium diphtheriae* grow on cystine-tellurite agar. Tellurite is reduced to black precipitate of tellurium metal in the colony.

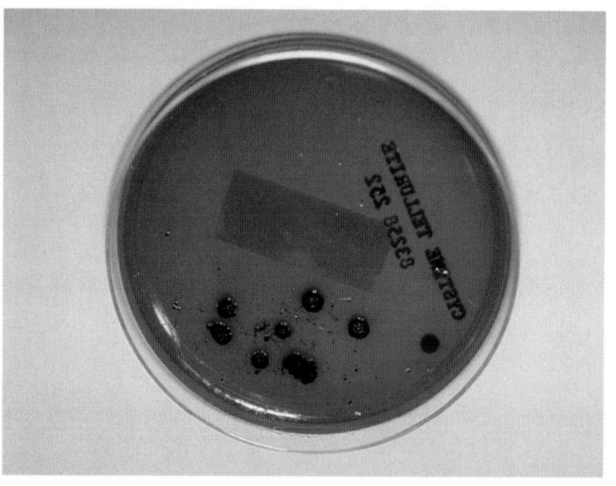

METHODS FOR DIAGNOSIS

DIRECT EXAMINATION

Culture Environments

- An atmosphere with 5 to 7% CO_2 and high humidity is beneficial for *primary growth* of many aerobic and facultative bacteria.
- *Anaerobic conditions* are provided by flushing with appropriate nitrogen and carbon dioxide mixtures or use of a hydrogen-generating compound and palladium catalyst to enhance water formation from O_2 and H_2 and monitored with a methylene blue indicator.
- Humidity and CO_2 must be provided.
- Although culture systems are often slow, the traditional media first devised to separate and screen for Enterobacteriaceae by pH indicator color changes are inexpensive to purchase as compared to molecular biologic methods.
  - The cost of the technologist's time spent working with slow culture systems must be considered.
  - The expense of rapid detection and identification of an infectious agent must be weighed against the cost of a delayed diagnosis for the patient and subsequent costs of hospitalization.

Cell Culture[30–32, 138, 141, 142]

- Obligate intracellular bacteria (e.g., *Chlamydia, Rickettsia, Coxiella,* and *Ehrlichia*) are usually isolated in appropriate cell cultures, the yolk sac of the embryonated hen's egg, and certain animals.
- Culture of these bacteria is detected with species- or genus-specific antibodies, immunofluorescent stains, and Giemsa staining of inclusions or elementary bodies.
- Viral isolation in cell culture is still the most frequently used method of diagnosis.
  - Cell culture detects a wide range of viruses, even though several cell lines and temperatures of incubation are necessary to rapidly recover most respiratory viruses.
  - Various virus detection systems such as cytopathogenic effect (CPE), hemadsorption, and antigen detection may be used to detect a virus.
  - This complex of procedures is time-consuming and very expensive.
  - Antigen detection systems for respiratory syncytial virus, influenzavirus, and parainfluenza viruses require as little as 2 to 3 hours and are less expensive than cell culture.
  - Reverse transcriptase (RT) and polymerase chain reaction (PCR) methods are available for detection of some of the respiratory viruses, which are mostly RNA viruses; these tests remain expensive and laborious.

METHODS FOR DIAGNOSIS

DIRECT EXAMINATION

Serologic Tests[33–35]

- Culture and antibody detection tests (serologic tests) have been the standard diagnostic methods for infectious agents.
- In general, immunoglobulin M (IgM) antibodies appear early in serum during infection, and IgG antibodies appear later, reaching a peak level in serum 4 to 6 weeks after infection.
  - The IgG antibodies may persist for life; the IgM antibody is generally transient.
  - If IgM antibody is present, this suggests recent infection.
  - However, the usefulness of IgM antibody for diagnosis is quite variable and must be evaluated for each infectious agent.
- In immunodeficiency the usefulness of immunoglobulin tests must be determined for each process.
  - The standard antibody tests require an acute phase serum, 5 to 7 days after onset of disease, and a convalescent serum 21 to 28 days after onset of disease.
  - A fourfold rise in IgG titer is considered evidence of recent or current infection.
  - Titration results are frequently markedly different from laboratory to laboratory.
- Diagnostic serologic tests, which are firmly based on clinical studies, should be used.
- The more commonly studied tests include complement fixation (CF), hemagglutination inhibition (HI), indirect immunofluorescence (IF), enzyme immunoassay (EIA), virus neutralization, Immunoblot or Western Blot (IB or WB).
- Tests for immune status or response to immunization are also useful.
- Single test solid phase immunoassay modules for detection of antigen are FDA-approved for respiratory syncytial virus and influenzavirus A and B.
  - These tests, which use monoclonal antibody, are as sensitive and specific as the immunofluorescence methods, detect a soluble viral antigen, and do not require host cells or infective virus.
  - Collection techniques are less stringent; performance and reading of the test requires less training and skill than the immunofluorescence tests.

Evaluation of Diagnostic Tests

- The performance of a particular test can be evaluated by determination of its sensitivity, specificity, and predictive values.
- The predictive value is the probability that the test will correctly indicate the presence or absence of a particular disease.
- Predictive values are affected by the prevalence of the disease process in the population studied (TABLE 7–2).

TABLE 7–2

Predictive Values

$$\%\ \text{Sensitivity} = \frac{\text{True positives}}{\text{True positives} + \text{false positives}} \times 100$$

$$\%\ \text{Specificity} = \frac{\text{True negatives}}{\text{False positives} + \text{true negatives}} \times 100$$

$$\%\ \text{Positive predictive value} = \frac{\text{True positives}}{\text{True positives} + \text{false positives}} \times 100$$

$$\%\ \text{Negative predictive value} = \frac{\text{True negatives}}{\text{True negatives} + \text{false negatives}} \times 100$$

METHODS FOR DIAGNOSIS

MOLECULAR DIAGNOSTICS[37]

- Systems for detection and identification of microorganisms based on gene structure or nucleic acid molecule interaction are being adopted.
- Knowledge of the chemistry of nucleic acid interaction upon hybridization led to the nucleic acid probe for identification.
- Hybridization may be limited when small amounts of nucleic acid are available for analysis.
- Nucleic acid amplification methods, such as the polymerase chain reaction (PCR), provide nucleic acid from agents that cannot be cultured or provide greater quantities from fastidious organisms.
- With the development of instruments such as thermal cyclers for PCR and sequencers for determining nucleic acid structure, more sensitive but more expensive diagnostic systems are available.
- Well-designed clinical studies must be done with the new test systems to demonstrate their clinical relevance, ease and time of performance, specificity, and sensitivity.

Nucleic Acid Probes[37, 38] (TABLES 7–3 and 7–4)

- Genomic sequences specific for an infectious agent are selected, cloned, synthesized, and used as a probe for identification.
- Generally cDNA for rRNA, which is present in large quantity, is used.
- Probes may be labeled with enzymes, antigens, or chemiluminescent molecules.
- Sensitivity of the probe is dependent upon the size and composition of the probe and the specimen target.
- Identification of pure cultures by probe is more clear-cut than detection in a primary specimen because there is less competing nucleic acid.
- Probes manufactured by Gen-Probe use a chemiluminescent hybridization-protection-assay to indicate probe identification.
  - The assay done in liquid phase requires 2 to 3 hours from the time of sufficient culture for analysis.
  - A luminometer is necessary.
  - Early identification of mycobacteria and fungi confirms appropriate selection of therapy.
  - The test is specific except for cross reactivity with very unusual mycobacteria.
  - Equivocal results may occur when inadequate culture is available for analysis.

TABLE 7–3

Nucleic Acid Probes for Identification of Respiratory Tract Isolates from Culture (Manufacturer: Gen-Probe)

Bacteria
- *Haemophilus influenzae*
- *Mycobacterium avium* complex
- *Mycobacterium avium*
- *Mycobacterium intracellulare*
- *Mycobacterium kansasii*
- *Mycobacterium tuberculosis* complex
- *Staphylococcus aureus*
- *Streptococcus agalactiae* (group B)
- *Streptococcus pneumoniae*
- *Streptococcus pyogenes* (group A)

Fungi
- *Blastomyces dermatitidis*
- *Coccidioides immitis*
- *Histoplasma capsulatum*

TABLE 7–4

Nucleic Acid Probes for Direct Detection in Clinical Samples (Manufacturer: Gen-Probe)

- *Mycobacterium tuberculosis,* direct (MTD) (smear positive samples)
- *Streptococcus pyogenes* (group A)

METHODS FOR DIAGNOSIS

NUCLEIC ACID PROBES

16S rRNA Gene Sequence for Identification of Bacteria[39]

- The small subunit (16S) ribosomal RNA gene contains several functionally different regions.
  - Some have conserved sequences, and other regions are highly varied.
  - These genotypic features can be used to indicate genotypic relationships and identify bacteria, sometimes not culturable, as to genus and species.
  - Broad-range PCR primers can be used to recognize conserved sequences and amplify highly variable regions in between.
- An analytical system "MicroSeq" (Perkin Elmer, Applied Biosystems Division) has been developed for identification.
  - It provides modules for DNA extraction, PCR, preparation for sequencing, cycle sequencing, and software for analysis of sequence.
  - As presently constituted, this system is expensive, requires at least 20 hours for analysis, and requires development of analytical software.
  - This system has considerable potential for the future.

Nucleic Acid Amplification[37, 40]

- The polymerase chain reaction (PCR) is based on the ability of DNA polymerase to copy a strand of DNA.
- The enzyme initiates elongation at the 3′ end of a short (primer) sequence bound to a longer (target) strand of DNA.
- When two primers bind to complementary strands of target DNA, the sequence between the two primer binding sites is amplified exponentially with each cycle of the PCR.
- By use of a programmable thermal cycler a detectable amount of target sequence originally present in less than 100 copies can be generated in 30 to 50 cycles for detection and analysis of microbial pathogens.
- The nucleic acid amplification techniques include three basic methodologies:
  1. Target amplification—PCR (Roche), transcription-mediated amplification (TMA-Gen-Probe) (NASBA-Organon-Teknika), strand displacement (SD-Becton-Dickinson)
  2. Probe amplification—Qbeta replicase (QBR-Vysis) and ligase chain reaction (LCR-Abbott)
  3. Signal amplification, branched DNA (bDNA-Bayer)
     - The bDNA probe method uses branched multiple probe–enzyme complexes to increase the signal in proportion to the amount of target in the reaction mixture.
     - All hybridization reactions occur simultaneously and the observed signal is proportional to the amount of target.
     - Target DNA can be quantified from a standard curve.
- Reverse transcriptase (RT)-PCR amplifies RNA targets.
  - RNA targets are converted to complementary DNA (cDNA) by RT and are then amplified by PCR.
  - RT-PCR has been used to detect RNA virus infection and *Mycobacterium* sp. and for determination of effectiveness of therapy in clearing an infectious agent.

TESTS FOR BACTERIAL INFECTIOUS AGENTS THAT CAUSE PNEUMONIA

GENERAL

- More than 100 different infectious agents are known to cause pneumonia. (See Chapter 3, Pathology.)
- New infectious agents are being found, such as *Chlamydia pneumoniae,* that account for a significant proportion of pneumonia (10 to 50%) that has not received an etiologic diagnosis.
- New laboratory tests are becoming available that enable rapid etiologic diagnosis by antigen detection (e.g., respiratory syncytial virus or influenza viruses, or nucleic acid amplification tests such as the PCR).
- As increasing antimicrobial resistance to common antimicrobial agents occurs, greater effort must be made to culture the microorganism so that susceptibility tests can be done.
- Eventually nucleic acid detection tests, which target antimicrobial resistance mechanisms, will be available.
- As specific laboratory tests become available, it is increasingly important for the physician to formulate a tentative specific etiologic diagnosis when possible (TABLE 7–5).

TABLE 7–5

Clues to Etiology of Pneumonia

Risk Group	Commonly Encountered Pathogens
Alcoholism or conditions that produce aspiration	Oral anaerobes, *S. pneumoniae,* gram-negative bacilli
COPD/smoker	*S. pneumoniae, H. influenzae, Branhamella (Moraxella) catarrhalis*
Exposure to parturient sheep, goats, other farm animals	*Coxiella burnetii*
Exposure to wild rodents or droppings	Sin Nombre virus (hanta virus)
HIV-1 infection, CD4 $< 200/\mu L$	*S. pneumoniae, H. influenzae, Legionella* spp., *M. tuberculosis, M. avium, M. kansasii, Cryptococcus neoformans, Histoplasma capsulatum, Pneumocystis carinii, Coccidioides immitis,* HSV, VZV
Householder had respiratory disease 2 weeks ago	*Mycoplasma pneumoniae*
Influenza in community	Influenza, *S. pneumoniae, S. aureus*
Neutropenia	*Klebsiella* spp., *E. coli, Enterobacter* spp., *S. pneumoniae, S. aureus, Aspergillus, Fusarium, Mucor, Candida*
Recent hospitalization	Gram-negative bacilli, *S. aureus, Legionella* spp.
Recent plumbing work or exposure to water	*Legionella* spp.
T-cell dysfunction	*Mycobacteria, Nocardia, Legionella, Cryptococcus, Histoplasma, Coccidioides, Pneumocystis, Strongyloides, Toxoplasma,* CMV, VZV, HSV
Travel or residence in southwestern United States	*Coccidioides*

TESTS FOR BACTERIAL INFECTIOUS AGENTS THAT CAUSE PNEUMONIA

ACUTE BACTERIAL PNEUMONIA

- The acute bacterial pneumonias are most often caused by bacteria that are part of the commensal bacterial flora of the upper respiratory tract.
- For this reason it is necessary that specimens be carefully collected and screened to ensure that the specimen represents expectorated sputum.
- The smear combined with clinical history can give valuable early information on the relative proportions of bacteria present and for comparison with the culture.
- Significant numbers of the prospective infectious agent should be seen on smear and culture.
- Because there is lack of homogeneity in specimen samples, culture sensitivity may vary.
- Respiratory specimens are regularly cultured on 5% sheep blood agar, chocolate agar which provides X (hemin) and V (NAD) growth factors and McConkey medium, which permits growth of many Gram-negative bacteria.
- Buffered charcoal yeast extract (BCYE) medium with supplements for *Legionella* and media for anaerobic bacteria are used when they are appropriate according to clinical history and when satisfactory specimens are collected.
- A large array of infectious agents cause pneumonia and respiratory tract infections.
- For discussion of the laboratory diagnosis of some of these agents, they are grouped according to their biologic classification and epidemiologic characteristics.

STREPTOCOCCAL PNEUMONIA[42–45]

- *Streptococcus pneumoniae* is the most common etiologic agent of community-acquired pneumonia.
- This organism may also cause otitis media, sinusitis, meningitis, and endocarditis.
- A capsular polysaccharide vaccine that contains 23 of the more common *S. pneumoniae* capsular antigens is available.
- Patients with HIV-1 infection and AIDS are highly susceptible to *S. pneumoniae* bacteremia.
- *S. pneumoniae* produces alpha-hemolytic colonies often with a depressed central portion or mucoid appearance.
- Pneumococci are distinguished from viridans streptococci, which also are alpha-hemolytic, by being both optochin-susceptible and bile-soluble.
  - An optochin 6-mm disk is placed on the secondary dilution streak of the respiratory specimen; a 14-mm or greater zone of inhibition of colonies resembling pneumococcus is positive.
  - The plate bile solubility test is done by dropping 10% sodium desoxycholate on colonies resembling pneumococcus; after 15 minutes of incubation at 35°C the *S. pneumoniae* colonies will be dissolved, and the agar surface will be flat.
- *S. pneumoniae* capsular antigen detection tests may be performed on clinical specimens by latex particle agglutination tests EIA and CIE.
  - Tests done on urine and blood culture supernatant are most sensitive.
  - There are cross-reactions between *S. pneumoniae* polyvalent "omniserum" (Statenseruminstitutet, Copenhagen) and antigens in rare viridans streptococcus and *E. coli.*
- There is a specific nucleic acid probe for *S. pneumoniae* (Gen Probe).
- Methods to detect *S. pneumoniae* resistance to penicillin have been defined (see discussion of antimicrobial susceptibility testing).

FIGURE 7-24

Streptococcus pneumoniae is a gram-positive diplococcus, which is 0.5 to 2.0 μm in diameter. It may be spherical, lanceolate, or elongated in pairs or short chains. It may lose its gram-positive nature in aged culture and upon exposure to β-lactam antibiotics and leukocyte lysozyme.

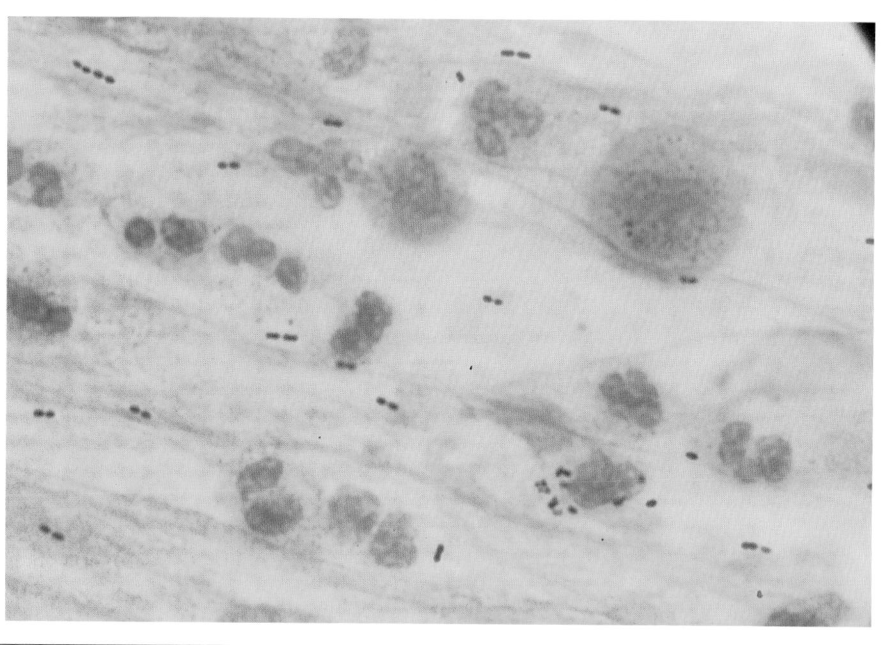

HAEMOPHILUS PNEUMONIA[47–54]

- *Haemophilus influenzae* can cause an acute pneumonia similar in clinical signs and predisposing factors to pneumonia caused by *S. pneumoniae.*
- *H. influenzae* can also cause otitis media, sinusitis, and epiglottitis.
- A polysaccharide vaccine against *H. influenzae* type b administered to children starting at age 2 months has been very effective in reducing invasive disease in this population.
- Upper respiratory tract colonization may be as high as 50% in humans with many of the isolates being unencapsulated (nontypable).
- In older children and adults nontypable strains may cause tracheobronchitis, pneumonia (sometimes with bacteremia), exacerbation of chronic bronchitis, and otitis media.
- Predisposing factors include malignancy, immunodeficiency as a consequence of therapy or HIV-1 infection, chronic obstructive pulmonary disease, pregnancy, and cystic fibrosis.
- *H. influenzae* is gram-negative and coccobacillary and therefore may be difficult to see on stained smear.
- Use of 0.05% basic fuchsin dye in place of safranin or use of nucleic acid stains (e.g., acridine orange or Giemsa) makes this organism more visible.
- Culture is the most sensitive, specific, and practical method for detection of *H. influenzae* at this time.
  - Specimens for culture should be collected while achieving minimal contact with colonized upper respiratory mucosa and streaked to give optimal distribution of small slow-growing colonies.
  - A culture medium providing factors X (hemin) and V (NAD), such as chocolate agar, must be used.
  - Incubation should be in a humid atmosphere with 5 to 10% CO_2.

H. influenzae is oxidase-positive and may form satellite colonies around *Staphylococcus* or *Pneumococcus* on deficient media.

- Some biotypes have an odor of mouse urine due to indol production.
- Identification of *H. influenzae* is done most conveniently with a quadrant plate containing Mueller-Hinton agar supplemented with X, V, X + V, horse blood + X + V.
- *H. influenzae* grow in the X + V and horse blood + X + V quadrants but do not cause hemolysis in the blood-containing quadrant.

(continued)

TESTS FOR BACTERIAL INFECTIOUS AGENTS THAT CAUSE PNEUMONIA

HAEMOPHILUS PNEUMONIA[47-54]

- Other identification systems use growth factors in filter paper strips, small tubes, or modules (API, HNID and RIM-H).
- A nucleic acid probe with high specificity is available to identify *H. influenzae* (Gen-Probe).
- Quellung tests can be done with type antisera to demonstrate encapsulated strains.
- Type b antigen detection tests on urine are available using an IgG-sensitized latex particle or a staphylococcal protein-A–mediated coagglutination test. For nonvaccinated patients these tests may still have value.

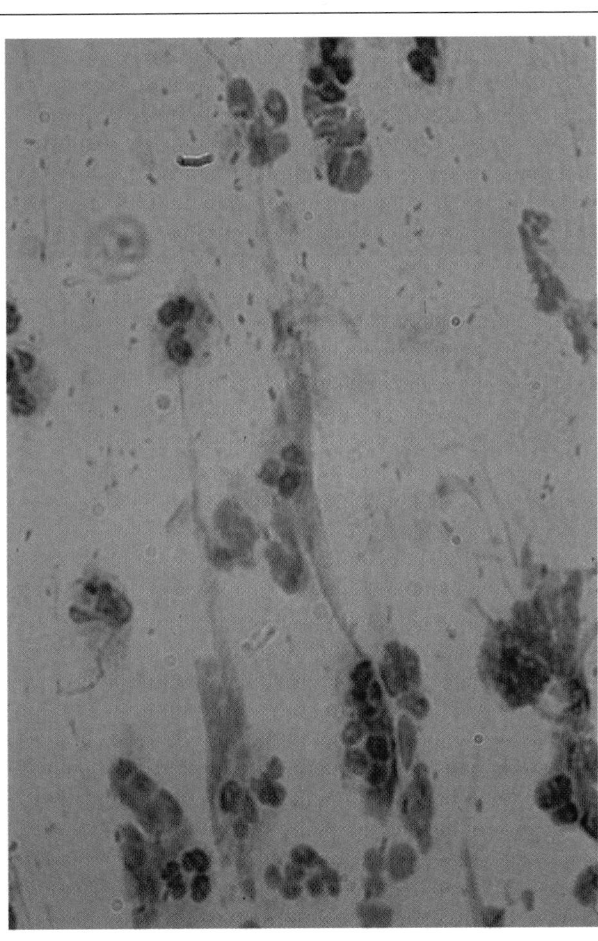

FIGURE 7–25

Haemophilus influenzae is gram-negative and coccobacillary, less than 1.0 μm in diameter. It elongates upon culture and on exposure to β-lactam antibiotics. (From Upjohn, GS-12.)

TESTS FOR BACTERIAL INFECTIOUS AGENTS THAT CAUSE PNEUMONIA

LEGIONELLA PNEUMONIA[55-58]

- Use of 0.05% basic fuchsin dye rather than safranin makes the bacteria more apparent.
- *Legionella* organisms are found in soil, in water, on plumbing surfaces, and in association with protozoa in water.
- Detection of *Legionella* infection can be accomplished by culture, direct fluorescent-antibody (DFA) staining (reagent available commercially only for *L. pneumophila*), antigen detection in urine (reagent available commercially only for *L. pneumophila* serogroup 1), nucleic acid amplification (FDA-approved environmental detection), or serologic indirect immunofluorescence test.
- Culture is recommended even if other detection methods will be used because it will detect most species and serogroups.
- DFA is not recommended when the prevalence of positive tests is less than 1% because the number of false-positive tests may exceed true-positive results.
- Culture should be done with lower respiratory tract specimens using acid buffer wash (pH 2.2) and culture on buffered charcoal yeast extract agar with L-cysteine, alpha-ketoglutarate, and an iron salt (BCYE); sputum screening and rejection should not be done on sputum specimens for *Legionella*.
- There is no relation between cell composition of sputum and recovery of *Legionella* organisms.
- Identification is determined by colony morphology, requirement for L-cysteine and serologic typing.

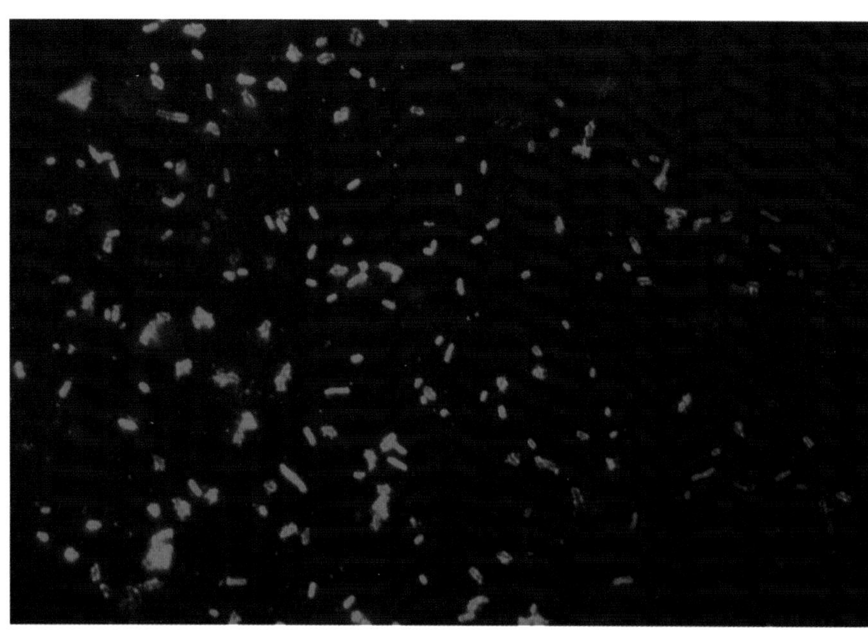

FIGURE 7–26

Legionella longbeachae DFA. Nineteen species of *Legionella* have been isolated from humans. *L. pneumophila* serogroups 1 and 6 and *L. micdadei* are more frequently recovered from human infections. Laboratories should determine species and serogroups recovered in their location as a guide to use of diagnostic tests. Legionellae are thin (0.3 to 0.9 μm), faintly staining gram-negative bacteria.

TESTS FOR BACTERIAL INFECTIOUS AGENTS THAT CAUSE PNEUMONIA

STAPHYLOCOCCAL PNEUMONIA[54, 59–63]

- The definitive test is a tube test done with EDTA rabbit plasma incubated 4 hours.
- The bound coagulase is detected by the rapid slide screening test.
- *S. aureus* is an opportunist organism that causes infections when the skin barrier is breached and when the mucociliary barrier is damaged by influenza and other respiratory infections opening the portal to pulmonary infection.
- *S. aureus* should be collected as directly as possible from the infected site, avoiding cutaneous and mucosal contamination.
  - It survives adverse conditions of transport well.
  - It grows well on 5% sheep blood agar.
  - Some strains require anaerobic conditions or elevated CO_2 atmosphere.
- Selective media that inhibit gram-negative bacteria (e.g., mannitol-salt agar, Columbia colistin-nalidixic acid agar) may be necessary for specimens such as sputum.
- Numerous commercial modules are available to identify *S. aureus* and coagulase-negative staphylococcus.
- The nucleic acid probe AccuProbe (Gen-Probe) is 100% specific.
- *S. aureus* may be responsible for nosocomial infections.
- Strain typing for epidemiologic study of infections can be done by phenotypic means using colony morphology, biotyping, and antibiogram.
- Genotypic typing can include pulsed-field gel electrophoresis of DNA fragments produced by restriction endonucleases or PCR of specific target sequences.
- Phage typing is not recommended. Reagents are rarely available.

FIGURE 7–27

Gram stain of *Staphylococcus aureus* in tracheal aspirate. It is a gram-positive coccus (0.5 to 1.5 μm in diameter), which forms irregular grape-like clusters. Colonies are cream, yellow to orange color. *S. aureus* is a commensal organism that inhabits the skin, especially the anterior nares, and may be found in the mouth and nasopharynx. *S. aureus* is identified by production of coagulase, which clots plasma.

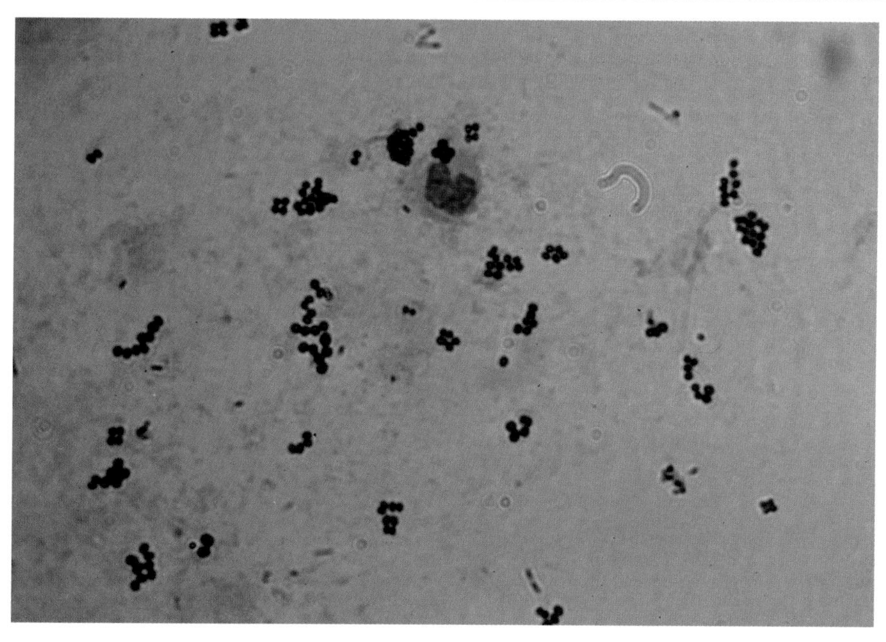

TESTS FOR BACTERIAL INFECTIOUS AGENTS THAT CAUSE PNEUMONIA

STREPTOCOCCAL PNEUMONIA

- *S. pyogenes*[64–66] is a facultative anaerobic, catalase-negative, beta-hemolytic organism that accounts for most of the group A streptococci (Lancefield classification).
  - It is a transient colonizer of mucous membranes.
  - It causes a wide variety of infections, including pharyngitis and occasionally pneumonia.
  - Some *S. pyogenes* infections cause a toxic shock–like syndrome, perhaps related to the pyrogenic exotoxins, which may act as superantigens.
- *S. pyogenes* is easily transported and withstands drying.
- It grows well on blood- or serum-supplemented media.
- On primary culture the candle jar enhances growth.
- *S. pyogenes* has large colonies over 0.5 mm in diameter; beta-hemolysis due to oxygen-labile streptolysin O is detected by stab inoculation into the agar medium.
- *S. pyogenes* is also PYR (pyrrolidonyl arylamidase) positive, and susceptible to bacitracin (0.04 IU bacitracin disk).
- Group A antigen can be demonstrated by fluorescein-conjugated antibody, EIA, latex particle agglutination (LPA), and nucleic acid probes. These tests can be used to identify group A streptococcus or to detect group A antigen.
- Serologic tests for antibody versus *S. pyogenes* antigens (e.g., antistreptolysin O, antihyaluronidase, or anti-DNAse B) detect evidence of *S. pyogenes* infection.
  - These tests may be useful for diagnosis of rheumatic fever or glomerulonephritis.
  - Because of the serious consequences of *S. pyogenes* infection and associated diseases, *S. pyogenes* is always identified and reported when found.

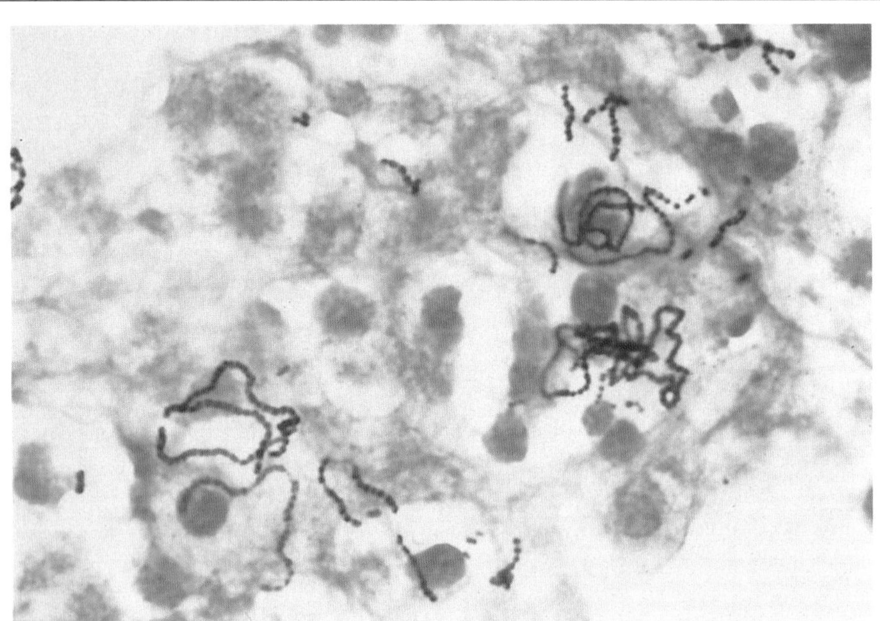

FIGURE 7–28

Streptococcus pyogenes is a spherical or ovoid coccus, 0.5 to 2.0 μm in diameter, which divides in only one plane, thus forming chains.

TESTS FOR BACTERIAL INFECTIOUS AGENTS THAT CAUSE PNEUMONIA

BRANHAMELLA (MORAXELLA) CATARRHALIS PNEUMONIA[67, 68]

- *Branhamella catarrhalis* grows in 5% sheep blood agar, chocolate agar, and nutrient agar at 22°C to 35°C.
- *B. catarrhalis* can be distinguished from *Neisseria cinerea* by its growth at 22°C on blood and chocolate agar, DNAase positivity, and nitrate reduction.
- Both *B. catarrhalis* and *N. cinerea* fail to utilize sugars with acid product as seen in the Quad-Ferm test used to identify *Neisseria.*
- Most *B. catarrhalis* isolates (85% or greater) produce beta-lactamase; however, in vitro the majority appear susceptible to cephamycins, cephalosporins, beta-lactamase–stable penicillins, and quinolones.

FIGURE 7–29

Branhamella (Moraxella) catarrhalis. Gram-negative diplococcus *B. catarrhalis* is occasionally carried in the throat of children and adults. It causes otitis media, sinusitis, bronchopneumonia, and acute purulent exacerbations of chronic bronchitis and pneumonia.

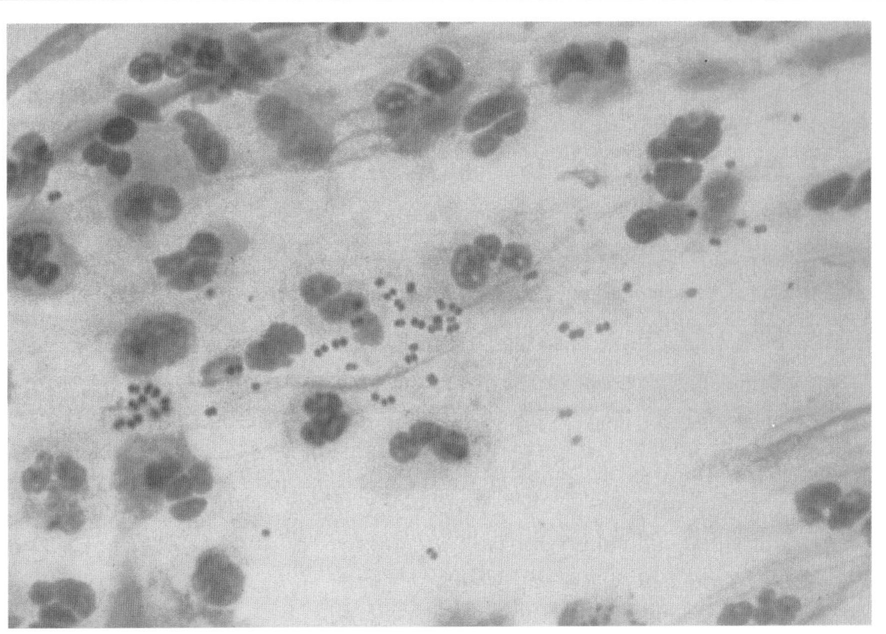

ANAEROBIC PLEUROPULMONARY PNEUMONIA[8, 69, 70] (TABLE 7–6)

- Anaerobic bacteria can survive and grow in locations where many bacteria are growing and thus reduce their environment.
- Such conditions are found in the gingival crevices, the oronasopharynx, and the lower gut.
- Infections by anaerobes occur by aspiration, dysphagia, or obstructive processes, which draw the bacteria inhabiting the upper respiratory tract into the lungs.
- Infections can also occur in the lungs through a hematogenous route through bacteremia, septic emboli and embolization with infarct.
- Anaerobic bacterial pneumonias are indolent; however, they may advance to form necrotizing pneumonia and abscess.
- From 80 to 95% of nontuberculous lung abscesses are caused by anaerobes.
  - These abscesses may advance to form a bronchopleural fistula and empyema.
  - Presumptive identification can be done by a series of simple tests, such as response to antibiotics, pigment, and fluorescence.
  - This testing can be done in large laboratories.
  - Definitive identification may require metabolic end product and whole cell fatty acid profiling by GLC and 16S-rRNA sequencing done in some reference laboratories (see discussion of antimicrobial susceptibility testing).

TESTS FOR BACTERIAL INFECTIOUS AGENTS THAT CAUSE PNEUMONIA

ANAEROBIC PLEUROPULMONARY PNEUMONIA

TABLE 7–6

Anaerobes Encountered in Pleuropulmonary Infections (Aspiration Pneumonia, Lung Abscess, Empyema)

Gram-negative bacilli
- Pigmented *Prevotella* and *Porphyromonas,* e.g., *Prevotella melaninogenica, Prev. intermedia Porphyromonas endodontalis* (pigmented and nonpigmented)
- Unpigmented bile-sensitive, e.g., *Prevotella oris, Prev. buccae*
- *Bacteroides urealyticus*
- *Campylobacter gracilis* (microaerophilic)
- *Bacteroides* (*B. fragilis* group), bile resistant
- *Fusobacterium nucleatum*
- *Fusobacterium necrophorum*

Gram-negative cocci
- *Veillonella* sp.

Gram-positive bacilli
- *Actinomyces* sp, forms filaments
- *Eubacterium* sp, fastidious anaerobe
- *Clostridium* sp, may form spores

Gram-positive cocci
- *Peptostreptococcus* sp
- viridans streptococcus (facultative, microaerophilic)

Data from Jousimies-Somer HR, Summanen PH, Finegold SM: *Bacteroides, Porphyromonas, Prevotella, Fusobacterium* and other anaerobic gram negative rods and cocci. In Murray PR (ed-in-chief): Manual of Clinical Microbiology, 7th ed. Washington, DC, ASM Press, 1999.

THE ATYPICAL PNEUMONIAS

- The atypical pneumonias are caused by unusual bacteria, which cannot be cultured on standard bacteriology culture media.
- Special media, cell culture, or yolk sac culture may be necessary to culture these bacteria.
- Because of the difficulty with culture diagnosis of infections by these agents, serologic antibody detection tests are usually used.
- Culture, antigen detection, and nucleic acid amplification (PCR) are under study.
- Multiplex-PCR tests may be useful for this complex of infections.
- Bacterial atypical respiratory infections are discussed in this section (Table 7–7).
- *Mycoplasma pneumoniae* is a bacterium that, by gene deletion, has permanently lost the capacity to form cell walls.
  - As a consequence, it is gram-negative and is not susceptible to beta-lactam antibiotics.
  - It is susceptible to tetracyclines and macrolides.
  - The EIA serologic test for antibody has replaced the complement fixation (CF) and indirect immunofluorescence (IFA) tests because of its ease of performance.
    - A fourfold seroconversion shows evidence of infection.
    - Tests specific for IgM are useful for detection of acute infection.
  - Cold agglutinins occur in about 50% of patients.
    - Titers of 1:64 or 1:28 or a fourfold rise in titer suggest recent infection.
    - Cold agglutinins occur as well in certain viral infections and autoimmune diseases.
  - *M. pneumoniae* can be cultured in SP4 (serum, yeast extract, glucose), but the yield is low and 1 to 4 weeks may be required.
  - Antigen detection tests cross-react with other mycoplasmas, which are inhabitants of mucous membranes.
  - PCR is sensitive, but positive results in patients who lack clinical evidence of disease suggests that prolonged colonization occurs.[33, 71, 72]
- Some atypical pneumonias are caused by *Chlamydia.*
  - *Chlamydia* organisms are gram-negative bacteria that are obligate intracellular parasites.
  - They use ATP produced by the host cell.
  - The elementary bodies (0.25 to 0.35 μm diameter) stain by Giemsa and species-specific fluorescein conjugated antibody.
  - They are susceptible to tetracyclines and macrolides.

(continued)

TESTS FOR BACTERIAL INFECTIOUS AGENTS THAT CAUSE PNEUMONIA

THE ATYPICAL PNEUMONIAS

- *C. pneumoniae* (TWAR) causes pharyngitis, bronchitis, and pneumonia in humans.
  - Seroprevalence is 40 to 50% at 30 to 40 years of age.
  - Antibody is very common around the world.
  - Micro-IF antigens can be purchased and are the basis of most serologic studies.
  - A fourfold rise in titer, an IgM titer of 1:16, or greater, or an IgG titer of 1:512 or more suggests recent infection.
  - Culture can be accomplished with difficulty using throat swabs or other respiratory specimens and HL or HEp-2 cell cultures.
  - There is no known animal reservoir.[32, 33, 73, 74]
- *C. psittaci* causes a pulmonary and systemic zoonosis transmitted from many avian species.
  - The organism infects the intestine of birds and is spread by contact and aerosol.
  - The agent is very stable in contaminated soil.
  - At one time it was the most common cause of laboratory-acquired infection. Laboratories must use a biosafety level 3 facility if the agent is to be cultured in cell culture.
  - Most diagnoses are made using micro-IF serologic tests.[75]
- *C. trachomatis* can infect the respiratory tract of the infant during passage through an infected birth canal.
  - Studies on different serologic tests for antigen and antibody, nucleic acid probes, and nucleic acid amplification tests are under way.[31]
- *Coxiella burnetii* is a gram-negative coccobacillus (0.2 × 0.7 μm) and is an obligate intracellular parasite. The organism can be cultured in Vero cells.
- *C. burnetii* infects a wide variety of arthropods, fish, birds, marsupials, and mammals.
- There is an acute reactivation of *C. burnetii* infection in pregnant cattle, sheep, and goats with large numbers of organisms in the placenta, uterus, and mammary glands (Q fever). Contact with such animals is the principal source of human infection.
- Acute Q fever is a febrile illness with pneumonia and hepatitis.
- Chronic disease may include endocarditis, osteomyelitis, and other systemic involvement.
- *C. burnetii* is highly infectious, so infected materials must be processed in a biosafety level 3 facility.
- *C. burnetii* undergoes a phase variation in lipopolysaccharide similar to smooth to rough variation in Enterobacteriaceae.
  - Phase I occurs in nature and in laboratory animals.
  - Phase II occurs after numerous passages in cell or embryonated egg culture.
  - An IFA test incorporating either phase I or phase II antigen is used for serologic diagnosis.
  - In acute Q fever the IFA titer with phase I antigen is usually 1:128 or less.
  - With phase II antigen the minimum diagnostic titer is 1:256.
  - In *C. burnetii* endocarditis, the diagnostic IgG titer with phase I antigens is 1:800 or greater.
- There are specific primers for *C. burnetii* PCR, and this detection system is more sensitive than culture.[33, 76, 77]

TABLE 7–7

The Bacterial Atypical Pneumonias

Etiologic Agent	Characteristics	Disease	Culture	Diagnostic Tests
Mycoplasma pneumoniae	Permanent loss of cell wall; not susceptible to antibiotics that inhibit cell wall	20% community-acquired pneumonia; tracheobronchitis; spreads through households	In vitro SP4; low yield; takes 1–4 weeks	EIA for IgM cold agglutinins, 50%; disease not specific; CF, IFA, PCR may detect prolonged colonization, antigen tests cross-react with other mycoplasmas
Chlamydia pneumoniae (TWAR)	Obligate intercellular; no animal reservoir	Infection very common; seroprevalence 40–50% at age 40; pharyngitis, bronchitis, mild pneumonia	Cell culture HL or Hep2	Microimmune fluorescence: • IgM titer ≥1:16 • IgG titer ≥1:512
Chlamydia psittaci	Obligate intracellular; zoonosis—birds, infects intestine; also infects domestic mammals	Pneumonia in persons in contact; all birds, abattoir, processing plants, turkeys; resistant to drying	Cell culture; culture not recommended; high incidence lab acquired infection	CF titer ≥1:64; fourfold increase in titer CF is genus-specific, not species-specific
Chlamydia trachomatis	Obligate intracellular; infects humans	Pneumonia in infants passing through infected birth canals	Culture; cyclohexamide treated; McCoy cells	Culture—mother, infant, or LCR (ligase chain reaction), PCR (polymerase chain reaction); antigen detection
Coxiella burnetii	Obligate intracellular; infects ticks, lice, flies, fish, birds, marsupials, and mammals; human infection most often from reactivating infection in placenta, uterus, mammary gland of pregnant sheep, goats, cattle	Q fever; pneumonia, hepatitis; chronic disease endocarditis, osteomyelitis	Cell culture; Vero cells; all infected material must be processed BSL-3	Indirect fluorescent antibody (IFA) phase I and II antigen

HOSPITAL-ACQUIRED PNEUMONIA[78–80]

- Hospital-acquired pneumonia (HAP) occurs in patients who have severe underlying disease and require a variety of procedures using catheters, intubation, and mechanical ventilation to bypass usual body defenses.
- 73% of critically ill patients have colonization by gram-negative bacilli (GNB).
- They may have microaspiration and resulting pneumonia (TABLE 7–8).
- Patients with more severe illness may have HAP due to *Pseudomonas aeruginosa,* mixed anaerobic bacteria, or *Legionella* spp. in hospitals with contaminated water systems.

TESTS FOR BACTERIAL INFECTIOUS AGENTS THAT CAUSE PNEUMONIA

HOSPITAL-ACQUIRED PNEUMONIA

TABLE 7–8

Most Likely Pathogens in Hospital-Acquired Pneumonia

Enterobacteriaceae	*Haemophilus influenzae*
– *Escherichia coli*	*Legionella* spp.
– *Enterobacter* sp.	*Staphylococcus aureus*
– *Klebsiella* sp.	*Streptococcus pneumoniae*
– *Proteus* sp.	
– *Serratia marcescens*	

- The Enterobacteriaceae are found widespread in nature.
- *Escherichia coli* colonizes the intestine of humans and animals.
- The *Enterobacter* sp., *Klebsiella* sp., *Proteus* sp., and *Serratia* sp. are present in soil, water, and vegetation and can colonize upper and lower respiratory and gastrointestinal tracts and skin.
- Most *K. pneumoniae* pulmonary disease is hospital-acquired bronchopneumonia or bronchitis, but it can also cause a community-acquired pneumonia in patients with alcoholism, diabetes mellitus, and chronic obstructive pulmonary disease.
- The *K. pneumoniae* capsule prevents phagocytosis and migration of phagocytes into infected sites.
- The enteric bacteria survive usual collection procedures and except for some growth-factor deficient strains grow well on the standard peptone or meat extract media.
- Standard identification and antimicrobial susceptibility tests (Microscan, Vitek, API) are satisfactory.

FIGURE 7–30

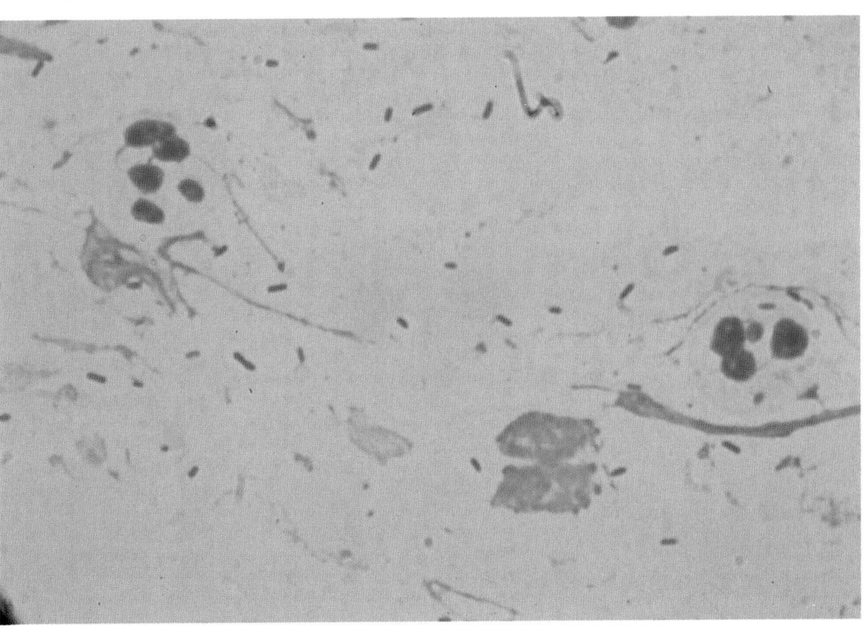

Klebsiella pneumoniae is a wide nonmotile gram-negative rod that often bears a polysaccharide capsule.

TESTS FOR BACTERIAL INFECTIOUS AGENTS THAT CAUSE PNEUMONIA

HOSPITAL-ACQUIRED PNEUMONIA

- *Pseudomonas aeruginosa* is found in moist environments such as water, soil, vegetables, and fruits.
- Solutions used in hospitals and some disinfectants may be contaminated by *P. aeruginosa.*
- Hospital equipment (e.g., respirators and tubing, nebulizers, bronchoscopes, and hydrotherapy equipment) cleaned but not completely decontaminated may be a source of *P. aeruginosa.*
- Failure to dry this equipment provides a location for growth of *Pseudomonas, Stenotrophomonas,* and related bacteria.
- Colonization increases in patients receiving antimicrobial or chemotherapeutic agents.
- Moist skin and mucosal surfaces may be colonized; 70 to 80% of adolescents with cystic fibrosis are colonized by *P. aeruginosa.*
- *P. aeruginosa* withstands usual collection systems and is cultured on standard agar media.
- The organism is identified by simple tests: motile by polar flagella; produces artificial grape odor; produces water-soluble yellow-green pyoverdin and blue pyocyanin; oxidase-positive; does not ferment glucose.
- Standard laboratory identification and susceptibility test systems (Microscan, Vitek, API) are satisfactory.[79, 80]

FIGURE 7–31

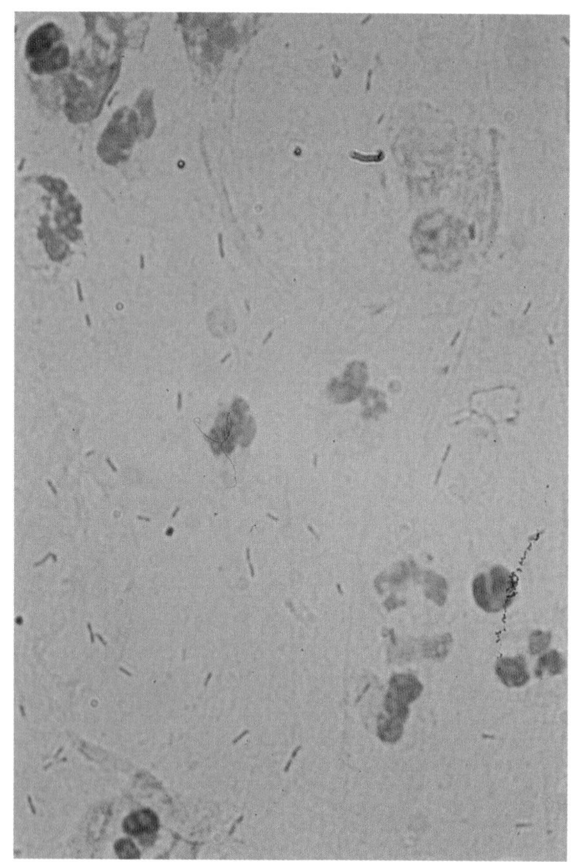

Pseudomonas aeruginosa is a thin, gram-negative rod 0.5 to 1.0 μm wide by 1.5 to 5.0 μm long. (From Upjohn, GS-12.)

AGENTS OF TERRORISM

- Most of the agents considered for biologic warfare are dispersed in the natural infection by aerosol, and the infective unit is relatively resistant to drying.
- Only simple aerosol devices are required for their dispersal; therefore, they may be used by terrorists.
- There is a high risk that the group generating biologic warfare agents will be infected by these agents, as occurred in an accident at the former Soviet Union biologic warfare facility in Sverdlovsk. Although self-exposure may be a deterrent to use of biologic warfare, it may not prevent use of these agents by terrorists.
- Stringent biosafety precautions are necessary when working with these agents, infected individuals, or specimens.
- Aside from the agents described below, agents for which aerosol is a concern and for which biosafety level 3 or 4 is recommended are of concern. These include *Coxiella burnetii, Chlamydia psittaci, Mycobacterium* sp., *Brucella* sp., dimorphic fungi, and others. Local public health facilities or the Centers for Disease Control and Prevention (CDC) should be consulted about precautions.

TESTS FOR BACTERIAL INFECTIOUS AGENTS THAT CAUSE PNEUMONIA

AGENTS OF TERRORISM

Anthrax[81–83]

- Anthrax[81–83] requires a large inhaled inoculum of more than 10,000 aerosolized spores to infect.
  - In 1 to 3 days after exposure there is a sudden acute illness lasting a few hours accompanied by massive septicemia (10^7 to 10^9 bacteria/mL).
  - Skin lesions with eschars may also occur.

FIGURE 7-32

Bacillus anthracis is a gram-positive spore-forming aerobic rod 0.5 to 2.0 μm wide by 1.2 to 10.0 μm long. Phase-contrast microscopy shows phase bright spores. Spores are carried by macrophages to the lymphatic system. **A,** Gram stain of *B. anthracis.* **B,** Culture with phase bright spores.

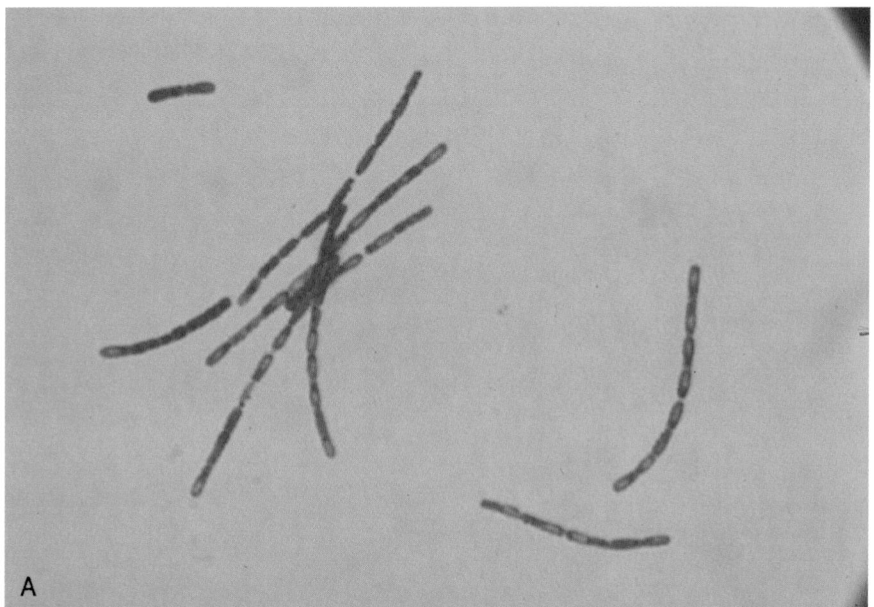

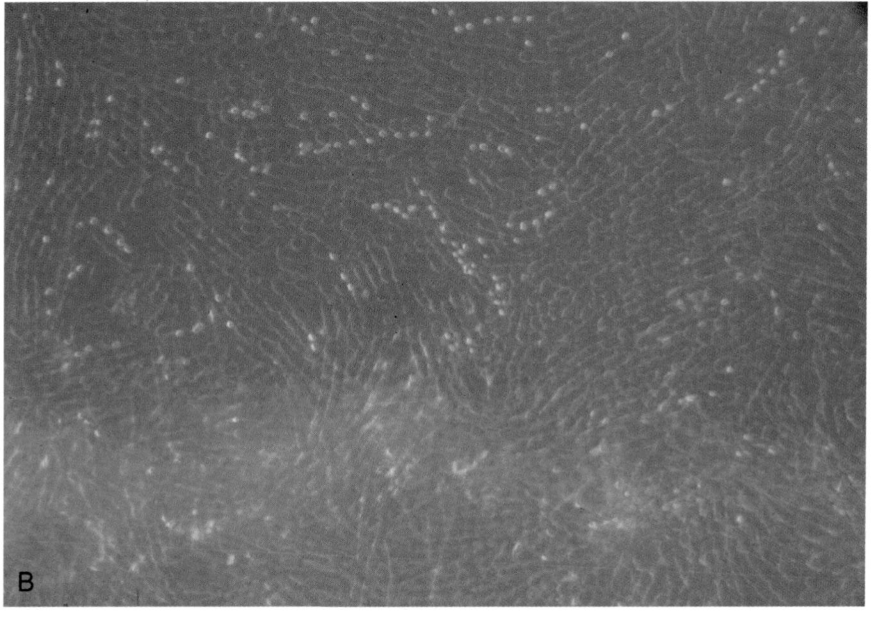

TESTS FOR BACTERIAL INFECTIOUS AGENTS THAT CAUSE PNEUMONIA

AGENTS OF TERRORISM

Smallpox

- Smallpox virus is thought to have been abolished by a large international effort to immunize the remaining susceptible human population with *Vaccinia* virus.
  - There is no animal reservoir.
  - The former USSR and United States by agreement retained the only known stocks of this virus in freezers at their national infectious disease institutions (CDC).
- This large virus is transmitted between humans by aerosol or direct contact.
- Initial signs are severe fever and prostration with an oral pox enanthem developing with lesions on the skin.
- The case fatality rate is 30 to 50%.

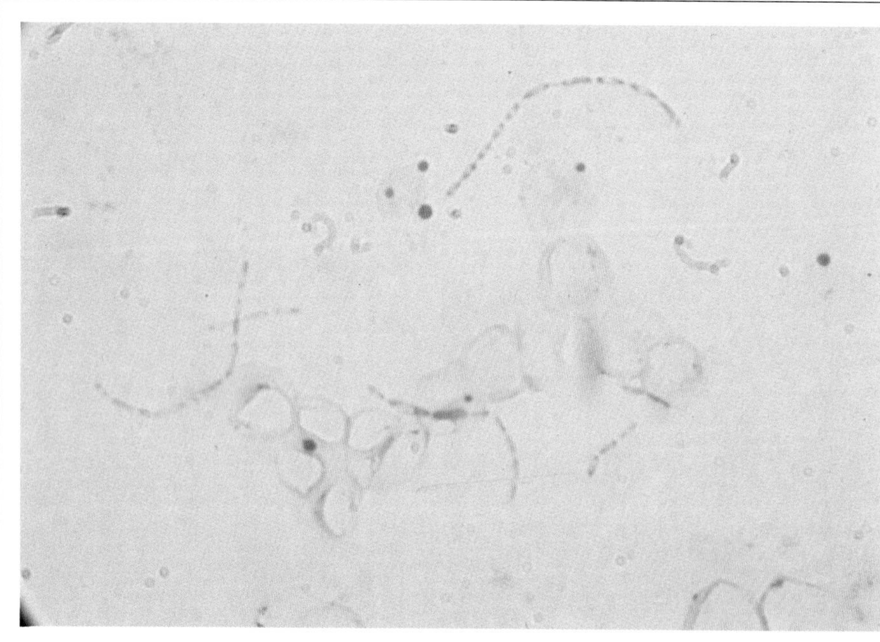

FIGURE 7–33

Yersinia pestis,[84–86] a rod-shaped gram-negative organism (0.5 to 0.8 μm in diameter by 1 to 3 μm in length), forms chains of bipolar-staining rods in broth cultures such as blood cultures. It is usually transmitted by means of fleas from infected rodents, i.e., rats, squirrels, and chipmunks. The fleabite transmits *Y. pestis,* producing bacteremia and enlarged spleen and lymph nodes (bubonic form). Individuals who do not receive treatment or are highly susceptible may develop hematogenous pneumonic plague, which is easily communicable from person to person through aerosols of respiratory secretions. Standard broth or solid media will grow *Y. pestis* in 24 to 48 hours. Direct fluorescent antibody stains of secretions and cultures and lytic phages are available for diagnosis by public health laboratories.

PULMONARY MYCOBACTERIOSES

- These mycobacteria are slow-growing, acid-fast bacteria.
- Gram-staining is weak or granular, sometimes with ghost boundaries visible against stained sputum exudate.
- *M. tuberculosis* is 0.3 to 0.6 μm by 1.0 to 4.0 μm.
- *M. avium* is usually filamentous in clinical specimens but may appear coccobacillary on culture.
- *M. kansasii* may form long, broad filaments with granules or bands in an acid-fast stain.

TABLE 7–9

Pulmonary Mycobacterioses
19, 24, 37, 38, 86a–91, 94

Mycobacterium tuberculosis complex
M. tuberculosis/M. bovis/M. africanum/M. microti
Mycobacterium avium complex
M. avium/M. intracellulare
Mycobacterium kansasii
Other nontuberculous mycobacteria in immunocompromised host

TESTS FOR BACTERIAL INFECTIOUS AGENTS THAT CAUSE PNEUMONIA

PULMONARY MYCOBACTERIOSES

FIGURE 7-34

M. tuberculosis stained with auramine/rhodamine fluorescent acid-fast stain. This stain can be read rapidly at low magnification.

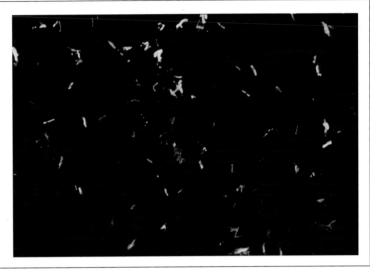

FIGURE 7-35

A, *M. tuberculosis* on Kinyon acid-fast stain. **B,** *M. tuberculosis* growing in BACTEC 12B broth medium showing marked cording growth on Kinyon acid-fast stain. **C,** *M. tuberculosis* colonies with "wavy" cording growth, which surround a single *M. avium* colony with clear translucent appearance. Growing on Middlebrook 7H10 medium. Solid media show mixed culture by different colonial growth. (Courtesy of Dr. David M. Yajko.)

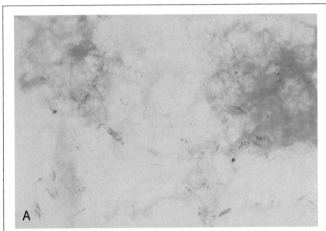

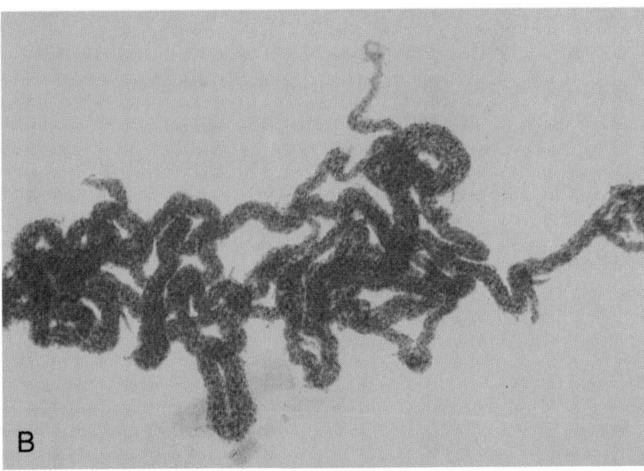

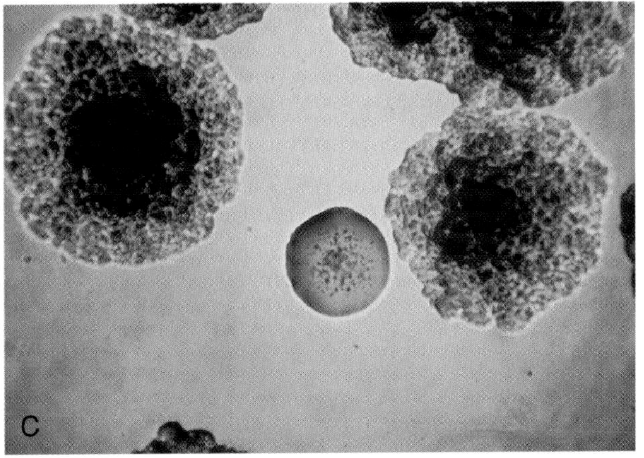

TESTS FOR BACTERIAL INFECTIOUS AGENTS THAT CAUSE PNEUMONIA

PULMONARY MYCOBACTERIOSES

- First-morning expectorated sputum, induced sputum, bronchoalveolar lavage, or biopsy specimens are most often used for diagnosis of pulmonary disease.
  - First-morning expectorated sputum specimens are more concentrated than later specimens.
  - Pooled 24- or 48-hour specimens are not useful because overgrowth by fungi and gram-negative bacteria resistant to the decontamination process prevents culture of *M. tuberculosis.*
- The sensitivity of expectorated sputum examination has been reported to increase with the number of specimens, up to five. However, the increase in yield from 3 to 5 is very small.
- In a study done at San Francisco General Hospital, 82% of positive specimens were obtained in the first specimen, 92% cumulative positive findings occurred in the second specimen, and 100% cumulative positive results in the third specimen (WK Hadley, unpublished observations, 1998).
  - Patients who had more than three specimens submitted accounted for 49% of the specimens in the study (210 specimens) and all were nondiagnostic.
- Digestion with *N*-acetyl-L-cysteine or dithiothreitol with 2% sodium hydroxide liquefies specimens containing mucous secretions so that the specimen can be concentrated by centrifugation at 3000 × to 3400 × *g*.
  - The specimen is neutralized by buffer.
  - Bacteria other than mycobacteria are killed by this treatment so that they do not overgrow the slow-growing mycobacteria.
  - The concentrated specimen is used for several purposes:
    1. It is smeared and stained by the acid-fast stain of choice; the auramine/rhodamine stain uses fluorescent dyes, which are brilliant against the black background of an epifluorescent microscope. As a consequence the stain yields high sensitivity. The Kinyon carbofuchsin stain is the most frequently used alternative acid-fast stain.
    2. Culture generally in broth medium and solid medium is necessary to identify the bacterium present and determine its antimicrobial susceptibility.
    3. In some cases a nucleic acid amplification method such as PCR will also be done to rapidly detect and identify the mycobacterium.
- Broth media labeled with ^{14}C in the BACTEC system (Becton-Dickinson) detect growth at an early stage.
  - An antimicrobial/growth stimulating mixture enhances growth of mycobacteria and inhibits other microorganisms.
  - A solid medium detects mixed cultures by their colony morphology.
- Mycobacteria can be identified by the conventional biochemical tests, HPLC or nucleic acid-probe (Gen-Probe) (see Table 7–9).
- Other broth-based culture systems detect mycobacterial growth by oxygen utilization resulting in less quenching of ruthenium complex fluorescence, lower pressure in headspace of culture bottle, and a colorimetric CO_2 sensor.
- Direct detection and identification by nucleic acid amplification and hybridization are available in the *Mycobacterium tuberculosis* Direct Test (Gen-Probe, MTD) (TABLE 7–10).
  - This test is based on transcription-mediated amplification of rRNA.
  - The Amplicor MTB PCR test (Roche, MTB) detects amplified DNA.
- These tests are approved by the FDA for performance on *smear-positive specimens.*
  - If the patient has not received therapy in up to 7 days the sensitivity of smear-positive specimens is over 95%, but sensitivity may be less than 50% with smear-negative specimens.
  - Nucleic acid amplification tests detect nucleic acid of live and dead bacteria.
  - They are not suitable for following the course of therapy.

TESTS FOR BACTERIAL INFECTIOUS AGENTS THAT CAUSE PNEUMONIA

PULMONARY MYCOBACTERIOSES

TABLE 7-10

Performance of Gen-Probe MTD and Roche Amplicor MTD Test Direct in AFB Smear-Positive Versus Smear-Negative Patients

	Overall (%)	Smear-Positive (%)	Smear-Negative (%)
Sensitivity	77/80	95/96	48/53
Specificity	96/99	100	96/99
PPV (positive predictive value)	57/85	100	24/58
NPV (negative predictive value)	99	86/90	99

Mycobacterium Avium Complex (MAC)[19, 24, 38, 86a, 86b, 87] (TABLE 7-9)

MAC occurs in water, soil, and vegetation. It may colonize respiratory or gastrointestinal tracts without producing disease. MAC is the most common nontuberculous mycobacterium (NTM) to cause human disease although it is a bacterium of low pathogenicity. MAC causes lung infection in males 40 to 60 years old who are chronic smokers, alcohol abusers, and who have chronic bronchopulmonary disease.

M. avium (the majority serovars 1, 4, 8) can produce disseminated disease in AIDS patients with CD4 $< 100/mm^3$ and in other patients with immunodeficiency. During dissemination the MAC is carried principally in the monocyte. The antimicrobials of first choice for therapy are azithromycin or clarithromycin.

FIGURE 7-36

Acid-fast stained *Mycobacterium avium* complex (MAC) in bone marrow from AIDS patient with disseminated disease.

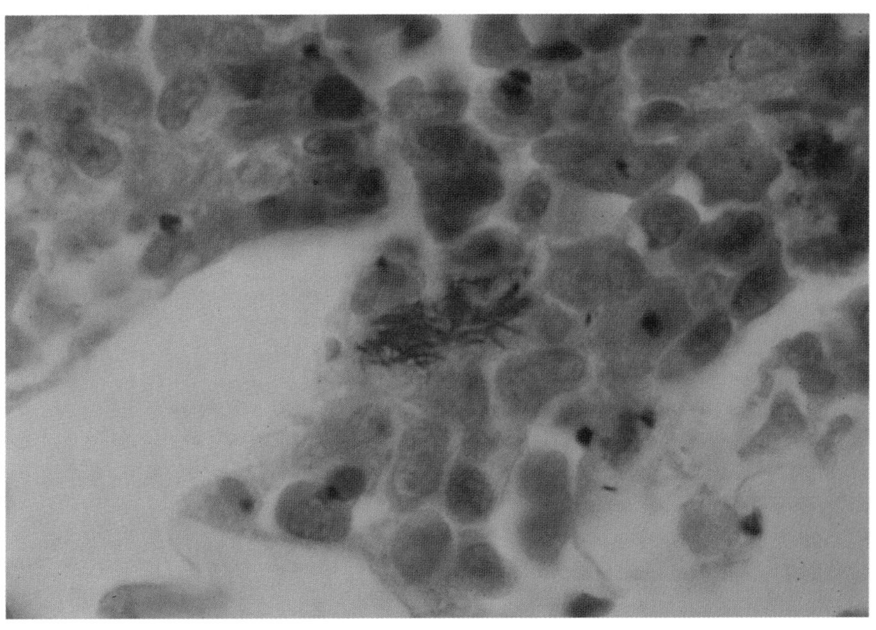

TESTS FOR BACTERIAL INFECTIOUS AGENTS THAT CAUSE PNEUMONIA

PULMONARY MYCOBACTERIOSES

Mycobacterium Kansasii[19, 37, 86a, 86c] (TABLE 7–9)

M. kansasii is a slow-growing (<7 days for mature colony) photochromogen (produces carotenoid yellow-orange pigment on exposure to light). The major reservoir is tap water. *M. kansasii* produces chronic lung disease resembling tuberculosis. Extrapulmonary infections of musculoskeletal, cutaneous, and lymph nodes are produced less often. Disseminated disease occurs in severe immunodeficiency such as AIDS and organ transplantation. Antimicrobials for primary consideration are rifampin, INH, and ethambutol.

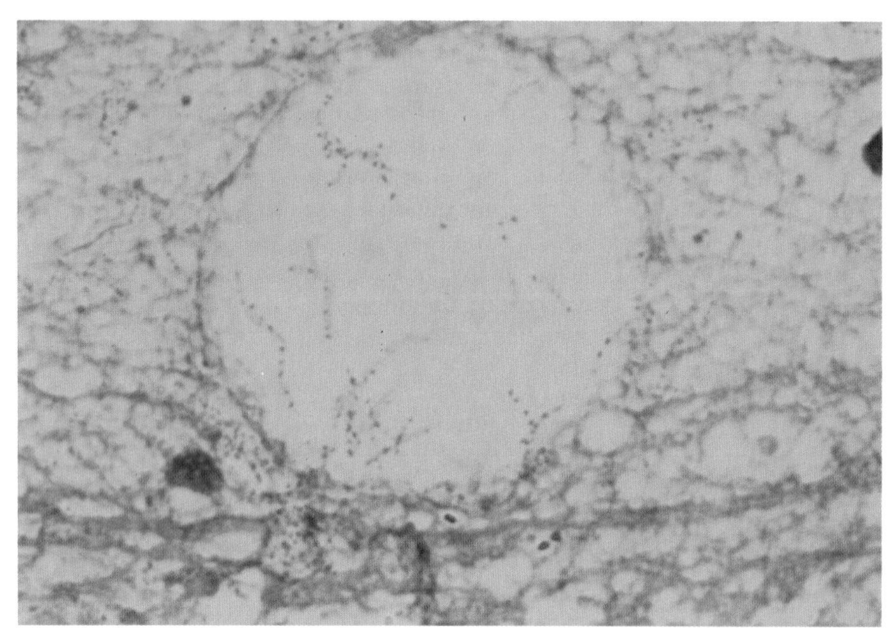

FIGURE 7–37

Acid-fast stained *Mycobacterium avium* in synovial fluid smear. Note long broad filaments with acid-fast staining granules and bands.

ANTIMICROBIAL SUSCEPTIBILITY TESTING

10, 13, 45, 52, 54, 59, 68, 92–94

GENERAL

- Performance standards for antimicrobial susceptibility testing are produced by the Subcommittee on Antimicrobial Susceptibility Testing of the National Committee on Clinical Laboratory Standards (NCCLS).
  - Members of the Subcommittee are professional, governmental, and industrial representatives.
  - The NCCLS membership through a process of consensus approves the Standards.
  - Commercial susceptibility testing devices are not described in these Standards.
  - The Standards serve as reference methods against which devices are compared.
- Bacteria that grow rapidly in aerobic cation-adjusted Mueller-Hinton medium (CAMHM) are tested by either the Performance Standards for Antimicrobial Disk Susceptibility Tests (M2-A6) or the Methods for Dilution Antimicrobial susceptibility tests for Bacteria that grow aerobically (M7-A4).
- The Enterobacteriaceae, *Staphylococcus* sp., *Pseudomonas aeruginosa,* and related bacteria would be tested by these methods.
- Automatic systems used in clinical laboratories for identification and antimicrobial susceptibility testing of bacterial isolates, e.g., Microscan and Vitek, are based on the microdilution standard.
- Microorganisms such as *Streptococcus pneumoniae, Haemophilus influenzae, Mycobacterium,* and fungi, which do not grow well in CAMHM, are tested with different media and reference standards.
  - Although standard laboratory methods have been developed, the clinical significance of the in vitro test may not be known.
  - Care in interpretation of in vitro data is essential.
- When resistance to a penicillin or cephalosporin is due to a beta-lactamase, bacteria can be tested for possession of a beta-lactamase by the nitrocefin chromogenic cephalosporin substrate test.
  - A portion of the bacterial culture is placed on a filter paper disk bearing nitrocefin.
  - The test reagent turns purple when the beta-lactam bond is broken by beta-lactamase.

STREPTOCOCCUS PNEUMONIAE

- *Streptococcus pneumoniae* is screened for resistance to penicillin by a 1.0 μg oxacillin disk on cation-adjusted Mueller-Hinton (CAMH) agar with 5% sheep blood using a direct colony suspension inoculum.
- An inhibitory zone size of over 20 mm is interpreted as susceptible and is equivalent to a minimal inhibitory concentration (MIC) breakpoint of 0.06 μg/mL.
- *S. pneumoniae* isolates, which produce a 19-mm zone, may be intermediate or resistant and rarely susceptible.
- The physician must be told that the isolate may be resistant to penicillin and that a lysed horse blood (LHB) CAMH broth dilution test will be set up with penicillin, cefotaxime, ceftriaxone, meropenem, and vancomycin in order to determine resistance.
  - LHB/CAMH broth medium supports the growth of *S. pneumoniae.*
- Strains that test in the intermediate category, MIC 0.12 to 1.0 μg/mL, may respond to usual doses of penicillin.
- When patients have meningitis, maximum doses of agents that enter the CSF will be required.[45, 54, 92, 93]

ANTIMICROBIAL SUSCEPTIBILITY TESTING

HAEMOPHILUS INFLUENZAE

- *Haemophilus influenzae* does not grow in Mueller-Hinton medium, the standard antimicrobial susceptibility test medium.
- In order to test the MIC for antimicrobials, the NCCLS recommends a specific test medium and standards.
- If a test is available to detect an inactivating enzyme, this can be used for determining resistant strains, such as beta-lactamase and chloramphenicol acetyltransferase.
- Resistance to penicillins and cephalosporins not due to beta-lactamase is detected by the high MIC of these isolates.[52, 54, 82, 93]

STAPHYLOCOCCUS AUREUS

- Most strains of *S. aureus* produce beta-lactamase and are resistant to penicillin.
- The prevalence of methicillin-resistant *S. aureus* (MRSA) (e.g., nafcillin or oxacillin resistance) is increasing in most hospitals.
    - As a consequence, the glycopeptide vancomycin has become the antibiotic of choice for treating MRSA.
    - Now vancomycin intermediate strains (MIC 8 to 16 μg/mL) are appearing in *S. aureus* and coagulase-negative staphylococcus.
- New drugs including oxazolidinones, new glycopeptides and glycylcyclines are under investigation.
    - Mupiricin when applied directly to anterior nares controls carriage and has diminished infections by *S. aureus* after dialysis and cardiac surgery.
    - Mupiricin-resistant *S. aureus* organisms have been found.[59, 93]

ANAEROBES

- An NCCLS agar-dilution standard for susceptibility testing of anaerobes has been established, but it is laborious and not economical.
- Other methods, broth microdilution and E-test (A-B Biodisk), are much less laborious, but major errors have been reported with penicillin and ceftriaxone among beta-lactamase-producing strains.
- It is suggested that anaerobes with known resistance such as *Bacteroides fragilis* group, *Prevotella* spp., *Fusobacterium* spp., *Clostridium* spp., and *Bilophila wadsworthia* be tested periodically to detect resistance developing within a hospital.
- Slow primary growth of anaerobic bacteria and prolonged time to isolate and test susceptibility of bacteria combined with variable use of empiric therapy and surgical therapy has led to limited correlation between clinical outcome and in vitro tests.

TESTS FOR FUNGAL RESPIRATORY TRACT INFECTIONS[95-104]

GENERAL

- Direct examination of specimens for fungi can yield a very rapid diagnosis. The time factor is especially important because culture, the main alternative system for detection and identification, may require as long as 6 to 8 weeks with some fungi, such as *Histoplasma capsulatum.*
- Use of optical methods, such as phase contrast, Nomarski, dark-field and reduced bright-field illumination, which increase contrast, will distinguish the cell walls of fungi as compared to the membranes without walls seen in animal cells.
  - The walls, which contain polysaccharide materials including chitin, can be stained by periodic acid–Schiff (PAS), Gomori methenamine silver (GMS), or calcofluor white (chitin).
  - Giemsa staining distinguishes the nuclei and cytoplasm of fungal eukaryotic cells and locates by contrast the cell wall that is not stained by Giemsa.
- Fungi often are present in small numbers in specimens. It is important to obtain as much of a tissue or fluid as possible and to release the organism for culture by mincing (into 1-mm squares), hemolysis or mucolysis (if necessary), and centrifugation to concentrate the specimen.
- Antigen detection by immunofluorescent staining is relatively rapid.
  - This technique has been most successful in detecting *Pneumocystis carinii.*
  - Antigen detection systems are successful using serum and cerebrospinal fluid for *Cryptococcus neoformans* and urine or serum for *Histoplasma capsulatum*
- Culture methods use three main groups of constituents: *nutrients* such as peptones, meat infusions (brain heart infusion-BHI), and sugars; *antimicrobials* against bacteria, such as gentamicin, ciprofloxacin, chloramphenicol; and *differential* constituents that distinguish fungi such as birdseed extract or caffeic acid to detect the phenol oxidase of *C. neoformans.*
- Cultures are incubated at 30°C or less and taken to a biosafety cabinet to open the cultures and make preparations for examination.
  - Yeasts can be identified by carbohydrate assimilation tests, tests for certain enzymes, morphology, and growth characteristics.
  - Molds are identified chiefly by morphology or growth factors.
- Nucleic acid probes (Gen-Probe) are available to identify dimorphic fungi *Blastomyces dermatitidis, Coccidioides immitis,* and *Histoplasma capsulatum* by a hybridization protection chemiluminescent assay, which can be completed in 2 hours.
- These same dimorphic fungi can be identified by an immunodiffusion test of fungal extractable antigen which may take 24 to 48 hours to complete (TABLES 7–11 and 7–12).

TABLE 7–11

Serologic Tests for Diagnosis of Fungal Diseases

Disease	CF	EIA	ID	LA
Aspergillosis	–	–	X	–
Blastomycosis	X	X	X	–
Coccidioidomycosis	X	X	X	–
Cryptococcosis	–	–	–	XA
Histoplasmosis	X	XA	X	–
Paracoccidioidomycosis	X	–	X	–
Sporotrichosis	–	X	–	X
Zygomycosis	–	X	X	–

Key: CF = complement fixation; ID = immunodiffusion; EIA = enzyme-linked immunoassay; LA = latex agglutination; XA = antigen detection.

TESTS FOR FUNGAL RESPIRATORY TRACT INFECTIONS

GENERAL

TABLE 7-12

Tests for Identification of Fungal Cultures

Fungus	Antibody vs. Exoantigen	Fluorescein Conjugated Antibody	Nucleic Acid Probe
Aspergillus spp.	X	–	–
Blastomyces dermatitidis	X	X	X
Coccidioides immitis	X	X	X
Cryptococcus neoformans	–	X	X
Histoplasma capsulatum	X	X	X
Paracoccidioides brasiliensis	X	X	–
Pneumocystis carinii	–	X	–
Pseudallescheria boydii	–	X	–
Sporothrix schenckii	X	X	–

CANDIDA sp.[98]

- Diagnosis is made by direct examination to identify oval yeasts with buds, which elongate to form pseudohyphae.
- *C. albicans* yeasts incubated in documented satisfactory serum 3 hours at 37°C form germ-tube progenitors of hyphae.
- *Candida* species can be identified by carbohydrate assimilation.
- *C. glabrata* and *C. krusei* are usually resistant to fluconazole.
- *C. lusitaniae* is often resistant to amphotericin B.

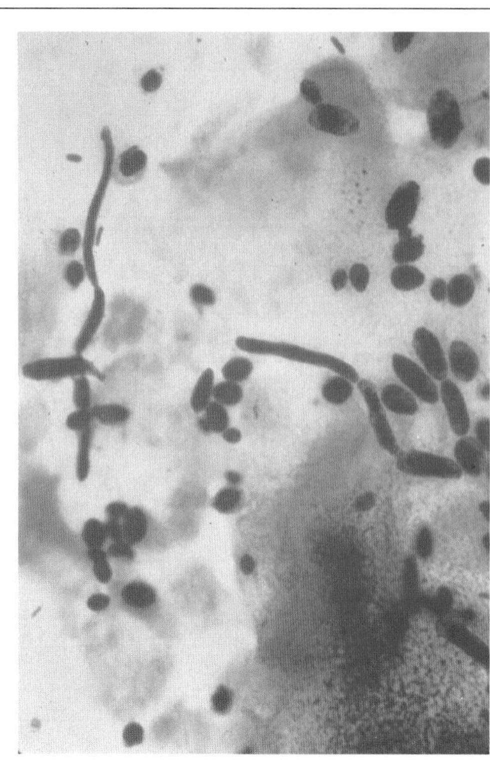

FIGURE 7-38

Scraping from thrush lesion on oral mucosa shows yeasts and pseudohyphae. Oval budding yeasts and filamentous periodically constricted pseudohyphae characteristic of *Candida* sp. are present. *Candida albicans, C. tropicalis, C. parapsilosis,* and *C. krusei* are most often seen on the human mucosal surfaces along with *C.* (*Torulopsis*) *glabrata,* which lacks pseudohyphae. Patients receiving immunosuppressive medication, antibiotic therapy, or who have immunodeficiency disease develop superficial ragged or plaque-like lesions on the oropharynx, sinus apertures, larynx, epiglottis, trachea, and bronchi. (From Koneman ZW: Color Atlas of Diagnostic Microbiology, 7th ed. Philadelphia, JB Lippincott, 1992.)

TESTS FOR FUNGAL RESPIRATORY TRACT INFECTIONS

CRYPTOCOCCUS NEOFORMANS[95, 99, 100]

- Hematogenous spread to meninges, bones, and joints may occur. Dissemination may be widespread in HIV-1 infection.
- Diagnosis is by detection of spherical to oval encapsulated yeasts in direct examination; culture of sputum, BAL, or CSF; and tissue biopsy. Blood or bone marrow culture may also be positive.
- Carbohydrate assimilation, growth at 37°C, and positive phenol/oxidase (birdseed agar test) identifies *Cryptococcus neoformans.*
- The nucleic acid probe (Gen-Probe, Accu-Probe) provides rapid identification (2 hours) after adequate culture is obtained.
- A sensitized latex particle agglutination test on CSF or pronase-treated serum is highly specific for diagnosis if rheumatoid factor is not present in serum.

FIGURE 7–39

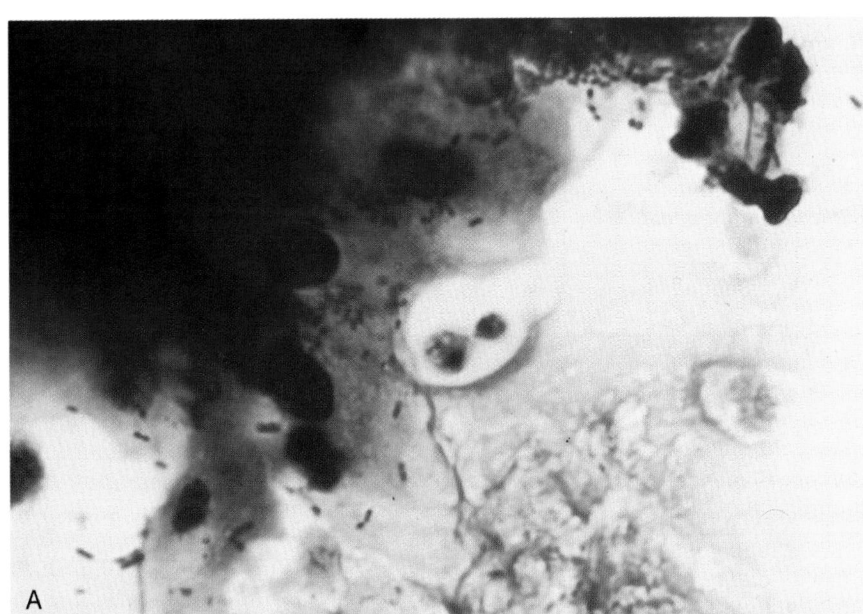

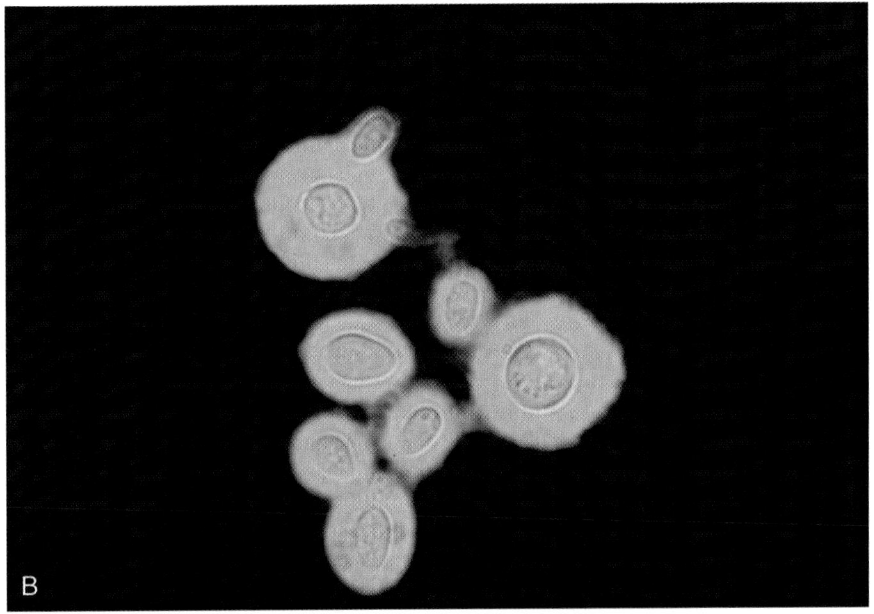

A, *Cryptococcus neoformans* encapsulated budding yeast from induced sputum stained by Giemsa. *C. neoformans* is found in aged pigeon droppings and *C. neoformans* var *gatti* is found in the flowers of the river red gum tree. Primary infection is pulmonary. Tissue response is by macrophages and lymphocytes. Capsules and vacuoles in macrophages, which contain capsular material, can be stained by mucicarmine and PAS. **B,** The large clear capsule of *C. neoformans* is demonstrated against the black background of India Ink.

TESTS FOR FUNGAL RESPIRATORY TRACT INFECTIONS

DIMORPHIC FUNGI[96, 98, 101, 102]

- The dimorphic fungi that cause systemic infections have a mycelial form (mold), which occurs in particular geographic areas and soil types and in culture.
- Microconidia or arthroconidia are 2 to 6 μm in diameter. When aerosolized and inhaled, can produce an infection.
- In infected tissues, a yeast form or spherule of characteristic form is produced inside infected cells.
- Laboratories that culture these fungi or process infected tissues must provide a biosafety cabinet and train their staff in safe practices.

TABLE 7-13

Characteristics of Dimorphic Fungi

Fungus	Epidemiology	Infectious Form	Tissue Form
Histoplasma capsulatum	Alkaline soil, high-nitrogen bird and bat guano throughout the world; U.S. states Mississippi, Missouri, Ohio river valleys	Microconidia 3–5 μm	Oval yeast 2–4 μm
H. capsulatum var. *duboisii*	Central Africa	Microconidia 3–5 μm	Thick-walled yeast 10–15 μm
Blastomyces dermatitidis	River and stream banks, Mississippi and Ohio river valleys	Microconidia	Thick-walled yeast 8–15 μm
Coccidioides immitis	Semiarid lower-Sonoran, Southwestern United States, Mexico, Central and South America	Arthroconidia 3–6 μm	Spherule 20–60 μm containing endospores 2–4 μm
Paracoccidioides brasiliensis	Central and South America	Microconidia	Thick-walled multiple budding yeasts 15–30 μm

Histoplasma Capsulatum[95, 96, 101,102]

- Infection occurs by inhalation of microconidia.
  - 95% of infections are self-limited and are detectable by complement-fixation (CF) and immunodiffusion serologic tests.
  - Disseminated disease may occur with a large primary inoculum.
  - Reactivation with dissemination may occur in elderly and immunocompromised patients.
- Serologic tests may be nonreactive in immunodeficient patients.
- Direct examination or culture of BAL, sputum, transbronchial lung biopsy, blood, bone marrow, other tissues, and mucosal lesions may yield *H. capsulatum.*
- The Isolator lysis centrifugation system (Wampole) is useful for culturing fungi from blood.
- Inhibitory mold agar or BHI media with antibacterial antibiotics are useful for culture.
- The nucleic acid probe (Gen-Probe, Accu-Probe) provides rapid (2 hours) identification of the culture.
- Alternatively, the culture may be extracted to yield cell-free exoantigens, which can be identified with specific antisera in an immunodiffusion test.
- *H. capsulatum* var. *duboisii,* found in Central Africa, has thick-walled yeasts (10 to 15 μm) in tissues.
- The *Histoplasma* antigen (HPA) test (Histoplasmosis Reference Laboratory, University of Indiana) is useful for the diagnosis of disseminated histoplasmosis.
  - The HPA test detects a heat-stable polysaccharide antigen with about 90% sensitivity in urine specimens.
  - False positive results have occurred with infection by other fungi, such as *Paracoccidioides*

(continued)

TESTS FOR FUNGAL RESPIRATORY TRACT INFECTIONS

DIMORPHIC FUNGI

Histoplasma capsulatum

brasiliensis, Penicillium marnefei, Blastomyces dermatitidis, and Coccidioides immitis.

- Culture is the definitive diagnostic system.
  - However, culture may take from 1 to 3 days with *Candida* to 3 to 8 weeks with some of the dimorphic fungi, such as *Histoplasma capsulatum.*
  - In order to speed culture, specimens should be concentrated by centrifugation prior to inoculation onto media.
- In order to obtain early clinically useful information, exudates and BAL should be examined directly with phase microscopy, and smears or tissue touch preparations should be stained by Giemsa and examined.
  - Diagnosis by antigen or antibody detection may be useful when culture is failing.
  - Delayed hypersensitivity skin tests may interfere with subsequent serologic tests. They are most useful for epidemiologic studies.
  - Nucleic Acid Probes. Tests for rapid identification of fungal cultures provide a more rapid report than culture based on morphologic tests.

FIGURE 7–40

A, *Histoplasma capsulatum* culture with infective microconidia and characteristic tuberculate macroconidia on hyphae. (From American Society of Clinical Pathologists, Publications Group. Chicago: ASCP Press.) **B,** *H. capsulatum* yeast from 2 to 4 μm in diameter in macrophage from bronchoalveolar lavage.

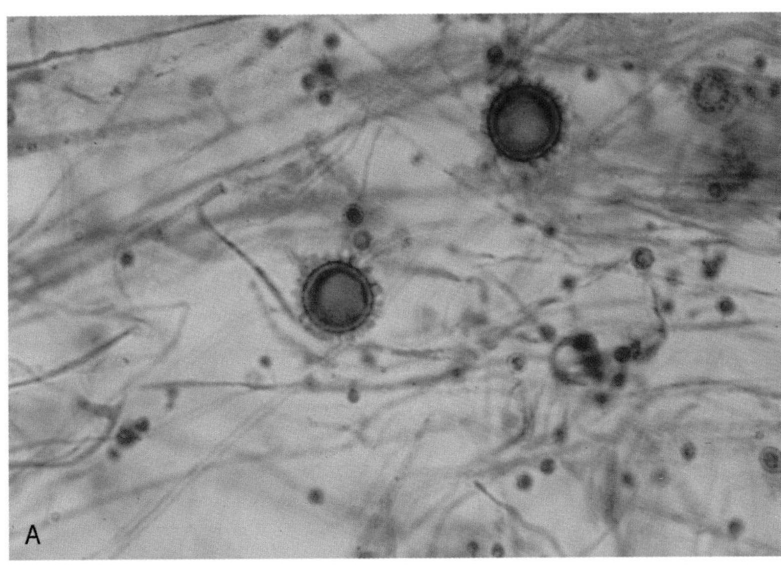

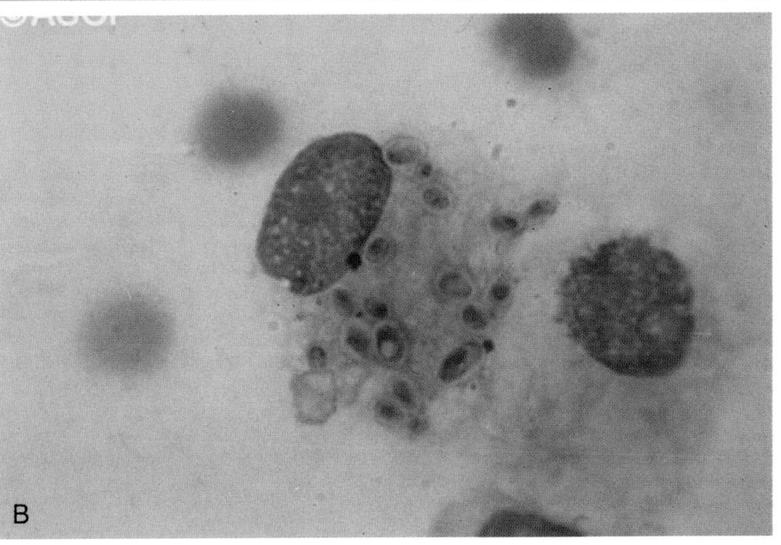

TESTS FOR FUNGAL RESPIRATORY TRACT INFECTIONS

DIMORPHIC FUNGI

Coccidioides immitis[95, 96, 101]

- *C. immitis*[101] with its characteristic spherule, which contains endospores, often can be identified in a few minutes of microscopic examination of exudate, BAL, body fluid, sputum, or fine-needle tissue aspirate.
  - Adjacent spherules, which can vary in size, may be confused for broad-based budding *Blastomyces dermatitidis* yeasts, especially in PAP stain.
  - This error can be avoided by looking for endospores in the spherules and avoiding dense stains.
- *C. immitis* grows within 3 to 5 days in the specimens listed here.
- Usually only 2 to 3 extra days of incubation yields enough culture for identification by nucleic acid probe.
- The CF test and the immunodiffusion analogues of the tube precipitin test have received extensive clinical study.
  - A rising CF test titer indicates dissemination or increasing severity of the disease in an immunocompetent patient.
  - CF test titers are variable from different laboratories.
  - Responsiveness in these serologic tests is variable in AIDS patients.

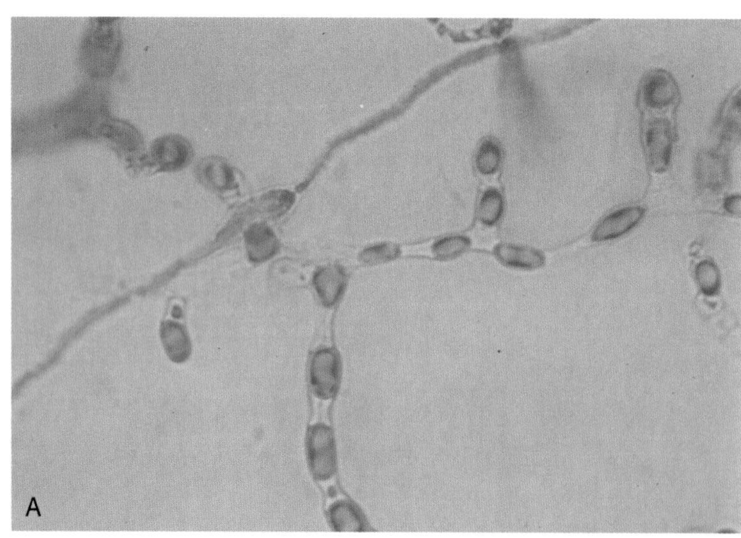

FIGURE 7–41

A, *Coccidioides immitis* with barrel-shaped arthroconidia in hyphal filament. **B,** Adjacent thick-walled spherules of *C. immitis* recovered from BAL. Spherules may be 20 to 60 μm in diameter. They may contain many endospores 2 to 4 μm in diameter.

TESTS FOR FUNGAL RESPIRATORY TRACT INFECTIONS

DIMORPHIC FUNGI

Aspergillus sp.[95, 103, 104]

- *Aspergillus* sp. are saprophytes in soil and dead and decaying plants and are found in air filtrates.
- They are frequently recovered in clinical specimens without clinical significance.
- Aspergillosis is, however, the second most common fungal infection requiring hospitalization.
- Invasive disease may occur in patients with granulocytopenia as a consequence of their disease, corticosteroid or cytotoxic therapy, immunosuppression for transplantation or as therapy for AIDS.
- Repeated culturing of the same *Aspergillus* sp. heightens significance.
- Colonization of the external auditory canal and pulmonary cavities (fungus ball) may occur without invasion.
- *Aspergillus* spp. most commonly found in invasive lesions or producing antibody are *A. fumigatus, A. flavus, A. niger,* and *A. terreus.*
- *Aspergillus* grows readily in commonly used fungal culture media. These fungi produce a hyaline, unpigmented mycelium.
- Morphology and pigmentation of conidiophores, conidial heads, and conidia are used to separate *Aspergillus* into "group" series.
- IgG antibody as measured by immunodiffusion is elevated in patients with allergic bronchopulmonary disease or persisting fungus ball.
  - There may be little or no antibody against *Aspergillus* sp. in patients with invasive disease.
  - So far, antigen detection tests have been specific but lack the sensitivity required for early diagnosis of invasion.
  - False negative results may be related to time of specimen collection as related to course of disease and antifungal therapy.
  - PCR-based assays with certain primers are still under investigation and they appear to be sensitive and specific.

FIGURE 7-42

Aspergillus sp. fungus ball in lung with superficial invasion of the lung.

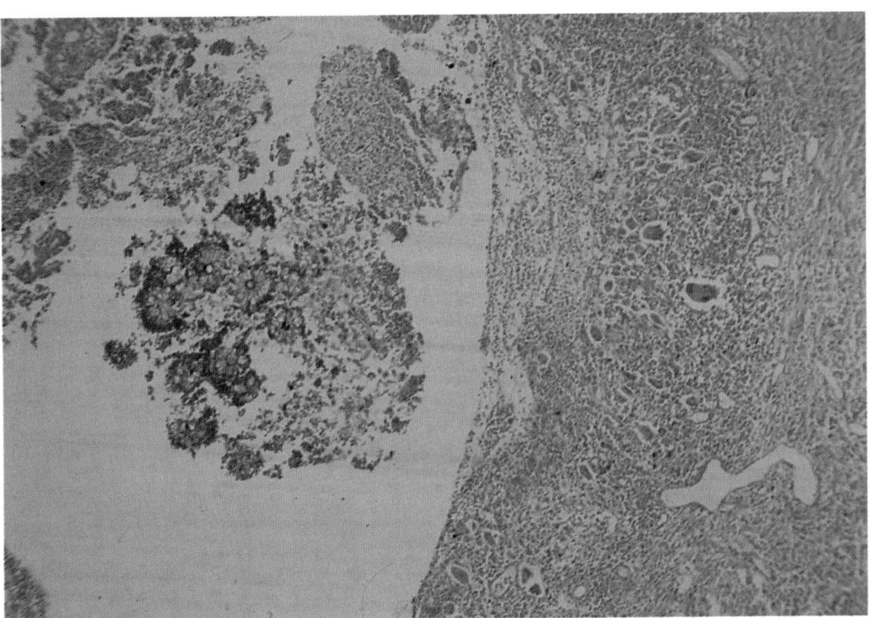

TESTS FOR FUNGAL RESPIRATORY TRACT INFECTIONS

DIMORPHIC FUNGI

Pneumocystis carinii[97]

- *Pneumocystis carinii,*[97] now recognized to be a fungus, cannot be cultured in vitro.
- There are no reliable serologic tests for antigen or antibody to *P. carinii.*
- The relationship between *Pneumocystis* recovered from humans and animal models of pneumocystosis is under study.
- *Pneumocystis* pneumonia and extrapulmonary disease are essentially diseases of immunocompromised patients.
- The diagnosis of *P. carinii* pneumonia (PCP) can be made using induced sputum in 75 to 85% of patients found to have PCP by the aggregate of induced sputum, BAL, or clinical response to treatment.
  - The induced sputum is generated by inhalation of aerosolized 3 to 5% saline by patients with sufficient respiratory reserve to cough.
  - The specimen is mucolysed with dithiothreitol concentrated by centrifugation, smeared and stained by a Giemsa-like stain (Diff-Quik).
  - Other stains, such as methenamine silver and toluidine blue O, produce similar results.
  - Direct immunofluorescent stains based on monoclonal antibodies are sensitive and specific; PCR tests using serum are under study.

FIGURE 7–43

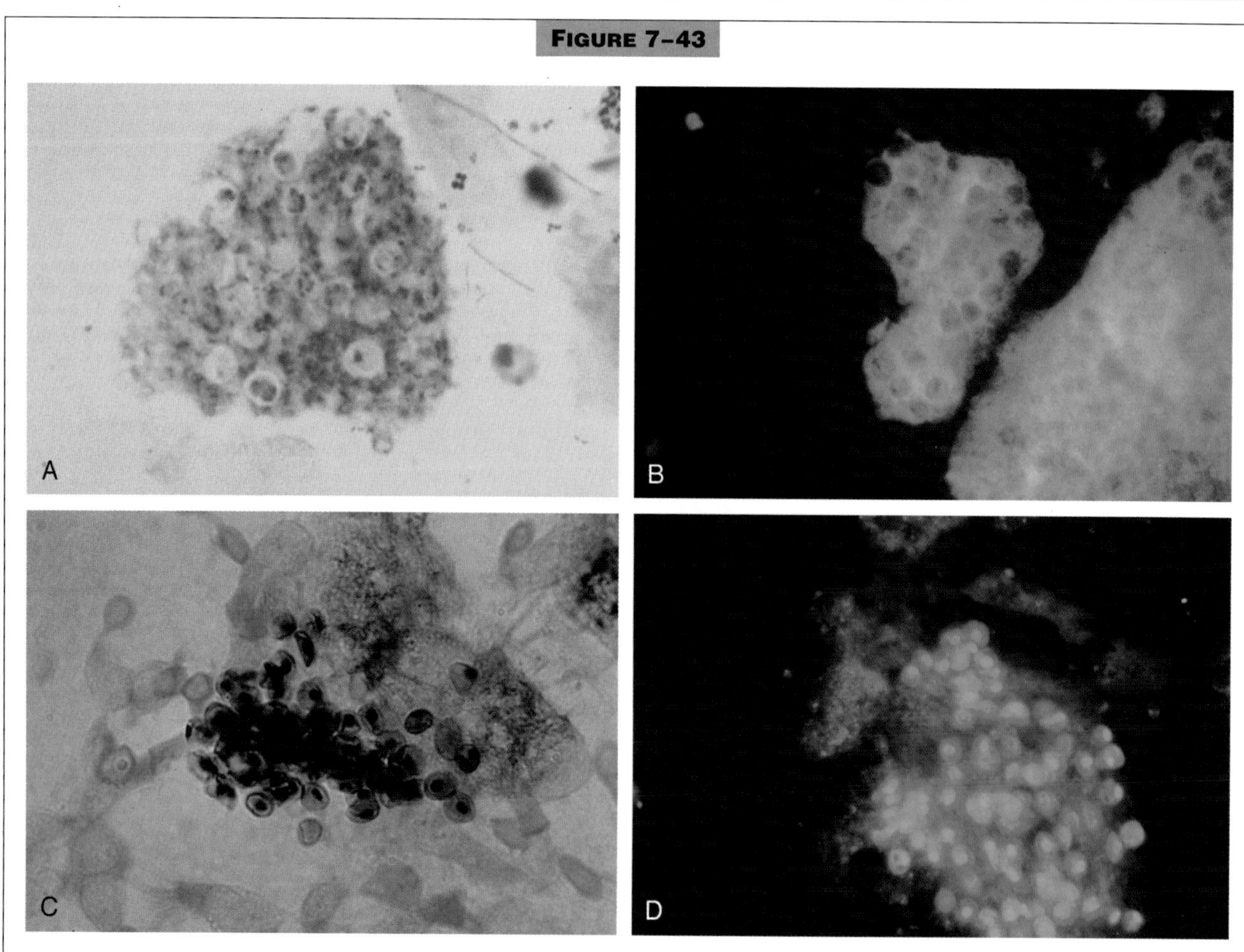

A, *Pneumocystis carinii* in adherent clump of cysts and trophic forms dislodged by sputum induction from respiratory system. Diff-Quik stain. **B,** Direct immunofluorescent stain of *Pneumocystis.* **C,** Gomori methenamine silver stain of *P. carinii.* **D,** Calcofluor stain of *P. carinii* with green filter. (**C,** from Hadley WK, Ng UL: *Pneumocysts. In* Murray PR (Ed-in-Chief): Manual of Clinical Microbiology, 7th ed. Washington, DC, American Society for Microbiology, 1999.)

TESTS FOR PARASITES[105, 106, 134]

NEMATODES

• Among the nematodes (round worms) some have a life cycle that includes larval migration through the right side of the heart and lungs, resulting in pneumonitis with blood and tissue accumulations of eosinophils.

• The extent of the pneumonitis is dependent upon the larval burden.

• In most cases the patient is asymptomatic and the pneumonitis is visible only as a radiographic infiltrate lasting 1 to 2 weeks.

TABLE 7–14

Helminths Associated with Respiratory Infections

Infecting Agent	Pulmonary Disease	Epidemiology	Laboratory Diagnosis
Ascaris lumbricoides Nematode	• Pneumonitis due to larval migration through lung • Peripheral eosinophilia (Loeffler's syndrome)	Moist warm sandy soil; poor sanitation; ingestion of human feces–contaminated soil with mature larvae	Examination of fecal sediment for typical *A. lumbricoides* ova
Hookworm *Necator americanus* *Ancylostoma duodenale* Nematode	• Pneumonitis and peripheral eosinophilia (Loeffler's syndrome) due to larval migration through lung	Moist warm sandy soil; poor sanitation; filariform larvae penetrate skin	Examination of fecal sediment for typical hookworm ova
Strongyloides stercoralis Nematode	• Primary infection • Filariform larval invasion of skin; autoinfection; hyperinfection: massive invasion by larvae through lung in patients with immunocompromised status: corticosteroids, HIV-1, malnutrition	Moist warm sandy soil; poor sanitation; free-living cycle in soil; filariform larvae penetrate skin; autoinfection may cause persisting infection for decades; hyperinfection may occur if patient becomes immunocompromised	Examination of fecal sediment for rhabditiform larvae; duodenal aspirate for rhabditiform larvae; sputum, tracheal aspirate for larvae in hyperinfection
Visceral larva migrans *Toxocara canis* Nematode	• Humans ingest mature ova from dog feces; larvae hatch in intestine, gain circulation, fail to break through capillary in lung and are carried to viscera	Pneumonitis and granulomatous reaction in liver, small intestine, brain, retina	EIA serologic test with larval stage antigen extract embryonated eggs
Echinococcus granulosus "Dog tapeworm" Cestode	• Hydatid cyst, contains scolices, daughter cysts, hooklets, "hydatid sand," 20% hydatid cysts in lung	Dogs develop tapeworm after ingesting infected organs from sheep and other animals; humans ingest ova from tapeworm in dog feces	Magnetic resonance imaging; surgical removal of hydatid cyst with "sand," screen for antibody by EIA or IHA, IB 8-kD band
Paragonimus westermani "Lung fluke" Trematode	• Fibrous capsule in lung containing two flukes, ova and exudate • Eosinophilia, hemoptysis, abscess	Metacercaria *P. westermani* in uncooked crabs, crayfish Central America, Equatorial Africa, Southeast Asia	Operculated ovum in sputum/fecal sediment; CF = sensitive/specific; IF = 8-kD band, 96% sensitivity, 1/210 false positive results

TESTS FOR PARASITES

ASCARIS LUMBRICOIDES AND HOOKWORMS[107-110]

- The clinical syndrome with transient low-grade fever was described by Loeffler who provided medical services to a population that used human feces to fertilize their crops.
- The acronym PIE (pulmonary infiltrates—eosinophilia) is sometimes used to identify this syndrome.
- This syndrome is seen with *Ascaris lumbricoides,* which is transmitted by ingestion of embryonated ova from fecal contaminated soil.
- The hookworms (*Ancylostoma duodenale* and *Necator americanus*) and *Strongyloides stercoralis* are transmitted by filariform larvae, which develop in fecal contaminated soil and burrow through the skin to the lymphatics and venules before reaching the right side of the heart and lungs.
- Diagnosis of the syndrome is usually based on a history of exposure to human feces–contaminated soil, radiographic evidence of a transient pneumonic infiltrate, and peripheral eosinophilia.
- The number of larvae in transit through the lungs is usually so small that examination of respiratory specimens for larvae do not yield a diagnosis.
- Diagnosis of the infecting worm can be made by examining concentrated stool sediments during the period from infection to discharge of ova by the mature female worm.

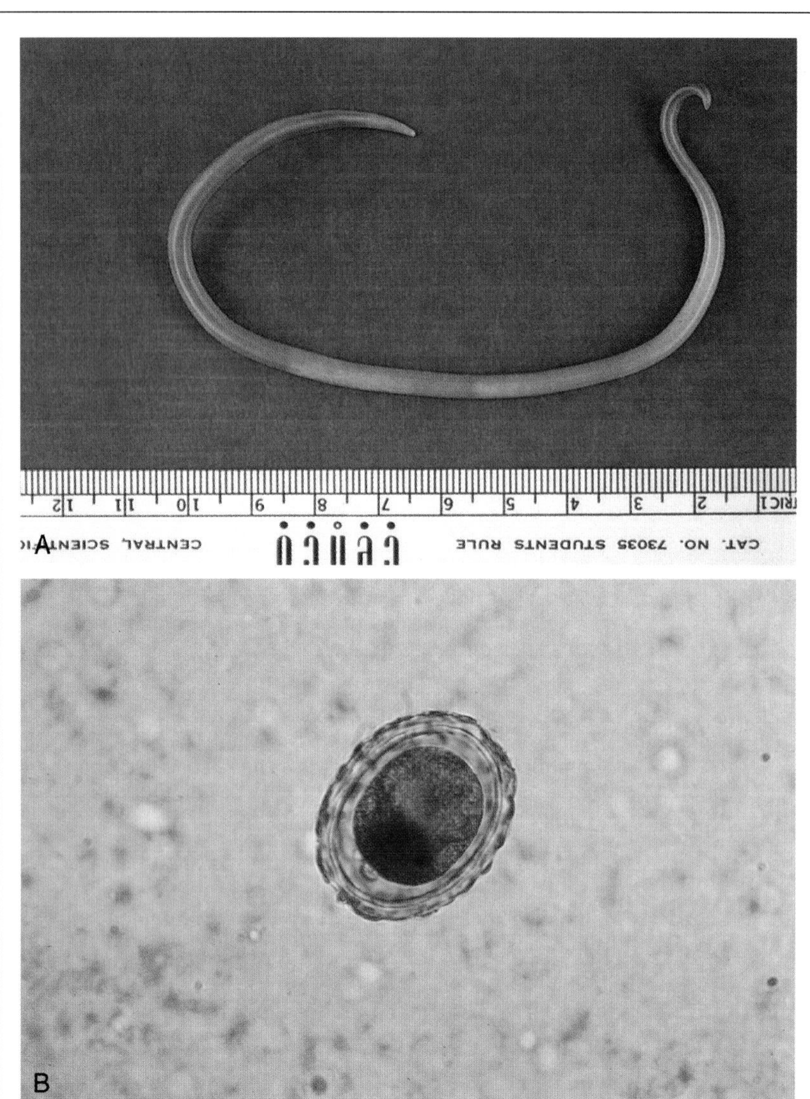

FIGURE 7–44

A, *Ascaris* adult worm. **B,** *Ascaris* ovum.

TESTS FOR PARASITES

ASCARIS LUMBRICOIDES AND HOOKWORMS

FIGURE 7–45

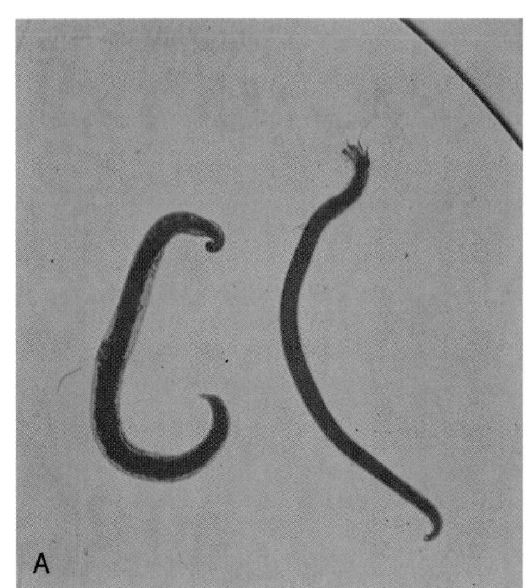

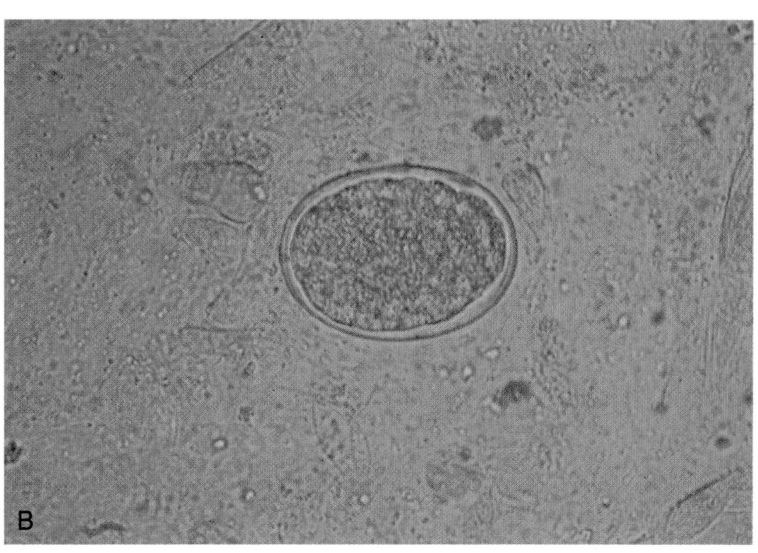

A, Adult hookworm. **B,** Hookworm ovum. (*A* and *B*, from Koneman EW, Richie L, Tiemann C: Laboratory Parasitology. MEDCOM, Inc., 1973.)

Strongyloides stercoralis[111–115, 134]

The eggs mature into rhabditiform larvae (250 × 20 μm), which can be found in stool sediment concentrates. Larvae may penetrate the colonic mucosa or perianal skin and maintain infection by autoinfection.

- *Strongyloides stercoralis* infection can persist in humans for decades after residence in endemic regions, which have warm moist sandy soil with poor sanitation.
- A process of autoinfection by larvae from the host is thought to maintain the infection without significant symptoms.
  - If the individual becomes immunosuppressed by corticosteroid or other therapy, cancer, malnutrition, or HIV-1 infection, hyperinfection syndrome may occur.
  - Hyperinfection is characterized by severe generalized abdominal pain, diffuse pulmonary infiltrates, ileus, shock, and sepsis with gram-negative bacteria.
  - Eosinophilia may be absent.
  - Abundant rhabditiform larvae and possible other stages can be seen in wet mounts or Gram-stained or Diff-Quik–stained sputum, tracheal aspirates, and BAL.
- *S. stercoralis* larvae break out of the pulmonary capillaries and migrate to the duodenum and upper jejunum where they penetrate the mucosa, mature, and deposit eggs in the mucosa that mature to form rhabditiform larvae.
- Diagnosis of infection can be accomplished by searching for rhabditiform larvae in aspirates or biopsies from the duodenal mucosa (sensitivity: 39 to 91%) or uptake on the string of the Enterotest capsule (sensitivity: 28%).
- Rhabditiform larvae are the stage passed in feces and can be seen in concentrated fecal sediments (sensitivity of one test 66%, sensitivity of two tests 84%). Serologic tests are available when the parasite cannot be found in duodenal aspirates or fecal sediments.
- EIA tests using filariform stage antigen have a sensitivity of 84 to 92%; some immunocompromised persons have detectable IgG antibodies against *S. stercoralis.*
- Crossreactions with other nematodes may occur; from 8 to 16% of *Strongyloides* carriers may have negative serologic tests.
- Immunocompetent individuals have markedly decreased antibody 6 weeks after successful chemotherapy.

TESTS FOR PARASITES

ASCARIS LUMBRICOIDES AND HOOKWORMS

Strongyloides stercoralis

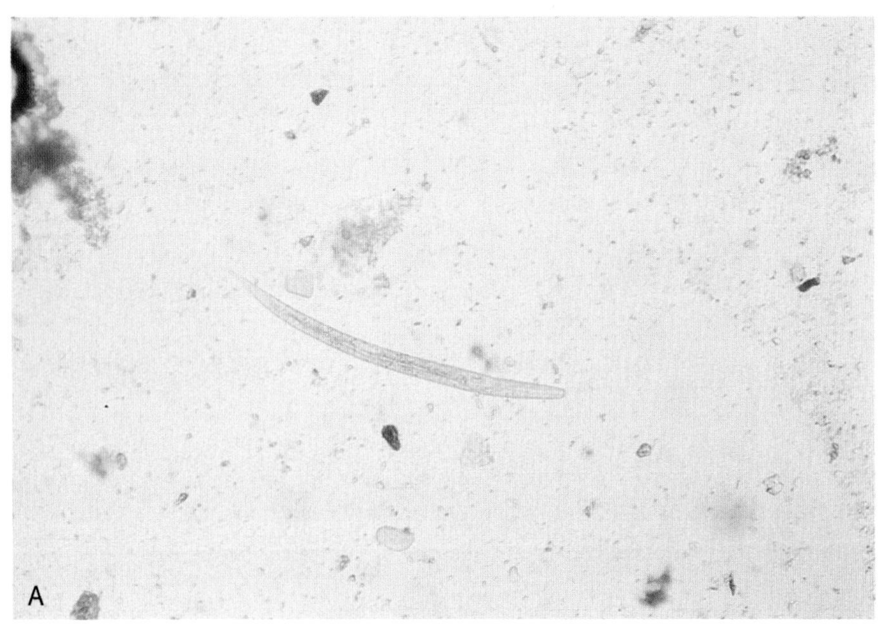

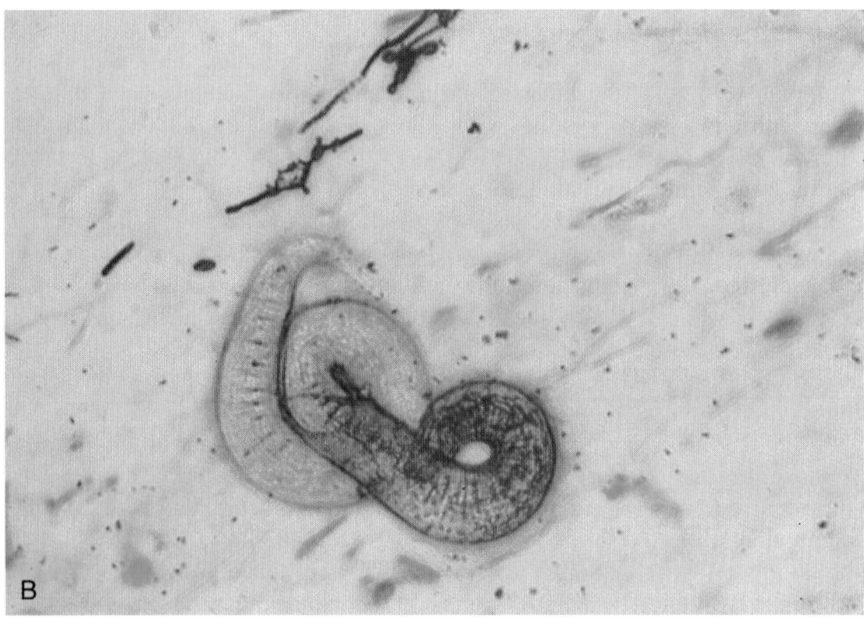

FIGURE 7–46

A, *Strongyloides stercoralis* rhabditiform larva from fecal concentrate. Filariform larvae penetrate the skin, pass through the right side of the heart, and break into the pulmonary alveolus. They are coughed up and migrate to the small intestine where the parthenogenic adult lays eggs in the mucosal epithelium. **B,** *Strongyloides* larva from sputum of patient with hyperinfection syndrome. Gram stain.

TESTS FOR PARASITES

TOXOCARA CANIS[116, 117, 134]

- The visceral larva migrans (VLM) syndrome is caused by migration of *Toxocara canis* as well as the larval form of other animal parasites.
- The syndrome is seen most often in young children.
- Although the larval form cannot complete its migration in humans leading to a mature nematode, it can produce lesions in the lungs, liver, and retina (ocular larva migrans).
  - The larvae may remain encapsulated in dense fibrous tissue.
  - Other larvae may continue migration, forming granulomas in the affected tissue.
- Peripheral eosinophilia from 20 to 40% may be the only detectable sign. Patients with a greater degree of eosinophilia usually have fever, hepatomegaly, pulmonary infiltrates, neurologic signs, and endophthalmitis.
- Antibody detection tests for *Toxocara* are generally the preferred means of confirming the diagnosis of VLM.
  - An EIA test, which uses a larval-stage antigen extracted from embryonated eggs, is used most often.
  - It is not possible to determine the true sensitivity and specificity of the EIA test because there is no other method of diagnosis.
  - Compared to presumptive diagnosis, the sensitivity is 78% at a titer of 1:32 or greater.
  - The titer does not indicate current infection; it is estimated that 2.8% of nearly 9000 persons studied had asymptomatic toxocariasis.

TROPICAL PULMONARY EOSINOPHILIA[118, 119]

- This syndrome is seen in persons who have lived in areas endemic for *Wuchereria bancrofti* or *Brugia malayi* filariasis.
- It is characterized by chronic nocturnal cough, low-grade fever, and eosinophilia.
- There may be high levels of IgG and IgE antibodies in the absence of peripheral blood microfilariae.
- Pulmonary function tests may show restrictive defects, and chest films may show reticulonodular opacities.
- The clinical diagnosis is confirmed by a clearance of symptoms by a therapeutic trial with diethylcarbamazine.

DIROFILARIA IMMITIS[120]

- The dog heartworm microfilariae are transmitted by mosquitoes common in many parts of the world including the southeastern United States.
- The adult worm develops in the heart and lungs of dogs but only rarely develops into the adult worm in humans.
- If maturation to the adult worm occurs, a pulmonary granuloma may form, sometimes appearing as a solitary nodule.

TESTS FOR PARASITES

ECHINOCOCCUS GRANULOSUS (HYDATID DISEASE)[121-124, 134]

- *Echinococcus granulosus,* which causes unilocular hydatid disease in humans, occurs wherever dogs or canines have free access to the viscera of infected animals such as sheep, goats, cattle, camels, and pigs.
- The dog becomes infected by ingesting the protoscolices present in the hydatid-infected animals.
- The protoscolices mature in the small intestine of the dog and form a small (4 cm) tapeworm with a scolex bearing suckers and hooklets.
- Proglottids mature and release fertile ova, which accumulate around the anus, tail, or coat of the dog.
- Ingestion of the ova leads to development of the hydatid cyst, principally in the liver and the lung.
  - In 15 to 30% of infected patients a lung hydatid cyst is formed.
  - Intact cysts in the lungs are usually asymptomatic until they cause cough, shortness of breath, and chest pain.
  - When cyst fluid leaks, recurrent urticaria, bronchospasm, and other signs of hypersensitivity may result.
- EIA and indirect hemagglutination serologic tests are available.
  - These tests have higher sensitivity in liver hydatid disease (50 to 80%) than with pulmonary hydatid disease.
  - A significant false positive test rate occurs.
- Most diagnoses are based on imaging procedures.
- Closed aspiration of hydatid cyst is not recommended because of the risk of a hydatid antigen leakage and hypersensitivity reaction.
- Surgical removal of the hydatid cyst is generally recommended.
- Hydatid sand made up of daughter cysts and scolices and hooklets identifies the hydatid cyst.
- Mebendazole or albendazole treatment may replace surgical treatment.

FIGURE 7–47

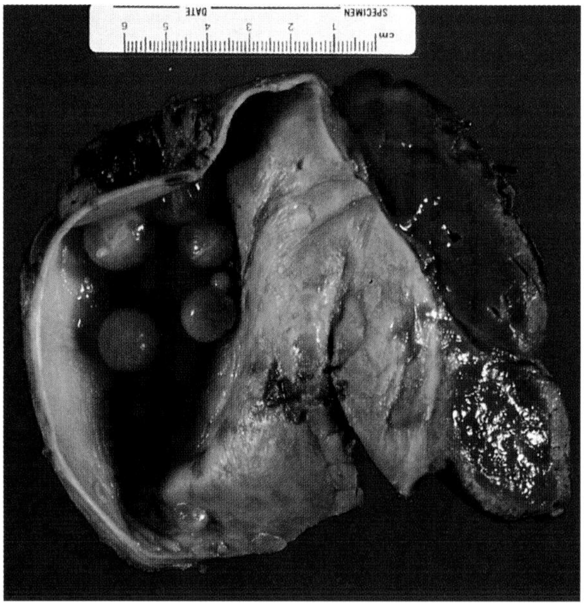

Hydatid cyst. (Courtesy of Dr. Kirk Jones.)

TESTS FOR PARASITES

PARAGONIMUS WESTERMANI (LUNG FLUKE)[126, 127, 134]

- The larval form matures in the lung surrounded by an eosinophilic and polymorphonuclear leukocyte exudate.
  - A fibrous capsule and mononuclear cells surround the mature flukes after 5 to 6 weeks.
  - The ova rupture into the bronchioles and appear in the sputum and eventually in the feces.
  - During this stage the patient may have cough with hemoptysis and mucoid sputum.
  - The disease may resemble bronchitis or tuberculosis.
- The ova are operculated with a raised shoulder and measure 80 to 120 μm by 45 to 65 μm.
- Diagnosis can be made by examination of the sputum and fecal sediment concentrates for typical ova.
- There often are few ova, and multiple examinations may be necessary.
- Serologic tests for antibody are available.
- The CF test has been used in the past. It is sensitive and specifically useful for assessing response to therapy.
- The CF test, which is laborious, is being replaced by an EIA test and an immunoblot (IB) test that uses a crude extract of the *P. westermani* fluke.
  - Positive reactions based on an 8-kDa antigen-antibody band have been obtained with sera from 96% of patients with proven infections.
  - A single false positive result occurred, out of 210 patients tested, from a patient with *Schistosoma hematobium* infection.
  - Cross-reactivity between *Paragonimus* spp. does occur but at varying levels with different species.

FIGURE 7–48

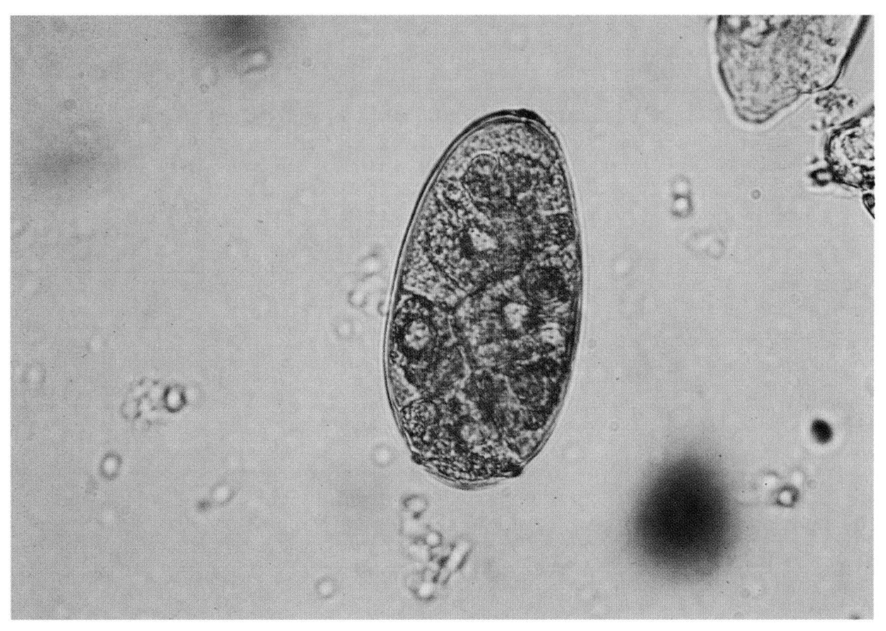

Egg of *Paragonimus westermani* recovered from sputum. This lung fluke infects humans through ingestion of fresh water crabs, or crayfish, which contain encysted metacercaria. Excystation takes place in the small intestine with penetration of the intestinal wall and migration through the peritoneal cavity, diaphragm, and pleural cavity and into the lung.

TESTS FOR PARASITES

SCHISTOSOMA (BLOOD FLUKES)[125, 126]

- Among the *Schistosoma,* three species can cause pulmonary diseases: *S. hematobium, S. japonicum,* and *S. mansoni.*
- Human infection is initiated by penetration of the intact skin by the freshwater infective stage, the cercaria.
  - This changes into a schistosomula, which migrates through the lungs and in 2 to 4 weeks settles in the liver to mature.
  - Its usual final habitat is the abdominal venous vasculature.
  - The mature worm deposits ova inside the host vasculature.
  - The eggs migrate toward the lumen of the gut or the urinary tract to be carried out by the excreta.
  - Some of the ova are retained in the host, producing a granulomatous response.
- During the initial schistosomula migration an acute febrile illness with cough, hepatosplenomegaly, adenopathy, and eosinophilia occurs.
- A chronic pulmonary schistosomiasis occurs when the *S. hematobium* ova reach the pulmonary vasculature through the inferior vena cava, producing granulomas and fibrosis in the pulmonary arteries and arterioles. This results in pulmonary hypertension and cor pulmonale.
- *S. japonicum* or *S. mansoni* can carry out a similar process by migration through anastomotic collaterals between the portal and systemic circulation.
- Diagnosis is confirmed upon biopsy, and surgical resection is performed.

TABLE 7–15

Protozoa and Microsporidia Associated with Respiratory Tract Infection

Infecting Agent	Clinical Presentation	Epidemiology	Diagnostic Specimens
Cryptosporidium parvum Protozoa-coccidian	Immunocompetent: self-limited diarrheal disease; immunocompromised: diarrhea, wasting syndrome, aspiration pneumonitis, tracheobronchitis	Worldwide distribution; found in unfiltered water; resistant to disinfectants; spread by contact with infected animals, direct person-to-person contact	Stool sediment concentrate; modified Kinyon acid-fast stain; tracheobronchial aspirate, biopsy
Entamoeba histolytica Protozoa-ameba	Lung abscess; 85% extend from liver abscess through diaphragm to lung; may also spread to lung by hematogenous route	All regions; more common in tropics with poor sanitation; ingestion of cyst form: amebic ulcers, liver abscess, lung abscess, asymptomatic	Stool specimens: *E. histolytica* EIA for *E. histolytica* ≥ 1:256 specific for liver and/or lung abscess; there may not be antibody, if restricted to intestine
Microsporidium Phylum-Microspora	Immunocompetent: self-limited, diarrhea, keratitis, and corneal ulcer; immunocompromised: diarrhea, wasting syndrome, cholangitis, keratoconjunctivitis, sinusitis, bronchitis, pneumonitis	Not certain; many animals infected; may be zoonosis; disease in immunocompromised, may be reactivation or primary infection	Direct observation; tissue biopsy, smears (thin) touch preparations; chromotrope 2R, calcofluor, PAS, silver, IFA, cell cultures, electron microscopy
Toxoplasma gondii Protozoa-coccidian	Immunocompetent: benign fever, enlarged lymph nodes, myocarditis, hepatitis, retinochoroiditis; Congenital toxoplasmosis; Immunocompromised: pneumonitis, encephalitis, and mass lesions	Worldwide distribution; infections by ingestion of oocysts present in cat feces; infection by ingestion of poorly cooked meat from animals which bear tissue cysts	Direct examination for tachyzoites, Giemsa-stained BAL and pleural fluid or biopsy touch-preparations, cell culture, EIA for IgG for past infection, EIA for IgM, in immunocompetent or congenital infection, EIA test variable in quality, IgM not useful in AIDS
Trichomonas tenax Protozoa-flagellate	Commensal in oropharynx	Oral indigenous flora; may be aspirated into lung with other agents which produce abscess	Characteristic flagellate with flagella and axostyle seen in smear stained by Giemsa or trichrome

TESTS FOR PARASITES

ENTAMOEBA HISTOLYTICA[105, 106, 132, 133, 134]

- *Entamoeba histolytica* trophozoites can be identified by iron-hematoxylin or trichrome stains.
- The trophozoites are 10 to 60 μm in diameter with a single nucleus containing fine, evenly distributed chromatin and a small central nucleolus.
- The cyst stage, 5 to 20 μm in diameter, contains one to four nuclei and may contain basophilic chromatoid bodies, which are made up of ribosomal particles in a crystalline array.
- The cyst is surrounded by a chitin-containing wall and transmits infection upon ingestion.
- The species *E. histolytica* is reserved to the invasive pathogenic ameba.
- This species was first distinguished from the nonpathogenic *E. dispar,* which has identical microscopic morphology, by isoenzyme electrophoresis.
- Less laborious EIA or immunofluorescent antibody tests for soluble amebic antigen distinguish *E. histolytica* from nonpathogenic *E. dispar.*
- Trophozoites, which are found in infected tissue or abscess or which contain erythrocytes, can be identified as *E. histolytica.*
- Pleuropulmonary amebiasis usually represents extension of an amebic liver abscess through the diaphragm and into the chest.
- Pulmonary abscess without liver involvement occurs in less than 15% of cases of thoracic amebiasis.
- Hepatobronchial fistula occurs in some patients.
- Diagnostic methods should include the following:

1. Imaging (CT, ultrasonography, MRI, and Gallium scans) demonstrates cystic lesions in liver and lung. Because amebic abscesses do not contain leukocytes centrally they appear as cold regions in Gallium scans, as compared to pyogenic abscesses.
2. Respiratory specimens and fecal sediment concentrates should be examined microscopically for *E. histolytica/dispar* in wet mounts and iron-hematoxylin–stained smears. The yield is often small when the lesion is hepatic or pulmonary abscess. *E. gingivalis,* a commensal ameba in the upper respiratory tract, may be difficult to distinguish from *E. histolytica/dispar.*
3. Serologic testing may be useful. The indirect hemagglutination (IHA) test has been standard. The IHA test detects antibody specific for *E. histolytica* at titers of 1:256 or greater in 95% of patients with extraintestinal amebiasis, 70% of patients with active intestinal disease, and 10% of asymptomatic persons who are passing cysts. Positive titers may persist for years after successful treatment. EIA tests, which are generally available now, are as sensitive and specific as the IHA test.

TRICHOMONAS TENAX[106]

Trichomonas tenax is pear-shaped, has one nucleus, four anterior flagella, one posterior flagellum that extends half-way down the body, and an axostyle that extends beyond the posterior end of the body.

FIGURE 7–49

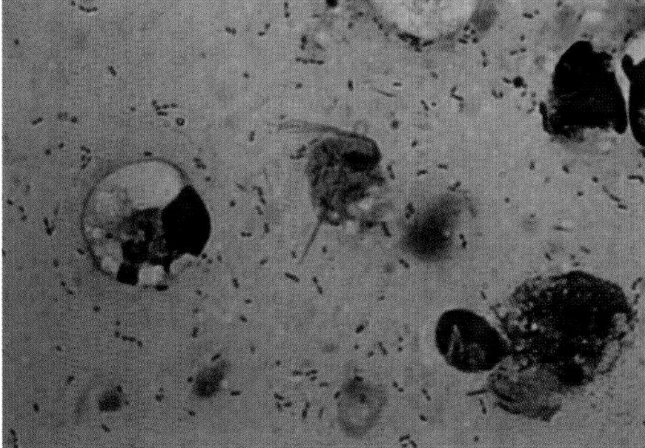

Trichomonas tenax present in Giemsa-stained aspirate from a pulmonary abscess containing many different anaerobic bacteria. *T. tenax* is a commensal organism found in the gingival crevice and dental tartar of patients with poor oral hygiene. It is best seen in wet mounts by use of phase or Nomarski microscopy or in stained smears.

TESTS FOR PARASITES

CRYPTOSPORIDIUM PARVUM[106, 128]

- This organism is usually transmitted by the oocyst (4 to 5 μm in diameter), which may contain four sporozoites.
- The oocyst is resistant to chlorinated water and most household disinfectants and cleaning agents.
- *C. parvum* is cleared from water supplies only by filtration.
- Tracheobronchial infection by *C. parvum* is usually transmitted by vomiting followed by aspiration.
- *C. parvum* causes a self-limited diarrheal disease in immunocompetent persons.
- Immunodeficient patients develop a persistent debilitating and sometimes fatal illness. This disease is especially apparent in HIV-1–infected persons with low numbers of CD4 lymphocytes.

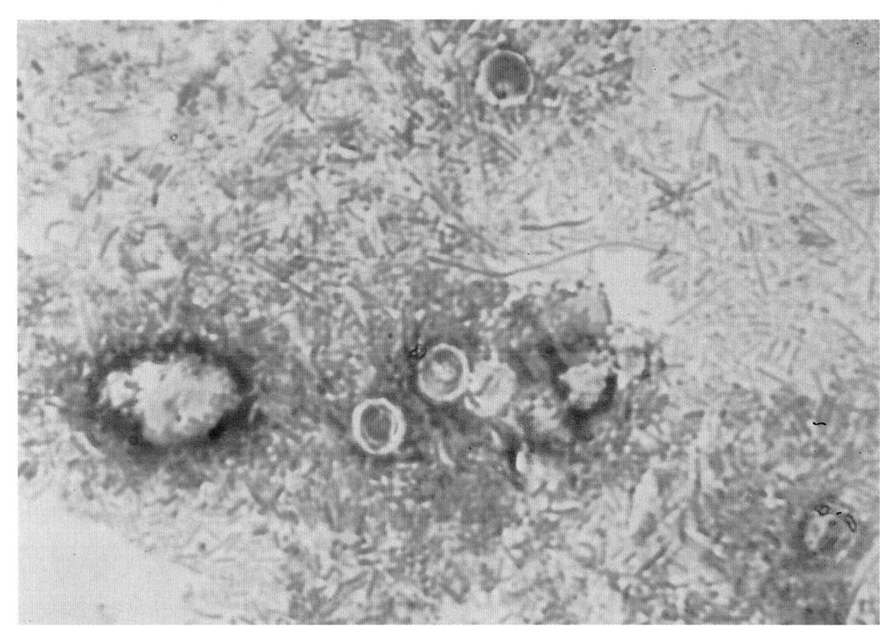

FIGURE 7–50

Cryptosporidium parvum oocyst, stained by modified Kinyon acid-fast stain, is a coccidian protozoan with an asexual and sexual cycle. It develops in the brush border of intestinal epithelial cells. *C. parvum* infects many domestic animals. Water supplies and the fecal-oral route have transmitted it.

TESTS FOR PARASITES

TOXOPLASMA GONDII[129-131]

- Infection can be acquired in several ways: accidental ingestion of oocysts which have developed in cat intestinal epithelial cells and are shed in cat feces; ingestion of raw or incompletely cooked meat containing tissue cysts; transmission in utero; or transmission by blood transfusion or organ transplant.
- Immunocompromised persons at risk for toxoplasmosis include those receiving corticosteroids or cytotoxic agents, those with malignancy or HIV-1 infection, and those with CD4 lymphocyte cell counts of 100/mm^3 or less.
  - In individuals with impaired immune response, a primary infection or recrudescent infection may follow a fulminant course.
- In patients with cancer, infection of lungs and heart by *Toxoplasma* is frequently noted at autopsy.
- In a study at San Francisco General Hospital on patients with AIDS, *T. gondii* organisms were found in transbronchial biopsy touch-preparations, BAL fluid, and pleural fluid (WK Hadley, unpublished observations, 1998). A minimally productive cough and increasing shortness of breath were noted. Chest roentgenographic appearance in these patients showed a diffuse interstitial pattern or a diffuse, coarse, nodular pattern.

FIGURE 7–51

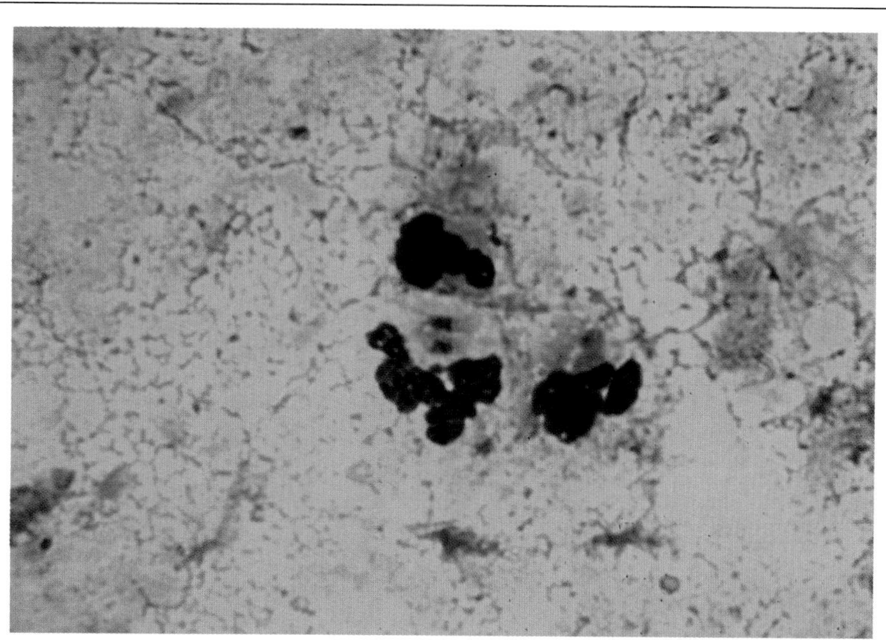

Toxoplasma gondii tachyzoites in bronchoalveolar lavage from a patient with HIV-1 infection and CD4 lymphocyte count of 48 cells/mm^3. Tachyzoites are 2 to 3 μm wide and 4 to 8 μm long. *T. gondii* is an obligate, intracellular protozoan that infects a large number of persons worldwide. It causes a benign self-limited disease in the normal host.

TESTS FOR PARASITES

TOXOPLASMA GONDII

Diagnosis of *T. gondii* infection requires the following:

1. Giemsa-stained BAL fluid, pleural fluid, or touch preparations of transbronchial biopsy specimens. Tachyzoites indicate acute infection or recrudescence.
2. Culture of specimens in cell cultures.
3. EIA test for IgG will indicate past infection.
4. EIA test for IgM antibodies is useful for congenital toxoplasmosis and for detection of acute infection of individuals who are immunocompetent. The IgM test is not useful for diagnosis of disseminated disease in HIV-1–infected patients.
5. The Sabin-Feldman dye test detects antibody against *Toxoplasma*. In the presence of immune serum, live *T. gondii* tachyzoites lose their affinity for methylene blue staining.

FIGURE 7–52

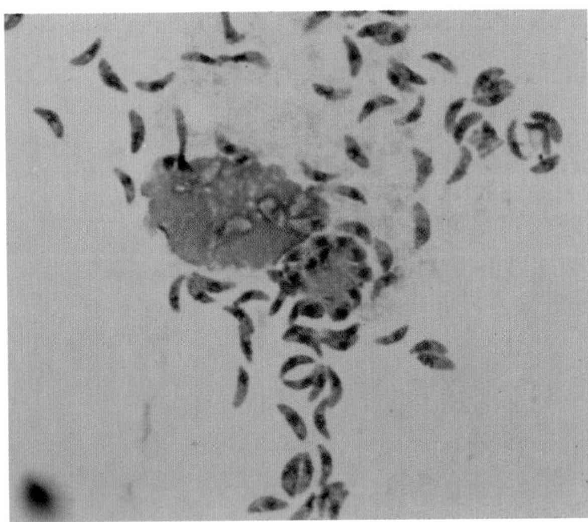

T. gondii tachyzoites multiplying in cell culture of BAL.

TESTS FOR PARASITES

MICROSPORIDIA[106, 135–137]

- These parasites have a unique life cycle with a proliferative merogonic stage followed by a sporogonic stage, which produces environmentally resistant spores. The spores bear a polar extrusion apparatus, which injects the infective spore into the host cell.
- Microsporidia organisms infect a wide variety of animals.
- Microsporidia have been recognized in human infection, particularly in HIV-1–infected patients.
  - It is not known whether the infection is a reactivation of a latent infection or a primary infection.
  - When the CD4 lymphocyte count is below 0.1×10^9/L, chronic diarrheal wasting syndrome, cholangitis, keratoconjunctivitis, sinusitis, bronchitis, and pneumonitis have been observed as well as other infections.
  - Infections in immunocompetent individuals produce a self-limited diarrheal disease, keratitis, and corneal ulcers.

Because of the small size of these microsporidia thin smears, touch preparations or thin plastic embedded tissue are necessary for diagnosis and require examination at 1000× magnification by light microscopy. Diagnosis may depend on the following:

1. Direct examination of tissue sections is best observed with PAS, acid-fast, silver, or Gram stains.
2. Smears of fecal, urine, or respiratory specimen sediment are fixed with formalin and stained by Chromotrope 2R modified trichrome or optical whiteners, such as calcofluor or uvitex. Alternatively, similar preparations are fixed with methanol and stained by Giemsa.
3. Indirect fluorescent antibody staining. Example: Rabbit antibody vs. microsporidia binds onto microsporidia in a human specimen. Localization of the rabbit antibody is accomplished with a fluorescent conjugated goat anti-rabbit immunoglobulin. Fluorescence on ultraviolet irradiation indicates the presence of microsporidia.
4. Cell cultures of human embryonic lung fibroblast (MRC5) or Madin-Darby canine kidney are used for culture.
5. Antigen detection and nucleic acid–based methods for detection and identification are under study.
6. Electron microscopy is definitive for identification of this unusual organism.

FIGURE 7–53

A microsporidium from maxillary sinus aspirate smear fixed with methanol and stained. The microsporidia are obligate intracellular protists, which are 1.0 to 2.0 μm in diameter. They are eukaryotes in the sense that they have a membrane-bound nucleus, but they have 70S ribosomes and lack mitochondria.

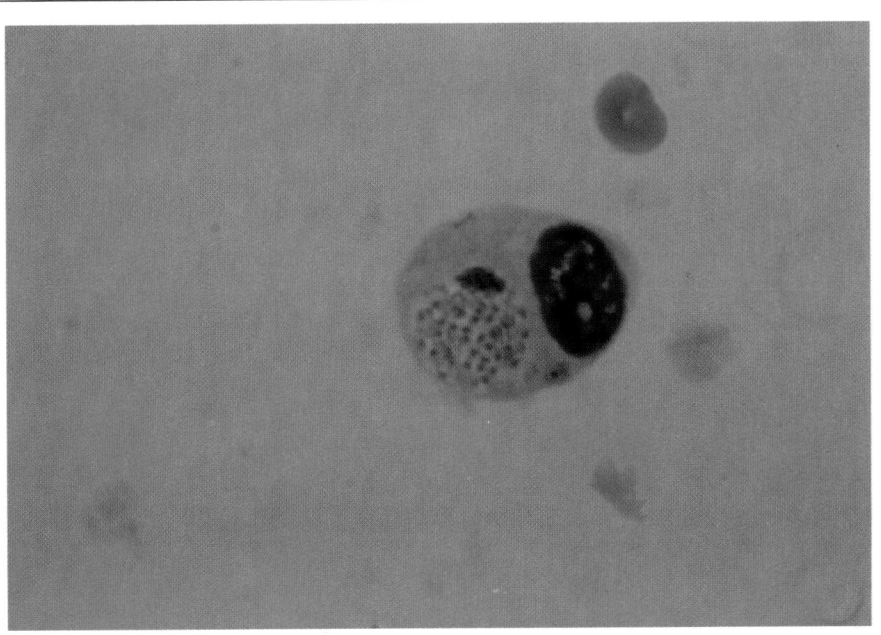

TESTS FOR VIRAL AGENTS[138–144] (TABLES 7–16 and 7–17)

CULTURE AND TRANSPORT

- The viruses that infect the respiratory tract are present within the epithelial cells and lymphoid tissue of the upper respiratory tract.
- Vigorous nasopharyngeal washing with saline using a bulb or aspiration trap or swabbing of the nasopharynx will release cells for diagnostic tests.
- Specimens obtained by bronchoscopy such as lavage, bronchial brush, and transbronchial biopsy also provide cells for diagnosis.
- Viral culture specimens must be placed in a viral transport medium that prevents drying and change in pH.
- Dacron or rayon swab culturettes, which provide a swab and a viral transport medium, are also useful.
- Temperature for holding specimens for viral culture is critical; respiratory syncytial virus (RSV) is especially thermolabile.
- Rapid transport of the specimens to the laboratory for culture is essential. If this cannot be done, the specimen should be refrigerated at 4°C.
- If prolonged storage is necessary, the specimen should be frozen at −70°C. Freeze-thaw cycles are destructive to virus infectivity, as is storage in a household type −20°C freezer.

TABLE 7–16

Detection of Respiratory Viruses

Virus	Cell Culture*	Shell Viral Cell Culture*	Direct Detection
Adenovirus	2–14	3–5	IF
Influenza A	1–7	2	EIA, IF
Influenza B	1–7	2	EIA, IF
Parainfluenza (1, 2, 3)	2–14	2	IF
Rhinovirus	2–14	–	–
Respiratory syncytial virus	2–14	2	EIA

* In days. EIA = enzyme-linked immunoassay; IF = immunofluorescent stain.

TESTS FOR VIRAL AGENTS

TABLE 7–17

Clinical Expression and Diagnosis of Viral Respiratory Infections

Virus	Clinical Expression of Infection	Diagnosis by Cell Culture	Other Diagnostic Test (FA, Antigen, PCR)	Diagnosis by Serology
Influenza A subtypes based on hemagglutinin and neuraminidase, e.g., H_3N_2; occurs in human, avian, swine, and equine; influenza B in humans only	Influenza A pandemics occur; tracheobronchitis, high-risk patients have high morbidity/mortality due to secondary bacterial infections; influenza B, no pandemics	Primary Rhesus or Cynomolgus monkey kidney; detect virus by CPE, hemadsorption, FA stain	EIA for A and B antigen test takes 30–60 minutes; FA staining exfoliated respiratory cells	HI, EIA, antibody IgM, IgG occur simultaneously
Parainfluenza viruses serotypes 1, 2, 3	Croup in children, laryngotracheobronchitis	Primary monkey kidney; detect virus by CPE hemadsorption, FA stain	FA stain of exfoliated cells	HI, EIA, fourfold rise IgG titer
Respiratory syncytial virus	Serious lower respiratory infection in children, also occurs in adults	H-Ep-2; virus thermolabile; detect by CPE, FA stain; requires 3–14 days	EIA for antigen as sensitive as culture; 30–60 minutes for tests; RT-PCR in trials	
Adenoviruses, 49 serotypes, in humans	1, 2, 5, 6, 7—respiratory disease in children 3, 4, 7—pharyngitis, bronchiolitis obliterans, infant diarrhea	Human embryonic kidney; HeLa, detect virus by CPE, group-specific FA stain, hemagglutination	FA stain infected cells; electron microscopy	CF, EIA, HI, fourfold rise in titer
Hantaviruses, transmitted by rodent urine, feces, tissues, Sin Nombre virus (SNV)	Pulmonary edema, shock, associated with *Peromyscus* (deer mouse); infects healthy young adults	Not cultured	RT-PCR	CDC-IgM capture ELISA vs. radiation-inactivated SNV (University of New Mexico) western blot

Key: CPE = cytopathogenic effect; EIA = enzyme-linked immunoassay; FA = fluorescein conjugated antibody; HI = hemagglutination inhibition; RT-PCR = reverse transcriptase polymerase chain reaction.

DIAGNOSTIC SYSTEMS

- Laboratory diagnosis of viral respiratory infections is in transition.
- The established diagnostic system consists of inoculation of multiple cell culture lines with a respiratory specimen followed by a variety of tests for cytopathic effect, hemadsorption, or immunofluorescence.
- The specimen must contain as much virus as possible with intact infectivity.
  - This system is likely to recover the largest number of different viruses.
  - However, the test system is slow, laborious, expensive, and not likely to yield results within the time needed for medical decisions.
- New test systems are more rapid and are expected to yield results in a time frame that can support medical decisions; however, reagent costs are likely to be expensive.
- Antigen detection tests for influenza viruses and respiratory syncytial virus, which make use of EIA methodology, take 30 to 60 minutes after receipt of nasopharyngeal washings or swabbings and require little training. They have a specificity and sensitivity similar to cell culture and immunofluorescent staining.
- Nucleic acid amplification tests have the potential for high specificity and sensitivity. However, respiratory tract specimens may have polymerase inhibitors.
- PCR-multiplex tests for a variety of respiratory viruses would be useful. For these tests the specimen should contain the maximum amount of virus, but infectivity is not necessary.

TESTS FOR VIRAL AGENTS

SPECIFIC AGENTS

- The rhinoviruses and the coronaviruses cause 25 to 50% and 10 to 30% of all "colds," respectively.
- Viral diagnosis of these agents is complicated and not usually pursued.
- The rhinoviruses have greater than 100 separate serotypes and require incubation of human diploid fibroblast cell lines at 33°C in order to recover the viruses.
- Coronaviruses have several serotypes and require tracheal ring, organ culture, or human embryonic kidney cell culture.
- Serologic reagents for coronavirus are not available commercially.
- Cytomegalovirus (CMV) recurrent infection commonly occurs outside the lung. CMV pneumonia is poorly defined.
- Pneumonia is best established by clinical and radiographic evidence of pneumonia in a patient with immunosuppression combined with virologic evidence of active primary infection. CMV viremia is a useful indication of active infection.
- Lung tissue or BAL sediment stained by Giemsa showing enlarged cells with basophilic intranuclear and acidophilic cytoplasmic inclusions is characteristic of CMV.
- Human diploid fibroblast shell viral cultures are more rapid than regular cultures. They show CMV by monoclonal immunofluorescent staining in 18 to 48 hours.
- A fourfold rise in antibody titer or elevation from seronegative to seropositive titer indicates active primary infection.
- CMV IgM antibody titer is not useful because IgM titer elevation also occurs in recurrent disease.
- Infection by herpes simplex virus (HSV) in immunosuppressed patients is usually evident on mucocutaneous regions.
- Lower respiratory tract involvement is rare.
- Consultation between the physician and laboratories on the selection of an appropriate test system is essential.

GENERAL REFERENCES

Murray PR, Baron EJ, Pfaller MA, et al (eds): Manual of Clinical Microbiology. 7th ed. Washington, DC, ASM Press, 1999.

Rose NR, Conway de Macario E, Folds JD, et al (eds): Manual of Clinical Laboratory Immunology. 5th ed. Washington, DC, ASM Press, 1997.

REFERENCES

1. Finegold SM: Anaerobic Bacteria in Human Disease. New York, Academic Press, 1977.

2. Johanson WG Jr, Pierce AK, Sanford JP, Thomas GD: Nosocomial respiratory infections with Gram-negative bacilli: The significance of colonization of the respiratory tract. Ann Intern Med 77:701–706, 1972.

3. Chartrand SA, Thompson KJ, Sanders C: Antibiotic resistant, gram negative bacillary infections. Semin Pediatr Infect Dis 7:187–203, 1996.

4. Sharp SE: Commensal and pathogenic microorganisms of humans. *In* Murray PR, Baron EJ, Pfaller MA, et al (eds): Manual of Clinical Microbiology. 7th ed. Washington, DC, ASM Press, 1999, chap. 3.

5. Shea YR: Specimen collection and transport. Section 1: Aerobic bacteriology 1.1.1–1.1.30. *In* Isenberg HD (ed in chief): Clinical Microbiology Procedures Handbook. Washington, DC, ASM Press, 1999.

6. Miller JM: A Guide to Specimen Management in Clinical Microbiology. Washington, DC, ASM Press, 1996.

7. Bartlett JG, Ryan KJ, Smith TF, Wilson WR: Cumitech 7A Laboratory Diagnosis of Lower Respiratory Tract Infections. Washington, DC, ASM Press, 1987.

8. Summanen P, Baron EJ, Citron DM: Wadsworth Anaerobic Bacteriology Manual. 5th ed. Belmont, CA, Star Publishing, 1993.

9. Hadley WK, Aronson SB: Quantitative conjunctival bacteriology. Arch Ophthalmol 90:386–388, 1973.

10. Chambers HF, Hadley WK, Jawetz E: Antimicrobials, disinfectants, antiseptics and sterilants. *In* Katzung B: Basic and Clinical Pharmacology. Norwalk, CT, Appleton & Lange, 1997.

11. Washington JA: Noninvasive diagnostic techniques for lower respiratory infections. *In* Pennington JE: Respiratory Infections: Diagnosis and Management. 3rd ed. New York, Raven Press, 1994.

12. Bartlett JG: Invasive diagnostic techniques in pulmonary infections. *In* Pennington JE: Respiratory Infections: Diagnosis and Management. 3rd ed. New York, Raven Press, 1994.

REFERENCES

13. Bartlett JB: Management of Respiratory Tract Infections. Baltimore, Williams & Wilkins, 1997.

14. Bartlett RC: Medical Microbiology Quality Cost and Clinical Relevance. New York, John Wiley, 1974.

15. Murray PR, Washington JA II: Microscopic and bacteriologic analysis of expectorated sputum. Mayo Clin Proc 50:339, 1975.

16. Geckler RW, Gremillion DH, McAllister CK, Ellenbogen C: Microscopic and bacteriological comparison of paired sputa and transtracheal aspirates. J Clin Microbiol 6:396–399, 1997.

17. Ingram JG, Plouffe JF: Danger of sputum purulence screens in culture of *Legionella* species. J Clin Microbiol 32:209–210, 1994.

18. Medici TC, Chodosh S: Nonmalignant exfoliative sputum cytology. *In* Duffano JJ (ed): Sputum, Fundamentals and Clinical Pathology. Springfield, IL, Charles C Thomas, 1973, chap 10.

19. Ng VL, Gartner I, Weymouth LA, et al: The use of mucolysed inducted sputum for the identification of pulmonary pathogens associated with human immunodeficiency virus infection. Arch Pathol Lab Med 113:488–493, 1989.

20. Kovacs JA, Ng VL, Masur H, et al: Diagnosis of *Pneumocystis carinii* pneumonia: Improved detection in sputum using monoclonal antibodies. N Engl J Med 318: 589–593, 1988.

21. American Thoracic Society: Clinical role of bronchoalveolar lavage in adults with pulmonary disease. Am Rev Respir Dis 142:481–486, 1990.

22. Smith RF: Microscopy and Photomicrography: A Working Manual. Boca Raton, FL, CRC Press, 1990.

23. Blumenfeld W, Wagar E, Hadley WK: Use of transbronchial biopsy for diagnosis of opportunistic pulmonary infections in acquired immunodeficiency syndrome (AIDS). Am J Clin Pathol 81:1–5, 1984.

24. Chapin KC, Murray PR: Stains. *In* Murray PR, Baron EJ, Pfaller MA, et al (eds): Manual of Clinical Microbiology. 7th ed. Washington, DC, ASM Press, 1999.

25. Chapin KC, Murray PR: Media. *In* Murray PR, Baron EJ, Pfaller MA, et al (eds): Manual of Clinical Microbiology. 7th ed. Washington, DC, ASM Press, 1999.

26. MacFaddin JF: Media for Isolation Cultivation Identification Maintenance of Medical Bacteria. Vol 1. Baltimore, Williams & Wilkins, 1985.

27. Blazevic DJ, Ederer GM: Principles of Biochemical Tests in Diagnostic Microbiology. New York, John Wiley, 1975.

28. MacFaddin JF: Biochemical Tests for Identification of Medical Bacteria. Baltimore, Williams & Wilkins, 1976.

29. Miller JM, O'Hara CM: Manual and automated systems for microbial identifiction. *In* Murray PR, Baron EJ, Pfaller MA, et al (eds): Manual of Clinical Microbiology. 7th ed. Washington, DC, ASM Press, 1999, chap. 11.

30. Landry ML, Hsiung GD: Primary isolation of viruses. *In* Spector S, Lancz G (eds): Clinical Virology Manual. 2nd ed. New York, Elsevier, 1992, chap. 3.

31. Ripa KT, Mardh PA: Cultivation of *Chlamydia trachomatis* in cyclohexamide-treated McCoy cells. J Clin Microbiol 6:328–331, 1977.

32. Cles LD, Stamm WE: Use of HL cells for improved isolation and passage of *Chlamydia pneumoniae.* J Clin Microbiol 28:938–940, 1990.

33. Mahony JB, Chernesky MA: Immunoassays for the diagnosis of infectious diseases. *In* Murray PR, Baron EJ, Pfaller MA, et al (eds): Manual of Clinical Microbiology. 7th ed. Washington, DC, ASM Press, 1999, chap. 12.

34. Tÿssen P: Practice and Theory of Enzyme Immunoassays. Amsterdam, Elsevier, 1985.

35. Kricka LJ: Chemiluminescence immunoassays. *In* Rose NR, deMacario EC, Folds JD, et al (eds): Manual of Clinical Laboratory Immunology. 5th ed. Washington, DC, ASM Press, 1997, chap. 7.

36. Annesley TM: Analytical test variables. *In* McClatchey KD (ed): Clinical Laboratory Medicine. Baltimore, Williams & Wilkins, 1994, chap. 3.

37. Tang Y-W, Persing DH: Molecular detection and identification of microorganisms. *In* Murray PR, Baron EJ, Pfaller MA, et al (eds): Manual of Clinical Microbiology. 7th ed. Washington, DC, ASM Press, 1999, chap. 13. pp 215–244.

38. Drake TA, Hindler JA, Berlin OG, Bruckner DA: Rapid identification of *Mycobacterium avium* complex in culture using DNA probes. J Clin Microbiol 25:1442–1445, 1987.

39. Greisen K, Loeffelholz M, Purohit A, Leong D: PCR primers and probes for the 16S rRNA gene of most species of pathogenic bacteria, including bacteria found in cerebrospinal fluid. J Clin Microbiol 32:335–351, 1994.

40. Persing DH, Smith TF, Tenover FC, White TJ (eds): Diagnostic Molecular Microbiology. Washington, DC, ASM Press, 1993.

41. Plouffe JF, McNally C, File TM Jr: Value of noninvasive studies in community acquired pneumonia. *In* Mandel A, Neiderman MD (eds): Lower Respiratory Tract Infections. Infect Dis Clin North Am 12(3): 689–699, 1998.

42. White B: The Biology of Pneumococcus: The Bacteriological, Biochemical and Immunological Characters and Activities of *Diplococcus pneumoniae.* A Commonwealth Fund Book. Cambridge, MA, Harvard University Press, 1938, reprinted 1979.

43. Watson DA, Musher DM, Jacobson JW: A brief history of the pneumococcus in biomedical research: A panoply of discovery. Clin Infect Dis 17:913–924, 1993.

REFERENCES

44. Munoz R, Fenoll A, Vicioso D: Optochin-resistant variants of *Streptococcus pneumoniae.* Diagn Microbiol Infect Dis 13:63–66, 1990.

45. Marshall KJ, Musher DM, Watson D, Mason EO Jr: Testing of *Streptococcus pneumoniae* for resistance to penicillin. J Clin Microbiol 31:1246–1250, 1993.

46. Hendolin PH, Markkanen A, Ylikoski Y, Wahlfors JJ: Use of multiplex PCR for simultaneous detection of four bacterial species in middle ear effusions. J Clin Microbiol 35:2854–2858, 1997.

47. Lauer BA, Reller LB, Mirrett S: Comparison of acridine orange and Gram stains for detection of microorganisms in cerebrospinal fluid and other clinical specimens. J Clin Microbiol 14:201–205, 1981.

48. Turk DC: Clinical importance of *Haemophilus influenzae. In* Sell SH, Wright PF (eds): *Haemophilus influenzae:* Epidemiology, Immunology and Prevention of Disease. New York, Elsevier, 1982.

49. Moxon ER: The carrier state: *Haemophilus influenzae.* J Antimicrob Chemother 18(Suppl A):17–24, 1986.

50. Rennie R, Gordon T, Yaschuk Y, et al: Laboratory and clinical evaluations of media for the primary isolation of *Haemophilus* sp. J Clin Microbiol 30:1917–1921, 1992.

51. Daly JA, Clifton ML, Seskin KC, Gooch WM III: Use of rapid nonradioactive DNA probes in culture confirmation tests to detect *Streptococcus agalactiae, Haemophilus influenzae* and *Enterococcus* spp. from pediatric patients with significant infections. J Clin Microbiol 29:80–82, 1985.

52. Doern GV, Brueggernan AB, Pierce G, et al: Antibiotic resistance among clinical isolates of *Haemophilus influenzae* in the United States in 1994 and 1995 and detection of β-lactamase-positive strains resistant to amoxicillin-clavulanate: Results of a national multicenter surveillance study. Antimicrob Agents Chemother 41:292–297, 1997.

53. Markowitz SM: Isolation of an ampicillin-resistant, non-β-lactamase-producing strain of *Haemophilus influenzae.* Antimicrob Agents Chemother 17:80–83, 1980.

54. O'Callaghan CH, Morris A, Kirby SM, Shingler AH: Novel method for detection of β-lactamases by using a chromogenic cephalosporin substrate. Antimicrob Agents Chemother 1:283–288, 1972.

55. Barbaree JM, Fields BS, Feeley JC, et al: Isolation of protozoa from water associated with a legionellosis outbreak and demonstration of intracellular multiplication of *Legionella pneumophila.* Appl Environ Microbiol 51:422–424, 1986.

56. Alary M, Joly JR: Factors contributing to the contamination of hospital water distribution systems by legionellae. J Infect Dis 165:565–569, 1992.

57. Buesching WJ, Brust RA, Ayers LW: Enhanced primary isolation of *Legionella pneumophila* from clinical specimens by low-pH treatment. J Clin Microbiol 17:1153–1155, 1983.

58. Joly JR: Monitoring for the presence of *Legionella:* Where, when and how. *In* Barbaree JM, Breimen RF, Doufor AP (eds): *Legionella:* Current Status and Emerging Perspectives. Washington, DC, ASM Press, 1993.

59. Cafferkey MT (ed): Methicillin-Resistant *Staphylococcus aureus.* New York, Marcel Dekker, 1992.

60. Archer GL: Coagulase-negative staphylococci in blood cultures: A clinician's dilemma. Infect Control 6:477–478, 1985.

61. Kluytmans J, Belkum A van, Verbrugh H: Nasal carriage of *Staphylococcus aureus:* Epidemiology, underlying mechanisms and associated risks. Clin Microbiol Rev 10: 505–520, 1997.

62. Bannerman TL, Hancock GA, Tenover FC, Miller JM: Pulsed field gel electrophoresis as a replacement for bacteriophage typing of *Staphylococcus aureus.* J Clin Microbiol 33:551–555, 1995.

63. Choi Y, Kotzin B, Herron L, et al: Interaction of *Staphylococcus aureus* toxin "superantigens" with human T cells. Proc Natl Acad Sci USA 86:8941–8945, 1989.

64. Kellog J: Suitability of throat culture procedures for detection of Group A streptococci and as reference standards for evaluation of streptococcal antigen detection kits. J Clin Microbiol 28:165–169, 1990.

65. Stevens DL: Streptococcal toxic-shock syndrome: Spectrum of disease, pathogenesis and new concepts in treatment. Emerg Infect Dis 3:69–78, 1995.

66. Ayob EM, Harden E: Immune response to streptococcal antigens: Diagnostic methods. *In* Rose NR, de Macario EC, Folds JD, et al (eds): Manual of Clinical Laboratory Immunology. 5th ed. Washington, DC, ASM Press, 1997.

67. Vaneechoutte M, Verschragen GK, Claeys G, et al: Respiratory tract carrier roles of *Moraxella (Branhamella) catarrhalis* in adults and children and interpretation of the isolation of *M. catarrhalis* from sputum. J Clin Microbiol 28:2674–2680, 1990.

68. Doern GV: *Branhamella catarrhalis*—An emerging human pathogen. Diagn Microbiol Infect Dis 4:191–201, 1986.

69. Finegold SM, Baron EJ, Wexler HM: A Clinical Guide to Anaerobic Infections. Belmont, CA, Star Publishing Co, 1991.

70. Finegold SM, Jousimies-Somer HR, Wexler HM: Current perspectives on anaerobic infections: Diagnostic approaches. Infect Dis Clin North Am 7:257–275, 1993.

71. Foy HM: Infections caused by *Mycoplasma pneumo-*

REFERENCES

niae and possible carrier state in different populations of patients. Clin Infect Dis 17(Suppl 1):37–46, 1993.

72. Cassell GH, Gambill G, Duffy L: ELISA in respiratory infections of humans. *In* Tully JG, Razin S (eds): Molecular and Diagnostic Procedures in Mycoplasmology. New York, Academic Press, 1996.

73. Tjhie JH, Roosendaal R, MacLaren DM, Vandenbroucke-Graules CM: Improvement of growth of *Chlamydia pneumoniae* on Hep-2 cells by pretreatment with polyethylene glycol in combination with additional centrifugation and extension of culture time. J Clin Microbiol 35: 1883–1884, 1997.

74. Gaydos CA, Roblin PM, Hammerschlag MR, et al: Diagnostic utility of PCR-enzyme immunoassay-culture and serology for the detection of *Chlamydia pneumoniae* in symptomatic and asymptomatic patients. J Clin Microbiol 32:903–905, 1994.

75. Schachter J, Sugg N, Sung M: Psittacosis: The reservoir persists. J Infect Dis 137:44–49, 1978.

76. Marrie TJ, Raoult D: Coxiella. *In* Murray PR (ed in chief): Manual of Clinical Microbiology, 7th ed. Washinton, DC, ASM Press, 1999.

77. Maurin M, Raoult D: Q Fever. Clin Microbiol Rev 12:518–553, 1999.

78. McEachern R, Campbell GD Jr: Hospital-acquired pneumonia: Epidemiology, etiology and treatment. Infect Dis Clin North Am 12:761–779, 1998.

79. Govan JRW, Deretic V: Microbial pathogenesis in cystic fibrosis: Mucoid *Pseudomonas aeruginosa* and *Burkholderia cepacia.* Microbiol Rev 60:539–574, 1996.

80. Relio J, Jubert P, Valles J, et al: Evaluation of outcome for intubated patients with pneumonia due to *Pseudomonas aeruginosa.* Clin Infect Dis 23:973–978, 1996.

81. Hilts PJ: US and Russian Doctors Tie Anthrax to Soviets. New York Times, March 15, 1993.

82. Logan NA, Turnbull PCB: Bacillus and recently derived genera. *In* Murray PR (ed in chief): Manual of Clinical Microbiology. 7th ed. Washington, DC, ASM Press, 1999.

83. Anthrax Vaccine. Med Lett 40:52–53, 1998.

84. Perry RD, Fetherston JD: *Yersinia pestis*—Etiological agent of plague. Clin Microbiol Rev 10:35–66, 1997.

85. Butler T: *Yersinia* infections: Centennial of the discovery of the plague bacillus. Clin Infect Dis 19:655–661, 1994.

86. Galimand M, Guiyoule A, Gerbaud G, et al: Multidrug resistance in *Yersinia pestis* mediated by a transferable plasmid. N Engl J Med 337:677–680, 1997.

86a. American Thoracic Society, Diagnosis and treatment of disease caused by nontuberculous mycobacteria. Am J Respir Crit Care Med Suppl 156:S1–S25, 1997.

86b. Inderlied C, Kempler C, Bermudez L: The *Mycobacterium avium* complex. Clin Microbiol Rev 6:266–310, 1993.

86c. Scherer R, Sable R, Sonnenberg M, et al: Disseminated infection with *Mycobacterium kansasii* in the acquired immunodeficiency syndrome. Ann Intern Med 105: 710–712, 1986.

87. Metchock BG, Nolte FS, Wallace RJ Jr: *Mycobacterium. In* Murray PR (ed in chief): Manual of Clinical Microbiology. 7th ed. Washington, DC, ASM Press, 1999.

88. Kaminski DA, Hardy DJ: Selective utilization of DNA probes for identification of *Mycobacterium* species on the basis of cord formation in primary BACTEC 12 B cultures. J Clin Microbiol 33:1548–1550, 1995.

89. Ichiyama SY, Inuma Y, Tawada Y, et al: Evaluation of GenProbe amplified *Mycobacterium tuberculosis* direct test and Roche-PCR microwell plate hybridization method for direct detection of mycobacteria. J Clin Microbiol 34: 130–133, 1996.

90. Burman WJ, Stone BL, Reves RR, et al: The incidence of false-positive cultures for *Mycobacterium tuberculosis.* Am J Respir Crit Care Med 155:321–326, 1997.

91. Trifiro S, Bourgault A-J, Lebel F, Rene P: Ghost mycobacteria on Gram-stain. J Clin Microbiol 28:146, 1990.

92. Hindler JA, Swenson JM: Susceptibility testing of fastidious bacteria. *In* Murray PR (ed in chief): Manual of Clinical Microbiology. 7th ed. Washington, DC, ASM Press, 1999.

93. National Committee for Clinical Laboratory Standards. Performance Standards for Antimicrobial Susceptibility Testing. Supplement M100-S9. Wayne, PA, National Committee for Clinical Laboratory Standards, 1999.

94. Inderlied CB, Salfinger M: Antimycobacterial agents and susceptibility tests. *In* Murray PR (ed in chief): Manual of Clinical Microbiology. 7th ed. Washington, DC, ASM Press, 1999.

95. Kaufman L, Kovacs JA, Reiss E: Clinical immunomycology. *In* Rose NR, de Macario EC, Folds JD, et al: Manual of Clinical Laboratory Immunology. 5th ed. Washington, DC, ASM Press, 1997.

96. Sandhu GS, Kline BC, Stockman L, Roberts GD: Molecular probes for diagnosis of fungal infections. J Clin Microbiol 33:2913–2919, 1995.

97. Hadley WK, Ng VL: *Pneumocystis. In* Murray PR (ed in chief): Manual of Clinical Microbiology. 7th ed. Washington, DC, ASM Press, 1999.

98. Walsh TJ, Chanock SJ: Laboratory diagnosis of invasive candidiasis: A rationale for complementary use of culture and nonculture-based detection systems. Int J Infect Dis 1(suppl 1):S11–S19, 1997.

REFERENCES

99. Hajjeh RA, Brandt ME, Pinner RW: Emergence of cryptococcal disease: Epidemiologic perspectives 100 years after its discovery. Epidemiol Rev 17:303–320, 1995.

100. Heelan JS, Corpus L, Kessimian N: False-positive reactions in the latex agglutination test for *Cryptococcus neoformans* antigen. J Clin Microbiol 29:1260–1261, 1991.

101. Larone DH, Mitchell TG, Walsh TJ: *Histoplasma, Blastomyces, Coccidioides* and other dimorphic fungi causing systemic mycoses. *In* Murray PR (ed in chief): Manual of Clinical Microbiology. 7th ed. Washington, DC, ASM Press, 1999.

102. Wheat J, Wheat H, Connolly P, et al: Cross-reactivity in *Histoplasma capsulatum* variety *capsulatum* antigen assays of urine samples from patients with endemic mycoses. Clin Infect Dis 24:1169–1171, 1997.

103. Andriole VT: *Aspergillus* infections: Problems in diagnosis and treatment. Infect Agents Dis 5:47–54, 1996.

104. Schonheyder H: Pathogenic and serological aspects of pulmonary aspergillosis. Scand J Infect Dis 51(suppl):1–62, 1987.

105. Mahmoud AAF (ed): Parasitic Lung Diseases. New York, Marcel Dekker, 1997.

106. Garcia LS, Bruchner DA: Diagnostic Medical Parasitology. 3rd ed. Washington, DC, ASM Press, 1997.

107. Salata RA: Intestinal nematodes. *In* Mahmoud AAF (ed): Parasitic Lung Diseases. New York, Marcel Dekker, 1997.

108. Löffler W: Zur Differential-Diagnose der Lungeniinfiltrierungen: Über flüchtig Succedan-Infiltraten (mit Eosinophilie). Beitr Klin Tuberkul specif Tuberkul-Forsch 79: 368–382, 1932.

109. Proffit RD, Walton BC: *Ascaris* pneumonia in a two-year-old girl. Diagnosis by gastric aspirate. N Engl J Med 266:931–934, 1962.

110. Gelpi AP, Mustafa A: Seasonal pneumonitis with eosinophilia in Saudi Arabia. Am J Trop Med Hyg 16:646–657, 1967.

111. Genta RM: Global prevalence of strongyloidiasis: Critical review with epidemiologic insights into the prevention of disseminated disease. Rev Infect Dis 11:755–767, 1989.

112. Liu LX, Weller PF: Strongyloidiasis and other intestinal nematode infections. Infect Dis Clin North Am 7:655–682, 1993.

113. Celedon JC, Mathur-Wagh U, Fox J: Systemic strongyloidiasis in patients infected with human immunodeficiency virus (HIV-1): A report of 3 cases and review of the literature. Medicine (Baltimore) 73:256–263, 1994.

114. De Kaminsky RG: Evaluation of three methods for laboratory diagnosis of *Strongyloides stercoralis* infection. J Parasitol 79:277–280, 1993.

115. Woodring JH, Halfill H III, Reed JC: Pulmonary strongyloidiasis: Clinical and imaging features. Am J Radiol 162:537–542, 1994.

116. Jacquier P, Gottstein B, Stingelin Y: Immunodiagnosis of toxocariasis in humans: Evaluation of a new enzyme-linked immunosorbent assay. J Clin Microbiol 29: 1831–1835, 1991.

117. Kazura JW: Visceral larva migrans and other tissue nematodes. *In* Mahmoud AAF (ed): Parasitic Lung Diseases. New York, Marcel Dekker, 1997.

118. Kazura JW: The filariases. *In* Mahmoud AAF (ed): Parasitic Lung Diseases. New York, Marcel Dekker, 1997.

119. Ottesen EA: Filarial infections. Infect Dis Clin North Am 7:619–633, 1993.

120. Ciferri F: Human pulmonary dirofilariasis in the United States: A critical review. Am J Trop Med Hyg 31: 302–308, 1982.

121. Jerray M, Benzarti M, Garrouch A, et al: Hydatid disease of the lungs: Study of 386 cases. Am Rev Respir Dis 146:185–189, 1992.

122. Blanton R: Pulmonary echinococcosis. *In* Mahmoud AAF (ed): Parasitic Lung Diseases. New York, Marcel Dekker, 1997.

123. Schantz PM, Gottstein B: Echinococcosis (hydatidosis). *In* Houba V (ed): Immunologic Investigation of Tropical Parasitic Diseases. Orlando, FL, Academic Press, 1986.

124. Force L, Torres JM, Carrillo A, Busc J: Evaluation of eight serological tests in the diagnosis of human echinococcosis and follow-up. Clin Infect Dis 15:473–480, 1992.

125. King CL: Schistosomiasis. *In* Mahmoud AAF (ed): Parasitic Lung Diseases. New York, Marcel Dekker, 1997.

126. King CH: Pulmonary flukes. *In* Mahmoud AAF (ed): Parasitic Lung Diseases. New York, Marcel Dekker, 1997.

127. Zhang Z, Zhang Y, Shi Z, et al: Diagnosis of active *Paragonimus westermani* infection with a monoclonal antibody-based antigen detection assay. Am J Trop Med Hyg 49:329–334, 1993.

128. Moore JA, Frenkel JK: Respiratory and enteric cryptosporidiosis in humans. Arch Pathol Lab Med 115:1160–1162, 1991.

129. Wilson M, Remington JS, Clavet C, et al: Evaluation of six commercial kits for detection of human immunoglobulin M antibodies to *Toxoplasma gondii.* J Clin Microbiol 35:3112–3115, 1997.

130. Schnapp L, Geaghan S, Campagna A, et al: *Toxoplasma gondii* pneumonitis in patients infected with the human immunodeficiency virus. Arch Intern Med 152: 1073–1077, 1992.

REFERENCES

131. Pomeroy C, Felice GA: Pulmonary toxoplasmosis: A review. Clin Infect Dis 14:863–870, 1992.

132. Ravdin J: Amebiasis. *In* Mahmoud AAF: Parasitic Lung Disease. New York, Marcel Dekker, 1997.

133. Ong SJ, Chang MY, Liu KH, Horng CJ: Use of the ProSpect microplate enzyme immunoassay for the detection of pathogenic and nonpathogenic *Entamoeba histolytica* in fecal specimens. Trans R Soc Trop Med Hyg 90: 248–249, 1996.

134. Wilson M, Schantz PM, Tsang VCW: Clinical immunoparasitology. *In* Rose NR, deMacario EC, Folds JD, et al (eds): Manual of Clinical Immunology. 5th ed. Washington, DC, ASM Press, 1997.

135. Schwartz DA, Bryan RT, Hewanlowe KO, et al: Disseminated microsporidiosis (*Encephalitozoon hellem*) and acquired immunodeficiency syndrome—autopsy evidence for respiratory acquisition. Arch Pathol Lab Med 116:660–668, 1992.

136. Didier ES, Orenstein JM, Aldra A, et al: Comparison of three methods for detecting microsporidia in fluids. J Clin Microbiol 33:3138–3145, 1995.

137. Weber R, Canning EU: Microsporidia. *In* Murray PR (ed in chief): Manual of Clinical Microbiology. 7th ed. Washington, DC, ASM Press, 1999.

138. Menegus MA: Laboratory diagnosis of infection with respiratory viruses. *In* Dolin R, Wright PF (eds): Viral Infection of the Respiratory Tract. New York, Marcel Dekker, 1999.

139. Connolly MG Jr, Baughman RP, Dohn MN, Linnemann CC Jr: Recovery of viruses other than cytomegalovirus from bronchoalveolar lavage fluid. Chest 105:1775–1781, 1994.

140. Ahluwalia G, Embree J, McNicol P, et al: Comparison of nasopharyneal aspirate and nasopharyngeal swab specimens for respiratory syncytial virus diagnosis by cell culture, indirect immunofluorescence assay and enzyme-linked immunosorbent assay. J Clin Microbiol 25:763–767, 1987.

141. Atmar RL, Englund JA: Laboratory methods for the diagnosis of viral diseases. *In* Evans AS, Kaslow RA (eds): Viral Infections of Humans. 4th ed. New York, Plenum Press, 1997.

142. McIntosh K: Diagnostic virology. *In* Fields BN, Knipe DM, Howley PM (eds in chief): Fields Virology. 3rd ed. Philadelphia, Lippincott-Raven, 1996.

143. Atmar RL, Baxter BD, Dominguez EA, Taber LH: Comparison of reverse transcription-PCR with tissue culture and other rapid diagnostic assays for detection of type-A influenza virus. J Clin Microbiol 34:2604–2606, 1996.

144. Jenison S, Yamada T, Morris C, et al: Characterization of human antibody responses to Four Corners hantavirus infections among patients with hantavirus pulmonary syndrome. J Virol 68:3000–3006, 1994.

Pulmonary Function Testing

Warren M. Gold, MD

MEASUREMENTS OF VENTILATORY FUNCTION

SPIROMETRY

General

- Spirometry records the volume of air inhaled and exhaled plotted against time during a series of ventilatory maneuvers (FIGURE 8–1).
- Abnormal spirometric patterns reflect obstructive, restrictive, or mixed ventilatory abnormalities; none of these patterns is specific, although most diseases cause a predictable type of ventilatory defect.
- Spirometry can be used to follow the course of many different diseases.
- Spirometric measurements are also useful to estimate the degree of exercise limitation due to a ventilatory defect (e.g., maximal voluntary ventilation can be predicted from the forced expiratory volume, exhaled in 1 second)[1] and to identify patients likely to develop ventilatory failure after pneumonectomy.[2] APPENDIXES 1 to 6 give equations for predicted normal values for spirometry.

FIGURE 8–1

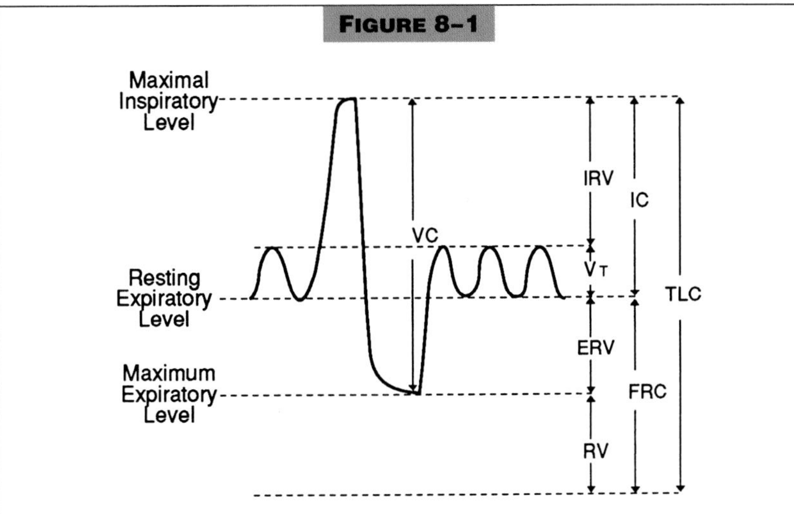

Volumes: There are four volumes, which do not overlap: (1) tidal volume (V_T) is the volume of gas inhaled or exhaled during each respiratory cycle; (2) inspiratory reserve volume (IRV) is the maximal volume of gas inspired from end-inspiration; (3) expiratory reserve volume (ERV) is the maximal volume of gas exhaled from end-expiration; and (4) residual volume (RV) is the volume of gas remaining in the lungs following a maximal exhalation.

Capacities: There are four capacities, each of which contains two or more primary volumes: (1) total lung capacity (TLC) is the amount of gas contained in the lung at maximal inspiration; (2) vital capacity (VC) is the maximal volume of gas that can be expelled from the lungs by a forceful effort following maximal inspiration, without regard for the time involved; (3) inspiratory capacity (IC) is the maximal volume of gas that can be inspired from the resting expiratory level; and (4) functional residual capacity (FRC) is the volume of gas in the lungs at resting end-expiration. (From Murray JF, Nadel JA (eds): Textbook of Respiratory Medicine. 3rd ed. Philadelphia, WB Saunders, 2000, p. 783.)

MEASUREMENTS OF VENTILATORY FUNCTION

SPIROMETRY

General

- The volumes of air inhaled and exhaled with relaxed and maximal effort can be measured easily with inexpensive equipment that meets recommended American Thoracic Society (ATS) criteria.[3]
- Results are performed and displayed as a spirogram (FIGURE 8–2).
- Spirometry should be obtained on all patients studied in a pulmonary function laboratory.
- Normal values have been established in a spectrum of subjects based on sex, age, size, and ethnic background,[4, 5] but few have been reported using standards of the ATS.[6–8]
- Measurements depend heavily on patient understanding and cooperation.
- Spirographic evaluation must be conducted by a well-trained technician who is able to communicate instructions clearly. (See following discussion of indications.)

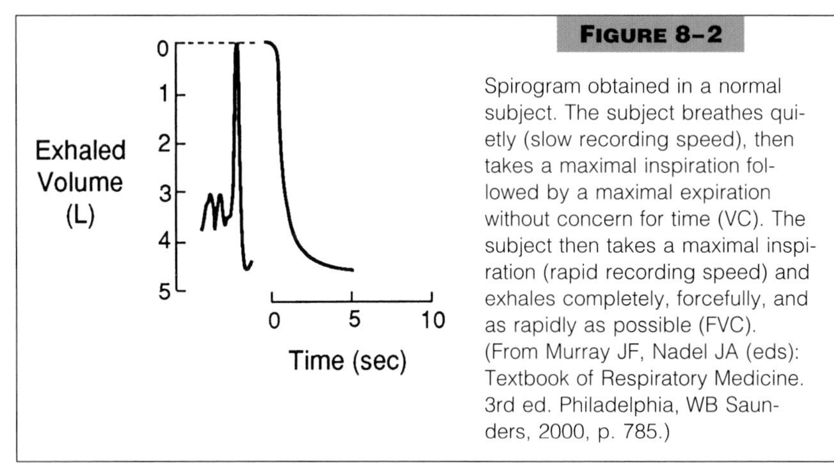

FIGURE 8–2

Spirogram obtained in a normal subject. The subject breathes quietly (slow recording speed), then takes a maximal inspiration followed by a maximal expiration without concern for time (VC). The subject then takes a maximal inspiration (rapid recording speed) and exhales completely, forcefully, and as rapidly as possible (FVC). (From Murray JF, Nadel JA (eds): Textbook of Respiratory Medicine. 3rd ed. Philadelphia, WB Saunders, 2000, p. 785.)

Indications

- *Occupational surveys:* In any potentially hazardous occupation, individual workers should be monitored periodically by spirometry to detect and quantitate evidence of pulmonary problems.
- *Indentifying high-risk smokers:* Spirometry offers the best method to identify smokers at risk for severe chronic airflow obstruction.[9–11]
- *Preoperative assessment:* Those findings can indicate the statistical risk of specific surgical procedures for a group of patients, but they are probably not very useful for the individual; arterial oxygen desaturation is a much better indicator than spirometry of the probability of a high risk associated with a major thoracoabdominal surgical procedure.[12]
- *Evaluation of treatment:* The effectiveness of treatment can be assessed for patients with asthma (e.g., peak expiratory flow, PEF, at home; FEV_1 in clinic) or other forms of chronic airflow obstruction as well as many restrictive disorders.
- *Evaluation of impairment:* Impairment caused by chronic bronchitis or emphysema, as well as pneumoconioses, pulmonary fibrosis, and other pulmonary disorders, can be quantitated.
- *Evaluation of the natural history of disease:* Spirometry is sensitive to progression of disease, especially if baseline values are available for comparison; serial tests much more sensitive than a single value to detect abnormal function because of large variation in the normal range.
- *Detection of disease:* It is an excellent screening test for chronic airflow obstruction and to detect restrictive disorders.
- *Baseline function:* Spirometry should be obtained for adult patients as part of baseline clinical examination; if abnormal (or if the patient has certain risk factors), it is then repeated regularly (every 1 to 5 years).

MEASUREMENTS OF VENTILATORY FUNCTION

SPIROMETRY

Forced Vital Capacity

- Subject inhales maximally to total lung capacity (TLC) and then exhales as rapidly and forcefully as possible.
- Volume is recorded on the ordinate and time on the abscissa of a graph called the FVC curve.
- Analysis of this curve permits computation of the volume exhaled during the time following the start of the maneuver (FEV_t), the ratio of FEV_t to total FVC, and average flow during different portions of the curve. (TABLE 8–1[13,14]).

TABLE 8–1

Terms Used for Spirometric Measurements

Term Used	Previously Used Terms	Description
Vital capacity (VC)		Largest volume measured on complete exhalation after full inspiration
Forced VC (FVC)	Timed VC, Fast VC	VC performed with forced expiration
Forced expiratory volume with subscript indicating interval in seconds (FEV_t, e.g., FEV_1)	Timed VC	Volume of gas exhaled in a given time during performance of FVC
Percentage expired in t seconds (FEV_t%, e.g., FEV_1%)	Timed VC	FEVt expressed as percentage of FVC $\frac{FEVt \times 100}{FVC}$
Forced mid-expiratory flow ($FEF_{25-75\%}$)	Average flow rate during middle two quarters of the FVC	Maximal midexpiratory flow
Forced expiratory flow with subscript indicating volume segment ($FEF_{V_1-V_2}$, e.g., $FEF_{200-1200}$)	Maximal expiratory flow rate	Average rate of flow for a specified segment of FVC, most commonly 200–1200 mL in adults
Maximal voluntary ventilation (MVV)	Maximum breathing capacity (MBC)	Volume of air a subject can breathe with voluntary maximal effort for a given time

Source: Modified from Kory RC: Clinical spirometry: Recommendation of the Section on Pulmonary Function Testing, Committee on Pulmonary Physiology, American College of Chest Physicians. Dis Chest 43:214, 1963.

MEASUREMENTS OF VENTILATORY FUNCTION

SPIROMETRY

Forced Expiratory Volume

- FEV at 1 second (FEV_1) is the measurement of dynamic volume most often used in conjunction with FVC in analysis of spirometry (FIGURE 8–3).
- FEV_1 incorporates the early, effort-dependent portion of the curve, but enough of the midportion to make it reproducible and sensitive for clinical purposes.
- FEV measurements taken at 0.5, 0.75, 2.0, and 3.0 seconds add little additional information to the FEV_1.

FIGURE 8–3

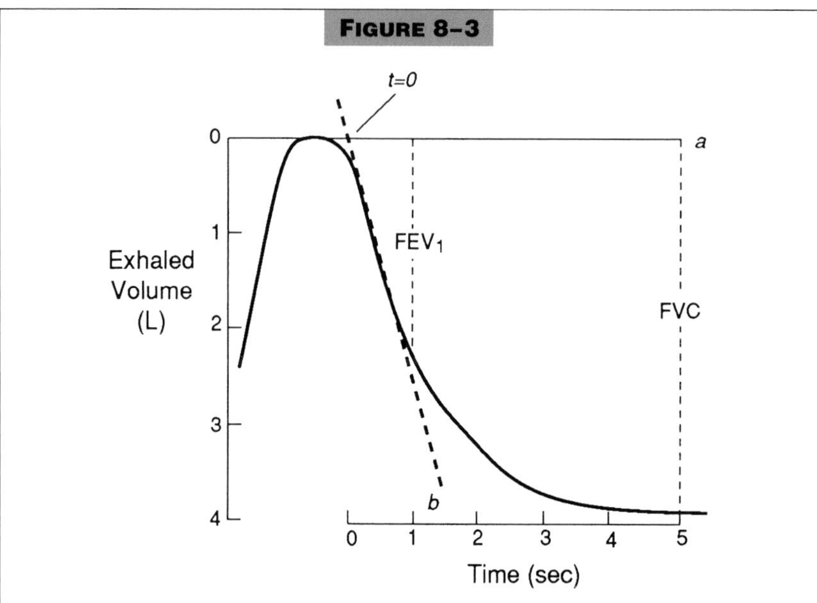

Back extrapolation to define time-zero. This diagram illustrates measurement of FEV_1 using the back extrapolation method to define time-zero, or the point during the FVC maneuver when the subject began to blow as hard and fast as possible. A solid, horizontal line (a) indicates the level of maximal inhalation. A heavy dashed line (b) passes through the steepest portion of volume-time tracing. The intersection point of these two lines becomes time-zero, as indicated, from which timing is initiated; 1 second after time-zero, the vertical dashed line is drawn, indicating FEV_1, and 5 seconds later, another vertical dashed line is drawn, indicating FVC. (From Murray JF, Nadel JA (eds): Textbook of Respiratory Medicine. 3rd ed. Philadelphia, WB Saunders, 2000, p. 786.)

MEASUREMENTS OF VENTILATORY FUNCTION

SPIROMETRY

Forced Expiratory Volume Over Time As a Percentage of Forced Vital Capacity (FEV_t/FVC)

- FEV_t/FVC has been defined precisely in healthy subjects.
- FEV_t/FVC declines with age,[15] but abnormally decreased ratios indicate airway obstruction.
- Normal or increased ratios do not exclude airway obstruction, particularly with decreased FVC.
- FEV_t/FVC ratios are increased when FVC is decreased by an interstitial process or chest wall restriction, and the airways are normal.
- FEV_t/FVC ratios may be increased in subjects who fail to make a maximal effort throughout the expiratory maneuver (see next item).
- The absence of an increased FEV_t/FVC ratio when expected, suggests the presence of concomitant airway obstruction.
- Interpretation of the spirogram in mixed ventilatory defects may be facilitated by examining exhaled volumes and flows as a percentage of predicted values.

Average Forced Expiratory Flow

- $FEF_{25-75\%}$ is the average flow (FEF) between 25% and 75% of FVC (FIGURE 8–4).
- This value reflects the most effort-independent portion of the curve, which is most sensitive to airflow in peripheral airways where diseases of chronic airflow obstruction are thought to begin.[16–20]
- There is a marked variability in studies of large samples of healthy subjects; 95% confidence limits are so large as to limit its sensitivity in detecting disease in an individual subject.[21, 22] (APPENDIX 5 gives the normal predicted values for bronchodilator response.)

FIGURE 8–4

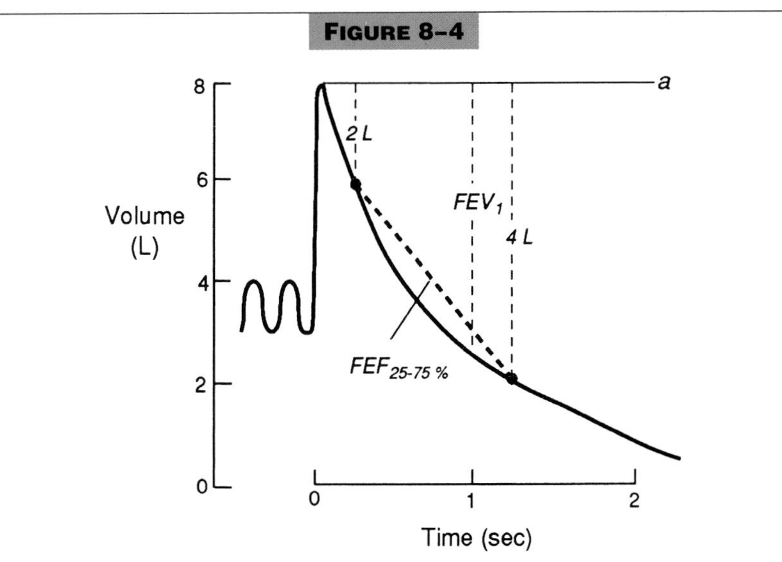

Determination of $FEF_{25-75\%}$. A heavy dashed line connects two points on the volume-time curve of the FVC maneuver. One point is marked when 25% of the FVC (2 L) has been exhaled; the other point is marked when 75% of the FVC (4 L) has been exhaled from the level of maximal inhalation indicated by the solid line (a). The elapsed time between these two points is 1 second; thus, the $FEF_{25-75\%}$ = 2 L/sec. (From Murray JF, Nadel JA (eds): Textbook of Respiratory Medicine. 3rd ed. Philadelphia, WB Saunders, 2000, p. 786.)

MEASUREMENTS OF VENTILATORY FUNCTION

SPIROMETRY

Peak Expiratory Flow Rate

- Peak flow occurs during a very effort-dependent portion of the expiratory maneuver as a transient peak; decreased values can result from even slightly submaximal effort rather than from airway obstruction.
- PEF is easily measured with an inexpensive, small portable device.[23]
- The PEF rate is useful to follow airflow obstruction on an ambulatory basis, in suspected occupational asthma, or in patients who are insensitive to the severity of bronchospasm.

Maximal Voluntary Ventilation

- Maximal volume of air moved by voluntary effort in one minute (MVV) originally was called maximal breathing capacity.
- The subject should perform several practice runs, and choose his or her own respiratory rate.
- Respiratory rate used in the MVV should be recorded as a subscript(e.g., MVV_{90} or MVV_{110}); maximal MVV usually achieved between 70 and 120 breaths per minute, but the choice of frequency does not greatly affect the test.[24]
- The MVV test has the following characteristics:
  - Its usefulness is heavily dependent on subject cooperation and effort.
  - This volume is decreased by loss of coordination of respiratory muscles, musculoskeletal disease of the chest wall, neurologic diseases, deconditioning from any chronic illness, and ventilatory defects.
  - MVV is decreased in airway obstruction, but less so with mild or moderate restrictive defects because rapid, shallow breathing can compensate effectively for the decreased lung volumes.
  - Results correlate well with subjective dyspnea; thus, it is useful in evaluating exercise tolerance.
  - MVV has prognostic value in preoperative evaluation, possibly because the extrapulmonary factors to which it is sensitive are also important for recovery from a surgical procedure.[25]
- MVV is a measure of respiratory muscle endurance; thus, it is useful to evaluate respiratory muscle fatigue.[26, 27]
- In myasthenia gravis, the patient can often produce maximal efforts for a short time (FVC and maximal inspiratory and expiratory pressures are normal), but cannot sustain an effort (MVV or repeated FVC values decrease, even within 12 to 15 seconds).
  - The respiratory crisis of myasthenia gravis may occur with great rapidity and lead to respiratory failure.
  - Evaluate treatment of patients with myasthenia gravis under carefully controlled circumstances.[28] (See APPENDIX 6 for predicted normal values for MVV.)

FLOW-VOLUME RELATIONSHIPS

General

- Computer-based electronic apparatus makes flow-volume curves as readily available in the doctor's office as spirometry.
- Indications for spirometry probably apply equally to the flow-volume curve.
- To measure flow and volume, the subject inspires and expires fully with maximal effort into an instrument that measures flow and volume simultaneously, and plots the results on the two axes of an *X-Y* recorder or oscilloscope (FIGURES 8–5 and 8–6).
- Maximal flow-volume envelope is approximated by having the subject make repeated trials of increasing effort (*left* in FIGURE 8–7), or by having the subject cough while recording flow-volume relationships (*right,* FIGURE 8–7).

(continued)

MEASUREMENTS OF VENTILATORY FUNCTION

FLOW-VOLUME RELATIONSHIPS

General

- The flow-volume curve and forced expiratory volume-time curve are mathematically interchangeable, and one can be derived graphically, or by computer analysis, from the other, providing an internal check on the accuracy of the tests.
- At volumes greater than 75% VC, respiratory muscles cannot contract forcefully and rapidly enough to achieve maximal $\dot{V}$.
  - At high lung volume, $\dot{V}$ is effort-dependent,
  - At middle and low lung volumes, $\dot{V}$ is effort-*independent* and reflects intrinsic properties of the lung (lung elastic recoil, dimensions of intrathoracic airways, and rigidity of airways subject to compression).

FIGURE 8–5

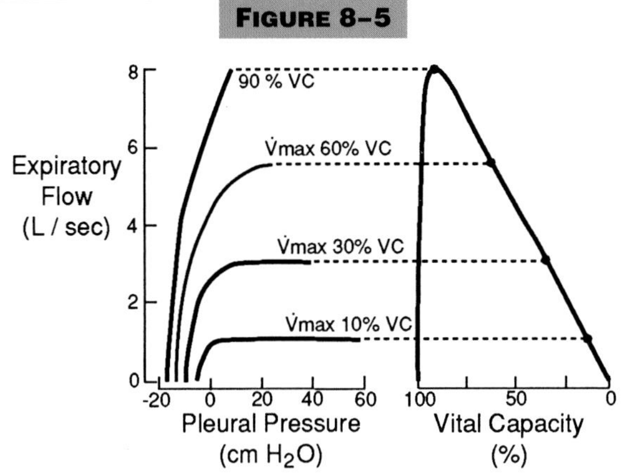

From a series of isovolume pressure-flow (IVPF) curves at varying vital capacities (*left*), it is possible to construct a maximal flow-volume curve (*right*). $\dot{V}$max = maximal expiratory flow. A similar flow-volume curve can be obtained by simply plotting expired flow against volume using an x-y recorder during a single forced expiratory vital capacity maneuver. (From Murray JF, Nadel JA (eds): Textbook of Respiratory Medicine. 3rd ed. Philadelphia, WB Saunders, 2000, p. 787.)

FIGURE 8–6

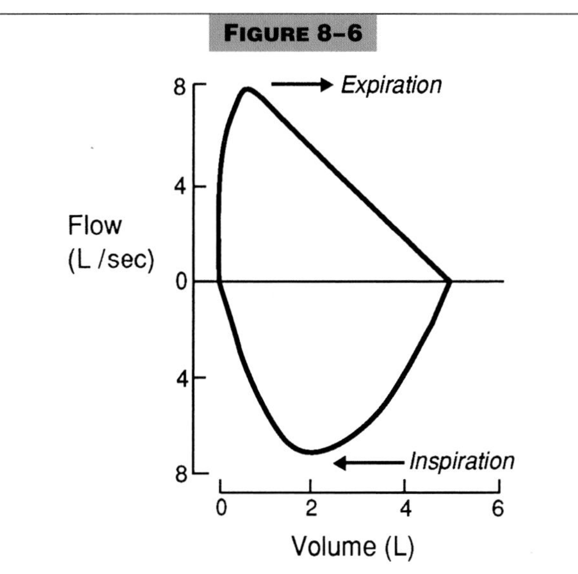

Flow-volume curve recorded during inspiration and expiration in a normal subject. (From Murray JF, Nadel JA (eds): Textbook of Respiratory Medicine. 3rd ed. Philadelphia, WB Saunders, 2000, p. 788.)

FIGURE 8–7

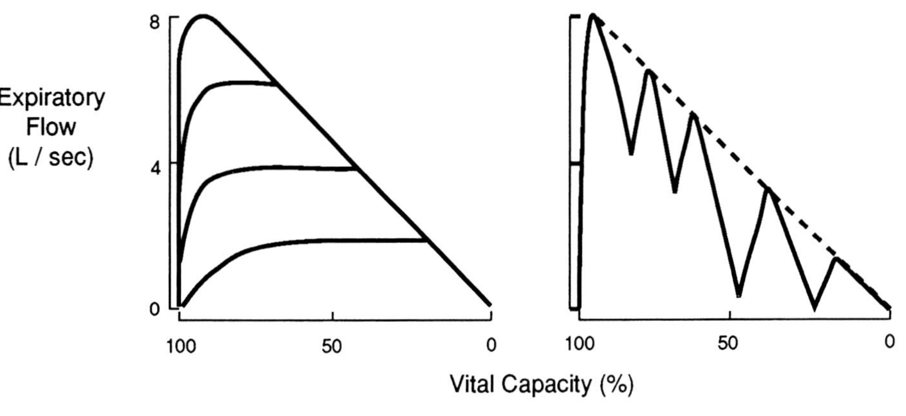

Expiratory flow-volume curve recorded during a series of expirations with increasing efforts, finally producing a maximal flow-volume envelope (*left*). Expiratory flow-volume curve (*right*) recorded during coughing (*solid line*), approximating the maximal flow-volume envelope (*dashed line*). (From Murray JF, Nadel JA (eds): Textbook of Respiratory Medicine. 3rd ed. Philadelphia, WB Saunders, 2000, p. 789.)

MEASUREMENTS OF VENTILATORY FUNCTION

FLOW-VOLUME RELATIONSHIPS

Shape During Exhalation

- The initial portion of the F-V curve (the first 25% to 33% of the vital capacity, VC, exhaled) depends on effort: subject exerts increasing effort during exhalation, associated with increasing intrathoracic pressure, generating increasing flow.
  - This portion of the curve has limited diagnostic use because its appearance depends primarily on the subject's muscular effort rather than on the mechanical characteristics of the lung.
- Following peak flow, the curve follows a reproducible, effort-independent envelope as flow diminishes in proportion to volume until RV (residual volume) is reached.
  - For each point on the volume axis, a maximal flow exists that cannot be exceeded regardless of the pressure generated by the respiratory muscles.
  - This portion of the curve is very reproducible in a given subject over time, but may be altered in a characteristic manner by the effect of diseases on the mechanical properties of the lungs.
- RV is usually determined by airway closure, so the flow-volume curve shows a progressive decrease in flow until RV is reached.
  - In young individuals, however, and perhaps in some patients with chest wall disease, RV is determined by chest wall rigidity, which limits maximal exhalation; thus, expiratory flow abruptly decreases to zero at low lung volumes.
- The shape of the inspiratory F-V curve is symmetric; flow increases to a peak midway through inspiration and then decreases as inhalation proceeds to TLC.
  - The inspiratory limb is more sensitive to tracheal obstruction than the expiratory limb, a situation in which ordinary spirometry reveals a nonspecific pattern (see discussion of flow-volume curves in Airway Obstruction).
  - The inspiratory limb is less influenced by diffuse airway or parenchymal disease.

Obstructive Ventilatory Defects

- Early asymptomatic obstructive disorders may be associated with decreased maximal flow at low lung volumes.[29]
- Limited numbers of anatomic studies correlate findings in patients with emphysema, and central and peripheral airway lesions.[17, 30–34] (See Chapter 3, Pathology.)
- The variability of the curve at low lung volumes makes it difficult to interpret individual curves, even when compared with studies of large populations.[35, 36]
- In patients with airflow obstruction, an initial sharp downward deflection (the effect of compression of major central airways or "tracheobronchial collapse") is followed by an exaggerated upward concavity of the descending limb of the curve.
- Emphysema has the greatest tendency to cause the descending limb of the curve to become concave upward; this loss of linearity relates to the severity of the obstruction as well as the type of disease.
- Decreased volume occurs in both obstructive and restrictive ventilatory defects, reflecting decreased VC.
- Decreased VC is relatively less in airway obstruction than in restrictive ventilatory defects:
  - F-V curve in obstructive ventilatory defects is oriented along the horizontal (volume) axis.
  - F-V curve in restrictive defects is oriented along the vertical (flow) axis.

MEASUREMENTS OF VENTILATORY FUNCTION

FLOW-VOLUME RELATIONSHIPS

Tidal Breathing vs. Maximal Effort

- The difference between flow during tidal breathing and flow during maximal effort is a measure of pulmonary reserve with respect to airflow.
- As airflow obstruction increases, the expiratory flow during the two maneuvers becomes superimposed, at first appearing low in the lung volume curve, but as the disease becomes more severe, it continues into the higher lung volumes.
- "Negative-effort dependence" is said to be present when expiratory airflow during quiet tidal breathing exceeds flow during maximal effort; this phenomenon suggests that the airways are less rigid than normal, as may be seen in emphysema and in some forms of chronic bronchitis.
  - When flow and volume are measured at the mouth, expiratory flow during tidal breathing may artifactually appear to exceed the flow observed during maximal effort because of compression of thoracic gas during the forced expiration.
- The relative positions of the two curves on the volume axis is a graphic demonstration of the amount of expiratory volume in reserve; as this reserve decreases owing to obesity, pregnancy, or ascites, the tidal volume loop moves closer to RV.

Upper Airway Obstruction

(See Chapter 6, Bronchoscopy)

- Central airway obstruction located within the thorax, proximal to the tracheal carina and distal to the thoracic outlet, produces a plateau during forced exhalation instead of the usual rise to and descent from peak flow (FIGURE 8–8).
- Relatively low in the lung volume, the curve then follows the normal flow-volume envelope to RV.
- In any patient with stridor, particular attention should be paid to the configuration of the inspiratory and expiratory portions of the flow-volume curve.
- Any lesion located below the thoracic outlet will cause decreased airflow during exhalation; during inhalation, the posterior tracheal membrane is pulled out so that increased effort increases airflow rates ($\dot{V}exhal < \dot{V}inhal$).
- Conversely, any lesion located between the vocal cords and the thoracic outlet will cause decreased airflow during inhalation, when the tracheal membrane is sucked in, and is usually associated with stridor ($\dot{V}exhal > \dot{V}inhal$).
- A critical orifice located at the thoracic outlet is not affected by pressure above or below the lesion if the orifice is narrow enough; airflow is limited equally during both inhalation and exhalation.[37]
- Estimate diameter of a critical orifice by analysis of the F-V curve with an accuracy of $\pm$ 1 mm; the length of the flow-limiting segment must be confirmed by tracheogram or computerized tomographic (CT) scan in order to properly plan surgical correction, if required. (See Chapter 4, Radiography and Imaging.)

MEASUREMENTS OF VENTILATORY FUNCTION

FLOW-VOLUME RELATIONSHIPS

Upper Airway Obstruction

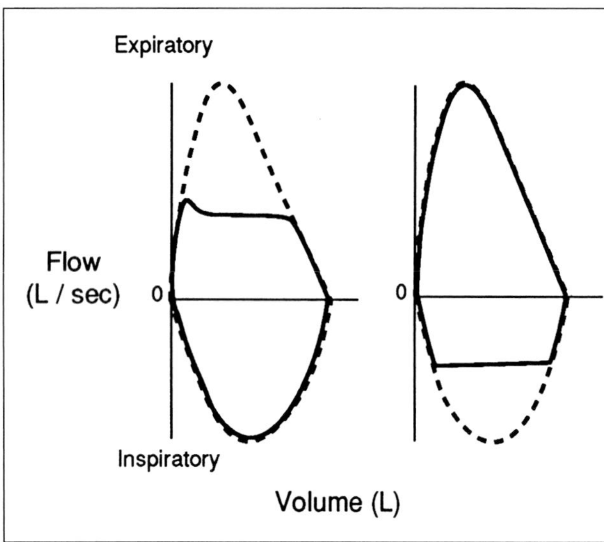

FIGURE 8-8

Flow-volume curves obtained in patients with upper airway obstruction. Dashed line represents a curve obtained in a normal subject with the same VC as observed in the patients. Solid line indicates a curve obtained in a patient with intrathoracic obstruction (*left*) and another patient with extrathoracic obstruction (*right*). (From Murray JF, Nadel JA (eds): Textbook of Respiratory Medicine. 3rd ed. Philadelphia, WB Saunders, 2000, p. 790.)

Gas Density

- Comparison of F-V curves obtained when the subject breathes air vs. low-density gas mixtures such as heliox (80% helium, 20% O_2) has been advocated to detect early or mild airway obstruction[38, 39] and to localize the site of airway obstruction.[17]
- During a forced exhalation, when flow limitation occurs in large central airways where flow is turbulent, low-density gas increases maximal flow, defined by the increased maximal flow at 50% VC ($\Delta\dot{V}\ max_{50\%}$).
- As lung volume decreases, the flow-limiting segment moves into small peripheral airways, where flow is laminar and density-independent.
- The lung volume at which flow becomes density-independent and where air and heliox flow-volume curves can be superimposed is called the volume of isoflow (Visoflow).

$\Delta\dot{V}max_{50\%}$ and Visoflow

- Theoretical analysis of reported observations has proved unsatisfactory.
- Differential diagnosis of central and peripheral airway lesions has not been successful.
- No studies have been performed that demonstrate the contribution to abnormal $\Delta\dot{V}max_{50\%}$ and Visoflow values by concomitant pathologic changes in central airways and emphysema as well as lesions in bronchioles.
- It has been difficult to interpret these measurements in healthy subjects and patients because of large intrasubject and intersubject variability.[40]
- Variability in interpretation of the same series of curves by different observers is also a problem.[41]
- Agreement has not been reached on these controversial issues and currently, these tests have little clinical usefulness[42] (FIGURE 8-9).

MEASUREMENTS OF VENTILATORY FUNCTION

FLOW-VOLUME RELATIONSHIPS

$\Delta\dot{V}max_{50\%}$ and Visoflow

FIGURE 8–9

Flow-volume curve (*solid line*) when the subject breathes air and flow-volume curve (*dashed line*) when the subject breathes heliox (80% helium, 20% oxygen). The volume at which maximal expiratory flow is the same in the two curves, regardless of the gas mixture breathed, is called the volume of isoflow (Visoflow). The difference in the maximal expiratory flow at 50% VC when breathing air vs. heliox is the $\Delta\dot{V}max_{50\%}$. (From Murray JF, Nadel JA (eds): Textbook of Respiratory Medicine. 3rd ed. Philadelphia, WB Saunders, 2000, p. 790.)

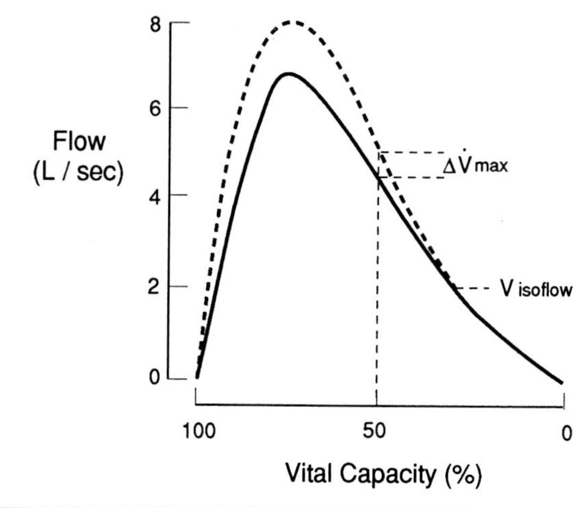

Restrictive Ventilatory Defects

- Increased lung elastic recoil accounts for the decreased VC of restrictive defects but also increases the force driving expiratory flow and pulling outward on airway walls; thus, the usual F-V curve in restrictive ventilatory defects is tall and narrow.
- PEF is relatively preserved and the descending portion of the expiratory limb is linear, decreasing rapidly from peak flow to RV.
- The loop often maintains a nearly normal shape but appears miniaturized in all dimensions.

LUNG VOLUMES

Vital Capacity

- The subject inhales as deeply as possible and then exhales fully, taking as much time as required. (Note that Figure 8–1 illustrates VC and the subdivisions of lung volume as defined by Pappenheimer and colleagues.[43])
- "Combined" VC = ERV + IC.
  - ERV (expiratory reserve volume) is obtained by having the subject exhale maximally from the resting end-tidal level.
  - IC (inspiratory capacity) is obtained by having the subject inspire fully from the resting end-tidal level.
- "Combined" VC = VC, provided that the resting end-tidal level is the same for the two component maneuvers.
- In severely obstructed patients, the "combined VC" is greater than VC, "slow VC" is greater than FVC, and "inspired VC" is greater than "expired VC."
  - These differences probably reflect poorly ventilated regions of lungs, or so-called "trapped gas," a result of increased transmural pressure, which tends to cause airway closure during a large portion of the single maneuver, but only during the portion near RV in the "combined VC" maneuver.
  - Increased transmural pressure also tends to cause airway closure during the forced FVC compared to slow VC and expired VC compared to inspired VC.
- VC can be decreased by a decrease in TLC or by an increase in RV, which can be differentiated only by measuring RV and TLC.
- Decreased VC alone is inadequate and nonspecific to assess decreased ventilatory reserve; measurement of FVC and its subdivisions as well as VC adds clarification of the mechanism and severity of a ventilatory defect.
- Measurement of RV provides convincing proof of the presence or absence of overinflation or underinflation of the lung.

MEASUREMENTS OF VENTILATORY FUNCTION

LUNG VOLUMES

Gas Dilution Methods

- The two most commonly used gas dilution methods to measure lung volume are the open-circuit nitrogen (N_2) method and the closed-circuit helium (He) method.
- Both methods take advantage of a physiologically inert gas that is poorly soluble in alveolar blood and lung tissues, and both are usually used to measure functional residual capacity (FRC), the volume of gas remaining in the lung at the end of a normal expiration.
- In the open-circuit method, all exhaled gas is collected while the subject inhales pure O_2:
  - Initial concentration of N_2 in the lungs is about 81%.
  - Rate of N_2 elimination from blood and tissues is about 30 mL per minute.
  - The total amount of N_2 washed out from the lungs is measured.
  - Thus, the volume of N_2-containing gas present in the lungs at the beginning of the maneuver may be calculated[44] (FIGURE 8–10).

FIGURE 8–10

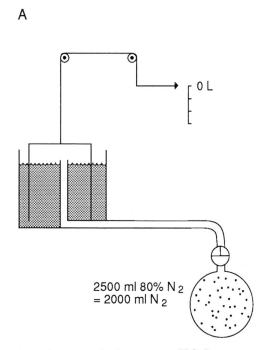

A

0 L

2500 ml 80% N 2
= 2000 ml N 2

B

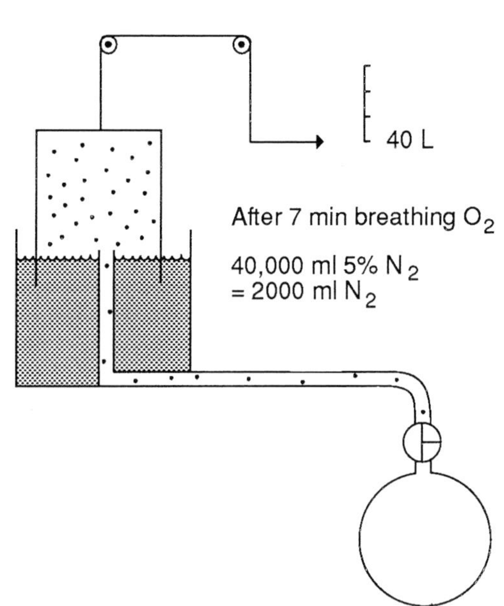

Open circuit nitrogen method to measure FRC. Dots represent N_2 molecules. Initially, all the N_2 molecules are in the lungs (as 80% N_2). When N_2-free oxygen is breathed, the N_2 molecules are washed out of the lungs and collected with the oxygen as expired gas in the spirometer. The spirometer contains 40,000 mL of mixed expired gas with a N_2 concentration of 5%. Thus, the spirometer contains 2000 mL (0.05 × 40,000) of N_2; the remaining 38,000 mL of gas is mainly O_2 used to wash the N_2 out of the lungs, plus some CO_2. The 2000 mL of N_2 was distributed within the lungs at a concentration of 80% N_2 when the washout began; therefore, the alveolar volume in which the N_2 was distributed was 100/80 × 2000 mL = 2500 mL. Corrections must be made for the small amount of N_2 washed out of the blood and tissue when oxygen is breathed and for the small amounts of N_2 in "pure O_2." (From Murray JF, Nadel JA (eds): Textbook of Respiratory Medicine. 3rd ed. Philadelphia, WB Saunders, 2000, p. 791.)

MEASUREMENTS OF VENTILATORY FUNCTION

LUNG VOLUMES

Open-Circuit N_2 Gas Dilution Method

Advantages of the open-circuit N_2 gas dilution method are as follows:

- The open-circuit method permits assessment of the uniformity of ventilation of the lungs in two ways:
  1. By analyzing the slope of the change in nitrogen concentration over consecutive exhalations
  2. By the conventions of measuring the end-expiratory concentration of N_2 after 7 minutes of washout,[45–48] and of measuring the total ventilation required to reduce end-expiratory nitrogen to less than 2%[49]
- This method is sensitive to leaks anywhere in the system (especially at the mouthpiece) and to errors in measurement of N_2 concentration and exhaled volume.
- If a pneumotachygraph is used to measure volume, attention must be paid to the effects of the change in viscosity of the gas exhaled, as it contains a progressively decreasing concentration of N_2.[50, 51]

The open-circuit N_2 gas dilution method also has several disadvantages:

- The volume of gas that is in poor communication with the airways (e.g., in lung bullae) is not measured.
- This method assumes that the volume at which the measurement was made corresponds to the end-expiratory point on the spirometry tracing used to calculate ERV and IC (needed for the computation of RV and TLC from the measured FRC). The assumption of a constant or reproducible end-expiratory volume can be eliminated by measuring spirometric volumes immediately before measuring FRC as a combined continuous sequence, using appropriate valves connected to the mouthpiece, available in many commercial systems.
- A long period of re-equilibration with room air is required before the test can be repeated.

Closed-Circuit Helium Dilution Method

- A gas mixture containing He, a physiologically inert tracer gas in a closed system, is rebreathed until equilibration occurs (FIGURE 8–11); if the volume and concentration of He in the gas mixture rebreathed are known, measurement of the final equilibrium concentration of He permits calculation of the volume of gas in the lungs at the onset of the maneuver (TABLE 8–2).
- He concentration: usually measured continuously by a thermal-conductivity meter, permitting return of the sampled gas to the system.
- CO_2 must be removed from a closed system, so a CO_2 absorber is added, resulting in a constant fall in the volume of gas in the closed circuit, as O_2 is consumed and the subject produces CO_2.
- An equivalent amount of O_2 is therefore introduced as an initial bolus or as a continuous flow.
- The subject must be "switched into" the system at the end-tidal point; it is possible to calculate the correction for an error in this point, but only if the subject is able to relax and exhale reproducibly to the actual end-tidal point while breathing from the circuit.
- In a cooperative subject IC, ERV, and VC can be measured from maneuvers recorded with the spirometer while the subject is switched into the system.
- The method is sensitive to errors from leakage of gas and alinearity of the gas analyzer.
- The volume of gas cannot be measured in lung bullae, and the procedure cannot be repeated at short intervals.
- Reproducible results (SD of repeated measurements is 90 to 160 mL)[52–54] and normal values are available from several studies of healthy subjects.[55–58] APPENDIX 7 gives the predicted normal values for TLC and RV.

MEASUREMENTS OF VENTILATORY FUNCTION

LUNG VOLUMES

Closed-Circuit Helium Dilution Method

TABLE 8–2

Functional Residual Capacity Calculated from Helium Closed-Circuit Method

Before Rebreathing Helium	After Rebreathing Helium
He in lung + He in spirometer	= He in lungs + He in spirometer
$V_L + V_S F_S$	$= (V_L + V_S)(F_L \text{ or } F_S)$
$0 + (2{,}000 \times 0.1)$	$= (V_L + 2000)(0.05)$
200	$= (0.05\ V_L + 100)$
2000	$= V_L$

F_L = fractional concentration of helium (He) in lungs; F_S = fractional concentration of He in spirometer; V_L = volume of gas in lungs; V_S = volume of gas in spirometer.

Source: Modified from Comroe JH Jr et al: The Lung: Clinical Physiology and Pulmonary Function Tests (2nd ed.). Chicago, Year Book Medical Publishers, 1962.

FIGURE 8–11

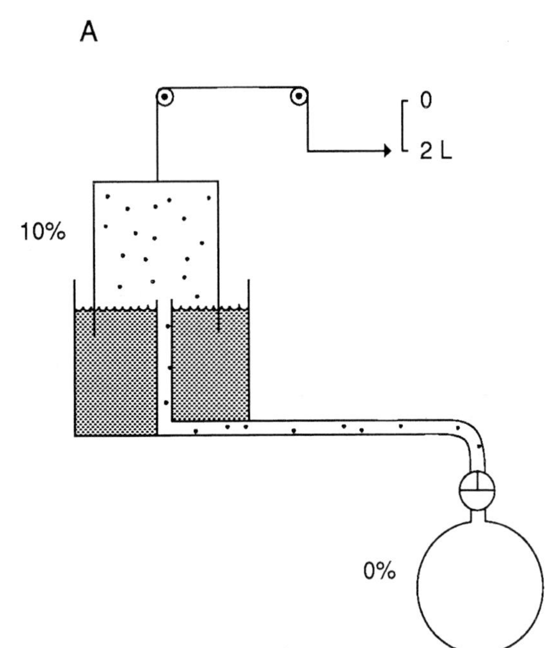

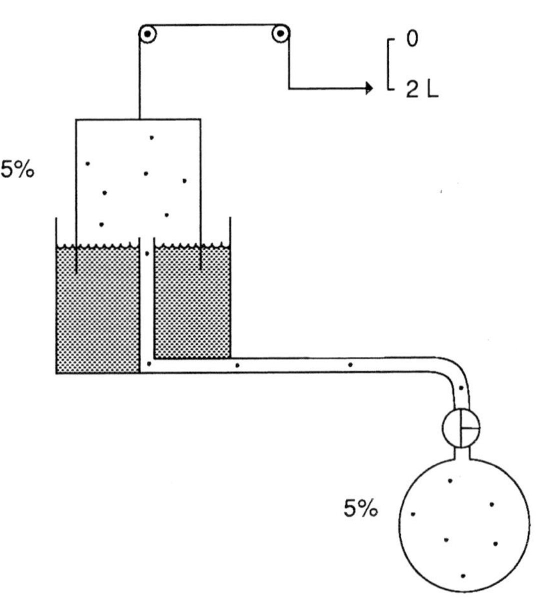

Closed-circuit helium (He) method to measure FRC. Dots represent molecules of He. Initially, all are in the spirometer (as 10% He) and none are in the lungs. If the spirometer contains 2000 mL of gas, of which 10% is He, then (2000 mL × 0.01) or 200 mL of He is present in the spirometer before rebreathing. Rebreathing results in redistribution of the He molecules until equilibrium occurs, at which time lung volume can be calculated. At the end of the test, the same amount of He (200 mL) must be redistributed in the lungs, tubing, and spirometer, assuming He is inert and not soluble in blood or tissues. Table 8–2 shows the calculation of FRC from these relationships, assuming the final concentration of He in the system was 5%. (From Murray JF, Nadel JA (eds): Textbook of Respiratory Medicine. 3rd ed. Philadelphia, WB Saunders, 2000, p. 792.)

MEASUREMENTS OF VENTILATORY FUNCTION

LUNG VOLUMES

Single-Breath Dilution Methods

- During the single-breath N_2 washout test of the distribution of ventilation, the single-breath N_2 dilution lung volume can be estimated from the mean concentration of N_2 in the air exhaled after the VC inspiration of pure oxygen.[59]
- During the single-breath measurement of the diffusing capacity for carbon monoxide (DL_{CO}), the lung volume is estimated for the change in concentration of the Ne, He, or CH_4 used as the inert tracer gas.[60]
- Alveolar volume achieved during performance of the standard diffusing capacity maneuver is approximately TLC and must be estimated in order to measure DL_{CO}.
- Values obtained correspond well with those obtained by body plethysmography in healthy subjects.[60, 61]
- Because the time for dilution of the tracer gas is short (10 seconds), true TLC will be underestimated in patients with severe airway obstruction or uneven distribution of ventilation. If FEV_1/FVC is less than 0.40, TLC may be underestimated by single breath dilution.[60] (APPENDIX 7 gives normal predicted values for TLC and RV.)

Roentgenographic Methods

(See Chapter 4, Radiography and Imaging)

- TLC and FRC can be estimated from chest roentgenograms.
- Planimetry method uses equations derived empirically from measurements of surface areas on chest roentgenograms and of TLC in the same subjects.[62]
- Mean planimetric values differ little from those determined by plethysmography.
- Large divergences are sometimes obtained in individuals because of the large effect of small errors in setting the distance between the subject and the x-ray film and because of failure of the subject to inhale to TLC.[24, 62a, 63, 64]
- Normal predictive values have not been established in adequate numbers of subjects.[65]
- Possible applications of roentgenographic evaluation include the following:
- To estimate retrospectively previous values of TLC in patients for whom old roentgenograms, but not the results of pulmonary function tests, are available.
- To estimate TLC in patients with lung bullae (when plethysmography is not available).
- To estimate lung volume in special cases, as in the patient with a tracheostomy.
- To manage patients with acute airway obstruction (e.g., asthma) in the emergency room. Spirometry, but not other pulmonary function tests, is usually available; roentgenographic measurement of overinflation (an important risk factor in asthma)[66] could be performed readily and could contribute to the proper care of the patient.

MEASUREMENTS OF VENTILATORY FUNCTION

LUNG VOLUMES

Pressure (Closed-Type) Plethysmograph

- Closed chamber with a fixed volume in which the subject breathes the gas in the plethysmograph (or body box) (FIGURE 8–12).
- Volume changes associated with compression or expansion of gas within the thorax are measured as pressure changes in gas surrounding the subject within the box.
- Volume exchange between lung and box does not directly cause pressure changes, although thermal, humidity, and CO_2-O_2 exchange differences between inspired and expired gas do cause pressure changes.
- Thoracic gas volume and resistance are measured during rapid maneuvers, so small leaks are tolerated or are introduced to vent slow thermal-pressure drift.
- The pressure plethysmograph is best suited for measuring small volume changes because of its high sensitivity and excellent frequency response; the chamber need not be leak-free, absolutely rigid, or refrigerated because the measurements are usually brief to study rapid events.

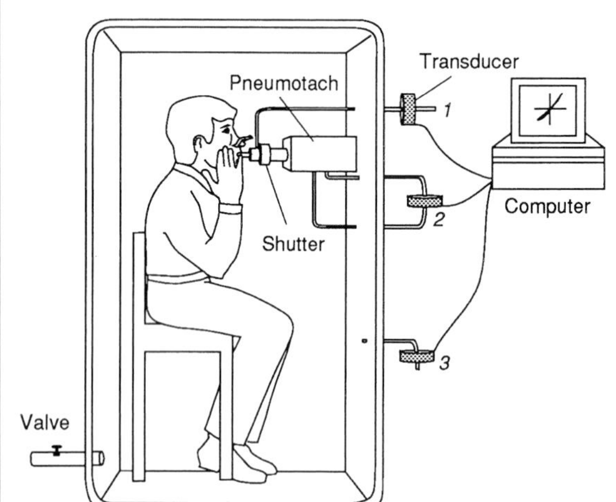

FIGURE 8–12

Pressure (closed-type) plethysmograph. The subject breathes through a shutter/pneumotachygraph. The shutter is open during tidal breathing and for measurements of airway resistance, and closed for measurements of thoracic gas volume. When the shutter is closed, mouth pressure (equal to alveolar pressure at no flow) is measured by a pressure transducer (top, 1). The pneumotachygraph measures airflow with another transducer (middle, 2), and the flow signal is integrated to volume electronically. The plethysmograph pressure is measured by a third transducer (bottom, 3). The signals from the three transducers are processed by a computer. Excess box pressure caused by temperature changes when the subject sits in the closed box is vented through a valve. (From Murray JF, Nadel JA (eds): Textbook of Respiratory Medicine. 3rd ed. Philadelphia, WB Saunders, 2000, p. 794.)

Volume (Open-Type) Plethysmograph

- This method uses constant pressure and variable volume (FIGURE 8–13).
- With thoracic volume changes, gas is displaced through a hole in the box wall and is measured either with a spirometer or by integrating the flow through a pneumotachygraph (or flowmeter).
- The open plethysmograph is suitable for measuring small or large volume changes.
- Gas displacement must be very small to attain good frequency response and requires:
  - Low-resistance pneumotachygraph, sensitive transducer, and fast, drift-free integrator
  - Meticulous utilization of special spirometers
  - Neither technique is applicable to a routine clinical laboratory.

MEASUREMENTS OF VENTILATORY FUNCTION

LUNG VOLUMES

Volume (Open-Type) Plethysmograph

FIGURE 8–13

Volume (open-type) plethysmograph. In this constant-pressure, variable-volume plethysmograph, the subject also breathes through a shutter/pneumotachygraph apparatus that usually is located outside the plethysmograph itself. The shutter is open for tidal breathing, measurement of airway resistance, and spirometry. It is closed for measurement of thoracic gas volume. In the closed-shutter mode, mouth pressure is measured by transducer (top, 1) and approximates alveolar pressure with no flow and small volume changes. The pneumotachygraph measures flow via another transducer (above pneumotach, 2). Flow is integrated electronically to obtain volume. Changes in volume of the plethysmograph, reflecting movement of the chest wall, are measured with a spirometer and a linear volume-displacement transducer, LVDT. The spirometer illustrated is a Krogh water-sealed spirometer with good frequency response and very small impedance to gas displacement. A low-resistance pneumotachygraph (flowmeter) with fast, drift-free integrator may be used instead. Processing is usually performed by computer and permits slow and FVC maneuvers as well. However, neither approach is routine. (From Murray JF, Nadel JA (eds): Textbook of Respiratory Medicine. 3rd ed. Philadelphia, WB Saunders, 2000, p. 794.)

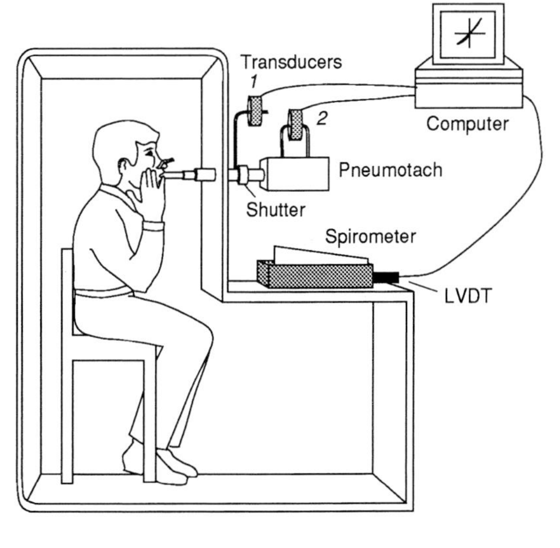

Pressure-Volume Plethysmograph (Fig. 8–14)

- The pressure-volume plethysmograph combines features of the closed and open types.
- Changes in thoracic gas volume compress or expand the air around the subject in the box and also displace it through a hole in the box wall.
  - Gas compression or decompression is measured as a pressure change; gas displacement is measured either by a spirometer connected to the box or by integrating airflow through a pneumotachygraph in the opening.
  - At every instant, the change in thoracic gas volume is accounted for by adding the two components (pressure change and volume displacement).
- This method permits all types of measurements with the same instrument (i.e., thoracic gas volume and airway resistance, spirometry, and flow-volume curves).
- Excellent frequency response, relatively modest requirements for the spirometer, and the integrated-flow version dispenses with water-filled spirometers and is tolerant of leaks.

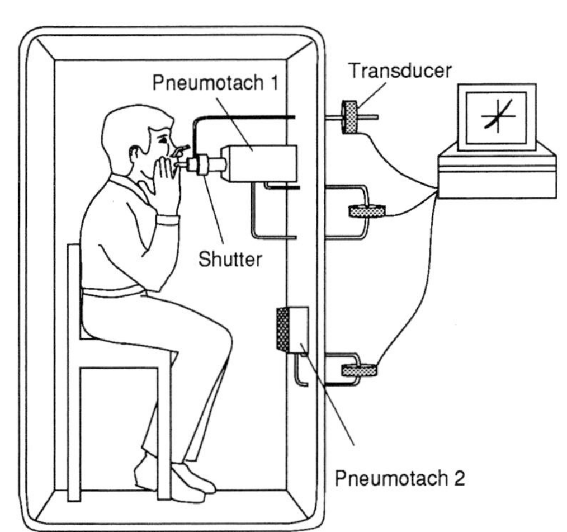

FIGURE 8–14

Pressure-volume (or flow) plethysmograph. This type of plethysmograph combines features of the closed and open types. The subject breathes through a shutter/pneumotachygraph apparatus. The shutter is open for tidal breathing, measurement of airway resistance, and spirometry. It is closed for measurement of thoracic gas volume. In the closed position, mouth pressure (alveolar pressure) is measured by a transducer (top). The pneumotachygraph (1) at the mouth measures airflow with another transducer (middle). This airflow at the mouth is integrated to obtain volume inhaled and exhaled at the mouth. Changes in plethysmograph or box volume resulting from movements of the chest wall are measured by a pneumotachygraph (2) in the wall of the plethysmograph with a third transducer (bottom) and this signal is integrated to obtain volume change of the thorax. The signals from all three transducers are now usually processed by computer to obtain slow and forced vital capacities as well as resistance and thoracic gas volumes. (From Murray JF, Nadel JA (eds): Textbook of Respiratory Medicine. 3rd ed. Philadelphia, WB Saunders, 2000, p. 795.)

MEASUREMENTS OF VENTILATORY FUNCTION

LUNG VOLUMES

Pressure-Volume Box Equations

$$\Delta V = (\text{Pbox})(\text{Kbox}) + \text{Pbox}/\text{Rbox} \int \dot{V}\text{box}$$

where

- Box pressure, Pbox, is multiplied by a constant, Kbox, which is proportional to the gas volume in the box (total box volume − patient volume);
- Box pressure, Pbox, is divided by the box flowmeter resistance, Rbox, and flow is integrated to obtain volume, Vbox.

Physical Principles of Pressure-Volume Plethysmograph

- Displacement volume, Pbox/Rbox $\int \dot{V}$box, is added to the plethysmograph compression volume, (Pbox) (Kbox), to produce the "true" volume (FIGURE 8–15*A*).
- Plethysmograph pressure increases abruptly and then decays exponentially (FIGURE 8–15*B*).
- Plethysmograph flow signal (*C*) has a similar shape as the pressure signal (*B*), if pneumotachygraph is linear.
- Plethysmograph flow signal is integrated to determine volume (*D*).
- The difference between *A* and *D* in FIGURE 8–15 is due to compression of the large volume of gas in the plethysmograph and is directly proportional to plethysmograph pressure.
- By adding a portion of the plethysmograph pressure to the integrated plethysmograph flow, the "true" volume event may be reconstructed accurately (*E*), $\Delta V = (\text{Pbox})(\text{Kbox}) + \int \dot{V}\text{box}$.

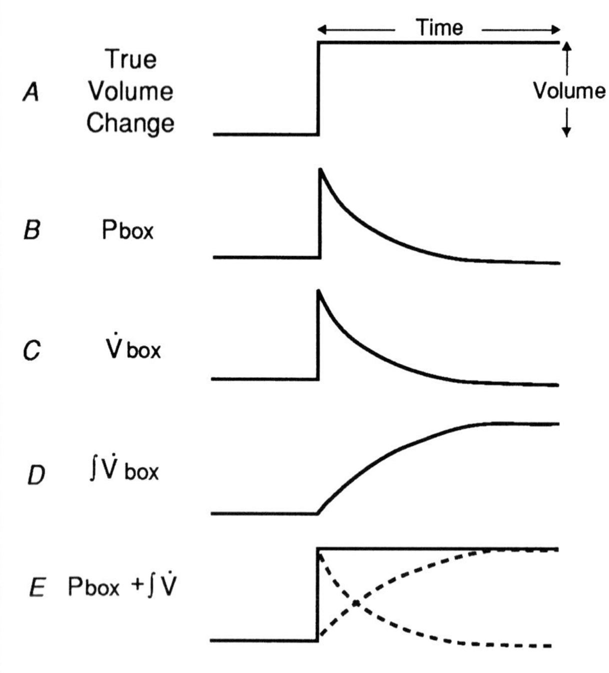

FIGURE 8–15

Physical principles underlying pressure-volume plethysmograph. The theoretical "true" instantaneous volume event is illustrated in *A*. During this event, plethysmographic pressure increases rapidly and then decays exponentially (*B*). If the plethysmograph pneumotachygraph is linear, the shape of the flow signal is similar to that of the pressure transducer (*C*). This flow signal is integrated to obtain volume (*D*) that reaches the same level as the true volume event, but the shape does not conform to the "true" event. The difference is a result of the compression of a large volume of gas in the plethysmograph and is directly proportional to the plethysmograph pressure. Therefore, by adding a portion of the plethysmograph pressure to the integrated plethysmograph flow (*E*), the true volume event is reconstructed accurately: $\Delta V = \text{Pbox} + \int \dot{V}\text{box}$. Thus, the true volume is obtained by adding the plethysmographic compression volume (Pbox) and the displacement volume ($\int \dot{V}$box). More precisely, (1) box pressure, Pbox, is multiplied by a constant, Kbox, a factor to correct pressure to volume that is proportional to the gas volume in the box (total box volume − patient volume); and (2) box pressure, Pbox, is also divided by the box flowmeter resistance, Rbox, to yield box flow, $\dot{V}$box, and integrated to obtain volume, Vbox. These two signals are added together to yield the change in lung volume: $\Delta V = \text{PboxKbox} + \int \dot{V}\text{box}$. Or, more accurately: $\Delta V = \text{PboxKbox} + \text{Pbox}/\text{Rbox} \times \int \dot{V}\text{box}$. (From Murray JF, Nadel JA (eds): Textbook of Respiratory Medicine. 3rd ed. Philadelphia, WB Saunders, 2000, p. 795.)

MEASUREMENTS OF VENTILATORY FUNCTION

LUNG VOLUMES

Thoracic Gas Volume

- Thoracic gas volume = compressible gas in the thorax, whether in free communication with airways or not.
- By Boyle's law, pressure × volume of the gas in the thorax is constant if its temperature remains constant ($PV = P'V'$).
- At end-expiration, alveolar pressure (Palv) = atmospheric pressure (P) because there is no airflow; V (thoracic gas volume) is unknown (FIGURE 8–16).
- Then, the airway is occluded and the subject makes small inspiratory and expiratory efforts against the occluded airway.
- During inspiratory efforts, the thorax enlarges (ΔV) and decompresses intrathoracic gas, creating a new thoracic gas volume ($V' = V + \Delta V$) and a new pressure ($P' = P + \Delta P$).
- The new pressure (P') is measured by a pressure transducer between the subject's mouth and the occluded airway.
- It is assumed that Pmouth = Palv during compression while there is no airflow at the mouth, because pressure changes are equal throughout a static fluid system (Pascal's principle).

FIGURE 8–16

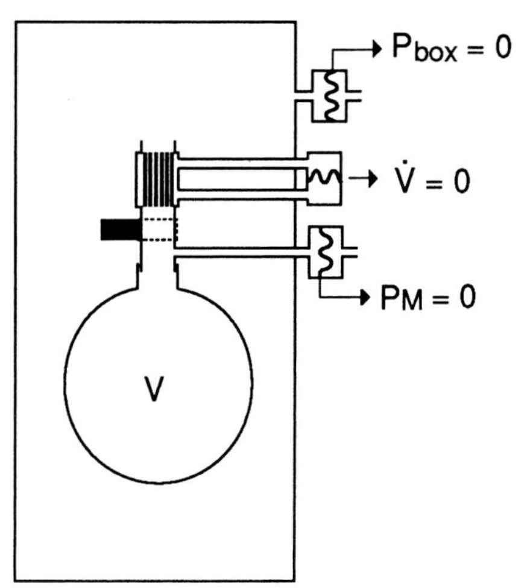

The rectangle represents a closed, constant-volume, variable-pressure whole-body plethysmograph. The subject is represented by a single alveolus and its conducting airway. V is the thoracic gas volume to be measured. The top pressure transducer measures pressure within the plethysmograph, or box pressure (Pbox). The middle pressure transducer measures the pressure drop across the pneumotachygraph connected in series with the open shutter to the airway. The bottom pressure transducer measures airway pressure (alveolar pressure during no flow). At end-expiration, airflow is zero and, at this instant, V = FRC and Palv = Pmouth = barometric pressure (P). (Modified from Comroe JH Jr, Forster RE, DuBois AB: The Lung: Clinical Physiology and Pulmonary Function Tests. 2nd ed. Chicago, Year Book Medical Publishers, 1962.)

Thoracic Gas Volume Equations

$$PV = P'V' = (P + \Delta P)\,(V + \Delta V)$$

$$0 = P\Delta V + \Delta P V + \Delta P\,\Delta V$$

$$\text{if } \Delta P \ll P, \text{ then } \Delta P\,\Delta V \sim 0$$

$$\text{so} \quad \boxed{V = -\frac{\Delta V}{\Delta P} P}$$

$$V = \frac{\Delta V(\text{mL})}{\Delta \text{Palv}(\text{cm } H_2O)} \times (P - 47 \text{ mm Hg}) \times (1.36 \text{ cm } H_2O/\text{mm Hg})$$

P = atmospheric pressure − water vapor pressure (mm Hg), assuming that alveolar gas is saturated with water vapor at body temperature.
ΔV = change in thoracic gas volume.
ΔP = change in mouth pressure = change in alveolar pressure.

MEASUREMENTS OF VENTILATORY FUNCTION

LUNG VOLUMES

Plethysmograph Methods

• If a closed plethysmograph is used, ΔV is detected by measuring increased plethysmographic pressure with a sensitive pressure transducer.

• If plethysmographic pressure is displayed on the *x*-axis and mouth pressure (alveolar pressure) on the *y*-axis of an oscilloscope, the slope of the line (α) is measured during panting efforts against the closed airways (FIGURE 8–17).

$$V = \frac{(P - 47 \text{ mm Hg})(1.36 \text{ cmH}_2\text{O/mm Hg} \times \text{box calibration (mL/cm)})}{\alpha \times \text{pressure calibration (cm H}_2\text{O/cm)}}$$

$$V \approx \frac{970 \times \text{box calibration}}{\alpha \times \text{pressure calibration}} (\text{mL})$$

Thoracic gas volume is usually slightly larger than FRC unless the shutter is closed precisely after a normal tidal volume is exhaled.

• Connecting the mouthpiece assembly to a valve and spirometer (or pneumotachygraph and integrator), or using a pressure-volume plethysmograph (see earlier discussion of types of plethysmographs) makes it possible to measure TLC and all its subdivisions in conjunction with the measurement of thoracic gas volume.

FIGURE 8–17

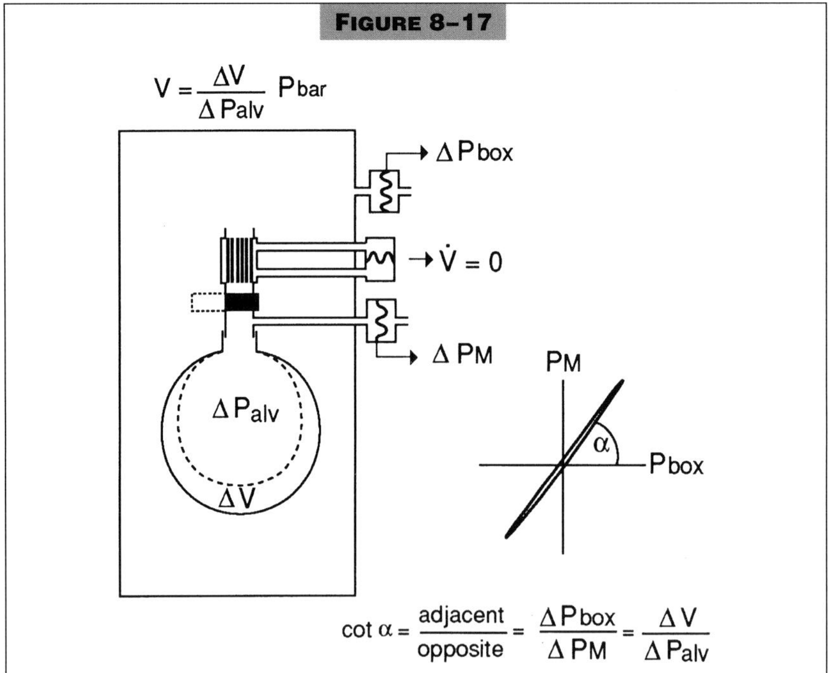

The rectangle represents a closed, constant-volume, variable-pressure whole-body plethysmograph, as shown in Figure 8–16. At end-expiration airflow is zero and, at this instant, V = FRC and Palv = Pmouth = barometric pressure (Pbar). When the subject inhales against an occluded shutter in the airway, airflow remains zero, but the thoracic gas volume (V) increases by ΔV to V, and mouth pressure (= alveolar pressure) increases by ΔP (P + ΔP = P′). When the PM is plotted against Pbox, the slope of the line (α) yields ΔV/ΔPalv, and V = ΔV/ΔP × Pbar. (Modified from Comroe JH Jr, Forster RE, DuBois AB: The Lung: Clinical Physiology and Pulmonary Function Tests. 2nd ed. Chicago, Year Book Medical Publishers, 1962.)

MEASUREMENTS OF VENTILATORY FUNCTION

LUNG VOLUMES

Effects of Heat, Humidity, and Respiratory Gas Exchange Ratio (R) on Plethysmography

- Heat, humidity, and R ($CO_2 - O_2$ exchange differences) cause unstable baselines.
- Heat production by the subject may be eliminated by creating a small leak in the chamber, by a pump, or by an electronic signal compensating for drift.
- Nonuniform and discontinuous effects of warming and humidifying inspired air and water vapor condensation of cooled expired air are reduced during shallow panting at 2 Hz.
- Signal-to-noise ratio is maximized by avoidance of thermal exchanges, or because thermal affects and inertance effects on the loop are balanced (i.e., equal and opposite in their effects on the transfer function).[67]
- Effects of heat, humidity, and R may be corrected electronically[68] or with an airbag to warm up and humidify respiratory air so that normal breathing patterns can be used.

Changes in Outside Pressure

- Outside pressure changes can make it difficult to detect the "signal" relative to "noise."
- Drift of chamber pressure due to heat output of the subject will still interfere, despite elimination of outside pressure effect.
- A simple method can be used to correct these problems[69]:
  - The box transducer is mounted inside the plethysmograph, with one side open to the box and the other side attached to a 1-L rigid container open to the plethysmograph via a 23-gauge needle.
  - The resistance of the needle permits thermally induced pressure changes to pass readily but impedes faster changes that are due to breathing efforts by the subject.
  - The slow thermal drift is present on both sides of the transducer and is thus nullified.

Cooling

- Refrigeration is required for many boxes.
- Cooling may cause a variety of problems related to vibration and localized cooling (e.g., a cool body and warm head result because of poor circulation currents in one type of commercial box).

Underestimation of Mouth Pressure

- Lung volume measured by plethysmograph in patients with asthma may be overestimated owing to an underestimation of alveolar pressure by measurements of mouth pressure.[70, 71]
- Results are free of error even in airway obstruction, as confirmed by roentgenographic estimation of lung volume, when esophageal pressure changes are used to estimate changes in alveolar pressure.
- "Trapped gas volume" estimated by the difference between plethysmographic and dilution measurements is not an accurate estimate of the volume of noncommunicating gas in the lungs, but is really the result of additive errors: overestimation of volume by traditional plethysmography using mouth pressure to measure alveolar pressure, and underestimation of volume by dilution in the presence of moderate-to-severe chronic airflow obstruction.[72]
- The discrepancies detected are usually small (maximal range: − 0.10 to 1.48 L) and do not account for the large increases in lung volume reported previously in acute and chronic asthma.
- The discrepancy can be eliminated by estimating changes in alveolar pressure with an esophageal balloon or, more simply, by having the subject pant at low and controlled frequencies (1 Hz rather than the more usual 2 Hz).

MEASUREMENTS OF VENTILATORY FUNCTION

LUNG VOLUMES

Compression Volume

- Measurement of compression volume can be used to assess the degree of effort, amount of "negative effort dependence," and true relationship between flow and lung volume when the pressure-volume plethysmograph is used in the transmural or flow mode.
- Some pressure-volume boxes measure volume change at the mouth relative to airflow, and simultaneously measure volume change of the thorax relative to airflow.
- The "compression-free" flow-volume loop (plethysmograph flow signal is integrated by computer to equal "true" volume change of the thorax) accurately reflects compression of thoracic gas during a forced expiratory maneuver.
- Compression volume is used to estimate alveolar pressure in order to measure airway resistance when the plethysmograph is used in the pressure mode.

AIRWAY RESISTANCE

General

- Airway resistance (Raw) is easy to measure repeatedly.
- Raw is always related to the lung volume at which it is measured.
- Raw is useful to detect diseases associated with increased airway smooth muscle tone (e.g., asthma).
- Raw may demonstrate an abnormally increased value relative to lung volume, or significant relaxation of bronchomotor tone induced by administration of bronchodilator drugs.
- Detects increased airway smooth muscle tone induced by provocative stimuli, e.g., pharmacologic agents, exercise, or cold air, or specific agents such as allergens or chemicals (e.g., isocyanates) associated with occupational asthma (see later discussion of bronchial provocation).
- Is useful in differential diagnosis of the type of airflow obstruction or localization of the major site of obstruction.

Methods for Measurement

- Airway resistance (Raw, during airflow) equals the driving pressure (between the alveoli and mouth)/ instantaneous airflow ($\dot{V}$).
- Inspiration of 500 mL of gas from the box into the lungs increases plethysmographic pressure (even if there are no effects of heat, humidity, or O_2-CO_2, exchange).
- At start of inspiration, thoracic gas volume enlarges and Palv (previously at atmospheric pressure) becomes subatmospheric throughout inspiration; thus, alveolar gas occupies a larger volume.
- Decompression of thoracic gas is equivalent to adding a small volume of gas to the plethysmograph so its pressure increases (measured by a sensitive transducer).
- Reverse occurs during exhalation when alveolar gas is compressed.
- $\dot{V}$ is measured continuously with a pneumotachygraph, Pmouth is measured with a pressure transducer connected to a side tap in the mouthpiece, and Palv is estimated continuously with the body plethysmograph (FIGURE 8–18).
- The slope (β) of plethysmograph pressure (x-axis) is displayed against airflow (y-axis) on an oscilloscope during rapid, shallow breathing through a pneumotachygraph within the plethysmograph.
- Then, with a shutter closed across the mouthpiece, the slope (α) of plethysmographic pressure (x-axis) is displayed against mouth pressure (y-axis) during panting under static conditions.
- Pmouth = Palv in a static system, so changes in plethysmographic pressure are related to changes in alveolar pressure.
- Palv is effectively measured during flow, provided that the ratio of lung to plethysmographic gas volume is constant, because Palv for a given plethysmographic pressure is the same, regardless of whether flow is interrupted.
- Raw is related to a particular thoracic gas volume.

MEASUREMENTS OF VENTILATORY FUNCTION

AIRWAY RESISTANCE

Methods for Measurement

FIGURE 8–18

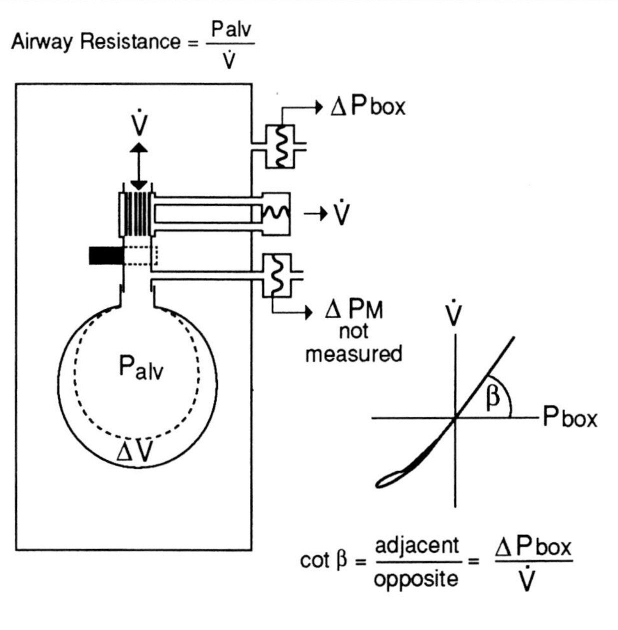

Measurement of airway resistance by plethysmography. The rectangle represents a closed, constant-volume, variable-pressure, whole-body plethysmograph, as shown in Figure 8–16. The subject is represented by a single alveolus and its conducting airway. The top pressure transducer measures pressure within the plethysmograph, or box pressure (Pbox). The middle pressure transducer measures the pressure drop across the pneumotachygraph connected in series with the open shutter to the airway, which yields airflow, $\dot{V}$. The bottom pressure transducer measures airway pressure (alveolar pressure during no flow). During inspiration, the alveolus has enlarged from the original volume (*broken line*) to a new volume (*solid line*); during expiration, the alveolus has returned to its original volume. Throughout inspiration, alveolar gas (previously at atmospheric pressure) is subatmospheric and therefore occupies more volume. This is the same as adding this increment of gas volume resulting from decompression of the plethysmograph, so Pbox increases and is recorded by the sensitive Pbox transducer. The reverse happens during expiration when alveolar gas is compressed. Thus, alveolar pressure can be monitored throughout the respiratory cycle. When $\dot{V}$ is plotted against Pbox, the slope of the line (β) yields the ratio of $\Delta P/\dot{V}$. (Modified after Comroe JH Jr, Forster RE, DuBois AB: The Lung: Clinical Physiology and Pulmonary Function Tests. 2nd ed. Chicago, Year Book Medical Publishers, 1962.)

Equations

$$\text{Raw} = \frac{\alpha}{\beta} \times \frac{\text{Pm calibration}}{\dot{V}\text{ calibration}} - \text{Rext}$$

$$\text{Raw} = \frac{\text{Pm}}{\Delta V} \times \frac{\Delta V}{\dot{V}} - \text{Rext}$$

$$\text{Raw} = \frac{\text{Pm}}{\dot{V}} - \text{Rext}$$

$$\boxed{\text{Raw} = \frac{\text{Palv}}{\dot{V}} - \text{Rex}}$$

where Pm calibration = mouth pressure calibration (cm H_2O/cm), $\dot{V}$ calibration = pneumotachygraph calibration ($L \cdot sec^{-1} \cdot cm$)
Rext = resistance of breathing through mouthpiece and pneumotachygraph (cm $H_2O \div L/sec$).

Physiologic Factors

The physiologic factors measured in assessment of ventilatory function are

- Airflow ($\dot{V}$)
- Volume (V)
- Lung elastic recoil (Pstl)
- Airway smooth muscle tone

MEASUREMENTS OF VENTILATORY FUNCTION

AIRWAY RESISTANCE

Airflow

- Raw is measured at low flows, when transmural compressive pressures across the airways are small and the relation to Palv is linear.
- During forced respiratory maneuvers, large transmural compressive pressures across the airways cause maximal dynamic airway compression limiting airflow rates and possible alterations in airway smooth muscle tone; Raw may be increased markedly.

Volume

- Near TLC, Raw is small; near RV, Raw is large.
- Lung volume may be changed voluntarily to evaluate Raw at larger and smaller volumes in health and disease.
- Airway conductance (Gaw = 1/Raw) is proportional to lung volume:

$$\text{Gaw} = 0.24\ \text{V (range: 0.13 V to 0.35 V)}$$

Lung Elastic Recoil

- Raw is related more directly to Pstl than to lung volume.
- Subjects with increased lung elastic recoil have a higher Gaw at a given lung volume than normal subjects because of increased tissue tension pulling outward on airway walls.[73]
- Loss of Pstl causes loss of tissue tension and decreased traction on airway walls, so that Gaw is decreased.
- This relationship may be used to analyze the mechanism of airflow limitation in different obstructive ventilatory defects (see discussion of bullous lung disease).[29, 74]

Airway Smooth Muscle Tone

- Airways, but not parenchyma, are affected markedly by smooth muscle tone, depending on the state of inflation and volume history.[75]
- Tone is increased in certain diseases (e.g., asthma) or at low lung volumes (e.g., during cough, or when pneumothorax is present).[76]
- Bronchoconstriction is not demonstrable temporarily after a deep breath or at TLC in healthy subjects.
- Raw in healthy subjects may be greater when a given lung volume is reached from RV than from TLC.

Panting

Panting serves several functions:

- It minimizes changes caused by thermal, water saturation, and CO_2-O_2 exchange differences during inspiration/expiration so they can be neglected.
- It improves the signal-to-drift ratio, because each respiratory cycle is completed in a fraction of a second.
- Panting makes gradual thermal changes and small leaks in the box insignificant compared with volume changes attributable to compression/decompression of alveolar gas.
- It keeps the glottis open, rather than partly closing and varying its position, as it does during tidal breathing.
- It minimizes abdominal pressure changes.

MEASUREMENTS OF VENTILATORY FUNCTION

LUNG ELASTIC RECOIL

General

Lung elastic recoil is

- Always increased in a restrictive ventilatory defect associated with decreased lung volumes.
- Probably decreased in almost all forms of airflow obstruction, although the shape of the curve may differ in emphysema and asthma.
- Measurement of lung elastic recoil is time-consuming, difficult to perform, expensive, and invasive.
- Useful to evaluate patients with isolated bullae and advanced emphysema to determine if they will benefit from resection of destroyed lung tissue.
- Useful in differentiating certain cases of emphysema from asthma or bronchitis.
- Useful to evaluate patients with mixed ventilatory defects (such as emphysema and fibrosis) to confirm the presence of both types of disorders.

Definitions

- Lung elastic recoil pressure (Pstl) equals the difference between the pressure inside the lungs (the alveolar pressure) and the pressure outside the lungs (the pleural pressure):

$$Pstl = Palv - Ppl$$

- To maintain a sustained inspiration at a volume of 75% of TLC with the mouth and glottis open, the muscles of inspiration must maintain a pleural pressure of about 12 cm H_2O below atmospheric pressure (Ppl = -12 cm H_2O).
- Under conditions of no flow, mouth, alveolar, and atmospheric pressures are equal; Pstl = 0 − (-12 cm H_2O).
- If the inspiratory muscles relax, allowing the chest wall to recoil inward, pleural pressure will rise from -12 to 0 cm H_2O and alveolar pressure from 0 to $+12$ cm H_2O at the instant before flow begins.
- Two principles underlie the measurement of lung recoil: (1) the pressure required to expand a lung to any volume is equal to the recoil pressure at that volume, and (2) under conditions of no flow, with the glottis open, alveolar pressure and mouth pressure are identical.
  - Mouth pressure is easy to measure, absolute lung volume can be measured by any of a variety of methods (see previous discussion), and the change in volume can be measured easily with a spirometer.
  - To measure lung elastic recoil pressure and lung compliance, it is necessary to measure pleural pressure in relation to lung volume.

Esophageal Pressure

- Because the esophagus passes through the pleural space, esophageal pressure generally approximates pleural pressure.
- These pressures are equal so long as the sphincters of the upper and lower esophagus are competent and there is no force compressing the esophageal lumen, such as active contraction of the esophageal muscles, or passive compression by surrounding mediastinal structures.
- Most of these conditions are met in subjects without esophageal disease who are sitting or standing upright.

MEASUREMENTS OF VENTILATORY FUNCTION

LUNG ELASTIC RECOIL

Protocol

- To preserve patency of a tube placed in the esophagus to measure esophageal pressure, the end of the tube is covered with a balloon.
- Intraballoon pressure is assumed to reflect intraesophageal pressure, which in turn is assumed to reflect the surrounding pleural pressure.
- Balloon artifacts may cause the measured pressure to be too positive, owing to the compression of the balloon by the walls of the esophagus (FIGURE 8–19).
- Balloon artifacts are reduced by using a long (10 cm), narrow (2.5 cm perimeter), thin-walled (0.04 cm), highly compliant latex balloon containing a small amount (0.2 to 0.4 mL) of air.[77]
- The volume of air to minimize artifact for each balloon is determined by suspending it vertically in water, with the top (proximal end) of the balloon at the surface, allowing it to empty before the tube is closed with a stopcock.[78, 79]
- The balloon is advanced to the gastroesophageal junction (identified by positive pressure caused by an inspiratory sniff) and then withdrawn 10 cm.

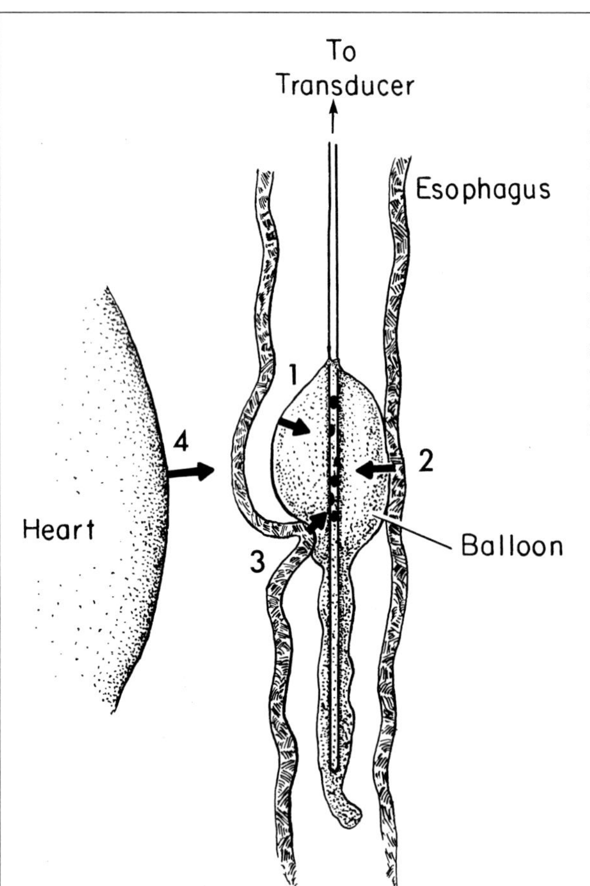

FIGURE 8–19

Schematic illustrating the position of an esophageal balloon in relation to adjacent structures. The balloon is made of latex (wall thickness 0.04 mm; length 10 cm; circumference 2.5 cm), tubing is polyethylene (inner diameter 0.14 cm; outer diameter 0.19 cm) with holes placed in a spiral arrangement in the portion inside the balloon. The balloon is filled with 0.2 to 0.4 mL of air and positioned in the lower third of the esophagus. Intraesophageal pressure recorded from the catheter within the balloon is affected by the following factors in addition to static transpulmonary pressure (Pstl): 1, retractile pressure of balloon wall; 2, pressure caused by resting esophageal tension; 3, pressure caused by mediastinal structures, including pulsations of the heart, 4. (From Murray JF, Nadel JA (eds): Textbook of Respiratory Medicine. 3rd ed. Philadelphia, WB Saunders, 2000, p. 800.)

MEASUREMENTS OF VENTILATORY FUNCTION

LUNG ELASTIC RECOIL

Analysis of Compliance

- Dynamic lung compliance (Cdyn) is the ratio of the change in volume to the change in pressure over a tidal breath with pressure measured at moments of zero flow during breathing.
  - Measurement of Cdyn at increasing respiratory frequencies allows determination of the degree of frequency-dependence of compliance.
  - A fall in Cdyn as frequency increases implies narrowing of some of the airways subtending alveoli.
  - In the absence of abnormalities in total airway resistance or in FEV_1 (which, as described previously, are largely determined by resistance in large airways) a decrease in Cdyn suggests possible narrowing of small, peripheral airways.[80]
- Static lung compliance (CL) is the slope of the pressure-volume curve of the lung as obtained during deflation from TLC, and is determined by a standardized protocol (FIGURE 8–20):
  - The pattern of breathing ("volume history") is standardized by having the subject inhale to TLC three times in a row to minimize changes due to the dynamics of the entry of surface-active material into the air-liquid interface.
  - On the third inhalation, the subject pauses at TLC for 3 to 5 seconds and then exhales slowly as flow is interrupted by closing the mouth shutter for 2 to 3 seconds at each of several volumes.
  - Repeating this maneuver four or five times provides enough data to characterize the relationship between the change in lung volume and the change in transpulmonary pressure over the entire VC (FIGURE 8–20).
  - Fixing the curve obtained on the volume axis requires knowing absolute lung volume at some transpulmonary pressure; absolute lung volume is easily measured directly if the curve is obtained with the subject in a body plethysmograph.
  - Alternatively, but less accurately, lung volume (TLC, FRC, or RV) measured at another time (by a gas dilution technique, for example) may be assumed to be the same at the time of measurement of lung compliance.

Physiologic Factors

- CL changes with lung volume, with the highest values at volumes around FRC and lower values prevailing as the lungs are expanded more nearly to TLC (FIGURE 8–20).
- Compliance equals the slope of the curve over the 0.5 L above FRC; when this convention is used, however, the value expressed for lung compliance is influenced by the determinants of FRC, rather than simply by the relationship between lung volume and distending pressure.
- Coefficient of retraction (Pstl at TLC divided by TLC).[81]
- Variability of CL is reduced by correction for height, predicted TLC, or measured FRC.[79, 81–86]
- Analyze the entire Pstl curve; for example, Pstl is plotted against lung volume and is expressed as a percentage of *predicted* TLC.[87]

FIGURE 8–20

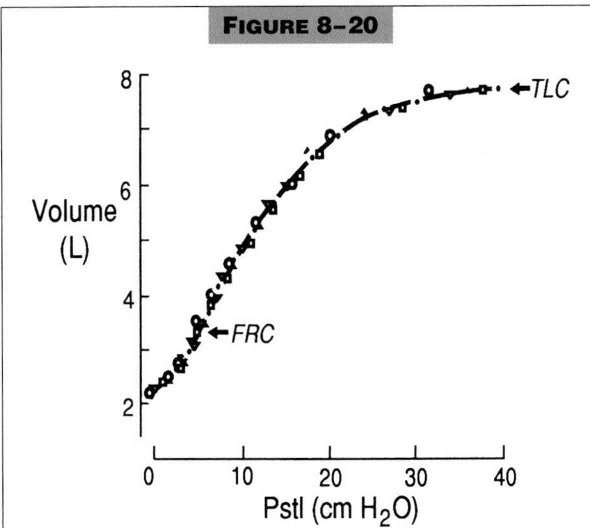

Static pressure-volume curve of the lungs during deflation in a normal subject. Measurements were obtained during five different maneuvers. Pstl = static transpulmonary pressure; TLC = total lung capacity. (From Murray JF, Nadel JA (eds): Textbook of Respiratory Medicine. 3rd ed. Philadelphia, WB Saunders, 2000, p. 801.)

MEASUREMENTS OF VENTILATORY FUNCTION

LUNG ELASTIC RECOIL

Exponential Analysis

- Exponential analysis is less affected by patient effort and lung size.
- Uses a greater range of the pressure-volume data.
- Mathematically describes the whole lung.[88–91]

$$V = Vmax - Ae^{-KP}$$

where V = lung volume, Vmax = maximal or extrapolated lung volume at infinite distending pressure, K is a constant describing the shape of the pressure-volume curve, and P = lung elastic recoil pressure.

- To describe the curve fully requires the two parameters, Vmax and A, which both have the dimensions of volume. $A = Vmax - V_0$, where V_0 equals the volume extrapolated to $P = 0$.
- This calculation is used to evaluate both restrictive and obstructive ventilatory defects (see discussion of these defects later in the chapter).[87, 91–93] (APPENDIX 8 gives normal predicted values for pressure-volume curves.)

Exponential Analysis in Fibrosis

- Exponential analysis differentiates restriction due to loss of volume from that due to increased elastic properties.[87, 91]
- Gibson and Pride[91] used this method to extrapolate the theoretical maximal volume of the lungs subjected to a limitless distending pressure.
  - If lung compliance is reduced because the alveoli are "stiffer" but not fewer in number (a pure increase in elastic forces), then the extrapolated volume should be normal. It would simply require greater distending pressure than the muscles of inspiration are capable of generating.
  - If lung compliance is reduced because of a loss of alveoli, then the extrapolated maximal volume should also be decreased; total compliance is reduced because fewer alveoli are able to expand.
- Elastic properties of the lungs in patients with diffuse interstitial fibrosis can be accounted for almost entirely by a loss of alveoli.[91] Fibrotic lungs are thought to consist of a population of completely obliterated, unventilated alveoli, and a population of surrounding normal alveoli.
- Thompson and Colebatch[94] concluded that the shape constant, K, correlated closely with airspace size; loss of lung distensibility reflected decreased airspace size, whereas the decrease in TLC reflected decreased inflatable lung tissue. (See Chapter 4, Radiography and Imaging.)

MEASUREMENTS OF VENTILATORY FUNCTION

LUNG ELASTIC RECOIL

Exponential Analysis in Emphysema

- In patients with a clinical diagnosis of emphysema, the constant K, describing the shape of the curve, fell outside the normal range (increased K in emphysema; decreased K in fibrosis).[95, 96]
- Morphologic emphysema and K in postmortem lungs correlated significantly.[97]
- In patients studied prior to surgical resection of an isolated peripheral pulmonary lesion,[93] emphysema was quantified by panel grading,[98] and pressure-volume data of the lung were fitted to an exponential. K was the best predictor of emphysema in individual subjects and was the only predictor that distinguished subjects with moderate emphysema (grade 20 or more) from those with mild (grade less than 20) or no emphysema, but did not distinguish those with mild emphysema from those without emphysema. Elastic recoil pressure correlated with emphysema and with FEV_1, suggesting that loss of elastic recoil is one determinant of airflow limitation in COPD.[99–101]
- Analysis of lung elastance (change in lung elastic recoil pressure to produce a given fractional change in lung volume) in normal and emphysematous lungs[102] showed that specific lung elastance and the change in specific elastance with lung elastic recoil were increased in emphysema compared to normal subjects.
  - No correlation was found between increased length of alveolar walls, specific lung elastance, and FEV_1.
  - Change in elastic properties of the lungs in emphysema does not appear to account for flow limitation.
  - Because of the decreased extensibility, these emphysematous regions are not only poorly perfused but also poorly ventilated; emphysema per se may not seriously disturb ventilation-perfusion relationships.

CLINICAL APPLICATIONS OF FLOW-VOLUME RELATIONSHIPS

NORMAL VALUES

Sources of Variability

- The American Thoracic Society (ATS) has recommended reference values and interpretative strategies for lung function tests including FVC, FEV_1, FEV_1/FVC, and criteria for response to a bronchodilator for adult white and black men and women.[103] (Tables of predicted normal values for these and other pulmonary function tests may be found in APPENDIXES 1 to 20 at the end of this chapter.)
- Laboratory control of technical sources of variation is critical and depends upon the following:
  - Strict adherence to ATS guidelines for equipment performance and calibration
  - Minimizing temperature-related errors
  - Careful validation of computer calculations when purchasing or changing equipment or software
  - Proper performance of the tests
- Sources of variation between individuals are critical to the choice of appropriate reference values.
- Environmental sources of variation pertinent to a given patient (in addition to other relevant clinical data) should be provided to the laboratory director to evaluate the clinical relevance of a given lung function report.

CLINICAL APPLICATIONS OF FLOW-VOLUME RELATIONSHIPS

NORMAL VALUES

Intraindividual Variation

Body position, head position, effort-dependence of maximal flows, and circadian rhythms cause the primary residual sources of variation when short-term variation caused by disease, drugs, environment, smoking, laboratory instruments, or submaximal efforts is excluded:

- **Body position:** FVC and VC are 7 to 8% higher in the sitting than in the supine position and 1 to 2% higher in the standing than in the sitting position.[104] In comparison studies, body position should be constant.
- **Head position:** Flexion of the neck may decrease peak expiratory flow rate and increase airway resistance.[105]
  - Hyperextension of the neck causes increased maximal expiratory flow.[106]
  - No corresponding changes in FEV_1 have been described.
  - These changes are thought to be due to the effects of the position of the head on tracheal dimensions.
- **Effort dependency of maximal flows:** Variable expiratory effort may contribute to the difficulty in evaluating small changes in maximal flows or timed volumes. For example, maximal effort is recommended for measurement of maximal expiratory flows, but FEV_1 may be 100 to 200 mL lower when compared with submaximal efforts because the airways are compressed in relation to the exhaled volume.[107]
  - When a flow-volume curve is available, peak expiratory flow may be an indicator of the degree of maximal expiratory effort.[108]
  - If measurements are made in a pressure-volume plethysmograph, the presence, magnitude, and duration of increased alveolar pressure related to the degree of compression of thoracic gas volume may be a useful measure of the degree of expiratory effort.
  - It is also important to recognize that some subjects with irritable airways may experience bronchospasm triggered by the repeated maximal efforts, resulting in progressive decrease in spirometric values.[109]
  - Thus, lack of reproducibility of forced spirometric efforts may be diagnostic of airway disease in some patients.
- **Circadian rhythm:**
  - Maximal expiratory airflow is highest at noon, and usually lowest in the early morning (4:00 to 6:00 AM).[97]
  - Similar circadian variations have also been described for airway resistance, TLC, and RV, but the mechanisms are unknown.[110–113]
  - Exaggerated circadian variations have been described in patients with asthma[114] and chronic bronchitis.[115]

Interindividual Variability

- **Host factors:** A number of individual factors must also be considered:
  - Sex difference accounts for up to 30% of the variability among adults. After correction for body size, girls have higher expiratory flow rates than boys, whereas adult men have larger volumes and flow rates than women.[116,117]
  - Size is measured in most laboratories as standing height.[118] Arm span may be substituted for standing height in subjects who cannot stand or for subjects with kyphoscoliosis.[119]
  - Age can be a significant factor. After adult height is attained, lung function either increases (young men) or shows little or no decrease (young women) for a period, and then decreases rapidly with increasing age.[120]
  - Race affects these measurements also.[121] When compared with white Europeans, most other races show similar or higher FEV_1/FVC ratios, but smaller static and dynamic lung volumes and lower forced expiratory flow rates. Diffusing capacity is also lower in some populations.[122] Regression equations for white populations based on standing height usually overpredict values in African-American subjects by 12% for TLC, FEV_1, and FVC and by about 7% for FRC and RV.[121] Mixed race individuals have intermediate values. Sitting height as an index of size to predict lung function values decreases but does not eliminate differences between whites and African-Americans.[117]
  - Past and present health can also be significant.

(continued)

CLINICAL APPLICATIONS OF FLOW-VOLUME RELATIONSHIPS

NORMAL VALUES

Interindividual Variability

Lung function at any particular time is the sum of all injuries sustained by the lung in the past, including those from prenatal and immediate postnatal periods.[123]

- **Environmental factors:** In addition to the enormous impact of tobacco smoke,[124, 125] geographic factors, general pollution, and socioeconomic status contribute to variation among individuals.
    - Geographic factors—Long-term residents at very high altitudes have larger lung volumes than do residents at low altitudes for unknown reasons.[126, 127] Short-term stays at altitude appear to have little effect on lung volumes, but decreased air density may increase flow rates and timed volumes.[128]
    - Pollution—Irritants such as ozone[129] or sulfur dioxide cause transient changes in lung function in controlled laboratory exposures and epidemiologic studies.[130–132] Increased responses are observed in subjects with hyperreactive airways during exercise.[133] Tobacco smoke affects lung function adversely whether exposure is active[134, 135] or passive.[136]
    - Socioeconomic status—Poor socioeconomic status adversely affects lung function as a result of complex interactions, including increased respiratory illness, increased indoor pollution, increased urban and industrial pollution, increased occupational exposure, and decreased access to health care.[137]

Statistical Considerations

- Distributions of FEV_1 and FVC in population studies are close to gaussian in the middle age range but not at the extremes.
- Distributions of flow rates and ratios (FEV_1/FVC) are not symmetric.[36]
- Reference populations should include not only the prediction equations but also a means to define their lower limits.
- In general, the lowest 5% of the reference populations may be considered as below the lower limit of normal for any spirometric value.[36]
- If the distribution of individual observations is close to gaussian, the value of the fifth percentile can be approximated[36]:

$$\text{Lower limit of normal} = \text{Predicted value} - 1.645 \times \text{SEE}^*$$

There is no statistical basis for using 80% of predicted normal for FEV_1 and FVC as the lower limit of normal in adults.[6]

- Individual laboratories should use published reference equations that most closely describe the populations tested in their laboratories.
- The results observed in 20 to 40 local subjects should be compared with those provided by the intended reference equations. These local subjects should be lifetime nonsmokers selected by age, ethnic group, and sex to match the population usually studied in the laboratory.

* Standard error of the estimate.

CLINICAL APPLICATIONS OF FLOW-VOLUME RELATIONSHIPS

NORMAL VALUES

Flow-Volume Curves

- Correlations with sex, age, and height are poor.
- Volume-correction of flow does not appear to decrease variability.[35, 125]
- Most published studies provide prediction equations for mean values only; a few report standard deviation (SD) or some other estimate of population variance, but this is of little use in predicting the lower limit of normal. (As discussed previously, a single value for the SD of the population also gives too low an estimate of the lower limit of normal if obtained by subtracting 1.645 × SD from the predicted mean.)
- Several investigators provide predicted mean values and estimates of the lower limit of normal values.[4, 22, 35, 36] (APPENDIX 9 gives the normal predicted values for maximal expiratory flow-volume curves.)
- A wide range of normal values limits the interpretation of spirometric and flow-volume curves.[21]
- Values in the very low normal range at a given time may represent normality for that subject, or significant functional derangement in a person whose VC and/or flow rates were much higher than average before the onset of the disease.
- A discrepancy between static and dynamic measurements, expressed as a percentage of predicted, may suggest significant dysfunction.
- Evalution of the results in the clinical context may help in interpreting the data.[25]
- Pulmonary function tests have precise reproducibility in the same subject.
    - Spirometry is reproducible within 5% of the initial values obtained; variability is 2% to 3% in cooperative subjects.[138]
    - Repeated measurements of spirometry over time provide a sensitive way of following disease.

PATHOPHYSIOLOGIC PATTERNS

General

- Most common application of flow-volume relationships is for the diagnosis and quantitation of airflow obstruction.
- Airway resistance is not measured directly by spirometry.
- Variables derived from spirometry and flow-volume curves may be used to infer increased airway resistance from expiratory airflow to be achieved with a maximum effort by the subject.
- Effort is not quantitated; thus, the observer can only presume that the decreased flow is due to increased resistance, rather than a decreased effort to produce the flow.
- Degree of effort can be determined using an intraesophageal balloon to estimate pleural pressure, or noninvasively, using compression volume estimated in a pressure-volume plethysmograph (see earlier discussion).

Obstructive Ventilatory Defects

- Reproducible patterns are obtained in normal subjects and in patients with obstructive ventilatory defects (FIGURE 8–21).
- In emphysema, decreased maximal expiratory flow is due to the effect of loss of lung elastic recoil on airway dimensions, which results in an increased resistance to flow owing to increased compliance and collapse of airway walls.
- Decreased expiratory flow is usually associated with decreased VC, from "air-trapping" associated with increased RV.
- Measurement of RV may be necessary to document this phenomenon and to rule out a mixed restrictive and obstructive ventilatory defect.

CLINICAL APPLICATIONS OF FLOW-VOLUME RELATIONSHIPS

PATHOPHYSIOLOGIC PATTERNS

FIGURE 8–21

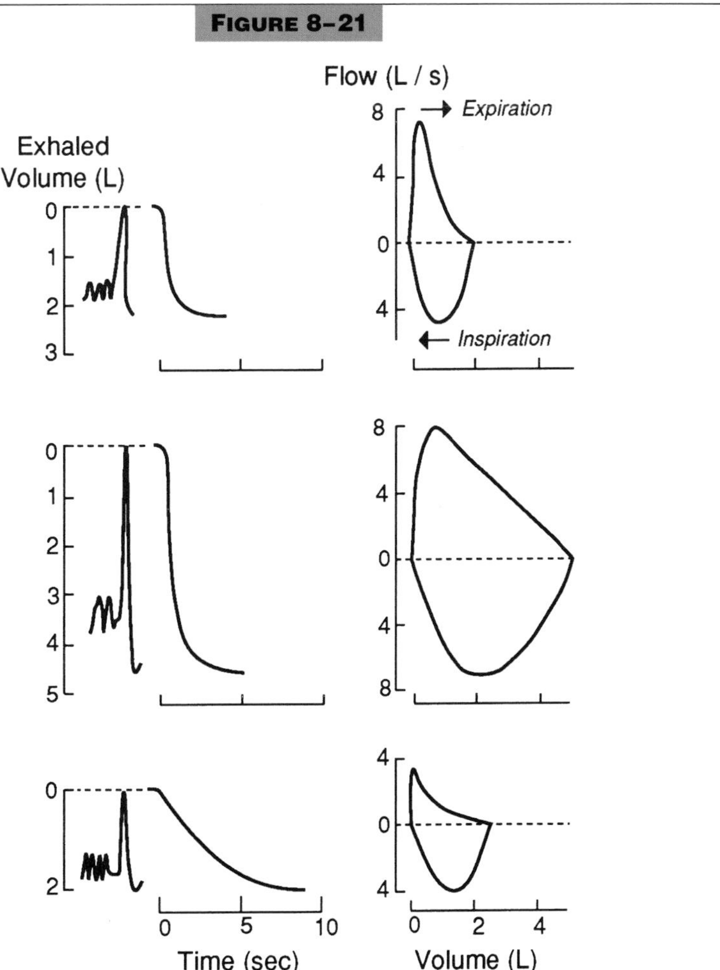

Spirograms and flow-volume curves obtained in a patient with a restrictive ventilatory defect (*top*), a normal subject (*middle*), and a patient with an obstructive ventilatory defect (*bottom*). (From Murray JF, Nadel JA (eds): Textbook of Respiratory Medicine. 3rd ed. Philadelphia, WB Saunders, 2000, p. 805.)

Restrictive Ventilatory Defects

Decreased VC reflects

- Limitation in chest excursion
- Little or no reduction in expiratory airflow
- Relative preservation of MVV (FIGURE 8–21)
- Increased volume-corrected flow and FEV_1/FVC ratios develop prior to development of decreased lung volumes:
  - The force pulling outward on airway walls is increased.
  - The airway diameters are increased relative to lung volume so that airflow rates are increased.
  - With increased severity, lung volumes become decreased.
  - If the restrictive process can be reversed, volumes return to normal first, followed by volume-corrected flows and a normal FEV_1/FVC ratio.

DISTRIBUTION OF VENTILATION

MEASUREMENTS OF DISTRIBUTION OF VENTILATION

General

Measurements of the distribution of ventilation are used as follows:

- To detect abnormalities in lung structure and function, although the tests are nonspecific.
- To detect the presence of abnormal function early when other tests are normal.
- To confirm the presence of airflow obstruction when other tests are only mildly abnormal.
- To evaluate patients with suspected upper airway obstruction to determine if there is associated disease of the airways distal to the trachea.
- To evaluate effects of smoking or air pollution in large populations.
- To assess the uniformity of gas distribution in the lungs and the behavior of the dependent airways.[17]

RESIDENT GAS, SINGLE-BREATH N_2 TEST

Protocol

- The single-breath N_2 test is used to measure the slope of phase III (alveolar gas plateau) in order to determine the uniformity of gas distribution.
- The subject inspires a single breath of pure O_2 from RV to TLC (inspiratory VC maneuver).
- N_2 concentration at the mouth during exhalation is measured with an N_2 analyzer or mass spectrometer.
- At end-inspiration, dead space is filled with O_2 that has just been inspired (FIGURE 8–22).
- At the beginning of the subsequent expiratory VC maneuver, the N_2 meter continues to record 0% N_2 because the first gas to leave the lungs is from the conducting airways—the so-called anatomic dead space (phase I) (FIGURE 8–22).
- Subsequently, the N_2 concentration increases in a sigmoid curve upward and reflects mixing of gas from dead space and alveoli (phase II).
- If inspired oxygen is distributed unevenly (as occurs to a small extent even in healthy subjects), the end-inspiratory N_2 concentrations are not equal throughout the lung, and the concentrations of exhaled nitrogen from different alveoli are not recorded as a horizontal line; the first portion of phase III usually contains a lower N_2 concentration than the last portion.
- In many but not all subjects, a sharp rise in N_2 concentration occurs during the final third of the VC, marking the onset of the closing volume (CV, or phase IV); during this fourth phase, it is assumed that dependent airways have closed, but gas continues to emerge from N_2-rich upper regions of the lung.[139]

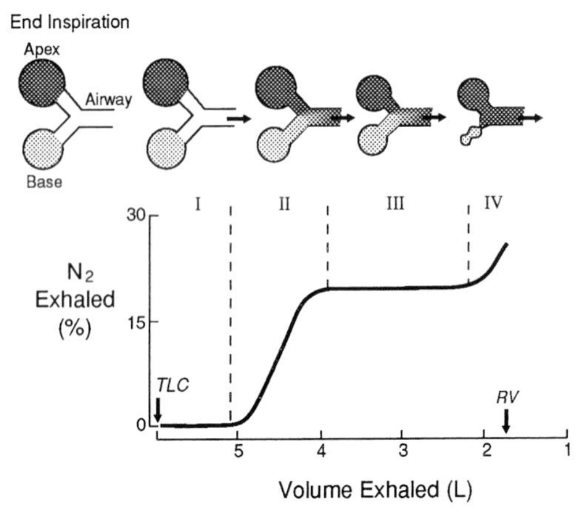

FIGURE 8–22

The relationship between N_2 concentrations in different regions of lung (*top*) and the single-breath N_2 washout test of distribution of ventilation (*bottom*). The figure at the top shows a ventilatory unit near the lung apex (*dark stipple*) and a ventilatory unit near the base (*light stipple*) subtended by a common airway. The intensity of stippling reflects the end-inspiratory concentration of the resident gas (N_2) at the end of a single maximal inspiration of pure O_2 (at TLC). The differences in N_2 concentration in each unit result from the effect of differences in regional RV and the distribution of inspired gas. At the start of exhalation, the gas (pure O_2) in the conducting airway empties first and 0% N_2 is recorded (*phase I, bottom*). As exhalation continues, gas from both ventilatory units mixes in the airway, and the N_2 concentration increases rapidly (*phase II, bottom*). With continued exhalation, mixed alveolar gas is recorded by the N_2 analyzer (*phase III, bottom*). Finally, dependent airways at the base of the lungs close near RV (*closing volume*), and exhalation continues from the apical ventilatory unit of the lung only, which contains a higher N_2 concentration than the basal unit (*phase IV, bottom*). (From Murray JF, Nadel JA (eds): Textbook of Respiratory Medicine. 3rd ed. Philadelphia, WB Saunders, 2000, p. 806.)

DISTRIBUTION OF VENTILATION

RESIDENT GAS, SINGLE-BREATH N_2 TEST

Interpretation

- N_2 concentration is higher at the end compared to the beginning of phase III in erect subjects.
- Because O_2 is inspired from RV, most of the dead space gas (79% N_2) is distributed to the upper zones of the lungs, a distribution due to gravity, which promotes closure of small airways in the dependent zone at RV and their opening as FRC is approached.
- Regional RV of the lower zone is smaller than regional RV of the upper zone; therefore, even if the same amount of O_2 were delivered to both zones, the dilution of the residual N_2 is greater in the smaller RV of the lower zone.
- Because at RV the alveoli in the lower zone are smaller than in the upper zone owing to gravity, the subsequent inspiratory VC maneuver causes a greater increase in volume of the dependent alveoli than of the nondependent alveoli.
- Dependent alveoli receive a larger portion of the inspired O_2, and have a lower N_2 concentration at end-inspiration than nondependent alveoli.
  - Subsequent exhalation produces preferential emptying of lower zones (lower N_2 concentration) initially, reflecting the decreased compliance of this region (FIGURE 8–23).
  - As RV is approached, closure of these airways leaves only the upper zones (higher N_2 concentration) to empty ("first in, last out" theory).
- In chronic airway obstruction, unobstructed units that fill early also empty early ("first in, first out" theory); because the N_2 concentration is lower in the unobstructed units that empty first, phase III has a steeper slope than in normal subjects.

FIGURE 8–23

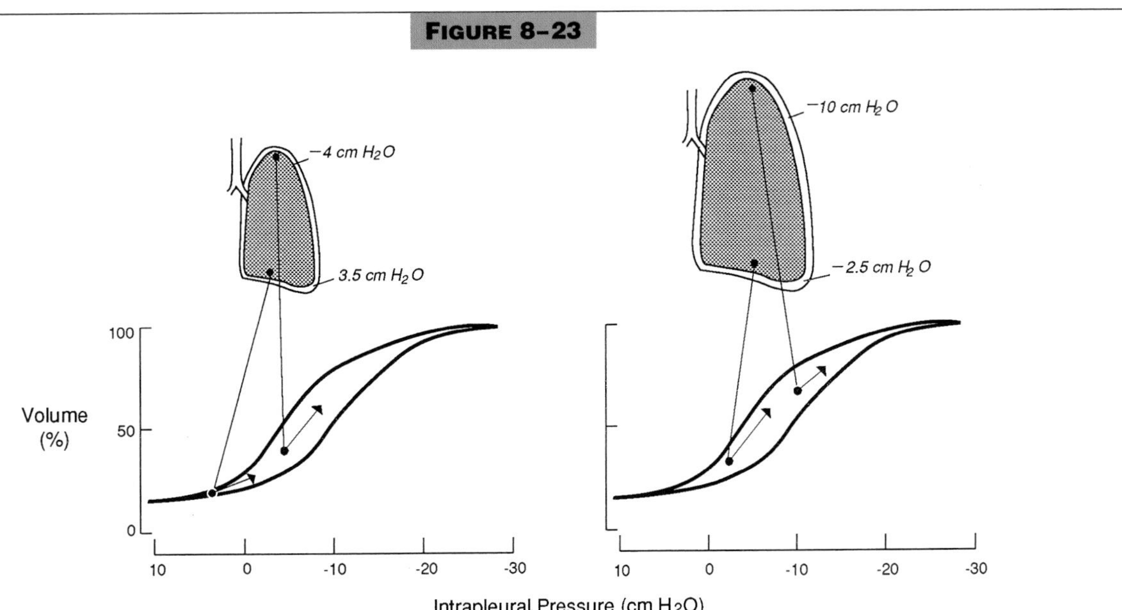

Variations in the relative volume of different regions of the lung in relation to the pleural pressure gradient caused by gravity in the upright posture. All regions of the lung are considered to have the same pressure-volume curve, but pleural pressure at the apex is about 8 cm H_2O more negative than the pleural pressure at the base. The two panels show the relative volumes of the apex and base at low and high lung volumes, respectively. The lengths of the arrows indicate the volume excursions for a change of 5 cm H_2O over the normal tidal breathing range. During deflation from TLC, the basal regions undergo a larger volume change, and near RV, they become stiffer and empty faster, contributing their lower N_2 concentration to the alveolar plateau early, whereas the apical regions undergo a smaller volume change and empty later, reflecting their higher compliance, contributing their higher N_2 concentration to the later portion of the alveolar plateau. (From Murray JF, Nadel JA (eds): Textbook of Respiratory Medicine. 3rd ed. Philadelphia, WB Saunders, 2000, p. 807.)

DISTRIBUTION OF VENTILATION

RESIDENT GAS, SINGLE-BREATH N_2 TEST

Analysis

- Analysis of these curves is not entirely objective.[140]
- In some cases, onset of phase IV cannot be determined easily; when the same observer reads such curves twice under "blind" conditions, agreement between the two measurements is poor.
- Such variability is due to differences between individual lungs; when a subject generates such a curve, usually all curves produced by that subject will be difficult to analyze.
- If a subject generates a curve that is easy to analyze, most curves produced by that subject will be easy to analyze.
- Some curves, although conforming to the criteria of acceptability, are unreadable and therefore should be ignored.
- Few satisfactory computer programs exist for the analysis of phase IV,[141] even though many programs have been developed to analyze phase III.

Normal Values

- In healthy nonsmokers, no significant differences exist between data obtained from men and women.[142]
- Age-related regression occurs in nonsmokers, and no significant differences exist related to geographic location, climate, air pollution, or occupation.[143–145]
- CV is expressed as a percentage of expired VC.
- Closing capacity (CC) is defined as CV + RV expressed as a percentage of TLC.
- Slope of phase III ($\Delta\%\ N_2/L$) is the line of best fit (by least squares linear regression) between 70% VC and the onset of phase IV; the range about the mean of three measurements of the slope of phase III should not be greater than $\pm$ 0.5% N_2/L.[146, 147]
- Standard deviation of repeated measurements of CV and TLC (both in liters) is large (approximately 0.13 L), so at least three measurements should be obtained.[146, 148]
- Variations are independent of the time of day.[146, 148]

Variability

- Variability in absolute values for CV in the same individual from test to test is attributable to variation in the lung volume at which airway closure occurs, variation in exhaled lung volume due to incomplete filling or emptying of the lungs,[148] and difficulties encountered in detecting the onset of phase IV.
- The volume at which phase IV occurs is influenced critically by expiratory flow,[147] and the slope of phase III depends on inspiratory flow[149]; thus, inability to control expiratory flow within acceptable limits is probably the major source of lack of precision in measurements of CV.
- The TLC measured by the single-breath N_2 test correlates well with that measured by helium dilution in a population of men and women free from abnormalities of gas distribution, for both smokers and nonsmokers with and without symptoms.[146]
- As expected, the measurement of TLC underestimates lung volume in patients with airway obstruction.[146] (APPENDIX 10 gives normal predicted values for the single-breath N_2 washout test.)

DISTRIBUTION OF VENTILATION

RESIDENT GAS, SINGLE-BREATH N_2 TEST

Other Tests

- Comparison of bolus and resident-gas techniques show close similarities in results or a systematic tendency for CV measurements determined by the resident-gas technique to be slightly lower than those determined by the bolus technique.[144, 150, 151]
  - Resident-gas method described here is a modification of the test described originally by Fowler.[152, 153]
- Residual N_2 following multiple-breath, open-circuit N_2 washout.[154, 155]
  - Continuous breath-by-breath measurement or N_2 concentration at the mouth during tidal breathing of pure O_2 is performed until end-tidal N_2 concentration falls to less than 1%.
  - End-tidal N_2 concentration on a breath-by-breath basis is related to the cumulative volume of ventilation or breath number.
  - Extending N_2 washout time to 30 minutes or more in subjects with severe chronic airway obstruction yields lung volume estimates that compare favorably with those by plethysmographic or roentgenographic methods.[156, 157]
- Helium mixing time during closed-circuit equilibration.[158, 159]

Exponential Analysis of the End-Tidal N_2 Concentration

- Cumulative ventilation, or breath number, reveals that in normal subjects, N_2 concentration decreases in a single exponential curve.
- In the presence of uneven distribution of ventilation, the curve can be described by two or more exponentials.
- This analysis permits estimation of the size of poorly ventilated regions of the lung, but these multiple-breath tests are cumbersome and time-consuming, may have no anatomic correlates, and cannot be repeated rapidly.[160, 161]

CLINICAL APPLICATIONS

- This test is useful in epidemiologic studies.
- In cigarette smokers and patients with mild airway obstruction, the single-breath N_2 washout test (phase III and phase IV) is often the most abnormal test of lung function and is sometimes the only abnormal test.
- The test may be used to detect effects of occupational hazards early.
- Findings are abnormal in both restrictive and obstructive ventilatory defects, reflecting abnormalities in the mechanical properties of the lungs. Some regions of lung fill and empty more slowly than others, resulting in an abnormal single-breath N_2 test.
- Despite its drawbacks, a test of distribution is indicated in a number of clinical evaluations:
  - In mild disease, spirometry and clinical evidence may be equivocal, but tests of distribution may provide a more sensitive indicator of the presence of disease and the response to treatment.
  - Degree of abnormality of the single-breath N_2 washout test is proportional to the amount of underlying lung disease.
  - When the closing volume (phase IV) is elevated above the FRC, it is likely to be associated with atelectasis and hypoxia, particularly when the drive to ventilation is depressed by narcotics or hypnotic drugs.
  - In patients with suspected upper airway obstruction, a test of distribution of ventilation (e.g., single-breath N_2 washout) may be the only way to assess whether there is associated disease of the airways distal to the carina. (See Chapter 4, Radiography and Imaging, and Chapter 5, Nuclear Medicine Techniques and Applications.)

DIFFUSION

MEASUREMENTS OF PULMONARY DIFFUSING CAPACITY

General

- The measurement of pulmonary diffusing capacity requires a gas that is more soluble in blood than in lung tissues.
- O_2 and CO are the only two such gases known that depend on the chemical reaction with hemoglobin for this unusual pattern of "solubility," and both molecules measure the same process.
- Diffusing capacity measured by CO can be converted to that for O_2 by multiplying by 1.23.

Carbon Monoxide

- A low concentration of CO is maintained in the airspaces by adding 0.3% CO to inspired air.
- Mixed venous CO is assumed to be zero for all practical purposes (unless the test is repeated frequently over a short time).
- Molecules of CO diffuse across the alveolar-capillary membrane, dissolve in the plasma, then combine with hemoglobin.
- CO has a marked affinity for hemoglobin, 210 times that of O_2; thus, any CO in the vicinity of a hemoglobin molecule binds avidly to it, and the partial pressure of dissolved CO remains very low.
- Available CO-binding sites are so numerous, except in severe anemia, that they cannot be saturated by the CO molecules diffusing from the airspaces to the capillary blood at the low CO concentrations used.
- Thus, CO transfer is not limited by pulmonary blood flow.
- CO transfer is limited primarily by the alveolar-capillary membrane diffusion rate and, to a lesser extent, by the red blood cell membrane diffusion rate and the chemical reaction rate between hemoglobin and CO.

Freon, Nitrous Oxide, Acetylene

In contrast to CO, these gases are used to measure pulmonary capillary blood flow to ventilated lung units, often as part of the measurement of CO transfer. They have several qualities in common:

- They are equally soluble in lung tissues and blood.
- They do not combine chemically with blood components.
- They diffuse across alveolar-capillary membranes and quickly saturate the plasma; further diffusion is prevented until fresh blood enters the pulmonary capillaries.

Carbon Monoxide and Oxygen

- There are marked differences in the transfer of CO and O_2.
- Both plasma and hemoglobin contain O_2 (but no CO) when mixed venous blood enters the pulmonary capillaries.
- O_2 diffusion rate into blood depends upon the alveolar-capillary PO_2 difference.
- As O_2 crosses the alveolar-capillary membranes, capillary PO_2 increases, narrows the alveolar-capillary PO_2 difference, and slows diffusion.
- Blood PO_2 must be known at every point along the capillary and can be obtained by a combination of certain measurements and mathematical computations.[162]

DIFFUSION

SINGLE-BREATH TEST[163]

$$DL_{CO} = \frac{\text{CO transferred from alveolar gas to blood (mL/min)}}{\text{mean alveolar CO pressure} - \text{mean capillary CO pressure (mm Hg)}}$$

- It is necessary to determine the amount of CO transferred from alveolar gas to blood per minute, mean alveolar CO pressure, and mean pulmonary capillary CO pressure.
- In the single-breath method, the patient inhales a gas mixture containing 0.3% CO and a low concentration of inert gas (0.3% Ne, 0.3% CH_4, or 10% He), then holds his or her breath for approximately 10 seconds, during which time CO leaves the airspaces and enters the blood; the larger the diffusing capacity, the greater the amount of CO that enters the blood in 10 seconds.

$$DL_{CO} = \frac{\dot{V}CO}{P_1 - P_2}$$

where $\dot{V}CO$ is carbon monoxide uptake per minute, P_1 is alveolar PCO, and P_2 is pulmonary capillary PCO (usually ignored).

- According to the Krogh[164] equation:

$$FA_{CO_t} = FA_{CO_0} \cdot e^{-kt}$$

where $FACO_t$ is alveolar CO concentration at time t, $FACO_0$ is initial alveolar CO concentration, and t is breath-hold time in seconds.

$$K = \frac{DL_{CO} \times (Pbar - 47)}{VA \times 60}$$

where Pbar is barometric pressure (mm Hg) and VA is alveolar volume (mL), (60 is the number of seconds per minute).

- After taking the logarithm and rearranging, the equation is

$$DL_{CO} = \frac{VA \times 60}{(Pbar - 47) \times t} \ln \frac{FA_{CO_0}}{FA_{CO_t}}$$

VA is obtained from the ratio of inspired and expired inert gas concentrations and inspired volume, and $FACO_0$ is the inspired CO concentration corrected for dilution by the RV as estimated by the ratio of inspired and expired inert gas concentrations.

Method

- Alveolar PCO is not maintained at a constant concentration, as it is in the steady-state method, because CO is absorbed during the period of breath-holding.
- Mean alveolar PCO is not the average of the PCO at the beginning and end of the breath-holding period.
- Using the Krogh equation (see preceding section), mean alveolar PCO can be estimated and diffusing capacity measured.
- The single-breath test requires little time or cooperation from the patient except to inhale and to hold the breath for 10 seconds.
- Analyses are performed with an infrared analyzer or gas chromatograph, and no blood samples are needed.
- The test can be repeated a number of times rapidly, if desired.
- Measurement of the patient's RV is required because a value for total alveolar volume during breath-holding must be calculated in order to measure CO uptake.
- Inert gas (e.g., He, CH_4, or Ne) must be inhaled with CO in order to correct for dilution of inspired CO.
- There are some disadvantages: CO is a nonphysiologic gas, breath-holding is not a normal pattern of breathing, and breath-holding may not be possible for patients with severe dyspnea or during exercise.

DIFFUSION

SINGLE-BREATH TEST[163]

Modifications

- Factors such as inhalation time, breath-holding time, breath-holding lung volume, exhalation time, and the size and portion of alveolar gas sampled have all been shown to change the single-breath CO diffusing capacity.
- Ogilvie and associates[163] proposed standardizations to correct for CO uptake during inhalation/exhalation.
- The diffusion equation is valid only for breath-holding.[165]
- Errors in calculation of single-breath DL_{CO} result from CO uptake during inhalation and exhalation.
- The Jones and Mead calculation method minimizes these errors, although it is difficult to implement because of the small size of alveolar gas samples and the precise timing needed for sample collection. This delay in collection of the alveolar sample causes an apparent increase in DL_{CO}.
- The American Thoracic Society's epidemiology standardization project[24] modified the Jones and Mead method by adding a strong emphasis on an automated system to standardize the maneuver.

Comparisons

- *Standard single-breath CO diffusing capacity* test is probably the most widely used and the best standardized method available. This parameter has been measured in the largest number of normal subjects, and values have been corrected for the effects of age, body size, sex, ethnic background, cigarette smoking, and physiologic factors that could affect results.
- *Three-gas iteration method* may actually be more reproducible and is unaffected by a wide variety of factors that alter the single-breath or intrabreath methods, especially for evaluation of abnormalities in distribution of ventilation. However, much more normal data is needed, as is validation in other laboratories.
- *Intrabreath method* requires a special, very rapid infrared analyzer, which is now commercially available. This method does not require a breath-hold; and expiratory flow may be controlled by a critical orifice so that it is probably easier for sick patients to perform than the first two tests.
  - By the use of proper filters, the same analyzer can be used to measure simultaneously CH_4, C_2H_2, as well as CO.
  - This method can be used during exercise to define distensibility of the capillary bed.
  - Extensive validation and establishment of predicted normal values are needed.
- *Oxygen method* to measure DL_{O_2}[166] largely has been displaced in clinical laboratories by CO methods[167] because it is difficult and time-consuming to perform. DL_{O_2} can be estimated by multiplying DL_{CO} by 1.23, as described previously.

Indications

- Results have not been standardized or well defined because of the variety of testing procedures in use and because of the complexity of the physiologic determinants of CO uptake.
- The most common clinical applications include evaluation of patients with diffuse interstitial lesions such as sarcoidosis or asbestosis, evaluation of patients suspected of having emphysema for which several structure-function studies are now available[29, 100, 168–171] and assessment of patients with pulmonary vascular obstruction.[172, 173]
- Results depend on hemoglobin concentration; decreased DL_{CO} caused by severe anemia must not be misinterpreted as secondary to nonexistent lung disease.

DIFFUSION

SINGLE-BREATH TEST[163]

Standardization

- ATS has recommended standardization of the test as follows:
  - At least two acceptable tests are produced with rapid inspiration.
  - Inspired volume is at least 90% of largest VC.
  - Breath-hold time is between 9 and 11 seconds.
  - Adequate washout and sample volumes are used.
- The mean of the acceptable tests is reported. If more than two tests are performed, the mean of all reported is used.
- Calculations are standardized for breath-hold time and adjusted for dead space, gas collection conditions, and CO_2.
- Reproducibility of the two acceptable tests should be within 10% or 3 mL $CO_{STPD} \times min^{-1} \times mm\ Hg^{-1}$, whichever is larger.
- When DL/VA is reported, DL is STPD and VA is BTPS.[103]

Hemoglobin

- Adjustment for hemoglobin is not mandatory but desirable.
- Unadjusted values must always be reported even if the adjusted value is also reported.
- The adjustment should be made on the observed, not predicted, value.
- Hemoglobin is reported in g/dL, and the method of Cotes[173] should be used to make the adjustment:

$$\text{Measured } DL_{CO} \times \frac{(14.6 \times DM/VC) + \text{hemoglobin}}{\text{hemoglobin } (1 + DM/VC)}$$

Carboxyhemoglobin

- Heavy smokers may have 10% to 12% carboxyhemoglobin in their blood, and therefore, backpressure of CO in mixed venous blood entering the pulmonary capillaries cannot be assumed to be zero in such individuals.
- The steady-state method is more sensitive to errors caused by this problem than the single-breath technique.
- Patients should be instructed not to smoke overnight prior to performance of DL_{CO} tests.
- CO backpressure may be estimated and DL_{CO} calculations may be corrected for backpressure of CO using the Haldane equation:

The subject rebreathes for 2 minutes from an anesthesia bag filled with pure O_2, and the CO is determined following washout from the lungs.

If

$$\frac{210 \times P_{CO}}{P_{O_2}} = \frac{\text{CO hemoglobin}}{O_2 \text{ hemoglobin}}$$

Then

$$P_{CO} = \frac{\text{CO hemoglobin}}{O_2 \text{ hemoglobin}} \times \frac{P_{O_2}}{210}$$

The latter value is subtracted from the fractional concentration of CO at the beginning of inhalation and at the end of breath-holding.

- Alternatively, CO hemoglobin may be measured directly.
- In either case, the measured D_{CO} is adjusted and both the unadjusted as well as the adjusted value are reported.
- DL_{CO} measurements should not be performed on patients who have been breathing O_2-enriched mixtures immediately before the test; at least 20 minutes of breathing room air should be allowed before measurement of DL_{CO}.

DIFFUSION

SINGLE-BREATH TEST[163]

Altitude

- As altitude increases and FI_{O_2} remains constant, PI_{O_2} will decrease and DL_{CO} will increase approximately 0.35% per mm Hg decrease in alveolar PO_2.
- Altitude-adjusted DL_{CO} = measured $DL_{CO} \times (1.0 + 0.0035[PAO_2 - 120])$
- If PAO_2 is not available, adjustments may be made for interpretative purposes, assuming a mean PI_{O_2} of 150 mm Hg at sea level:

$$\text{Altitude-adjusted } DL_{CO} = \text{measured } DL_{CO} \times (1.0 + 0.0031[PI_{O_2} - 150])$$

Assume

$$PI_{O_2} = 0.21\ (\text{Pbar} - 47).$$

Interpretation

- *Normal values for pulmonary diffusing capacity:* APPENDIX 11 gives predicted normal values for DL_{CO} and KCO. A number of factors probably affect normal values.[163, 174–183]
- *Body size:* Diffusing capacity has been found to vary with body surface area according to the following equation derived by Ogilvie and associates[163]:

$$DL_{CO} = 18.85 \times \text{BSA}\ (m^2) - 6.8$$

where BSA is the body surface area in square meters (m^2). A better prediction[174] is based on height and age:

Males:

$$DL_{CO} = 0.416\ \text{height (cm)} - 0.219\ \text{year (age)} - 26.34$$

Females:

$$DL_{CO} = 0.256\ \text{height (cm)} - 0.144\ \text{year (age)} - 8.36$$

  - Values for DL_{CO} measured by analyzing the gases with a chromatograph yield results approximately 6% higher than values obtained with infrared meters.[175]
  - Maximal diffusing capacity for O_2 (DL_{O_2} during maximal exercise) has been found to decrease with increasing age according to the following equation:

$$\text{Maximal } DL_{O_2} = 0.67\ \text{cm (height)} - 0.55\ \text{year (age)} - 40.9$$

- *Lung volume:* Diffusing capacity determined by the single-breath technique measured between FRC and TLC is relatively independent of lung volume in the same individual, although diffusing capacity varies with lung volume between individuals, reflecting differences in alveolar-capillary surface with lung volume.[29]

$$DL_{CO} = 13.67 + 4.36\ \text{BTPS (TLC)} - 0.2\ \text{year (age)}$$

- *Body position:* DL_{CO} is 15% to 20% greater in the supine than in the sitting position and about 10% to 15% greater in the sitting than in the standing position because of the effects of changes in posture on pulmonary capillary blood volume.
- *Alveolar oxygen pressure:* Alveolar O_2 pressure affects DL_{CO} because of its effect on the CO reaction with hemoglobin.
  - For example, diffusing capacity measured at alveolar O_2 pressures of 40 and 600 mm Hg will be approximately 45 and 18 mL/min per mm Hg, respectively (FIGURE 8–24).
  - Changes in DL_{CO} caused by variations in alveolar PO_2 in the physiologic range are much smaller.
  - In patients with severe hypoxia ($PaO_2 < 40$ mm Hg), increased pulmonary blood flow and dilation of the pulmonary capillaries may increase DL_{CO}.
  - Hypoxia may also increase DL_{CO} as a result of its effect on the reaction rate between CO and hemoglobin.[184]
- *Alveolar carbon dioxide pressure:* Addition of 6% to 7.5% CO_2 to inhaled gas for some minutes before measuring DL_{CO} increases the value by 5% to 25%. When 6% CO_2 is added for the 10-second breath-holding period required for the single-breath test, only a 5% increase occurs.
- *Intrathoracic pressure:* Valsalva's maneuver is reported to decrease DL_{CO} by as much as 17%, whereas a Mueller maneuver may increase it by approximately 15%.[163]

DIFFUSION

SINGLE-BREATH TEST[163]

Interpretation

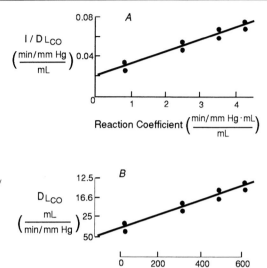

FIGURE 8–24

A plot demonstrating how experimental values of the diffusing capacity for CO obtained at different alveolar P_{O_2} values (*bottom, B*) can be analyzed mathematically to obtain the subdivisions of total diffusing capacity (DL_{CO}): the diffusing capacity of the membrane (DM) and pulmonary capillary blood volume (Vc). As the alveolar P_{O_2} was increased from 40 mm Hg to 600 mm Hg, the duplicate measurements of DL_{CO} decreased from approximately 45 to 15 mL/min/mm Hg. Changing alveolar P_{O_2} changes the reaction coefficient (Θ) reflecting the change in hemoglobin affinity for CO. The reaction coefficient is plotted against $1/DL_{CO}$ in the top diagram (*A*). There is a linear relationship between $1/DL_{CO}$ and 1/Θ such that $1/DL_{CO} = 1/\Theta V_C + 1/D_M$. Under these conditions, DM is derived from the value of the *y*-intercept and Vc from the slope of the line. (From Murray JF, Nadel JA (eds): Textbook of Respiratory Medicine. 3rd ed. Philadelphia, WB Saunders, 2000, p. 810.)

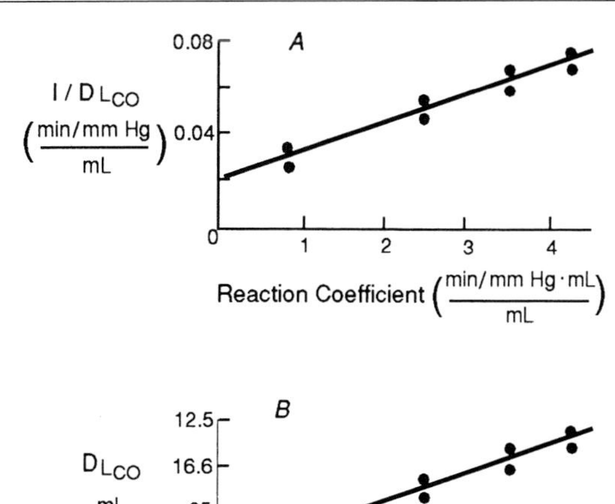

Exercise

- Exercise raises DL_{CO} and DL_{O2}, through an enlargement of the surface area of functioning alveoli in contact with pulmonary capillaries, due primarily to recruitment of capillaries (FIGURE 8–25).
- Exercise doubles pulmonary diffusing capacity and pulmonary capillary blood volume.[163, 176]
- An upper limit to DL_{CO} with respect to O_2 uptake during exercise was observed by Stokes et al.,[177] using the intrabreath CO method, but Hsia found no upper limit to DL_{CO} in normal subjects or patients following pneumonectomy with respect to cardiac output.
    - Similar results have been reported in dogs following pneumonectomy.[178]
    - Maximal values attained during exercise in patients following pneumonectomy were less than those attained by normal control subjects, because the patients were chronic smokers and probably had emphysema in the remaining lung.
- Whether DL_{CO} reaches a true plateau during exercise appears to depend on the method used and the level of exercise attained by the subjects.[179, 180]
- These findings are consistent with studies of capillary perfusion patterns in single alveolar walls visualized through a transparent thoracic window implanted in anesthetized dogs.[181]
    - When inflating a balloon in the left atrium increased left atrial pressure, capillaries were maximally perfused.
    - With repetitive increases and decreases in left atrial pressure, the same capillary segments were perfused 79% of the time, a strong indication that a reproducible combination of individual segmental resistances determined the predominant pattern of pulmonary capillary perfusion.
    - The residual inconsistency of capillary perfusion may be of benefit physiologically by ensuring that long-term tissue nutrient requirements of the alveolar walls are met.
    - Results of this study agree with a computer model of capillary flow developed by West et al.[182]

DIFFUSION

SINGLE-BREATH TEST[163]

Exercise

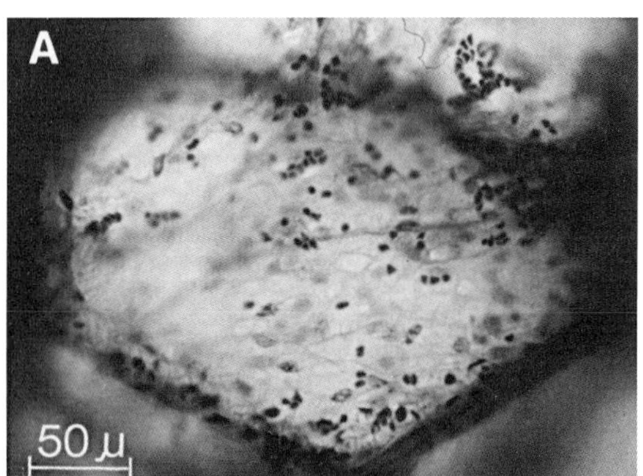

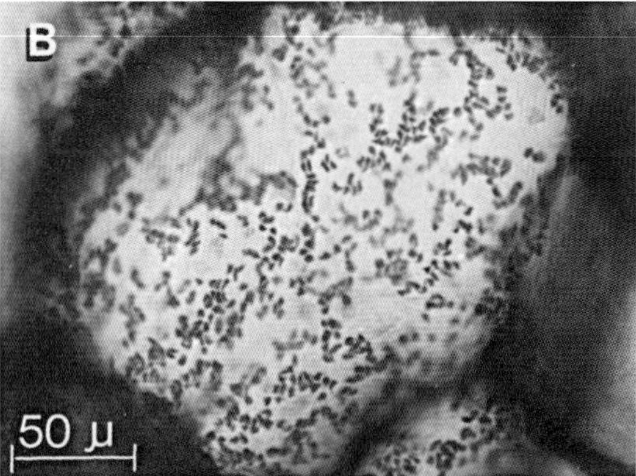

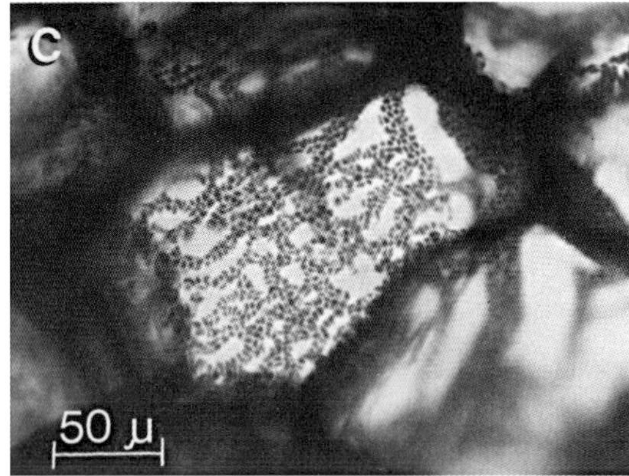

FIGURE 8–25

Face-on view of freeze-dried, stained alveolar walls (200-μm thick section) showing the distribution of the pulmonary capillary bed in anesthetized cats. **A,** Zone I lobe. **B,** Zone II lobe. **C,** Zone III lobe. Morphometric analysis showed that 21% of the alveolar walls were occupied by red blood cells in Zone I lobes, 43% in Zone II lobes, and 61% in Zone III lobes. Independent changes in pulmonary arterial or venous pressure were associated with changes in pulmonary capillary blood volume over a threefold range. (From Vrierm CE, Staub NC: Pulmonary vascular pressures and capillary blood volume changes in anesthetized cats. J Appl Physiol 36:275–279, 1974.)

DIFFUSION

CLINICAL APPLICATIONS OF DL_{CO}

Obstructive Ventilatory Defects

(See Chapter 4, Radiography and Imaging, and Chapter 5, Nuclear Medicine Techniques and Applications.)

- Association of an obstructive pattern with a normal single-breath diffusing capacity argues against the presence of emphysema.[29]
- A normal or increased single-breath DL_{CO} associated with airflow obstruction is often associated with asthma.[185, 186]
- Single-breath DL_{CO} may be abnormal in emphysema when there is no evidence of airflow obstruction and may become progressively more abnormal much more rapidly than tests of airway function, even when they do become abnormal.[187]
- Airway obstruction associated with decreased diffusing capacity usually reflects the presence of significant anatomic emphysema; several studies have now demonstrated a correlation not only with the presence of emphysema but also with the amount of emphysema based on the severity of the diffusion defect.[29, 100, 168, 188–191]
- Destruction of the airway wall may be seen in cigarette smokers, preceding the development of either increased airspace size, or anatomic evidence of emphysema.[192]
- In one laboratory, single-breath DL_{CO} was correlated with emphysema grade by panel grading[98] from grade 1 to grade 100 (r = 0.73) in 50 patients whose lungs were studied at surgical resection, which was performed within 1 week of their pulmonary function tests (FIGURE 8–26).
  - Single-breath DL_{CO} showed no significant correlation when patients had emphysema of grades 30 or less.
  - Intrabreath DL_{CO} showed a significant correlation with emphysema of grade 30 or less (r = 0.70),[193] suggesting that this test is more sensitive and specific than the single-breath DL_{CO}.

FIGURE 8–26

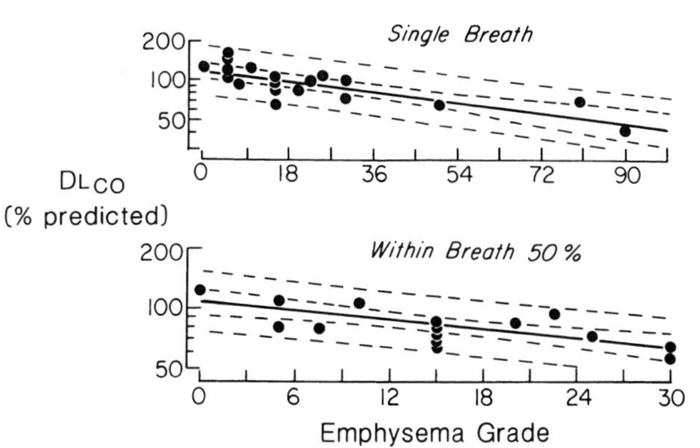

Correlation between DL_{CO} and emphysema grade. *Top,* The single-breath DL_{CO}, expressed as the log of the percentage of predicted normal, is displayed on the ordinate. Emphysema grade is displayed on the abscissa and was determined by the panel grading method on lung tissue resected from these patients within 1 week of pulmonary function testing. The *solid line* is the line of best fit (R = −0.73), the *outer dashed lines* show the 95% confidence limits for the points, and the *inner dashed lines* show the 95% confidence limits for the line. The single-breath DL_{CO} correlates with the presence and amount of emphysema except when emphysema is mild (grades 0 to 30); when single-breath DL_{CO} was plotted against emphysema for patients with minimal disease (grades 0 to 30), there was no significant correlation. *Bottom,* the intrabreath DL_{CO}, expressed as the log of the percentage of predicted normal at 50% exhaled vital capacity, is displayed on the ordinate. Emphysema grade is displayed on the abscissa and was determined by the panel grading method on lung tissue resected from these patients within 1 week of pulmonary function testing. The *solid line* is the line of best fit (R = −0.77), the *outer dashed lines* show the 95% confidence limits for the points, and the *inner dashed lines* show the 95% confidence limits for the line. Thus, the intrabreath DL_{CO} correlates with the presence and amount of emphysema even when emphysema is mild (grades 0 to 30) and cannot be detected or quantified by the single-breath method. (From Murray JF, Nadel JA (eds): Textbook of Respiratory Medicine, 3rd ed. Philadelphia, WB Saunders, 2000, p. 816.)

DIFFUSION

CLINICAL APPLICATIONS OF DL_{CO}

Pulmonary Vascular Obstruction

(See Chapter 4, Radiography and Imaging, and Chapter 5, Nuclear Medicine Techniques and Applications.)

- In the presence of precapillary vascular obstruction, single-breath DL_{CO} may be decreased, normal, or even increased, depending on the relationship between pulmonary artery pressure, pulmonary venous pressure (or left atrial pressure), and bronchial collateral blood flow.
- In every patient studied in the author's laboratory who had decreased single-breath DL_{CO}, pulmonary capillary blood volume was also decreased.[172]
- Although DL_{CO} is often decreased in patients with pulmonary vascular obstruction,[194, 195] it may be normal in other patients with proven pulmonary vascular obstruction.[195, 196]
- In the presence of pulmonary vascular obstruction, the DL_{CO} value will depend on the size of the obstructed vessel, bronchial collateral blood flow, and the effects of relative pressures affecting pulmonary capillaries.
  - Thus, if pulmonary capillaries are obstructed, no carbon monoxide transfer will occur in the vessels, so DL_{CO} must be decreased.[191, 194]
  - Bronchial arterial pressure may distend capillaries via collateral channels, even if pulmonary arteries are obstructed, so that DL_{CO} may be maintained.

Pulmonary Capillary Obstruction

- DL_{CO} depends on the relative effects of pulmonary arterial, pulmonary venous, and pulmonary alveolar pressure, which may vary in different parts of the lung (FIGURE 8–27).
- According to the West model of the zones of lung perfusion,[197] capillaries at the lung base are distended by pulmonary arterial and pulmonary venous pressures.
- The capillaries will be distended by pulmonary venous pressure even if the arteries are obstructed, and DL_{CO} will be maintained; DL_{CO} will decrease in this zone if the capillaries are occluded or if pulmonary venous pressure is decreased.
- Capillaries in the middle zone of the lung are distended by pulmonary artery pressure only; they are not affected by pulmonary venous pressure.
  - Pulmonary artery obstruction will decrease DL_{CO} unless pulmonary artery pressure increases and distends apical capillaries that were not perfused previously; this situation would result in a normal DL_{CO} despite arterial obstruction.
  - Alternatively, if pulmonary venous pressure increases, pulmonary capillaries will remain patent despite pulmonary artery occlusion in this zone.
- Pulmonary capillaries in the lung apex may not be distended because alveolar pressure exceeds both pulmonary arterial and venous pressure (assuming the lung ever is in this condition).[198]
- Obstruction of pulmonary arteries would not affect DL_{CO} in this situation.
  - Changes in alveolar pressure would affect the analysis and might affect DL_{CO}.[199]
  - Changes in posture may alter DL_{CO} in the presence of pulmonary vascular obstruction.
- Decreased DL_{CO} may support the diagnosis of pulmonary vascular obstruction, but a normal DL_{CO} does not rule out this diagnosis.[172]

DIFFUSION

CLINICAL APPLICATIONS OF DL_{CO}

Pulmonary Capillary Obstruction

FIGURE 8-27

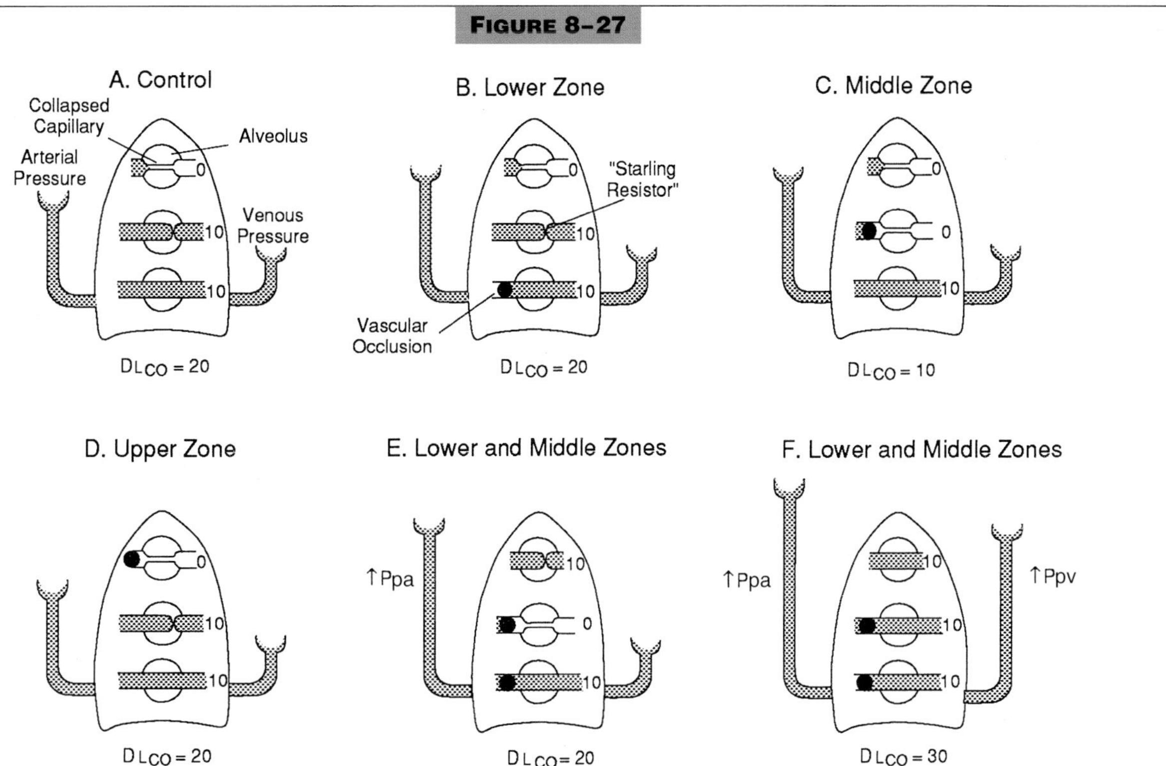

Theoretical model showing effect of pulmonary arterial pressure (Ppa) and pulmonary venous pressure (Ppv) on pulmonary capillaries at different levels of the lungs. Magnitude of Ppa and Ppv are indicated by height of fluid columns. For simplicity, in the example, pressure in alveoli is atmospheric. Single-breath carbon monoxide diffusing capacity (DL_{CO}) is given in arbitrary units indicating relative contribution of various zones of lung. In control state (*A*), at the bottom of the lung both Ppa and Ppv are greater than Palv and both keep the capillaries open. In the middle zone, Ppa is greater than Palv and Ppv, so Ppa holds capillaries open. (The exact anatomy of capillaries in the zone in which alveolar pressure is greater than pulmonary venous pressure is unknown; in the diagram, the compressed segment at the end of the capillary is meant to suggest a "Starling Resistor" effect.) In the upper zone, Palv is greater than Ppa and Ppv and capillaries are "collapsed." When arterial inflow is occluded to the lower zone (*B*) (indicated by dark solid sphere), Ppv is greater than Palv, so the capillaries in this zone remain distended and DL_{CO} is unchanged. When arterial inflow to the middle zone is occluded (*C*), Palv is greater than Ppv so that capillaries in this area collapse and no change in DL_{CO} occurs. When arterial inflow to the upper zone is occluded (*D*), the capillaries are already collapsed, so no change in DL_{CO} occurs. When arterial inflow to the lower and middle zones are occluded simultaneously (*E*), capillaries in the middle zone may collapse. However, if Ppa increases, capillaries in the upper zone may become distended and the net result may be no change in DL_{CO}. Under these circumstances, if Ppv also increases (*F*), DL_{CO} may actually increase. (After Nadel JA, Gold WM, Burgess JH: Early diagnosis of chronic pulmonary vascular obstruction. Value of pulmonary function tests. Am J Med 44: 16–25, 1968.)

DIFFUSION

CLINICAL APPLICATIONS OF DL_{CO}

Restrictive Ventilatory Defects

- DL_{CO} is reduced in interstitial pulmonary fibrosis and correlates with anatomic findings in resected lung tissue or high-resolution CT scans.
- DL_{CO} is reduced at rest in at least half of these patients, but the test may be normal in at least one third more who have abnormal responses to exercise (tachypnea above 50 breaths per minute associated with hypoxemia and ventilation-perfusion mismatching) and documented fibrosis by lung biopsy or CT scan.[200, 201]
- DL_{CO} is decreased in patients with asbestos-induced pleural fibrosis who have a restrictive ventilatory defect without evidence of associated parenchymal abnormalities as documented by chest roentgenogram, bronchoalveolar lavage, and high-resolution CT scan.[202]

Rejection of Transplanted Lungs

- DL_{CO} is decreased abnormally in most patients reported with single lung, double lung, or heart and lung transplants.
- Great emphasis has been placed on the importance of detection of bronchiolitis obliterans in these patients as a potentially lethal but reversible manifestation of rejection if treated inadequately or too late.[203–214]
- Despite the frequency of diffusion defects and bronchiolitis obliterans in patients with lung transplants, serial evaluation of DL_{CO} to detect rejection early has not proved useful to detect this lesion.[203–214]

REGULATION OF VENTILATION

MEASUREMENTS OF REGULATION OF VENTILATION

General

- Rebreathing assessment of the response to hypoxia and hypercapnia has been used widely and is less time-consuming and tiring than classic steady-state methods.
- Steady-state techniques do not appear to provide significant additional information, but the equipment and method described by Severinghaus and colleagues[215] allows rapid step changes in the patient's PO_2 while PCO_2 is stabilized and offers the advantage of a brief stable period of hypoxia.
- Measurement of inspiratory occlusion pressure at 100 msec (0.1 second) is thought to reflect the entire neural output of the respiratory center.
  - This pressure is not influenced by conscious muscle effort and is less influenced by abnormal mechanical properties of the respiratory system than is measurement of ventilation.
  - Other methods, including electromyographic (EMG) measurements of the diaphragm, the measurement of isometric inspiratory loads, and the use of drugs that stimulate the carotid body, have not been used enough to establish their clinical utility.[216]

REGULATION OF VENTILATION

MEASUREMENTS OF REGULATION OF VENTILATION

General Protocol

- The subject should be prepared for these tests according to the recommendations of the American Thoracic Society Workshop on Assessment of Respiratory Control in Humans.[217]
- At a minimum, the subject should be screened from the meters, monitors, and manipulators; preferably, the subject's eyes should be closed during the test procedure.
- Ventilatory responses to hypoxia and hypercapnia, even in normal individuals, vary considerably.
- To prevent extraneous influences from further increasing this variability, the following is recommended:
  1. Studies should be performed in the fasting state with the bladder empty.
  2. The subject should be comfortable and should rest for at least 30 minutes before the test.
  3. The room should be quiet.
  4. Body temperature should be determined.
  5. Tests may be performed in either the sitting or semisupine position.
  6. Preliminary evidence suggests that normal subjects may have greater (presumably exaggerated) hypoxic responses when using nose clip and mouthpiece than when using masks.
  7. Tests should be performed in duplicate with at least 10 minutes of rest between tests.
- Ventilatory responses to hypoxia and hypercapnia are potentially hazardous. The clinical condition of the patient should be considered when evaluating the potential hazardous effects of the test procedure, and the usual precautions for safety of the patient used in any stress test should be taken.

Breath-Holding Time

- With nose clips in place, the subject exhales to RV, inhales to TLC, and holds his or her breath as long as comfortably possible.
- Analyses of expired gases can be made to estimate end-tidal CO_2 concentrations.
- Breath-holding time equals the average time in seconds from the end of inspiration to TLC until the first expiration.
- The test is repeated until the breath-holding times or end-tidal CO_2 concentrations are reproducible.
- The mean value for predicted breath-holding at TLC is 78 seconds.[218]
- In six normal subjects studied by Davidson and associates,[219] reproducibility of the test at TLC was 75 ± 3 seconds at sea level (mean $\pm$ SEM); subjects were trained until the expired end-tidal CO_2 was reproducible within 2 mm Hg.

REGULATION OF VENTILATION

HYPERCAPNIC RESPONSE

Protocol

- A reservoir bag is filled with a volume equal to the subject's VC plus 1 L with a mixture containing 7% CO_2 and 93% oxygen.[220]
- The subject breathes room air and exhales into the room; expired flow and end-tidal CO_2 are recorded.
- After a period to establish a stable baseline, valves are turned so that the subject breathes in and out of the reservoir bag.
- The test is continued until the subject stops because of dyspnea, until the end-tidal P_{CO_2} equals 9%, or until 4 minutes have elapsed.

Analysis

- The ventilation in L/min (BTPS), either breath-by-breath or averaged over 5 to 10 breaths, is plotted on the ordinate, and the mean end-tidal CO_2 (mm Hg) is plotted on the abscissa for the same periods (FIGURE 8–28).
- The slope (change in $\dot{V}_E[\Delta\dot{V}_E]$/change in end-tidal P_{CO_2}) is determined for all the periods, preferably by linear least-squares regression analysis, eliminating the first 30 seconds of rebreathing.
- The variability between normal subjects is large. (APPENDIX 12 lists predicted normal values for responses to hypercapnia.)[220, 221]
- The hypercapnic response correlates with weight, height, and VC.[222]
- In subjects studied on two occasions 15 minutes apart, the mean ± SEE of the slope of the first test was 2.60 ± 0.11, and for the second test it was 2.46 ± 0.10.
- The mean ± SEE of the intercept on the CO_2 axis was 32.42 ± 0.67 mm Hg for the first test and 31.17 ± 0.71 mm Hg for the second test.
- When 10 of the same subjects were retested as long as 2 years later, the differences in slopes from earlier values varied from 0.04 to 3.57 L/min · mm Hg and the differences in intercepts on the abscissa varied from 0 to 7.6 mm Hg.

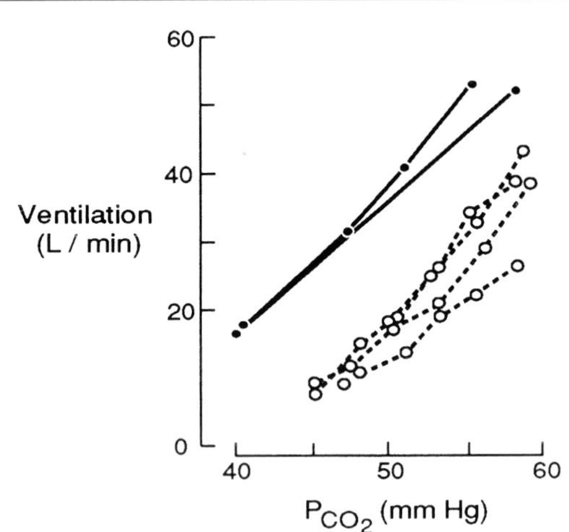

FIGURE 8–28

Comparison of rebreathing and steady-state hypercapnic response curves. Response lines defined by the steady-state method (*solid symbols*) and by the rebreathing method (*open symbols*) are shown for two experiments on the same subject. In one experiment, the steady-state points were defined by inhalation for 20 minutes of each of four CO_2 mixtures without intervening periods of air breathing. In the other experiment, the steady-state points were defined by inhalation for 30 minutes of each CO_2 mixture, with an intervening rest of 30 minutes. The figure illustrates a difference in position of the response lines due to a smaller P_{CO_2} gradient between arterial blood and chemoreceptor tissue during the rebreathing method. The close agreement in slope implies that the ratio, Δ end-tidal P_{CO_2}/Δ chemoreceptor P_{CO_2}, is the same in the two methods. (Modified after Read DJC: A clinical method for assessing the ventilatory response to carbon dioxide. Australas Ann Med 16:20–32, 1967.)

REGULATION OF VENTILATION

HYPOXIC RESPONSE

Protocol

- A reservoir bag is filled with a volume equal to the VC of the subject plus 1 L with a mixture containing approximately 7% CO_2, 70% N_2, and the balance O_2.[223]
- The subject breathes from and exhales into the room.
- Values for expired volume, end-tidal PO_2, end-tidal PCO_2, and O_2 saturation are recorded; when the end-tidal PCO_2 values stabilize, appropriate valves are then turned so the subject rebreathes from the bag.
- The subject then takes three deep breaths to facilitate mixing; after these three breaths, the CO_2 value is recorded.
- CO_2 is maintained at this level by manually adjusting flow through the carbon dioxide absorber.
- Rebreathing is continued until end-tidal PO_2 decreases to 45 mm Hg, the O_2 saturation decreases to 75%, or the subject becomes distressed.
- If ventilation increases too rapidly, addition of O_2 at a rate of 125 to 200 mL/minute will slow the rate of change.

Analysis

- Ventilation in L/min, BTPS (breath-by-breath or averaged over five to ten breaths) is plotted on the ordinate, and the mean oxygen saturation percentage is plotted on the abscissa for the same periods (FIGURE 8–29).
- The slope (change in $\dot{V}E[\Delta\dot{V}E]/1\%$ desaturation) is calculated, preferably by linear least-squares regression analysis, and reported in terms of the mean end-tidal PCO_2 during the test.
- The variability of the hypoxic response during eucapnia in normal subjects is large. (APPENDIX 13 gives the predicted normal values for response to hypoxia.)[223, 224]
- The difference in slopes indicates that the hypoxic response is very sensitive to the level of end-tidal PCO_2 selected.
- Repeated measurements in five subjects from day to day showed a variance within individuals of 0.76 and between individuals of 7.75.[223]

FIGURE 8–29

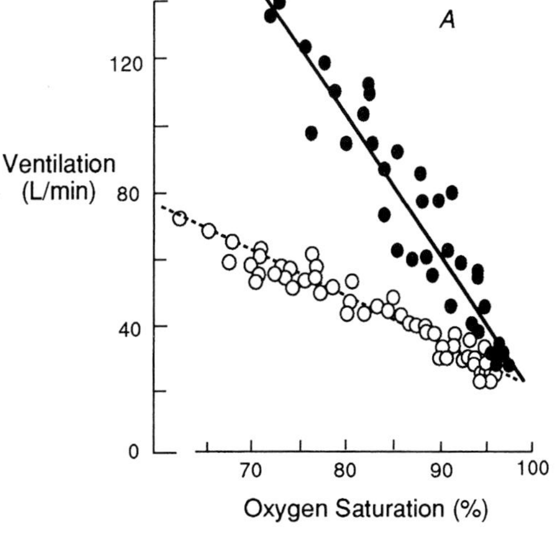

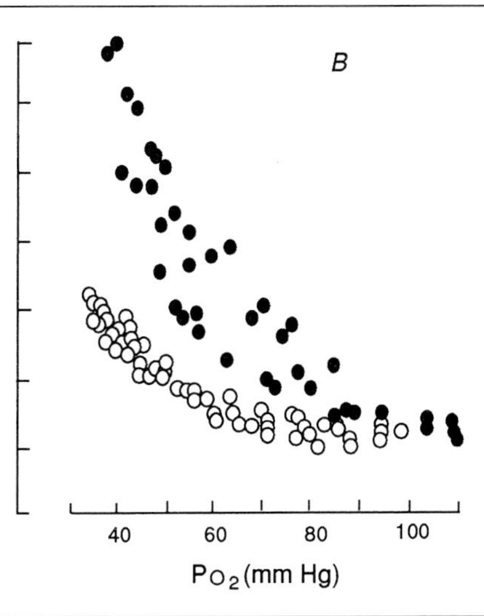

Hypoxic response curves. Pooled results of four studies in two subjects. In **A,** ventilation is plotted against O_2 saturation, producing linear responses. In **B,** the more traditional hyperbolic relationship is obtained by plotting ventilation against alveolar PO_2. (Modified after Rebuck AS, Campbell EJM: A clinical method for assessing the ventilatory response to hypoxia. Am Rev Respir Dis 109:345–350, 1974.)

REGULATION OF VENTILATION

INSPIRATORY OCCLUSION PRESSURE

Protocol

- Mouth pressure at 100 msec (0.1 second), $P_{0.1}$, or the maximum rate of inspiratory pressure change, (DP/DT)max, can be measured when the patient is breathing room air or while the hypercapnic or hypoxic response is being tested.
- Brief inspiratory occlusion should be performed randomly, always preceded by three or more tidal breaths[225] and should be measured every minute and at the same time after the inspiratory effort begins (for example, 100 ± 10 msec).
- Starling resistor method: out of view of the subject, the operator compresses a syringe during expiration to close a Starling resistor arranged in series with the inspiratory channel so that the channel is occluded.
  - The syringe is decompressed as soon as possible after the inspiratory attempt is initiated.
  - Recorder speed should be 50 mm/second during the subject's inspiratory attempt.
- Inspiratory valve method: alternatively, mouth pressure and its differential (the change in pressure) can be measured in the 10 to 50 msec before the inspiratory valve opens. This approach takes advantage of the inherent resistance of the valve and can be measured at a slow recorder speed for every breath without requiring use of a Starling resistor or other maneuvers by the operator.[226]

Analysis

- The $P_{0.1}$ measured during single partially occluded breaths, or the average (DP/DT)max of several breaths is determined directly from the recording and plotted on the ordinate.
- On the abscissa, mean $\dot{V}E$ calculated from three or more breaths preceding inspiratory occlusion, end-tidal P_{CO_2}, or arterial O_2 saturation is displayed (FIGURE 8–30).

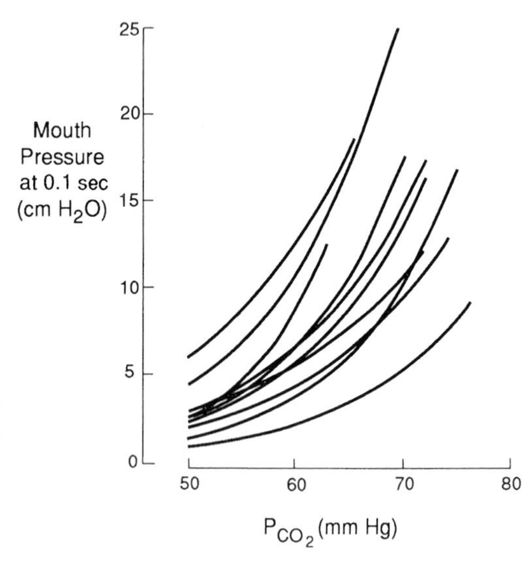

FIGURE 8–30

Inspiratory occlusion pressure at 100 msec (0.1 sec) in response to hypercapnia. Each curve is the mean regression of $P_{0.1}$ against CO_2 for one subject. Inspiratory occlusion pressure may be used to measure the output of the respiratory center in response not only to hypercapnia, but also to hypoxia, exercise, and other factors. (Modified after Whitelaw WA, Dernne J, Milic-Emili J: Occlusion pressure as a measure of respiratory center output in conscious man. Respir Physiol 23:181–199, 1975.)

REGULATION OF VENTILATION

INSPIRATORY OCCLUSION PRESSURE

Normal Values

- Kryger and associates[227] found a mean $P_{0.1}$ of 2.6 cm H_2O (range, 1.5 to 5.0 at $PaCO_2$ of 39 to 42 mm Hg).
- Gelb and coworkers[228] found a mean ± SD increase of 0.52 ± 0.19 cm H_2O/mm Hg PCO_2 during increasing hypercapnia.
- Whitelaw and colleagues[225] found a mean $P_{0.1}$ ± SD of 13.2 ± 0.76 cm H_2O during constant hypercapnia (end-tidal PCO_2 56 mm Hg).
- Matthews and Howell[226] found $(DP/DT)_{max}$ to vary during quiet breathing from 12.5 to 25 cm H_2O/second. During hypercapnia, the increase in $(DP/DT)_{max}$ ranged from 0.6 to 4.6 cm $H_2O \cdot sec^{-1} \cdot$ mm Hg CO_2, and end-tidal PCO_2 increased from 50 to 60 mm Hg.

CLINICAL APPLICATIONS

CO_2 Responses

There are three clinical conditions associated with abnormal CO_2 responses: (1) decreased central chemoreceptor CO_2 response, (2) neuromuscular disease preventing normal response to CO_2, and (3) patients with abnormal mechanical properties of the respiratory system.

- Patients with abnormal medullary or pontine CO_2 chemoreceptors have decreased CO_2 responses, as do patients with congenital abnormalities, trauma, or inflammatory lesions in the CNS.
  - Chronic CO_2 reduction with associated increased bicarbonate levels and increased buffer capacity of blood and other tissue fluids may cause decreased central CO_2 response.
- Patients with neuromuscular disease have normal output from the ventilatory centers but an inadequate peripheral response. *Myasthenia gravis* patients cannot respond because of the defective neuromuscular junction, and patients with poliomyelitis cannot respond because of damaged anterior horn cells. These patients have decreased inspiratory work and diminished maximal inspiratory force in response to inhaled CO_2. Tests of respiratory muscle strength will diagnose these kinds of patients with neuromuscular weakness.
- Chronic airflow obstruction or pulmonary restriction or deformities of the chest wall may inhibit adequate ventilatory response to inhaled CO_2 whereas the diaphragmatic EMG, the $P_{0.1}$, or the work of breathing is appropriate for the CO_2.

Hypoxic Responses

There are few clinical indications for evaluation of hypoxic responses.

- It is used in patients with carotid body denervation to test the degree of depressed sensitivity to oxygen.
- Patients born at altitude or patients with cyanotic congenital heart disease may have diminished response to hypoxia. The degree of abnormality can assessed by administration of low oxygen mixtures to breathe, but this is largely a research procedure.
- This evaluation can be used in patients with chronic CO_2 retention because their ventilation may be driven primarily by hypoxemia.
- Hypoxic response is assessed by measuring the level of ventilation when the patient breathes room air and again when the patient breathes O_2.
  - Normal subjects will show a brief small decrease in ventilation, and some patients with chronic CO_2 retention may show a marked decrease in ventilation.
  - Although this response is unusual in patients with chronic airflow obstruction who are treated with oxygen, it is important to be aware that this response does occur in some patients who may require intubation and assisted ventilation.

VENTILATION-PERFUSION RELATIONSHIPS

RESTING VENTILATION

Protocol

- Resting ventilation is defined as the amount of air exhaled per minute ($\dot{V}E$).
- It is measured readily using a recording spirometer equipped with a CO_2 absorber. (The measured expired volume must be corrected for the amount of absorbed CO_2.)
  - Many laboratories use a mouthpiece equipped with valves that separate inhaled and exhaled gases, permitting collection of exhaled air in a plastic bag or meteorologic balloon in preference to the use of a spirometer.
  - The volume of exhaled gas collected is then measured with a 120-L (Tissot) spirometer or with a dry-gas meter.
- For use at the bedside, a Wright respirometer[229] is preferred and is used commonly in surgical recovery rooms and critical care units.
- From $\dot{V}E$, it is possible to estimate alveolar ventilation using an assumed value for dead space:

$$VD(mL) \approx \text{weight (lb)}$$

Analysis

- Measurement of resting $\dot{V}E$ usually plays a minor role in routine assessment of pulmonary function because patients with advanced disease of the lungs often breathe with a normal tidal volume and respiratory frequency.
- The attending physician may wish to obtain an accurate record of resting $\dot{V}E$ if hypoventilation or an abnormal respiratory pattern is suspected, such as that associated with central nervous system lesions or psychogenic disorders.
- Resting $\dot{V}E$ in normal subjects has been studied in detail: men breathe at an average rate of 16 breaths/minute, women at 19 breaths/minute, although there is much individual variation, and sighs occur at an average of 10 per hour.[230, 231]
- Because the attempts to measure $\dot{V}E$ change an automatic, unconscious process to one of concern to the subject, it is difficult to obtain accurate measurements of the rate and pattern of resting $\dot{V}E$.
- In addition to making measurements when the subject is unaware, investigators have used magnetometers attached to the chest wall and impedance plethysmography[231–234] to measure ventilation and pattern of breathing accurately.
- Measurement of resting $\dot{V}E$ plays an important, but previously neglected part in management of patients in danger of developing respiratory failure from hypoventilation (e,g., patients with obesity and sleep disorder syndromes).[235]
- In such patients, or in patients in postoperative states, with drug intoxication, or with neuromuscular disease, measurement of $\dot{V}E$ is as important as measurement of the usual vital signs (heart rate and blood pressure) and should be obtained at frequent intervals.

VENTILATION-PERFUSION RELATIONSHIPS

DEAD SPACE MEASUREMENT

Bohr's Equation for Respiratory Dead Space

- Bohr's equation, applied to a particular gas X, is as follows: Total volume of expired gas (V_E) = volume of alveolar gas (V_A) + volume of dead space (V_D)
  - Expired gas is the total volume of gas leaving the nose and mouth between the beginning and the end of a single exhalation (V_E).
  - V_A is the volume of alveolar gas contributed to the exhaled gas and does *not* refer to the total volume of gas in the alveoli.
  - Amount of gas X in V_E, V_A, or V_D = fractional concentration (F_x) times the volume in which gas X is contained.

$$F_{E_X}V_E = F_{A_X}V_A + F_{D_X}V_D$$

Gas in the dead space or conducting airways at the beginning of exhalation is inspired gas:

$$F_{D_X} = F_{I_X}$$

$$F_{E_X}V_E = F_{A_X}V_A + F_{I_X}V_D$$

Because $V_A = V_E - V_D$,

$$F_{E_X}V_E = F_{A_X}(V_E - V_D) + F_{I_X}V_D$$

Solving,

$$\boxed{V_D = \frac{[F_{A_X} - F_{E_X}]V_E}{[F_{A_X} - F_{I_X}]}}$$

Inspired air contains little CO_2 ($F_{A_{CO_2}} = 0.0005$), and the Bohr equation becomes

$$V_D = \frac{[F_{A_{CO_2}} - F_{E_{CO_2}}]V_E}{F_{A_{CO_2}}}$$

Single-Breath Measurement of Anatomic Dead Space

- Measurement of anatomic dead space requires continuous analysis of the gas concentration in the exhaled breath (with an N_2 meter or mass spectrometer) plus simultaneous measurement of exhaled gas flow or volume.[236, 237]
- FIGURE 8–31 shows N_2 concentration and exhaled volume at the mouth recorded during exhalation following a single inhalation of N_2-free gas (O_2).
  - If a square wave front were maintained during exhalation between the dead space gas (0% N_2) and alveolar gas (about 60% N_2 because of dilution by oxygen), the exhaled N_2 concentration would remain zero until a volume equal to the dead space had been exhaled; then, the exhaled N_2 concentration would rise suddenly (dashed vertical line FIGURE 8–31) to equal the N_2 concentration of alveolar gas.
  - Dead space volume = volume exhaled up to the point at which alveolar gas suddenly appeared.
- Alveolar gas actually mixes with dead space gas during exhalation; nevertheless, it is still possible to construct a "square wave front" on the record by numerical methods.
- A vertical line (dashed vertical line in FIGURE 8–31) is placed so the amount of N_2 in the shaded area A exactly equals the amount of N_2 contained in the shaded area B; (The amount of N_2 equals the concentration of N_2 times the total volume of expired gas; in the example in FIGURE 8–31) where expiratory flow is constant, equal amounts of N_2 are contained in equal areas of the recording from the N_2 analyzer.)
- Once the square front is constructed, V_D equals the volume exhaled up to that point. Bohr's equation can also be applied to these data and N_2 is measured instead of CO_2. At the end of the single breath of O_2, the dead space is filled with N_2-free O_2. Therefore, $F_{I_{N_2}} = 0$, and the equation simplifies to

$$V_D = \frac{[F_{A_{N_2}} - F_{E_{N_2}}]V_E}{F_{A_{N_2}}}$$

$F_{A_{N_2}}$ is obtained from the N_2 meter record of expired alveolar gas.
- V_E is computed from the pneumotachygraph or volume recording.
- $F_{E_{N_2}}$ is the volume of N_2 exhaled (obtained from measuring the area under the curve of N_2 concentration divided by the total volume of expired gas, V_E).

VENTILATION-PERFUSION RELATIONSHIPS

DEAD SPACE MEASUREMENT

Single-Breath Measurement of Anatomic Dead Space

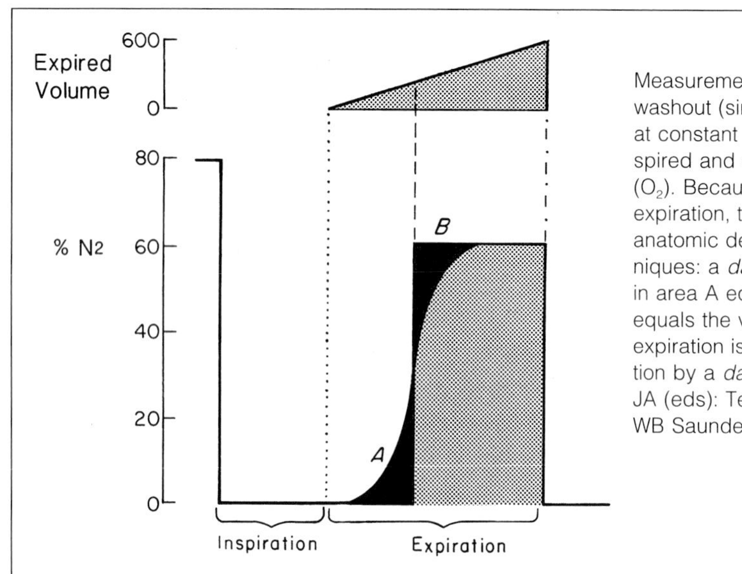

FIGURE 8–31

Measurement of anatomic dead space from single breath N_2 washout (single-breath O_2) test. *Top,* Expired volume is recorded at constant flow. *Bottom,* Recording of N_2 concentration of inspired and expired gas following a single breath of N_2-free gas (O_2). Because alveolar gas mixes with dead space gas during expiration, the exact point at which a volume is equal to the anatomic dead space must be constructed by numerical techniques: a *dashed vertical line* is placed so that the amount of N_2 in area A equals that in area B; thus, the dead space volume equals the volume expired up to that point. The beginning of expiration is indicated by a *dotted vertical line,* the end of expiration by a *dashed and dotted vertical line.* (From Murray JF, Nadel JA (eds): Textbook of Respiratory Medicine. 3rd ed. Philadelphia, WB Saunders, 2000, p. 823.)

Physiologic Dead Space

- In Bohr's equation, FE_{CO_2} and $\dot{V}E$ can be measured easily, but FA_{CO_2} is difficult to obtain, and V_D cannot be calculated unless the correct value for FA_{CO_2} is known.
- Arterial P_{CO_2} represents a mean alveolar P_{CO_2} over several respiratory cycles, provided that arterial blood is sampled over this same period and the patient does not have a significant venous-to-arterial shunt.
- Arterial P_{CO_2} can replace alveolar P_{CO_2} as follows:

$$V_D = \frac{[Pa_{CO_2} - PE_{CO_2}]V_E}{Pa_{CO_2}}$$

Ideally, anatomic and physiologic dead space are equal. In patients with uneven ventilation/blood flow ratios, the physiologic dead space is larger than the anatomic dead space, because regions with increased alveolar ventilation in relation to blood flow act as regions of wasted ventilation or respiratory dead space.[238]

- Physiologic dead space includes anatomic dead space and alveolar dead space ventilation.
- Alveolar dead space ventilation includes ventilation of alveoli without perfusion; alveoli with decreased perfusion and increased, normal, or slightly decreased ventilation; and alveoli with normal perfusion and marked overventilation.
- Physiologists assume the lung behaves as if it comprised two compartments: one with perfusion and one without perfusion.
  - Overventilation relative to perfusion wastes ventilation with respect to oxygen transfer because of the shape of the oxygen-hemoglobin dissociation curve.
  - Little oxygen is added to blood by increasing alveolar P_{O_2} from 100 to 140 mm Hg..
  - This excess ventilation is not wasted with respect to CO_2 elimination because increased ventilation decreases arterial CO_2.
  - Regions with excess ventilation are usually accompanied by other regions with diminished ventilation and increased P_{CO_2}.
  - Ventilation is still "wasted" with respect to CO_2, because it is not distributed proportionately to perfusion.

VENTILATION-PERFUSION RELATIONSHIPS

ALVEOLAR AIR EQUATION[162]

Principle

- Measurement of alveolar PO_2 and PCO_2 from analysis of a single sample of exhaled alveolar gas is subject to considerable error, but mean alveolar PO_2 can be calculated accurately.
- The underlying principle is based on the fact that at sea level, the total pressure of gases (O_2, CO_2, N_2, and H_2O) in the alveoli equals 760 mm Hg; thus, if the partial pressures of any three of these four are known, the fourth can be obtained by subtraction.

$$760 \text{ mm Hg} = PO_2 + PCO_2 + PN_2 + PH_2O$$

$$PO_2 = Pbar - PH_2O - PN_2 - PCO_2$$

$$\begin{aligned} PO_2 &= 760 \text{ mm Hg} - 47 \text{ mm Hg} \\ &\quad - 563 \text{ mm Hg} - 40 \text{ mm Hg} \\ &= 110 \text{ mm Hg} \end{aligned}$$

PH_2O at 37°C is 47 mm Hg.

- Arterial PCO_2 is used to represent mean alveolar PCO_2, because arterial blood coming from all the alveoli approaches an integrated value of alveolar PCO_2 with respect to different regions of the lung and to different times during the respiratory cycle.
- PN_2 = 563 mm Hg.
- This is true if the respiratory gas exchange ratio (R) were 1 (i.e., the amount of CO_2 added to the alveoli equals the amount of O_2 removed from the alveoli per minute).

Effect of R

Actually, however, more O_2 is removed per minute than CO_2 is added, and R is usually 0.8.

$$\text{The usual R} = \frac{200 \text{ mL } CO_2/\text{min}}{250 \text{ mL } O_2/\text{min}} = 0.8$$

- When R = 0.8, N_2 molecules are slightly more concentrated, because the same number of N_2 molecules are present in a smaller volume. If alveolar N_2 concentration increases to 81%, alveolar PN_2 increases to 577 mm Hg and alveolar PO_2 falls to 96 mm Hg. Thus, it is essential to measure R in order to calculate alveolar PN_2 accurately.
- The precise formula (assuming inspired PCO_2 is zero) is as follows:

$$PA_{O_2} = PI_{O_2} - PA_{CO_2}\left[FI_{O_2} + \frac{1 - FI_{O_2}}{R}\right]$$

(unknown) (known) (measured) (correcting factor)

PI_{O_2} is inspired O_2 pressure (moist) at sea level; 20.93% of (760 − 47 mm Hg) = 149 mm Hg

- PA_{CO_2} is alveolar CO_2 pressure and is assumed to be equal to arterial PCO_2, which can be measured accurately.

VENTILATION-PERFUSION RELATIONSHIPS

ALVEOLAR AIR EQUATION[162]

Correcting Factor

- The "correcting" factor introduces no correction when R is 1; if R = 1, the correcting factor is:

$$\left[F_{I_{O_2}} + \frac{1 - F_{I_{O_2}}}{R}\right] = 0.2093 + \frac{1 - 0.2093}{1} = 1$$

Usually, R < 1 (the volume of O_2 absorbed exceeds that of CO_2 exhaled), so the volume of exhaled gas is slightly less than the volume of inhaled air; if R = 0.8, the correcting factor becomes:

$$\left[F_{I_{O_2}} + \frac{1 - F_{I_{O_2}}}{R}\right] = 0.2093 = \frac{1 - 0.2093}{0.8} = 1.2$$

If R = 1, Pa_{CO_2} = 40 mm Hg, and the correcting factor is 1, then $P_{A_{O_2}}$ = 109 mm Hg.

- If R = 0.8, $P_{A_{CO_2}}$ = 40 mm Hg, and the correcting factor is 1.2, then $P_{A_{O_2}}$ = 101 mm Hg.

Approximation for Clinical Use

- Alveolar air equation is approximated for clinical purposes as follows:

$$P_{A_{O_2}} = P_{I_{O_2}} - \frac{Pa_{CO_2}}{R}$$

- Alveolar-arterial O_2 difference has been shown to be larger in older subjects than in younger ones.[239–241]
  - The Mellemgaard regression with age is (A − a) D_{O_2} = 2.5 + 0.21 × age in years.[242]
  - The increase in alveolar-arterial O_2 differences is due almost entirely to a decrease in arterial P_{O_2} with age.

ALVEOLAR VENTILATION AND PULMONARY BLOOD FLOW

Calculations

- CO_2 in exhaled gas must all come from alveolar gas.
- The volume of CO_2 leaving the alveoli and entering the exhaled gas per unit time ($\dot{V}_{CO_2}$) equals the volume of alveolar ventilation in that same time ($\dot{V}_A$) × ($F_{A_{CO_2}}$).

$$\dot{V}_{CO_2} = \dot{V}_A \times F_{A_{CO_2}}$$

$$\dot{V}_A = \frac{\dot{V}_{CO_2}}{F_{A_{CO_2}}}$$

$$F_{A_{CO_2}} = \frac{\%\ \text{alveolar}\ CO_2}{100}$$

$$\dot{V}_A = \frac{\dot{V}_{CO_2}}{\%\ \text{alveolar}\ CO_2} \times 100$$

$\dot{V}_A$ and $\dot{V}_{CO_2}$ must be corrected to BTPS.

- $\dot{V}_A$ is usually corrected to BTPS, but $\dot{V}_{CO_2}$ to STPD; in this case, the right side of the equation must be multiplied by a factor of 1.21 (or the left by 0.863).
- To use with alveolar P_{CO_2}:

$$\dot{V}_A\ (\text{mL/min}) = \frac{\dot{V}_{CO_2}\ (\text{mL}) \times 863}{\text{alveolar}\ P_{CO_2}}$$

VENTILATION-PERFUSION RELATIONSHIPS

ALVEOLAR VENTILATION AND PULMONARY BLOOD FLOW

Principles

- In any steady state, the quantity of CO_2 leaving venous blood to enter the alveoli and the amount of CO_2 leaving the alveoli to enter exhaled gas must be equal.
- CO_2 leaving pulmonary capillary blood each minute equals pulmonary capillary blood flow (in mL/min) times the arteriovenous difference (in mL of gas per mL of blood):

$$\dot{V}CO_2 = \dot{Q}C(C\bar{v}_{CO_2} - Cc'_{CO_2})$$

where
$\dot{Q}c$ = pulmonary capillary blood flow
$C\bar{v}_{CO_2}$ = CO_2 concentration in mixed venous blood
Cc'_{CO_2} = CO_2 concentration in the end-pulmonary capillary blood

- To determine the quantity of CO_2 washed out of the alveoli by alveolar ventilation:

$$\dot{V}_{CO_2} = \dot{V}A \times FA_{CO_2}\, 0.83$$

Because the CO_2 concentrations in both equations are equal,

$$0.83\dot{V}A \times FA_{CO_2} = \dot{Q}c(C\bar{v}_{CO_2} - Cc'_{CO_2})$$

$$\frac{\dot{V}A}{\dot{Q}c} = \frac{(C\bar{v}_{CO_2} - Cc'_{CO_2})}{FA_{CO_2} \times 0.83}$$

$$\frac{\dot{V}A}{\dot{Q}c} = \frac{863(C\bar{v}_{CO_2} - Cc'_{CO_2})}{PA_{CO_2}}$$

Effect on PCO_2

- Because the mixed venous blood distributed to all pulmonary capillaries has the same CO_2 concentration, and because end-pulmonary capillary blood has the same PCO_2 as alveolar gas, alveolar PCO_2 is determined by the ratio $\dot{V}A/\dot{Q}c$.
- West analyzed a ten-compartment lung with changing mixed venous composition reflecting arterial blood with decreased O_2 and increased CO_2 as well as $\dot{V}A/\dot{Q}c$ imbalances.[243]
- As $\dot{V}A/\dot{Q}c$ imbalance increases, arterial PO_2 decreases rapidly and progressively; PCO_2 increased gradually initially, but then quite rapidly.
- $\dot{V}A/\dot{Q}c$ imbalance can cause significant hypercapnia in patients with pulmonary disease, particularly when the disease is so severe that hyperventilation of some regions of lung no longer compensates for regions that have decreased PO_2.[243]

VENTILATION-PERFUSION RELATIONSHIPS

VENOUS-TO-ARTERIAL SHUNT

Principle

- When a venous-to-arterial shunt is patent, arterial blood contains some mixed venous blood that has bypassed the lungs and some well-oxygenated blood that has passed through the pulmonary capillaries (TABLE 8–3).
- This relationship for blood is analogous to Bohr's equation for calculation of respiratory dead space.
- Amount of O_2 in arterial blood = amount of O_2 in blood that has traversed pulmonary capillaries plus the amount of O_2 in shunted blood.

Key: $\dot{Q}_s$ = shunt blood flow; $\dot{Q}$ = total blood flow; $\dot{Q}c$ = pulmonary capillary blood flow.

$$Ca_{O_2}\,\dot{Q} = Cc'_{O_2}\,\dot{Q}c + C\bar{v}_{O_2}$$

$$\dot{Q}c = \dot{Q} - \dot{Q}_S$$

$$Ca_{O_2}\,\dot{Q} = Cc'_{O_2}\,(\dot{Q} - \dot{Q}_S) + C\bar{v}_{O_2}\,\dot{Q}_S$$

$$\dot{Q}s = \frac{Ca_{O_2} - Cc'_{O_2}}{C\bar{v}_{O_2} - Cc'_{O_2}} \times \dot{Q}$$

TABLE 8–3

Causes of Hypoxia, Their Effect on Alveolar-Arterial Po_2 Differences and Arterial Pco_2

Cause	Effect on Pao_2	Effect on (A–a) Po_2	Effect on $Paco_2$
Normal lungs/inadequate oxygenation			
• Deficiency of O_2 in atmosphere	↓	↔	↓
• Hypoventilation (neuromuscular disorder)	↓	↔	↑
Pulmonary disease			
• Hypoventilation (airway/parenchymal disorder)	↓	↔	↑
• Diffusion abnormality	↓*,†	↑*	↓
• Ventilation/perfusion imbalance	↓†	↑	↓, ↔, or ↑
• Right-to-left shunts	↓	↑	↓, ↔, or ↑
Inadequate transport/delivery of O_2			
• Anemia	↔	↔	↔
• General/localized circulatory insufficiency	↔	↔	↔
Inadequate tissue oxygenation			
• Abnormal tissue demand/poisoned enzymes/edema	↔	↔	↔

Key: ↑ = increased; ↔ = no change; ↓ = decreased.

* Infrequently observed at rest, but more likely during exercise.

† Unless patient is hyperventilating.

Source: Adapted from Comroe JH Jr., Forster RE II, DuBois AB, et al: Arterial blood oxygen, carbon dioxide and pH. *In* The Lung: Clinical Physiology and Pulmonary Function Tests (2nd ed.). Chicago, Year Book Medical Publishers, 1962, pp. 140–161.

VENTILATION-PERFUSION RELATIONSHIPS

VENOUS-TO-ARTERIAL SHUNT

Using Pure O_2

- Ca_{O_2} and $C\bar{v}_{CO_2}$ can be measured as follows:
  - Quantity of blood flowing through the shunt can be determined by having the patient breathe pure O_2 for a sufficient time to wash all the N_2 from the alveoli.
  - Alveolar PO_2 will then be 760 − PA_{H_2O} − PA_{CO_2}, or approximately 673 mm Hg.
  - Under these conditions, end-capillary blood can be assumed to contain an amount equal to the O_2 capacity of hemoglobin plus 2.0 mL of dissolved O_2 per 100 mL.
- The normal amount of blood flowing through anatomic shunts (2% of cardiac output) results in a decrease in O_2 in PO_2 of 35 mm Hg below the theoretic maximal value for arterial PO_2 when the patient is breathing pure O_2.

VENOUS ADMIXTURE OR PHYSIOLOGIC SHUNT

Using 12% to 14% O_2

- Venous admixture or physiologic shunt can be estimated by the method of Lilienthal and colleagues.[166]
- "Shunt" means decreased $\dot{V}A/\dot{Q}c$ ratios and includes perfused alveoli without ventilation; very poorly ventilated alveoli with normal, increased, or slightly decreased perfusion; and ventilated alveoli with markedly increased perfusion.
- In this situation, the physiologist assumes two compartments: one with and one without a complete shunt.[244]
  - When the subject breathes 20.93% O_2, the PO_2 difference at the beginning of the pulmonary capillary is about 60 mm Hg, the transfer of O_2 across the membranes to hemoglobin is initially rapid, and equilibrium with alveolar gas is attained quickly.
- When breathing air, a healthy subject has virtually no difference between alveolar and end-capillary PO_2.
- When 12% to 14% O_2 is breathed, the PO_2 difference at the beginning of the capillary is only 25 mm Hg, the initial O_2 transfer rate is slower, and a measurable PO_2 difference persists at the end of the capillary.
- Decreasing alveolar PO_2 increases the alveolar–to–end-capillary PO_2 difference, whereas increasing alveolar PO_2 decreases the alveolar–to–end-capillary PO_2 difference (TABLE 8–4).

TABLE 8–4

Effect of Oxygen Breathing on Alveolar-Arterial PO_2 Differences

	12–14% O_2	20.93% O_2*	50–100% O_2
Total alveolar-arterial PO_2 difference (mm Hg)	10	9	35–50
Venous admixture	1	8	35–50
Alveolar-to-end-capillary difference (mm Hg)	9	1	0

*Room air. *Source:* Adapted from Comroe JH Jr, Forster RE II, DuBois AB, et al: The Lung: Clinical Physiology and Pulmonary Function Tests (2nd ed). Chicago, Year Book Medical Publishers, 1962, pp. 111–139.

VENTILATION-PERFUSION RELATIONSHIPS

VENOUS ADMIXTURE OR PHYSIOLOGIC SHUNT

Analysis

- Pulmonary capillary blood PO_2 can be estimated but not measured.
- Samples of arterial blood can be obtained and its PO_2 measured accurately, but its PO_2 is less than that of end-pulmonary capillary blood because of "physiologic shunt" or venous admixture.
- PO_2 difference between alveolar gas and arterial blood is caused by (1) incomplete equilibration between PO_2 in alveolar gas and end-capillary blood and (2) venous admixture, which can be eliminated by having the subject breathe 12% to 14% O_2.
  - The elimination of the PO_2 difference by breathing 12% to 14% O_2 depends on the shape of the O_2-hemoglobin dissociation curve.
  - Breathing room air causes arterial PO_2 and O_2 saturation to fall on the flat portion of the curve, where a small decrease in O_2 saturation caused by shunted blood is associated with a large decrease in arterial PO_2.
  - Breathing 12% to 14% O_2 causes arterial PO_2 and O_2 saturation to be reduced and fall on the steep slope of the O_2-hemoglobin dissociation curve: under these conditions, the same decrease in arterial O_2 saturation caused by the same degree of venous admixture is associated with a very small decrease in arterial PO_2 (FIGURE 8–32).
- The response to inhaling 12% to 14% O_2 permits not only differential diagnosis of arterial hypoxemia but also estimation of DL_{O_2}.

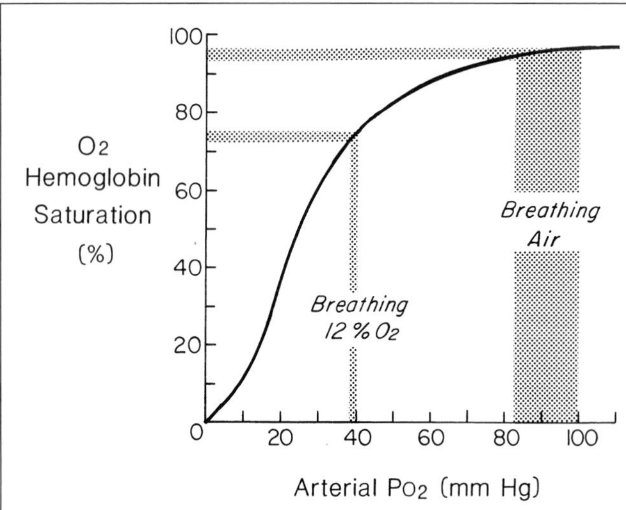

FIGURE 8–32

Effect of venous-to-arterial shunt on arterial PO_2. If 10% of mixed venous blood bypasses the lungs, arterial PO_2 is decreased by 19 mm Hg when the patient breathes room air, but only by 1.2 mm Hg when the patient breathes 12% O_2. In each case, the arteriovenous O_2 saturation difference is 22%, and the 10% shunt causes a 2.2% decrease in arterial O_2 saturation (breathing air, 97 −94.8%; breathing 12% O_2, 75 −72.8%). (From Murray JF, Nadel JA (eds): Textbook of Respiratory Medicine. 3rd ed. Philadelphia, WB Saunders, 2000, p. 826.)

VENTILATION-PERFUSION RELATIONSHIPS

METHODS OF MEASUREMENT

Using Pure O_2

• If a patient is given pure O_2 to breathe, it is possible to distinguish a right-to-left shunt from a ventilation-perfusion abnormality. The alveolar and arterial Po_2 values expected in an ideal lung, with $\dot{V}A/\dot{Q}c$ ratio imbalance, and with right-to-left shunt, are given in TABLE 8–5.

• Pure O_2 replaces N_2 with O_2 in all gas exchange units that have patent airways, even in the presence of severe airway obstruction or pulmonary restriction; this leaves only O_2, CO_2, and H_2O in the airspaces.

$$PA_{O_2} = PA_{TOTAL} - PA_{CO_2} - PA_{H_2O}$$

• Total pressure and water vapor pressure are the same in all patent gas exchange units; thus, alveolar Po_2 differences between units exist only when there are differences in Pco_2.

• In ideal lungs or lungs with $\dot{V}A/\dot{Q}c$ imbalance, the high alveolar Po_2 corrects the ventilation-perfusion imbalance; arterial Po_2 values are also high, provided all N_2 is washed out of communicating units by O_2.

• In most normal subjects, the right-to-left shunts are distal to the gas exchange units, so-called post-pulmonary shunts.

  • These shunts involve bronchial veins, mediastinal to pulmonary veins, and thebesian vessels (left ventricular muscle to left ventricular cavity).

  • In some patients, intracardiac shunts, pulmonary arteriovenous malformations, or perfusion of non-ventilated gas exchange units produce pulmonary shunts.

  • Most shunts in patients with pulmonary disorders involve the latter.

• For clinical purposes, the amount of right-to-left shunt may be estimated from the fall in arterial Po_2 below the expected value of 673 mm Hg, as long as Po_2 is sufficient to saturate hemoglobin (>200 mm Hg): For every 2% shunt, Po_2 decreases 35 mm Hg. (See Chapter 5, Nuclear Medicine Techniques and Applications.)

TABLE 8–5

Effect of Breathing 21% and 100% Oxygen on Mean Po_2 Values in Alveolar Gas, Arterial and Mixed Venous Blood in Two-Compartment Lung with Ideal Gas Exchange, $\dot{V}A/\dot{Q}c$ Abnormality, and Right-to-Left Shunt

	Ideal Gas Exchange		$\dot{V}A/\dot{Q}c$ Ratio Imbalance		Right-to-Left Shunt*	
	21%	100%	21%	100%	21%	100%
Mixed venous Po_2 (mm Hg)	40	51	40	51	40	42
Alveolar Po_2 (mm Hg)	101	673	106	675	114	677
Arterial Po_2 (mm Hg)	101	673	89	673	59	125
Alveolar-arterial Po_2 difference (mm Hg)	0	0	17	2	55	552

*Right-to-left shunt equals one-third of the cardiac output.

Source: Murray JF: The Normal Lung (2nd ed). Philadelphia, WB Saunders, 1986, p. 194.

VENTILATION-PERFUSION RELATIONSHIPS

METHODS OF MEASUREMENT

Ventilation

Radioactive Xenon

- Radioactive xenon (^{133}Xe) is a relatively insoluble gas with a blood gas partition coefficient of about 0.13.[245]
- When inhaled, ^{133}Xe can be used to measure regional ventilation in volume, and when dissolved in saline and injected intravenously, it can be used to measure regional blood flow.[246–249]
- When either of these procedures is followed by rebreathing in a closed circuit, a plateau is obtained that reflects the product of lung volume seen by the counter and the geometric factor for ^{133}Xe; for this purpose, the subject is switched into a closed circuit at the end of the injection.
- Typical measurements are illustrated in FIGURE 8–33.

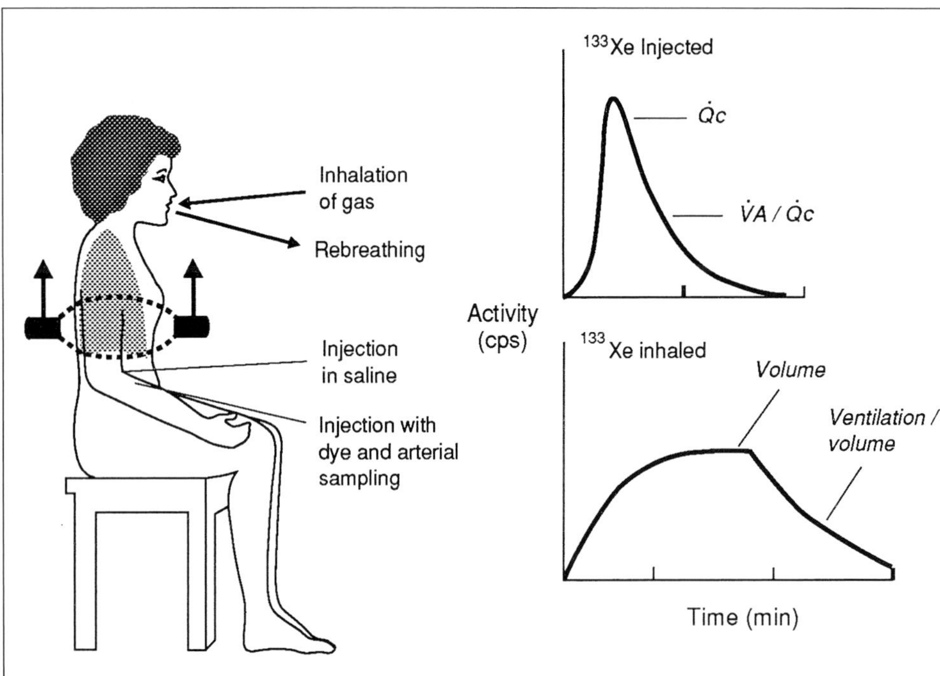

FIGURE 8–33

Assessment of regional lung function using ^{133}Xe. *Top tracing.* After injection, the initial peak reflects the regional blood flow Q̇c; the isotope then passes into the gas phase, in which the clearance during normal breathing reflects the ventilation of lung tissue that is perfused. A slow washout indicates a low ventilation/perfusion ratio (V̇A/Q̇c). *Bottom tracing,* During rebreathing, the plateau count rate when mixing is complete reflects the volume of lung gas in the field of counting. The slopes of the washin and washout curves indicate the ventilation per unit volume. (Modified after Cotes JE: Lung Function. 4th ed. Oxford, Blackwell Scientific Publications, 1979.)

Perfusion

Radioactive Xenon

- Following intravenous injection, peak activity reflects appearance of the isotope distributed in proportion to pulmonary blood flow; because of its low blood gas partition coefficient, about 85% of the isotope passes into the alveolar gas, where it remains as long as the subject holds his or her breath. On resumption of breathing, distribution reflects ventilation of perfused tissue.
- Slow clearance implies units with a relatively low ventilation-perfusion (V̇A/Q̇c) ratio.
- Because of the overlap of many units (at least 10^7) with a single counting field, functional definition of V̇A/Q̇c ratio in this manner is more closely related to pulmonary gas exchange than a V̇A/Q̇c ratio obtained by dividing a measurement of regional ventilation by a separate measurement of regional perfusion.

VENTILATION-PERFUSION RELATIONSHIPS

METHODS OF MEASUREMENT

Using Insoluble Gases

Variations in Protocol

- The lower quadrant of FIGURE 8–33 shows a wash-in of ^{133}Xe in a closed circuit followed by a washout.
  - The equilibration plateau is evidence that the isotope concentration is the same in all alveoli.
  - Local count rates then reflect the volume of alveolar gas in the counting fields.
  - Perfusion per unit volume is obtained by dividing the peak counts for any region by the counts at equilibrium after intravenous injection.
- Both measurements should be made at the same lung volume, so that geometric factors in the chest wall and differences in detector sensitivity do not influence the results.
- If several vital capacity breaths are taken at the beginning of the test, healthy subjects reach equilibration after rebreathing for 1 to 2 minutes or less. Patients with airway obstruction may not reach full equilibration in 20 minutes because isotope is accumulated in the blood and chest wall; rebreathing may then be terminated at 4 minutes.
- Ventilation per unit of lung volume may be obtained from the initial slope or half-life ($t_{1/2}$) of the wash-in or washout of ^{133}Xe (FIGURE 8–33). Beyond the $t_{1/2}$ the washout curve cannot be interpreted because of activity in the chest wall and in the recirculating blood.
- Ventilation per unit of lung volume may also be obtained from the activity during a breath held subsequent to taking in a tidal volume of ^{133}Xe; activity is divided by the plateau level at the same lung volume.

^{133}Xe Bolus

- Alternatively, a bolus of ^{133}Xe may be injected close to the mouthpiece just before the start of inhalation, which is then continued until full inflation. Under these circumstances, the bolus is distributed in a pattern reflecting the early phase of inspiration starting at end-expiration.
- Because ventilation tends to be sequential, it is preferable to label the whole tidal breath. A bolus given at the beginning of inspiration after a maximal exhalation to residual volume is distributed preferentially to the lung apex and is the basis for measuring closing volume (see previous discussion of distribution of ventilation).
- An inspiratory capacity breath of ^{133}Xe reflects regional compliance, not regional ventilation, and measures the regional inspiratory capacity; thus, it is possible to use the gas dilution principle to calculate regional inspiratory capacity or regional vital capacity using a variety of radioisotopes.[247, 250]

Using Microspheres and Microaggregates

- The most widely used radioisotope study of the lung is the perfusion scan following intravenous injection of human serum albumin microspheres or microaggregates labeled with technetium-99m (^{99m}Tc).[251]
- Particles are 20 to 50 μm in diameter and lodge in small pulmonary vessels in proportion to local perfusion: Regional perfusion is measured, not perfusion per unit volume, so the volume of lung in the counting field will influence the measurement.
- Calculations suggest that from 1 mg of protein, particles of 500-, 100-, and 30-μm diameter will obstruct, respectively, 0.12%, 0.31%, and 0.26% of the vascular bed.[252]
- On this basis, injection is potentially hazardous in patients with severe pulmonary vascular disease, and deaths in this situation have been recorded; however, with reasonable precautions, the risk is minimal.[253]
- Passage of particles into systemic circulation through right-to-left intrapulmonary or intracardiac shunts appears not to be accompanied by side effects.
- Radiation dose from most pulmonary isotopic procedures is low and confined primarily to the lungs, being about 0.2 to 0.4 rads (the annual permitted dose is 5 rads).

VENTILATION-PERFUSION RELATIONSHIPS

METHODS OF MEASUREMENT

Multiple Inert Gas Method (Wagner)

Distribution of Ventilation of Perfusion Ratios

- Distribution of perfusion in relation to ventilation of the lung may be analyzed on the basis of a region or lobe or for the lung as a whole and expressed in terms of physiologic shunt, physiologic dead space, and other compartments, or as ventilation-perfusion ratios.
- In an approach developed by Wagner and associates,[254] the lung is assumed to consist of a large number of homogeneous compartments in parallel, each with its own ventilation, blood flow, and appropriate gas concentrations.
- Distribution of ventilation-perfusion ratios is evaluated with six inert gases of different solubility dissolved in saline and infused intravenously and concurrently at a constant rate.
- Under these circumstances in the steady state, the amount of any gas exchanging between alveoli and pulmonary capillary blood is identical to that exchanging between alveoli and atmosphere.
- For each compartment, the quantity of gas is a function of the ventilation-perfusion ratio and the blood gas partition coefficient for the gas in question, expressed as a fraction of that in the mixed venous blood. This may be expressed in the form:

$$\frac{P_A}{P_{\bar{v}}} = \frac{Pc'}{P_{\bar{v}}} = \frac{\lambda}{\lambda + \dot{V}_A/\dot{Q}c}$$

where the three partial pressure terms refer to alveolar gas (P_A), mixed venous blood ($P_{\bar{v}}$), and blood leaving alveolar capillaries (Pc'), λ is the blood gas partition coefficient of the inert gas in question, and $\dot{V}_A/\dot{Q}c$ is the ventilation-perfusion ratio for the particular compartment.

- For the lung as a whole, the mixed arterial concentration is a blood-flow-weighted mean of the values for several compartments, whereas the mean expired level is similarly a ventilation-weighted mean of the compartmental values.
- These parameters are measured directly together with the cardiac output and the minute volume of ventilation; they are used to calculate the corresponding mixed venous and alveolar concentrations and then a distribution of ventilation-perfusion ratios that is compatible with the arterial and alveolar concentrations of all gases concurrently (FIGURES 8–34 and 8–35).

Limitations

- The limitations of the method include the limited accuracy of current chromatographic techniques for gas analysis.
- In addition, it does not provide a unique solution, because the same arterial and alveolar gas concentrations could result from other distributions of ventilation and perfusion in the lung.
- However, these limitations are no greater than for other methods that attempt to describe in simple terms the complex gas-exchanging function of the lung.
- Wagner and colleagues have also reported a modification of the multiple inert gas method that permits estimation of the levels of inert gases in peripheral venous blood, rather than arterial blood.
- This method is a relatively noninvasive approach to measuring $\dot{V}_A/\dot{Q}c$ inequalities that can also be repeated frequently and may prove to be of considerable clinical interest.[255] (See Chapter 5, Nuclear Medicine Techniques and Applications.)

VENTILATION-PERFUSION RELATIONSHIP

METHODS OF MEASUREMENT

FIGURE 8–34

Lower panel, Continuous distribution of ventilation/perfusion ratios as found in a semirecumbent young (22-year-old) normal subject by means of the inert gas elimination method. Note the narrow dispersion and the absence of shunt. Dashed line = ventilation; solid line = blood flow. *Upper panel,* The retention (arterial/venous, solid line) and excretion (expired/venous, dashed line) data points together with the curves for a homogeneous lung. (Modified after West JB: Ventilation/Blood Flow and Gas Exchange. 3rd ed. Oxford, Blackwell Scientific Publications, 1977.)

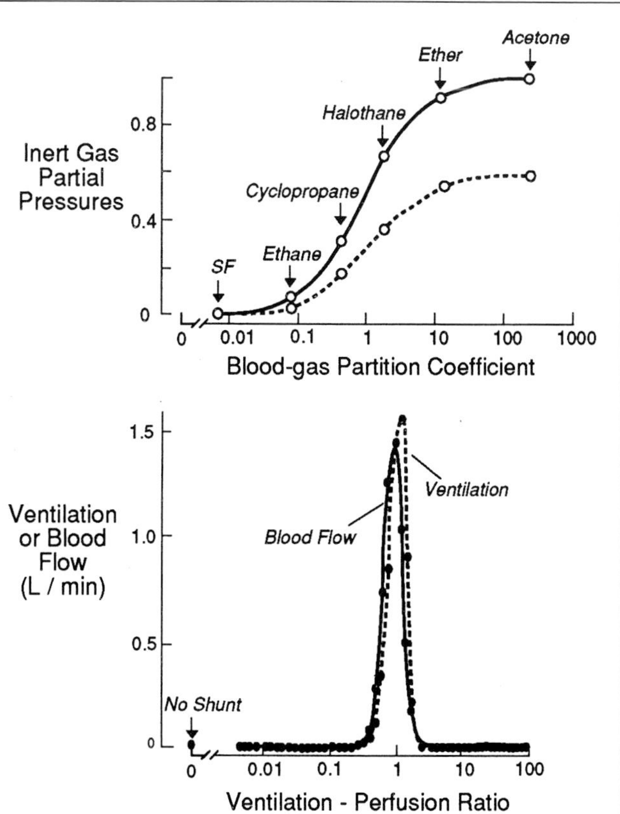

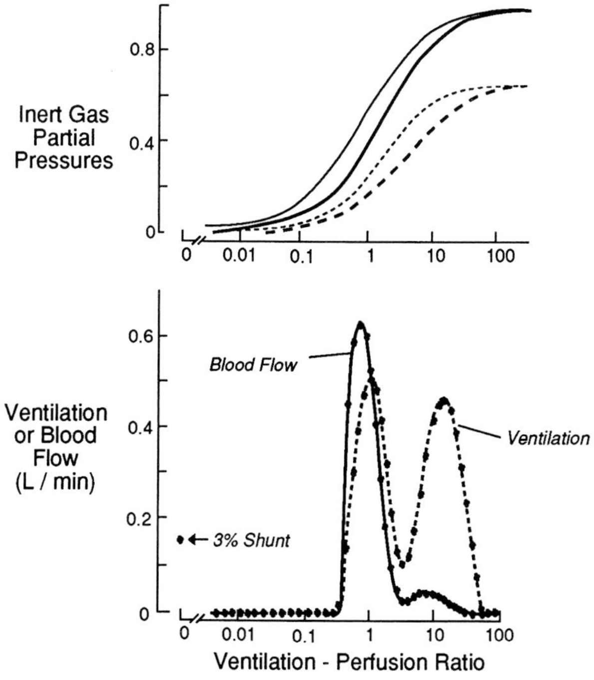

FIGURE 8–35

Lower panel, Continuous distribution of ventilation/perfusion ratios in a 60-year-old patient with chronic airway obstruction, predominately emphysema (dashed line = ventilation; solid line = blood flow). Note the broad bimodal distribution with the large amount of ventilation going to lung units with very high ventilation/perfusion ratios. *Upper panel,* Retention and excretion-solubility curves. (heavy lines = patient; fine lines = data from normal subject). (Modified after West JB: Ventilation/Blood Flow and Gas Exchange. 3rd ed. Oxford, Blackwell Scientific Publications, 1977.)

ARTERIAL BLOOD GASES

INVASIVE MEASUREMENTS

pH Measurement

• The pH of blood is now measured almost entirely by the use of the pH electrode (FIGURE 8–36) in which an electrical potential difference exists across a special type of glass membrane placed between solutions of different pH; by maintaining one side of the membrane at a known pH with a buffer solution (pH = 6.84), the pH of the solution placed on the other side of the membrane can be calculated from the potential difference generated, using the Nernst equation.

• The modern pH electrode is made up of two cells: the measurement half-cell consists of a fine capillary tube of pH-sensitive glass separating the introduced sample (as little as 25 μL) from the buffered solution, and a silver/silver chloride electrode to conduct the generated potential difference to the electronic circuitry. The reference half-cell usually contains a calomel (mercury/mercurous chloride) electrode in an electrolyte solution to provide a constant reference voltage and is connected to the measurement half-cell by a contact bridge to complete the circuit. These two cells are together enclosed in a sealed jacket and are maintained at a constant temperature (FIGURE 8–36).

• The potential difference generated across the glass membrane is a linear function of the pH.
  • Thus, the electrode is usually calibrated with two buffered solutions of known pH that span a significant portion of the range expected in the samples to be measured.
  • The normal range for arterial pH at sea level is 7.35 to 7.45 units.[256]
  • Deviations from this range can be interpreted only by also examining the PCO_2, using the Henderson-Hasselbalch equation, to infer whether the deviation in pH is due primarily to a metabolic or respiratory cause and whether it is due to an acute or chronic disturbance.

$$pH = 6.10 + \frac{\log (HCO_3^-)}{0.03 \times PCO_2}$$

Accuracy and Precision

• Accuracy depends on the integrity of the differential permeability of the glass membrane to hydrogen ions.
  • Permeability may be altered by the deposition of protein or by the development of cracks on the membrane surface.
  • Proper quality control requires that pH calibration be checked at one point before each series of pH determinations and at two major points every 4 hours.
  • A number of different standard phosphate buffer solutions are suitable for routine calibrations and are available commercially.
  • Protein contamination of the membrane can be minimized by flushing the electrode with a cleaning solution at regular intervals (every ten samples) and by taking care to follow injections of blood with injections of saline rather than distilled water.

• Precision of measurements of a single sample by the same instrument fall within a narrow range of ± 0.02 unit (± 2 SD),[256] and there generally is good agreement among the values obtained on unknown samples by the different instruments used by laboratories enrolled in quality control programs (SD = 0.014 pH unit obtained in more than 800 laboratories).[257]

FIGURE 8–36

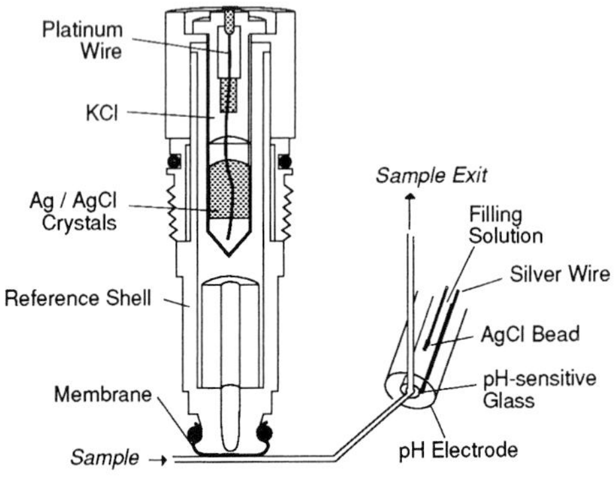

pH electrode. There are two cells, the measurement half-cell consists of a fine capillary tube of pH-sensitive glass separating the introduced sample of 25 μL from the buffered solution, and a silver/silver chloride electrode to conduct the generated potential difference to the electronic circuitry. The reference half-cell usually contains a calomel (mercury/mercurous chloride) electrode in an electrolyte solution to provide a constant reference voltage and is connected to the measurement half-cell by a contact bridge to complete the circuit. Both cells are enclosed in a sealed jacket and maintained at a constant temperature. (From Murray JF, Nadel JA (eds): Textbook of Respiratory Medicine. 3rd ed. Philadelphia, WB Saunders, 2000, p. 831.)

ARTERIAL BLOOD GASES

INVASIVE MEASUREMENTS

PCO_2 Measurement

- Early chemical methods for measuring gas concentrations in blood were laborious and demanding, involved liberating chemically bound O_2 and CO_2 in blood by adding chemical agents to a sample kept in a closed vessel.[258]
- The breakthrough in measurements of CO_2 came with the development of the membrane-covered CO_2 electrode (FIGURE 8–37).
- This device exploits the principles of the pH electrode and the known relationship between PCO_2 and pH in a buffered solution. The sample to be analyzed is separated from a buffer solution by a membrane permeable to CO_2.
- CO_2 molecules that diffuse through the membrane alter the concentration of carbonic acid, and therefore the concentration of hydrogen ion (H^+) in the buffered solution:

$$CO_2 + H_2O \leftrightarrow H_2CO_3 \leftrightarrow H^+ + HCO_3^-$$

A pH meter reads the resulting change in pH with the output scaled in terms of PCO_2.

- Response time of the CO_2 electrode depends on
  - The concentration and volume of buffered solution
  - The diffusion properties of the artificial membrane
  - The thickness of a second "stabilizing membrane" placed over the pH-sensitive glass
- With silicone-rubber membranes, the 95% response time has been reduced to as little as 10 seconds (FIGURE 8–37).

Accuracy and Precision

- Because it incorporates a pH electrode in its design, the PCO_2 electrode also has the advantages of precision and dependability, if calibrated regularly.
- A one-point calibration should be checked before each series of blood gas measurements, and two-point calibrations should be checked every 4 to 8 hours, or whenever the one-point calibration indicates the need for readjustment of more than 2 mm Hg PCO_2.
- The range of repeated measurements of samples of blood tonometered to PCO_2 of 20 to 60 mm Hg is ± 3.0 mm Hg,[256] and tests with commercially available, sealed buffer solutions with different PCO_2 values show similar reproducibility with a variety of different blood gas measuring devices.
- Normal range of values for PCO_2 varies with altitude. At sea level, it ranges from 36 to 44 mm Hg[256]; in Salt Lake City, Utah (elevation 1340 to 1520 m), the range is reported to be 30 to 40 mm Hg.[259]

FIGURE 8–37

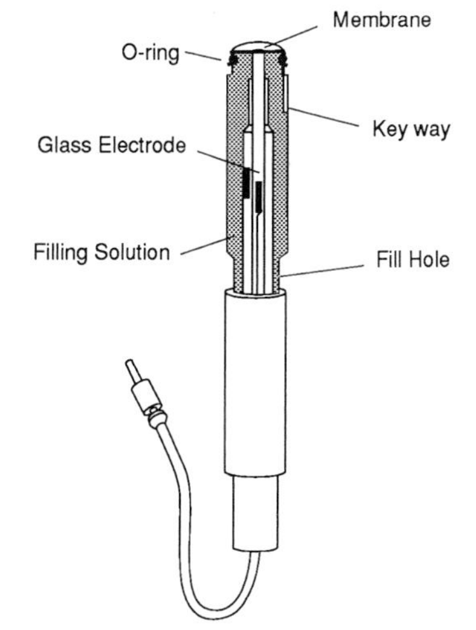

CO_2 electrode. This electrode uses the combination of the relationship between PCO_2 and pH in a buffered solution and the pH electrode. The sample is separated from a buffer solution by a membrane permeable to CO_2 permitting the CO_2 molecules to diffuse through the membrane, alter the concentration of carbonic acid and therefore the hydrogen ion concentration in the buffered solution. The change in pH is read by a pH meter with output scaled in terms of PCO_2. (From Murray JF, Nadel JA (eds): Textbook of Respiratory Medicine. 3rd ed. Philadelphia, WB Saunders, 2000, p. 832.)

ARTERIAL BLOOD GASES

INVASIVE MEASUREMENTS

Po_2 Measurement

- Development of an accurate, stable electrode has almost entirely supplanted the use of older chemical methods for measuring total blood O_2 content and then back-calculating Po_2.
- The principle of the O_2 electrode differs from that of the pH and Po_2 electrodes in that the O_2 electrode measures a current generated by the presence of the relevant molecule, rather than a potential difference.
- The device consists of platinum and silver electrodes placed in potassium chloride solutions, a polarizing voltage of 0.5 to 0.6 volt, and an electrolyte bridge to complete the circuit.
  - Oxidation takes place at the silver electrode, where silver reacts with chloride ions to form silver chloride.
  - This reaction produces electrons, which are consumed by the reduction of O_2 at the platinum electrode.
  - Electron flow (current) is thus proportional to the concentration of O_2 at the platinum electrode (FIGURE 8–38).
- Development of a useful electrode from this principle was achieved by Clark.[260] Important features of the Clark electrode are minimization of O_2 consumption by the use of a thin platinum electrode and the ensurance of a constant diffusion distance between the surface of the electrode and the sample by covering the electrode with an O_2-permeable membrane.
- The surface area of the platinum electrode and the permeability of the membrane to O_2 determines sensitivity and response times of the electrode.
- The larger the electrode and the more permeable the membrane, however, the more rapidly O_2 is consumed, causing Po_2 to fall in small samples as the measurement is made. For most available devices, the compromises made result in a 95% response time of about 50 seconds.

Practical Problems

- Slightly different currents are generated when gases and liquids at the same Po_2 are introduced in the oxygen electrode. The magnitude of the difference is usually about 3% to 4% but depends on electrode diameter, the nature and thickness of the membrane, and the flow of the sample around the electrode.
- A correction factor is sometimes introduced into calculation of arterial Po_2 when gases are used for calibration. These factors, however, may not be related linearly to Po_2, resulting in errors when high O_2 pressures are measured, as in samples obtained from a patient to whom pure O_2 is given to estimate the magnitude of a right-to-left shunt.
- The simplest approach would seem to be to calibrate the electrode with solutions, rather than gases. This is probably true, but large differences have been found for the same machine using samples of different test solutions tonometered to the same Po_2.[261] In general, the more the O_2-carrying capacity of the solution approximates that of blood, the smaller the error.
- Thus, the large interinstrument variability of O_2 pressure values reported for blind samples tested in a quality-control program may not reflect the variability that would be achieved if all tests were run with tonometered blood.[262]
- For a single machine, the range of repeated measurements of Po_2 in blood is 3.0 mm Hg for Po_2 values ranging from 20 to 150 mm Hg.[256]
- In normal seated adult subjects, the predicted Po_2 can be obtained from Mellemgaard's data[242] with an SD around the regression line of approximately 6.0 mm Hg:

$$Po_2 = 104.2 - 0.27 \times \text{age (in years)}$$

A final problem for some highly automated blood gas machines appears only when samples of very high or very low Po_2 are tested.

- This problem is due to the error introduced by "contamination" of the sample chamber by the rinsing fluid.[262]
- If the Po_2 of the rinsing fluid is similar to that of room air, then the persistence of a small amount of fluid will not much alter the Po_2 measured for blood samples with O_2 at 60 and 100 mm Hg, but it will affect the values recorded for samples with O_2 pressures at either extreme.
- If the design of the machine permits, this source of error can be reduced by flushing the sample chamber with a fluid with Po_2 near the estimated value of the sample or by introducing consecutive specimens without flushing the chamber.

ARTERIAL BLOOD GASES

INVASIVE MEASUREMENTS

Po_2 Measurement

FIGURE 8-38

O_2 electrode. This electrode consists of platinum and silver electrodes placed in potassium chloride solutions, a polarizing voltage of 0.5 to 0.6 volt, and an electrolyte bridge to complete the circuit. Oxidation at the silver electrode is secondary to silver reacting with chloride ions to form silver chloride to produce electrons that are consumed at the platinum electrode by reduction of oxygen. The flow of electrons (current) is thus proportional to the concentration of oxygen at the platinum electrode. (From Murray JF, Nadel JA (eds): Textbook of Respiratory Medicine, 3rd ed. Philadelphia, WB Saunders, 2000, p. 832.)

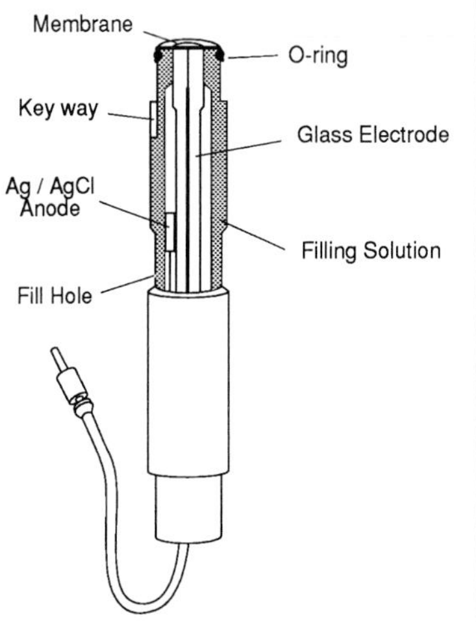

O_2 Content

Accuracy and Precision

- O_2 content, the sum of the O_2 bound to hemoglobin and of the O_2 dissolved in plasma, can be measured directly by chemical or galvanic cell methods and can be estimated from the Po_2, the total hemoglobin concentration, and the percentage of oxyhemoglobin.
- The O_2 content is required for calculating cardiac output by the Fick equation and for estimating the "shunt equivalent" in hypoxemic patients.
- Van Slyke method: ferricyanide liberates chemically bound O_2 and CO_2 from blood, and the total quantity of displaced gas is measured before and then after absorbing the CO_2 with sodium hydroxide. This has been the reference method for many years, but now is used infrequently because of its demands on time and technical skill.[263]
- Galvanic call method: O_2 is chemically liberated from blood and transferred to a fuel cell, where a current is generated in proportion to the amount delivered. The accuracy and precision are similar to those obtained by the Van Slyke method.[264]
- The most commonly used current method measures total hemoglobin by the cyanmethemoglobin method,[265] percentage of oxyhemoglobin by a spectrophotometric method, and dissolved O_2 as the product of Pao_2 and oxygen's solubility coefficient (0.003 mL/100 mL blood).

ARTERIAL BLOOD GASES

INVASIVE MEASUREMENTS

Spectrophotometry

- Spectrophotometry is based on the discovery that different wavelengths of light are differentially absorbed by different substances.
- In the absence of other materials that absorb light at the same wavelength, the concentration of a substance in a solution is proportional to the amount of light absorbed.
- Various forms of hemoglobin (oxy-, reduced, carboxy-, sulf-, and methemoglobin) have characteristic spectra of light absorption.
- Three-wavelength instruments can simultaneously measure oxyhemoglobin and carboxyhemoglobin; a four-wavelength instrument permits measurement of methemoglobin.[256]
- Measurement of carboxyhemoglobin permits quantifying correctly the proportion of nonreduced hemoglobin actually available for carrying O_2, but also in identifying a cause of a shift in the position of the O_2-hemoglobin dissociation curve.
  - Carboxyhemoglobin increases the affinity for O_2 of adjacent hemoglobin molecules, shifting the curve to the left; thus, less oxygen is unloaded from oxyhemoglobin at normal tissue P_{O_2}.
  - Similar disorders result from inherited abnormalities in hemoglobin structure, e.g., Chesapeake—50% desaturation does not occur until the P_{O_2} is lowered to 19 mm Hg, as opposed to the normal 50% unloading point of 27 mm Hg.

P_{50} Oxygen

- P_{50} requires measuring hemoglobin saturation after the blood sample is tonometered at three O_2 pressures spanning the expected range (P_{O_2} values from 20 to 35 mm Hg would be typical).[256]
- Measurement of P_{50} is rarely needed in clinical practice, however, and with the important exception of conditions in which carboxyhemoglobin is likely to be present in appreciable quantities (as in victims of fires or of exposure to closed-space combustion, and heavy cigarette and cigar smokers), the estimation of blood O_2 content from measurements of Pa_{O2} and hemoglobin concentration will usually provide sufficient information for decisions about clinical management.

Technical Issues

- It is important to avoid contamination with room air or an excessive amount of anticoagulant when the sample is obtained, and to prevent leakage, diffusion, or consumption of gases while the sample is being transported and stored.
- Samples should be obtained with minimal discomfort and hazard.
- Samples are best obtained with a sterile glass syringe with a close-fitting plunger and a small (23- to 25-gauge) needle.
- The quantity of heparin left in the barrel and needle hub after the syringe is flushed and rinsed with a 1000 U/mL solution is adequate for anticoagulation of samples up to 5 mL and will not alter pH or P_{CO_2} significantly in samples as small as 1 mL.

ARTERIAL BLOOD GASES

INVASIVE MEASUREMENTS

Choice of Sites

- *Adults:* The radial artery is preferable for blood samples because of the adequacy of collateral flow in the event of occlusion of the sampled artery. In elderly patients, however, and in patients with arteriosclerotic vascular disease, the adequacy of ulnar flow should be confirmed by the Allen test (appearance of palmar flush when the ulnar artery alone is decompressed).[266]
- *Infants:* The temporal or umbilical artery is preferred for samples. If radial and femoral arterial cannulation cannot be accomplished, then the brachial, axillary, or dorsalis pedis artery should be considered.
- Brachial artery:
  - Physicians have been mistakenly advised to avoid percutaneous cannulation of the brachial artery because of a lack of collateral vessels and the anatomic proximity to the median nerve.
  - Aneurysm formation, thrombosis with loss of radial arterial pulse, and permanent median nerve neuropathy caused by hematoma have all been reported as complications of brachial cannulation.
  - Literature associated with left-sided heart catheterization states that percutaneous cannulation of the brachial artery is as "safe and effective" as surgical cutdown and arteriotomy.[267, 268]

NONINVASIVE MEASUREMENTS

Arterialized Samples

- An alternative to arterial puncture is to obtain a sample of "arterialized" capillary or venous blood.
- This method is based on the assumption that the vasodilatation produced by heat or by application of vasodilator cream to a region with low metabolic activity will result in delivery of such an excess of arterial blood that local metabolism causes only small changes in P_{O_2}, P_{CO_2}, and pH so that analysis of capillary or venous blood will give close estimates of arterial values.
- The most common sites are the earlobe in adults and children, and the lateral margin of the foot in infants; for sampling of arterialized venous blood, a dorsal hand vein is most commonly used.
- From any of these sites, the values obtained should correlate well with arterial pH and P_{CO_2}.[269]
- The values for P_{O_2} are also accurate, except in patients with arterial hypotension or local reductions in flow to the sample site (as may occur with the vasoconstrictive response to severe hypoxemia), in newborns, and in patients with high arterial P_{O_2} (i.e., breathing oxygen-enriched gas mixtures).
- Once the sample is obtained, it should be analyzed promptly or placed on ice to minimize the effects of continued cell metabolism on O_2 consumption.
- This care is especially important for samples with very high white blood cell or platelet counts and in samples with P_{O_2} values greater than 100 mm Hg.[270]
- However the sample is obtained, clinical interpretation of blood gas values is possible only if the condition of the patient at the time of sampling is noted.
  - Most important is description of the O_2 pressure of the inspired gas mixture, but position, activity level, habitus, diet, and other factors can also influence arterial blood gas values.
  - Clearly, an excited or frightened patient may hyperventilate or breath-hold during arterial puncture, but apprehension does not routinely cause a change in alveolar ventilation.[271]

ARTERIAL BLOOD GASES

NONINVASIVE MEASUREMENTS

Oximetry

- The principles of spectrophotometry can be applied to transcutaneous measurement of O_2 saturation in capillary blood by measuring the quantities of light at different wavelengths transmitted through or reflected from the earlobe.
- With dilation of local arterial vessels through application of heat or a vasodilating chemical (e.g., nicotine, alcohol), capillary O_2 saturation should approximate arterial oxygen saturation.
- Early ear oximeters were reported to give accurate data but were not accepted widely because of the practical difficulties in operating cumbersome instruments that were hard to calibrate, sensitive to changes in position, and likely to give unpredictable, unstable values.[271]

Beer's Law

- Amount of light absorbed by a solute in solution is related to the concentration of the unknown solute.

$$\text{Log}\,\frac{I_{IN}}{I_{TR}} = C_A \times d \times \epsilon_A$$

where
I_{IN} = quantity of incident light
d = distance through which light passes
C_A = concentration of the solute (e.g., hemoglobin)
ϵ_A = absorption coefficient
I_{TR} = amount of light transmitted through A, the substance containing the solute.

- When light passes through tissue from the oximeter, most of the light is absorbed by the tissues.
- Amount of light absorbed does not vary with the cardiac cycle.
- During the cardiac cycle, however, a small increase in arterial blood causes an increase in absorption of light.
- By comparing absorption at the peak and trough of the arterial pulse, the nonarterial sources of absorption become irrelevant (FIGURE 8–39).

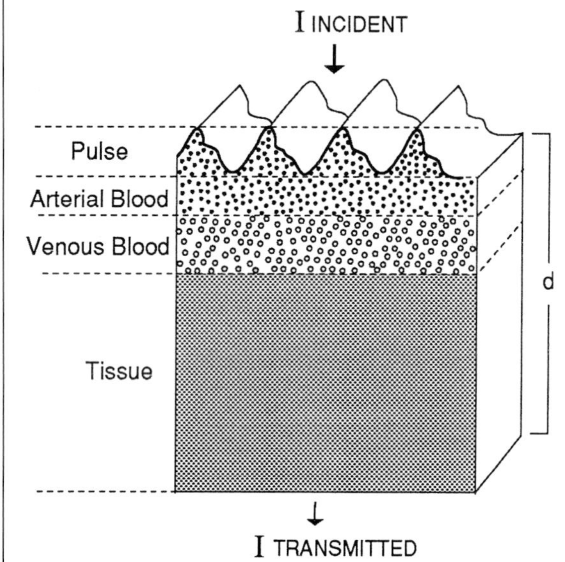

FIGURE 8–39

Factors influencing detection by pulse oximetry of light absorption through a pulsatile vascular bed. (IINCIDENT = incident light, ITRANSMITTED = transmitted light, d = distance through tissue that absorbs incident light.) Stippled zone represents absorption by tissue. Open circles represent light absorption by venous blood. Solid circles represent light absorption by arterial blood and by the pulse of arterial blood. (From Murray JF, Nadel JA (eds): Textbook of Respiratory Medicine. 3rd ed. Philadelphia, WB Saunders, 2000, p. 835.)

ARTERIAL BLOOD GASES

NONINVASIVE MEASUREMENTS

Oximetry Probes

- Probe has two light-emitting diodes that emit light at specific wavelengths, usually 660 nm and 940 nm (FIGURE 8–40).
- At these wavelengths, the light absorption by oxyhemoglobin and reduced hemoglobin are markedly different.
- A photodetector is placed across a vascular bed (finger, nose, earlobe) from the light source.
- When the ratios (R) of pulsatile and baseline light absorption are compared at these two wavelengths, the ratio of oxyhemoglobin to reduced hemoglobin may be calculated.

$$R = \frac{\text{Pulsatile absorbance (660)/Baseline absorbance (660)}}{\text{Pusatile absorbance (940)/Baseline absorbance (940)}}$$

The relationship between R and O_2 saturation was determined experimentally because there is no known function relating these two variables.

- A calibration curve was created by having healthy subjects with previously measured amounts of methemoglobin and carboxyhemoglobin breathe different hypoxic gas mixtures designed to produce O_2 saturations between 70% and 100%.[272]
- An arterial blood sample was obtained with each gas mixture, O_2 saturation was measured using a CO oximeter (spectrophotometric hemoximeter), and the R value measured by the pulse oximeter were compared.

- By using only two wavelengths, the pulse oximeter can measure only two substances, so it determines "functional saturation."

$$\text{Functional saturation} = \frac{\text{oxyhemoglobin}}{\text{oxyhemoglobin + reduced hemoglobin}}$$

Pulse oximeters are accurate when O_2 saturation is between 70% and 100%,[273, 274] but may be inaccurate below that range.

- These devices may be misleading in the presence of abnormal hemoglobins (methemoglobin, carboxyhemoglobin, fetal hemoglobin), dyes (methylene blue, indocyanine green), increased bilirubin, low perfusion states, anemia, increased venous pulsations, and external light sources.[275]

FIGURE 8–40

Absorption spectrum of reduced hemoglobin (Hb) and oxyhemoglobin (HbO_2). Readings are made at 660 nm (red) and 940 nm (infrared) wavelengths. (From Murray JF, Nadel JA (eds): Textbook of Respiratory Medicine. 3rd ed. Philadelphia, WB Saunders, 2000, p. 835.)

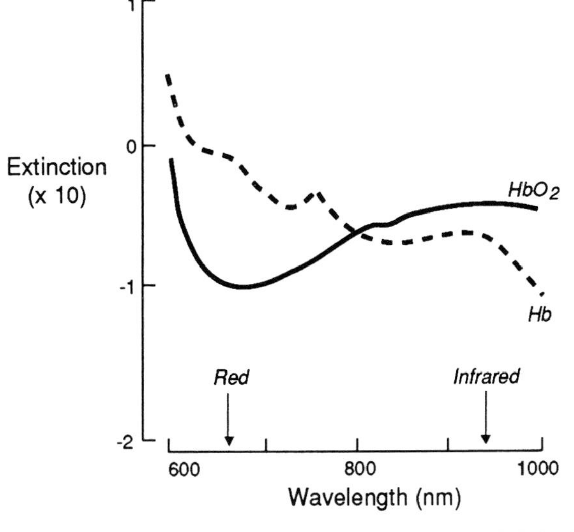

ARTERIAL BLOOD GASES

NONINVASIVE MEASUREMENTS

Clinical Applications of Oximetry

- Continuous monitoring of O_2 saturation is the standard of care in operating rooms and recovery rooms.[276]
- It is also used widely in intensive care units, and during cardiac catheterization or when detecting hypoxemia is important (e.g., in patients with respiratory failure, during sleep studies, during bronchoscopy, at different levels of exercise, after delivery of supplemental O_2).
- The flattened shape of the upper portion of the O_2-hemoglobin dissociation curve means that large changes in PO_2 result in small changes in arterial O_2 saturation.
- Oximetry is insensitive to changes in PO_2 from the normal range that have diagnostic and clinical significance even if they do not result in an important decrease in O_2 delivery.
- Actual 95% confidence limits of ±5% for arterial oxygen saturation have been reported for oximetry and make this limitation all the more important.
- Availability of oximetry did not wholly diminish the interest in transcutaneous measurement of PO_2.

Trancutaneous Oxygen Electrode

- The basic idea behind this method is that a small polarographic electrode can measure the O_2 pressure in a bubble of gas trapped over the skin.
- Because the PO_2 at the surface of unwarmed skin is near zero, the success of the transcutaneous O_2 electrode depends on producing enough local vasodilatation to compensate for the arterial-capillary gradient and also for the further loss of O_2 due to skin metabolism and to imperfect diffusion of oxygen through the skin layer.
- This degree of vasodilatation is achieved by warming the skin to 42°C.
- The increase in temperature causes local vasodilatation and displaces the O_2 hemoglobin dissociation curve to the right so that O_2 pressure is increased for any blood O_2 pressure, partially correcting for the losses of O_2 between the arterioles and the skin surface.
- The skin surface electrode was developed by Huch and associates[277] in 1973 and has proved accurate in continuous measurement of transcutaneous PO_2 ($tcPO_2$) in both healthy and sick newborns.
- $tcPO_2$ most severely underestimates arterial PO_2 when skin perfusion is decreased from hypotension and in infants treated with tolazoline for pulmonary hypertension, possibly because the general peripheral vasodilatation caused by the drug overcame the preferential local vasodilatation intended from local heating of the skin.
- Transcutaneous oxygen electrode measurements are used widely for regulating O_2 therapy or ventilatory assistance to infants with neonatal respiratory distress syndrome, for monitoring apnea, for sleep studies, or for analyzing the impact of nursery procedures on oxygenation.
- This method is not so well accepted for estimating PO_2 in adults, in whom the greater thickness of skin impairs O_2 diffusion, although it appears reliable for measuring the direction of change in PaO_2 in adult patients performing exercise.[278–283]

ARTERIAL BLOOD GASES

NONINVASIVE MEASUREMENTS

Capnography

- Measurement of CO_2 during the respiratory cycle is called capnometry, and the display of the analog waveform is called a capnogram (FIGURE 8–41).
- This measurement is made using an infrared spectrometer, which is widely available.
- The spectrometer must be calibrated regularly, and interference by nitrous oxide, acetylene, and CO must be avoided.[284, 285]
- Mass spectrometers can measure all the respiratory gases (CO_2, O_2, and N_2) as well as many anesthetic gases. The procedure is very rapid, but very expensive. It is used most commonly in pulmonary and exercise laboratories and operating rooms.

FIGURE 8–41

Normal capnogram. During inspiration, P_{CO_2} is zero. At the start of exhalation, P_{CO_2} remains zero as gas from the anatomic dead space leaves the airway (comparable to phase I in the single-breath N_2 distribution test). Then, P_{CO_2} rises rapidly as alveolar gas mixes with gas from the dead space (comparable to phase II in the single-breath N_2 distribution test), and then P_{CO_2} levels stabilize as gas from the dead space decreases and all the gas comes from alveoli containing CO_2. The P_{CO_2} at the end of the "alveolar plateau" is called the end-tidal P_{CO_2} (comparable to phase III in the single-breath N_2 distribution test). (From Murray JF, Nadel JA (eds): Textbook of Respiratory Medicine. 3rd ed. Philadelphia, WB Saunders, 2000, p. 836.)

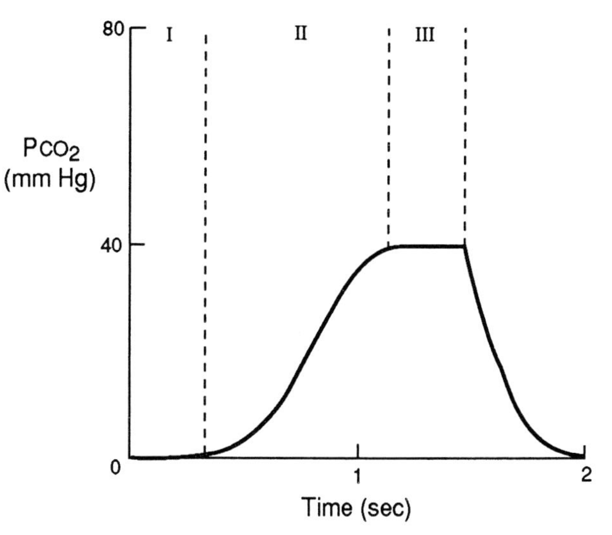

Applications of Capnography

- The end-tidal CO_2 may be misleading when dead space is increased (increased anatomic dead space, dead space added in series to the airway of the patient, or the respiratory rate is abnormally increased).
  - In these situations, there is an increased difference between arterial and end-tidal CO_2 and the end-tidal level does not plateau.
- When wasted ventilation is increased because of regional increased ventilation relative to perfusion (e.g., restrictive or obstructive ventilatory defects), parallel dead space, or pulmonary vascular obstruction, arterial–end-tidal CO_2 differences are also increased.
  - In these situations, the alveolar plateau is present but abnormally reduced; the shape of the waveform may be diagnostic of pulmonary vascular obstruction (FIGURE 8–42).

ARTERIAL BLOOD GASES

NONINVASIVE MEASUREMENTS

Applications of Capnography

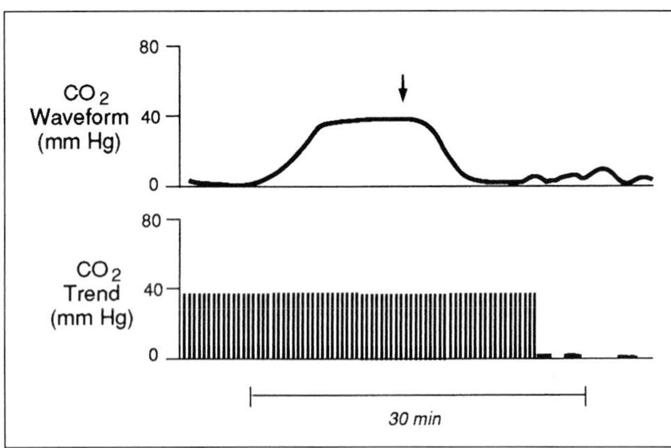

FIGURE 8–42

Abnormal capnogram. A sudden decrease in end-tidal P_{CO_2} suggests a life-threatening situation in which the capnograph no longer detects CO_2 in the exhaled gas. This capnogram suggests the possibility of esophageal intubation, obstructed endotracheal tube, disconnected airway, or ventilator malfunction; these possibilities must be excluded before assuming the capnograph is malfunctioning. (From Murray JF, Nadel JA (eds): Textbook of Respiratory Medicine. 3rd ed. Philadelphia, WB Saunders, 2000, p. 836.)

Single-Breath CO_2 Test

- An abnormal single-breath N_2 washout test (also called single-breath O_2 test) result indicates that ventilation is asynchronous and inhaled gas is distributed nonuniformly.
- An abnormal single-breath CO_2 test result indicates that the lung empties asynchronously and ventilation-perfusion abnormalities are present.
- Exhaled gas is analyzed continuously by a CO_2 analyzer or mass spectrometer; if the CO_2 concentration increases throughout exhalation, different regions of lung must have different CO_2 concentrations at end-inspiration, and the lung must empty asynchronously during exhalation.
- If the CO_2 concentration is constant during exhalation, $\dot{V}_A/\dot{Q}_C$ ratios must be equal, or blood flow may be nonuniform when ventilation is uniform. In the latter condition, even if regional end-inspiratory CO_2 concentrations vary, synchronous exhalation will result in mixing of CO_2 in constant proportions from different regions of lung, yielding a constant exhaled alveolar CO_2 concentration. (Even in this case, arterial P_{CO_2} would exceed mixed alveolar P_{CO_2}.)
- The single-breath CO_2 test result will be abnormal only when the single-breath N_2 washout test is abnormal, but the latter result indicates uneven ventilation only, whereas the abnormal CO_2 test result indicates that there must be uneven perfusion in relation to ventilation.
- This test appears to be sensitive to the presence of ventilation-perfusion abnormalities. Although it is not quantitative, the typical capnogram in these cases should warn the observer of the presence of potentially life-threatening changes in pulmonary perfusion (FIGURE 8–43).
- Schwardt and colleagues analyzed a single-path model of lung airways and demonstrated that cardiac output and pulmonary arterial P_{CO_2} strongly affect the height of phase III of the CO_2 washout curve.[286]

FIGURE 8–43

This abnormal capnogram shows an exponential decrease in end-tidal P_{CO_2}. Note the progressively more sloping alveolar plateau reflecting both abnormal distribution of ventilation, but also uneven perfusion relative to ventilation. This pattern suggests a potential life-threatening situation such as cardiac arrest, severe pulmonary hypoperfusion, or pulmonary embolism. (From Murray JF, Nadel JA (eds): Textbook of Respiratory Medicine. 3rd ed. Philadelphia, WB Saunders, 2000, p. 837.)

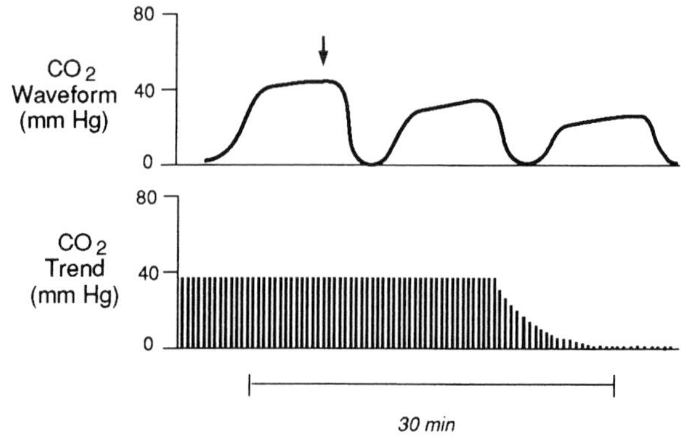

ARTERIAL BLOOD GASES

NONINVASIVE MEASUREMENTS

Colorimetric Methods

- Colorimetric measurement of end-tidal CO_2 is being used in critical care units, recovery rooms, and operating rooms to monitor end-tidal CO_2 instead of capnography or other devices.
- Colorimetry is as accurate and sensitive as capnography.
- Both techniques appear to be useful in the management of critically ill patients:
  - They detect successful tracheal intubation vs. esophageal intubation and in monitoring cardiopulmonary resuscitation.
  - They detect a variety of problems in ventilated patients including obstructed endotracheal tube, disconnected airway, ventilator malfunction, severe pulmonary hypoperfusion, and pulmonary embolism.[287–289]
  - They are used increasingly in ventilated patients to assist in weaning while minimizing repeated arterial punctures. Wasted ventilation is measured and P_{CO_2} is correlated with end-tidal P_{CO_2}; acute rises suggest hypoventilation and prompt further study with blood gas measurements.

Transcutaneous Carbon Dioxide Electrode

- A device for transcutaneous measurement of P_{CO_2} has also been developed and involves trapping gas above the skin layer, measuring CO_2 pressure by photometric analysis with infrared light.[290]
- The device has a long time-constant, and skin preparation requires stripping of the stratum corneum.
- Although the values for tcP_{CO_2} correspond closely to those for Pa_{CO_2} in healthy subjects, erroneous values occur with decreased skin perfusion, edema, and obesity.[281–283, 291]

EXERCISE

PHYSIOLOGIC RESPONSE TO EXERCISE

Energy Production

- The amount of O_2 consumed during exercise depends on the amount of external work done by the exercising muscles.
- Even in patients with disease, mechanical efficiency is about 21%; thus, almost 79% of the calories produced in the muscle are lost as heat.
- Oxidative energy production is derived from (1) lactic acid and anaerobic mechanisms and (2) transfer of molecular O_2 from atmosphere to the exercising muscle.
- Initially, most of the energy comes from internal sources, but subsequently energy production depends upon O_2 delivered from the atmosphere.
  - The fraction obtained from nonatmospheric sources increases with work intensity but decreases with time.
  - Conversion of pyruvate to lactate increases during heavy work.
  - Transfer of molecular O_2 from atmosphere to exercising muscle depends on both circulatory and respiratory systems.
- Thus, circulation and ventilation must be linked to the demands of the exercising muscle.

EXERCISE

PHYSIOLOGIC RESPONSE TO EXERCISE

Cardiovascular Response

- Cardiac output increases in proportion to the severity of exercise, and stroke volume increases during light to moderate exercise with maximum values at about 45% of $\dot{V}O_{2\,max}$; thereafter, cardiac output increases as heart rate increases.
- Blood flow to specific tissues is regulated in proportion to metabolic activity.
- Maximum O_2 uptake is determined by maximum cardiac output and maximum arteriovenous O_2 difference.
- Systolic blood pressure also increases in proportion to O_2 uptake and cardiac output.
- The amount of O_2 extracted per heart beat (O_2 pulse) increases only when work rate increases, suggesting that blood flow distribution depends on work intensity.

Respiratory Response

- Initially, ventilation increases linearly with exercise (FIGURE 8–44).
- Perfusion of the upper region of lung increases markedly with exercise, VD/VT falls to 0.15 to 0.20, and pulmonary perfusion increases without increased pulmonary vascular resistance.
- During heavy exercise when O_2 is no longer transferred in sufficient amounts to meet the needs of the exercising muscle, metabolic acidosis develops, increasing the ventilatory drive.
- Lactic acid increases, bicarbonate decreases, arterial PO_2 rises in response to alveolar hyperventilation, and arterial PCO_2 falls in response to H^+-mediated ventilatory drive that buffers the fall in pH.
- Thus, ventilation increases nonlinearly late in exercise, and there is a delay in establishing a steady state.

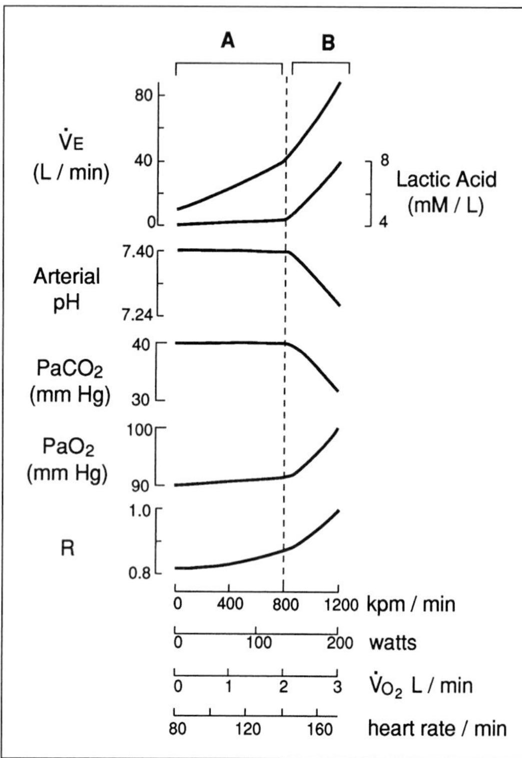

FIGURE 8–44

Schematic of the ventilatory response to exercise. During phase A, ventilation increases linearly with exercise (hyperpnea of muscular exercise) without significant changes in arterial blood gases, pH, or lactic acid. During phase B, molecular O_2 can no longer be supplied in sufficient quantities to the exercising muscle, lactic acidosis develops, pH falls and stimulates ventilation, PCO_2 decreases in response to alveolar hyperventilation and buffers the fall in pH, and PO_2 increases. This ventilatory response is plotted against the corresponding external work rate (kpm/min and watts), O_2 consumption ($\dot{V}O_2$), and heart rate. (From Murray JF, Nadel JA (eds): Textbook of Respiratory Medicine. 3rd ed. Philadelphia, WB Saunders, 2000, p. 839.)

EXERCISE

TYPES OF EXERCISE TESTS

TABLE 8-6

Relationships Between Work Rate and Various Physical Activities

Power		Oxygen Uptake						
KPM/MIN*	WATTS*	L/MIN	MET†	ENERGY (KCAL/MIN‡)	WALKING (MPH)	RUNNING (MPH)	ATHLETIC ACTIVITY	WORK ACTIVITY
300	50	0.9	4–5	5	3.0	—	Golf	Housework, clerical
600	100	1.5	7–8	8	4.5	—	Tennis, dancing	Farming, mining
900	150	2.1	8–10	11	5.0	5.5	Basketball, skiing	Very heavy manual labor
1200	200	2.8	12	14	—	7.0	Squash, cross-country skiing	
1500	250	3.5	14	17	—	8.0	Competition endurance	
1800	300	4.2	16	20	—	10.0	—	
2100	350	5.0	18	24	—	—	—	

**Force* is defined in newtons which is the unit of force acting on 1 kg to accelerate it at 1 m/sec^2. The force of gravity acting on a stationary mass of 1 kg is 9.8 newtons, which equals 1 kilipond. *Work* is the force of 1 newton acting through 1 m, or 1 newton-meter, which equals 1 joule. One kilogram moving through a vertical distance of 1 m against gravity requires 9.8 joules or 1 kilipond-meter (kpm). The actual exercise performed is expressed in terms of power or the work performed by the muscles per unit of time. The unit of power is the joule/sec or watt. Many physiologists prefer to use kilipond-meters per minute as the unit of power. This equals 9.8 divided by 60 watts, or 0.1635 watt. (An easy conversion: 600 kpm/min is about 100 watts). No agreement has been reached regarding which of these two units to use.

† MET = a multiple of resting O_2 consumption equal to 3.5 mL O_2/min/kg.

‡ 1 kcal/min = 427 kpm/min, or 72 watts, which equals 0.2 L O_2/min.

Walk Tests

- Useful clinical evaluation of exercise can be done without sophisticated equipment.
- At a minimum, the subject may be asked to walk up stairs or down a hallway or along a course of predetermined length.
- Data sufficient for analysis may be obtained by observing the subject while walking (respiratory pattern, speaking pattern, pulse rate, distance covered, and time required).
- The 12-minute (or 6-minute) walking distance test in which the subject is instructed to walk as far as possible in 12 minutes, regardless of rate and rest periods, is a popular approach.[292]

EXERCISE

TYPES OF EXERCISE TESTS

Simple Ergometer and Treadmill Tests

- A more sophisticated system permits measurement of heart rate, electrocardiogram, inspired or expired minute volume, tidal volume, respiratory rate, and external work rate.
- Equipment required includes a cycle ergometer (mechanical or electromechanical) or treadmill.
- A mechanical cycle, braked by a strap and weight whose position is controlled by the operator, is portable, reliable, and inexpensive.
  - Pedaling frequency must be controlled carefully using a metronome to obtain accurate work rates.
  - Electromechanical cycles allow variation in pedaling frequency and a finer adjustment of power.
- A treadmill, equipped with side platforms and handrails for safety, should be adjustable in speed from 1.5 to 10 kph and in grade from 0% to 30%.
- Other equipment includes stopwatch, metronome, and an electrocardiogram with chest electrodes.

Complex Ergometer and Treadmill Tests

- A still more sophisticated system permits the measurements described from the preceding system as well as measurement of O_2 uptake, CO_2 output, ventilatory equivalents for O_2 and CO_2, O_2 pulse, and efficiency of work at several work rates.
- Equipment required, in addition to that already described, includes the following:
  - Plastic balloons or bags are required for direct collection of expired gas. Balloons should be rinsed with expired gas before use and checked for leaks and rate of loss of CO_2 in the event that analysis of gas concentration must be delayed.
  - Gas samples from bags or balloons can be stored for hours in an oiled 100-mL glass syringe with three-way stopcocks (stored plunger-up until analysis so the weight of the plunger places the gas content under pressure).[293]
  - Analysis of gas samples using a Scholander or Haldane apparatus provides great accuracy but is time-consuming.
  - A 120-L (Tissot) spirometer is ideal for measurement of volume of bag contents and calibration of other volume and flow devices, but a dry-gas meter may be used instead.
  - Appropriate humidified tubing and low-resistance valves with minimal dead space can be used.
- Expired gas may be passed through a mixing chamber,[294] from which mixed expired gas is sampled continuously by a gas analyzer.
  - A mass spectrometer allows rapid analysis of CO_2 and O_2 as well as other gases.
  - Zirconium fuel cells, polarographic O_2 analyzers, and some infrared CO_2 analyzers may prove to be satisfactory for analysis of gases rapidly.
- A multichannel recorder is desirable for calibration of equipment, electrical integration of flow to volume, and recording all physiologic variables simultaneously (volume, flow, gas concentrations, electrocardiogram, and heart rate).

EXERCISE

TYPES OF EXERCISE TESTS

Automated Exercise Tests

- Automated commercial systems[295, 296] permit repetitive measurements of gas flow, volume, and concentrations; calculations from these values, and graphic or tabular displays.
- Breath-by-breath analysis permits measurement of end-tidal CO_2 and O_2, peak flow, and expiratory flow pattern, in addition to the data provided by the systems described previously.
- Breath-by-breath analyses allow the operator to follow the changes of rapidly incremental exercise more accurately than analysis of samples from a mixing chamber.
- Additional equipment required includes pneumotachygraph and differential pressure transducer; and a calculator or computer with a minimum of a four-channel analog-to-digital (A-D) converter, oscilloscope, and printer.
- Airflow, O_2 and CO_2 concentrations, and heart rate signals may be transmitted by the A-D converter to a desktop calculator or computer for storage, retrieval, and analysis.
- The oscilloscope permits data, calculated breath-by-breath or averaged over several breaths, to be displayed during the test.
- A printer is required for data output, and graphics capability is useful.

Additional Equipment

- An indwelling arterial cannula is useful for sampling blood, with an appropriate transducer for measuring systemic blood pressure.
- An arterial cannula permits blood gas and blood pressure measurements.
  - Measurements of arterial CO_2 and O_2 pressure, arterial O_2 saturation, pH, arterial O_2 content, bicarbonate, and lactate may be obtained; and alveolar-arterial oxygen difference and wasted ventilation (i.e., physiologic dead space) may be calculated.
  - Because arterial punctures during exercise are difficult, an indwelling catheter with stopcock and slow or intermittent heparin infusion at a concentration of 1000 units/mL of diluent should be used.
- Nasal prongs, gas regulator, and source of O_2 can be used (with or without an ear oximeter) to evaluate O_2 therapy.
- Equipment to measure venous blood, pulmonary artery pressures, cardiac output, and stroke volume may be needed.
- Multiple-lead electrocardiogram (ECG) is recommended for reliable evaluation of cardiac rhythm abnormalities and ST-segment changes, if exercise testing is intended to evaluate patients with cardiac disease.

EXERCISE

PROTOCOLS FOR EXERCISE TESTING

Contraindications

Exercise testing may be contraindicated in a number of situations:

- Chest pain
- Severe dyspnea
- Recent myocardial infarction
- Resting hypertension
- Ventricular or atrial arrhythmias
- Congestive heart failure
- Aortic valve disease
- Severe pulmonary hypertension

Preparations

- Prior to exercise testing, the subject should have a complete history and physical examination, 12-lead ECG to exclude unsuspected cardiac disease, and routine pulmonary function studies (including lung volumes, maximal airflow rates, maximal voluntary ventilation, single-breath CO diffusing capacity, and arterial blood gas analysis as well as response of airflow rates to inhaled bronchodilators).
- The choice of exercise test will depend on available equipment and the need for diagnosis, quantitation of disease, or evaluation and response to treatment.
- In most cases, an effort should be made to familiarize the subject with the equipment before initiating the actual test.
- The subject should practice cycling at the correct pedaling frequency at a low work rate.
- If a treadmill is used, the subject needs to practice getting on while the treadmill is moving, walking without support of the guard rails, and stopping as the treadmill is slowed gradually; initially, the subject should practice without the mouthpiece, then become accustomed to the mouthpiece, and then several trials should be conducted so that the subject feels comfortable starting and stopping on the treadmill.

Criteria for Cessation of Exercise

Several signs and symptoms are an indication that the exercise test must be stopped immediately:

- Severe chest pain with or without ECG changes
- Severe dyspnea
- Marked apprehension, lightheadedness
- Sudden pallor or cyanosis, significant cardiac rhythm disturbances
- Progressive depression of ST segments
- Systolic blood pressure decrease in excess of 20 mm Hg or a rise to over 300 mm Hg
- Diastolic blood pressure rise above 140 mm Hg
- Maximal heart rate should be limited to 85% of maximum predicted values in subjects with known or suspected heart disease
- Emergency drugs and equipment suitable for cardiopulmonary resuscitation (CPR) should be on hand, and technicians should be certified in CPR.

Arterial Catheterization

If pulmonary vascular obstruction or interstitial lung disease is suspected, arterial catheterization is desirable for the following purposes:

- To obtain arterial P_{CO_2} values.
  - To calculate wasted ventilation.
  - To determine if alveolar hypoventilation occurs.
- To obtain arterial P_{O_2} values to determine whether oxygen transfer becomes abnormal during stress.
  - To reveal abnormalities missed by following oxygen transfer with an ear oximeter because of the shape of the O_2-hemoglobin dissociation curve.
  - To evaluate the effect of O_2 therapy at rest and during exercise.

EXERCISE

PROTOCOLS FOR EXERCISE TESTING

Estimation of Mixed Venous CO_2 Content and Cardiac Output

- Rebreathing techniques estimate mixed venous CO_2 pressure at rest.
- Rebreathing methods estimate cardiac output during exercise.[294]
- Other gas uptake techniques, using exogenous tracer gases, permit estimation of pulmonary blood flow.[297]

Steady-State Measurements

- For quasi-steady-state measurements, the subject should be at rest for 5 minutes with expired gas volumes and concentrations measured for the last 2 minutes.
- Samples of blood and exhaled gases should be collected over complete ventilatory cycles.
- Minimum of three levels (bracketing the anaerobic threshold) are sampled, with each level lasting for 6 minutes and samples of exhaled gas and blood taken during the final 2 minutes at each level.

Incremental Work Loads

- Work rates are increased by a fixed amount (on a bicycle in watts, on a treadmill in percentage of grade or speed) every minute until the subject is exhausted.
- Increase exercise load rapidly enough so that the subject becomes exhausted in 6 to 10 minutes.
- The highest minute ventilation, O_2 consumption, and heart rate recorded are peak or maximal values.
- In general, the test begins at 15 watts and then the work rate is increased in 15-watt increments.
- With rapid incremental increases, the subject will recover quickly, and the study can be repeated in 30 to 45 minutes with supplemental inhaled O_2, if desired.

(APPENDIXES 14 to 20 give predicted normal values for incremental exercise testing in healthy adults.)

Ramp

- Maximal O_2 uptake, anaerobic threshold, time constant for oxygen kinetics, and work efficiency can be determined from a single test in which the work rate increases continuously at a constant rate.[298]
- Valid assessment of the parameters of aerobic function may be obtained with ramp slopes between 20 and 50 watts/minute; no further information is gained by ramps lower than 20 watts/minute.
- The subject exercises for 6 minutes at a work rate of 50 watts and a pedal frequency of 60 rpm; then the work rate is increased continuously with a ramp slope between 20 and 50 watts/minute.

EXERCISE

PROTOCOLS FOR EXERCISE TESTING

Exercise-Induced Asthma

- FEV_1 by spirometry or airway resistance by body plethysmography should be measured before exercise and again every 5 minutes for 20 to 30 minutes beginning promptly after cessation of exercise.
- A decrease in FEV_1 of 20% or in specific airway conductance (SGaw) of 40% compared with the pre-exercise value is considered significant.[299, 300]
- Inhaling dry room air (e.g., from a meteorologic balloon filled with room air obtained from a cylinder of compressed gas) will enhance the chances of inducing asthma in a patient with hyperirritable airways, but will not affect the results obtained in other patients or healthy subjects.

During Oxygen Administration

- In patients who have significant hypoxemia, assess the advantages of reducing the degree of hypoxemia and the possible complications of decreased ventilatory drive by administering O_2 during rest and exercise with concurrent measurements of oximetry, arterial blood gases, and minute ventilation.
- If O_2 is administered by nasal prongs at 2 to 4 L/minute, it is possible to determine the effect of O_2 on maximal work rate, blood gases, and symptoms, but not on ventilation.
- Although the error in O_2 consumption tends to increase as the fractional concentration of inspired O_2 increases, measurements of ventilation and CO_2 production remain accurate.
- If measurements of ventilation while breathing O_2 are needed, consider using tanks of either 40% O_2 (which is about the highest concentration that can be delivered practically and economically at home) or pure O_2.
- With pure O_2 during exercise, it is possible to estimate other factors, including the percentage of right-to-left shunt, the symptomatic effect of suppressing ventilation in individuals limited by effort dyspnea, and carotid body function (by measuring change in ventilation 15 to 30 seconds after onset of oxygen breathing).
- With 40% O_2 it is still possible to measure all the usual parameters of interest, except for oxygen uptake.

CALCULATIONS

Gas Concentrations and Volumes

- Fractional concentration of nitrogen (F_{N_2}) is considered to include all the inert gases (N_2 plus rare gases).
- Scholander and Haldane analysis values can be used directly; with other analyzers, values displayed or recorded need to be adjusted so that dry-gas fractions total 1.000.
- Volume values should also be adjusted for volumes removed for O_2 or CO_2 analyses.
- Valve dead space should be included in calculating $\dot{V}_E$ and V_T but excluded in calculating $\dot{V}_E/\dot{V}_{O_2}$, $\dot{V}_E/\dot{V}_{CO_2}$, and V_D/V_T.

$$V_{BTPS} = V_{ATPS} \times \frac{(273 + 37)\ (Pbar - P_{H_2O} \text{ at t})}{(273 + t)\ (Pbar - 47)}$$

where t is ambient temperature in degrees centigrade; BTPS is body temperature and pressure, saturated; ATPS is ambient temperature and pressure, saturated with water vapor; and Pbar is barometric pressure.

EXERCISE

CALCULATIONS

Temperature Corrections of Volumes

- At a temperature t of 10°C to 40°C,

$$P_{H_2O} = 10 - 0.3952t + 0.03775t^2$$

$$V_{STPD} = \frac{V_{ATPS} \times (P_{bar} - P_{H_2O} \text{ at } t)}{760(1 + 0.00367t)}$$

where STPD is standard temperature and pressure, dry.[293]

$$\dot{V}_E = \frac{\dot{V}_I \cdot F_{I_{N_2}}}{F_{E_{N_2}}}$$

$$V_T = \frac{\dot{V}_E}{f}$$

where $F_{I_{N_2}}$ is the fraction of inspired N_2, $F_{E_{N_2}}$ is the fraction of expired N_2, f is the breathing frequency per minute, and F_{ICO_2} is 0.0005.

O_2 consumption

$$\dot{V}_{O_2(STPD)} = \dot{V}_{E(STPD)} \times [0.265(1 - F_{E_{O_2}} - F_{E_{CO_2}}) - F_{E_{O_2}}]$$

where $F_{I_{O_2}}$ is 0.2093.

O_2 Pulse

The amount of O_2 extracted per heart beat is termed the O_2 pulse and is calculated by this equation:

$$O_2 \text{ pulse} = \frac{\dot{V}_{O_2} \text{ (mL/min)}}{\text{heart rate (beats/min)}} = O_2 \text{ extraction per beat (mL/beat)}$$

This relationship is based on the Fick principle for determination of cardiac output:

$$\text{Cardiac output} = \frac{\dot{V}_{O_2}}{Ca_{O_2} - C\bar{v}_{O_2}}$$

$$\dot{V}_{O_2} = SV \cdot HR \cdot (Ca_{O_2} - C\bar{v}_{O_2})$$

$$\frac{\dot{V}_{O_2}}{HR} = SV \cdot (Ca_{O_2} - C\bar{v}_{O_2})$$

$$O_2 \text{ pulse} = SV(Ca_{O_2} - C\bar{v}_{O_2})$$

where SV is stroke volume and HR is heart rate.

- O_2 extracted per beat in the peripheral circulation depends on stroke volume and arterial and mixed venous O_2 concentrations.
- With a normal heart, O_2 pulse may be decreased by arterial hypoxemia, or failure to decrease mixed venous O_2 (as in arteriovenous fistula, maldistribution of oxygenated blood to nonessential tissues not involved in exercise, or metabolic abnormality in muscle).

Respiratory Gas Ratio

$$R = \frac{\dot{V}_{CO_2}}{\dot{V}_{O_2}}$$

where R is the respiratory exchange ratio.

Ventilatory Equivalents

The minute ventilation required for each liter of gas (CO_2 or O_2) exchanged is a measure of the efficiency of the lung as a gas exchanger.

$$VE_{CO_2} = \frac{\dot{V}_E \text{ (BTPS)}}{\dot{V}_{CO_2} \text{ (STPD)}}$$

or

$$VE_{O_2} = \frac{\dot{V}_E \text{ (BTPS)}}{\dot{V}_{O_2} \text{ (STPD)}}$$

Efficiency

Efficiency is defined by the power output (in watts) near anaerobic threshold produced by the O_2 consumed above basal levels.

$$E\ (\%) = 0.3t/(y - z)$$

where
t is power in watts near anaerobic threshold
y is O_2 consumption in L/minute at t watts
z is O_2 consumption in L/minute at 0 watts[301]

EXERCISE

CALCULATIONS

Gas Pressures

Calculation of alveolar PO_2:

$$PA_{O_2} = PI_{O_2} - PA_{CO_2}\left[FI_{O_2} + \frac{1 - FI_{O_2}}{R}\right]$$

where $PACO_2 = PaCO_2$ (see discussion of alveolar air equation earlier in chapter). Alveolar-arterial O_2 difference:

$$(A - a)PO_2 \text{ (in mm Hg)} = 10 + 0.43\ (y - 20)$$

where y is age in years.

For these relationships, the standard deviation (SD) is 4.1 (where $PCO_2 = 40$ mm Hg, and r = 0.8).[302]

Wasted Ventilation

- Physiologic dead space (VD) is the critical measurement for the evaluation of pulmonary vascular obstruction.

$$PE_{CO_2} = FE_{CO_2} \times (Pbar - 47)$$

$$VD = \left[VT \times \frac{(Pa_{CO_2} - PE_{CO_2})}{(Pa_{CO_2} - PI_{CO_2})}\right] - VD \text{ of valve}$$

$$\frac{VD}{VT} = \frac{(Pa_{CO_2} - PE_{CO_2})}{(Pa_{CO_2} - PI_{CO_2})} - \frac{VD \text{ of valve}}{VT - VD \text{ of valve}}$$

VD/VT at rest is usually below 0.40, but during exercise it decreases below 0.30 as the lung becomes more efficient at gas exchange.

$$\frac{VD}{VT} < 0.40$$

excluding the dead space of the valve.

$$VD(mL) = 0.859Y + 1.32H + 0.264\ VT - \frac{905}{f} - 179$$

where Y is age in years, H is height in centimeters, VT is tidal volume in milliliters, and f is breathing frequency per minute.

- SD = 28 mL.[303]

Reproducibility

- Healthy subjects who underwent exercise testing twice, 2 to 10 days apart, in the author's laboratory showed an average difference at 10 watts, 60 watts, and maximum exercise:
- Minute ventilation: 13%, 12%, and 10%
- O_2 consumption: 14%, 8%, and 6%

EXERCISE

CONTROVERSIAL ISSUES

Treadmill vs. Cycle Ergometer

- From the viewpoint of the subject, most subjects appear to consider walking to be more natural than cycle riding, and most individuals find that the bicycle seat produces considerable discomfort with prolonged exercise testing.
- All subjects require orientation and training to learn to get on a moving treadmill safely.
- With a mouthpiece in place, subjects may have difficulty signaling when they are exhausted and wish to stop walking or running on the treadmill. Therefore, a signal code should be arranged prior to the test procedure.
- Formerly, many treadmills did not have speeds slow enough to accommodate very dyspneic subjects, but this is no longer the case.
- On the other hand, most individuals are capable of pedaling a bicycle after practice (if necessary, uncoordinated subjects' feet may be strapped to the pedals); on a cycle, the subject has the advantage of stopping at will.
- For quantitation of work rate, cycle riding is preferred to the treadmill.
- Efficiency of walking and running improves measurably with practice on a treadmill. Efficiency also varies with grade and speed and produces marked variability in results.
- For the cycle, there is little or no increase in efficiency of pedaling with training; work rates can be incremented rapidly and predictably. With mechanical cycles, the subject must pedal at a constant rate (50 to 60 rpm), whereas with an electromechanical cycle, the work rate will be within 5% of a given setting even when pedal frequency varies between 40 and 80 rpm.
- Maximum O_2 uptake is usually about 10% to 15% lower on a cycle ergometer than on a treadmill.
- When arterial or venous catheters are to be used for sampling blood, pressure measurements, or during infusions, the cycle is preferred over the treadmill because on a cycle, the site of withdrawal is relatively fixed, and manipulation of a stopcock and syringe is easier.

Steady-State vs. Maximum Tests

- Steady-state exercise can be performed with simpler equipment than incremental exercise.
  - Allows estimation of cardiac output by rebreathing techniques.
  - Needs to be repeated at several work rates of 6 minutes in duration in order to estimate anaerobic threshold or maximum O_2 uptake.
- In contrast, when work rate is increased every minute until exhaustion or cessation of exercise, a single 6 to 10 minute incremental exercise (preferably on a cycle) gives the same information as a steady-state study but in a shorter time.[304]
  - Incremental exercise to exhaustion is less tiring than several bouts of steady-state exercise at different work rates to exhaustion.
  - Recovery is quicker and the test can be repeated again with a variable such as O_2 breathing if desired.
- The least invasive procedure necessary for clinical diagnosis or management is preferable.

EXERCISE

CONTROVERSIAL ISSUES

Assessing Subjective Responses[305]

- *Borg Scales:* Ratings of perceived exertion[306] correlate well with external work intensity.
  - In many studies, correlations with heart rate ranged from 0.80 to 0.90, and close correlations have been found with other physiologic variables as well.
  - Scale has been modified with ratio properties so that comparisons can be made between subjects or between different forms of exercise.
  - A similar approach has been used to quantify symptoms such as breathlessness, fatigue, and the degree of respiratory effort so that better correlations can be obtained between the physiologic changes during exercise and what the patient perceives.
- *Specific word descriptors:* An important new approach has been to try to define the sensation of dyspnea more precisely. Specific phrases characterizing the sensation of dyspnea have been identified and correlated with specific stimuli driving ventilation in experiments with healthy subjects.[307]
- *Visual analog scale* is used to quantitate both perceived exertion and symptoms.[308]
  - In its simplest form, a horizontal line is labeled "not at all breathless" and "very breathless" at either end.
  - Patients mark the line to show how they feel.
  - Good correlation has been found between the Borg scale and the visual analog scale.[292, 309–311]

Anaerobic Threshold

- Whether or not the anaerobic threshold is due to inadequate O_2 delivery to the muscles or inadequate O_2 utilization has not been resolved. Circumstantial evidence is abundant, but measurement of PO_2 in the microenvironment of the mitochondria at the anaerobic threshold in exercising humans is impossible currently.
- A more recent debate concerns the ability to measure accurately and reliably the anaerobic threshold by noninvasive methods and whether or not anaerobic threshold estimated by gas exchange is a useful indicator of an abrupt increase in blood lactate concentration or the onset of lactic acid production.
- There is enough evidence to question the routine clinical use of the anaerobic threshold and the determination of the anaerobic threshold by inexperienced investigators.
  - Whether or not experienced investigators using sophisticated techniques are able to measure the anaerobic threshold accurately and reliably is still a matter of dispute.
  - Further refinement of the criteria for threshold determinations along with the use of computer programs raises the possibility of improving the quality of these measurements.
- The concept that nonmetabolic CO_2 production is due to buffering of lactic acid by bicarbonate during exercise may be too simplistic.
  - The rise of lactate may result from excess production or decreased clearance from the blood unrelated to oxygenation of the muscle.[312–314]
  - Acid efflux from contracting muscle can exceed lactic acid efflux and may also have a different time course.
  - Increases in blood lactate concentration and ventilation during incremental exercise are not necessarily causally related, and can be explained by factors other than hypoxia.[315]
- A study by Richardson and associates[316] provides convincing data against the theory of local muscle hypoxia and, instead, suggests that catecholamines released during exercise are responsible for lactate accumulation.
  - Intracellular PO_2 remains constant (about 3 mm Hg) during graded incremental exercise in humans (FIGURE 8–45) and is unrelated to the linear fall in intracellular pH and concomitant linear rise in net muscle lactate efflux (FIGURE 8–46).
  - With low respired O_2, despite the same O_2 delivery at any given muscle $\dot{V}O_2$, there was a significant reduction in intracellular PO_2, which again remained constant during graded incremental exercise (FIGURE 8–45).
  - Under these hypoxic conditions the rate of fall in pH and rate of muscle lactate efflux, both in

(continued)

EXERCISE

CONTROVERSIAL ISSUES

Anaerobic Threshold

relation to absolute $\dot{V}O_2$, were increased (FIGURE 8–46).

- These data demonstrate that during incremental exercise, skeletal muscle cells do not become anaerobic as lactate levels suddenly rise, because intracellular PO_2 is well preserved at a constant level even at maximum exercise and there is a lack of relationship between intracellular PO_2, lactate efflux, and muscle pH.
- There is a strong positive correlation between blood lactate concentration, epinephrine concentration, exercise intensity, and O_2 saturation. Net muscle lactate efflux is closely related to arterial epinephrine and is independent of inspired O_2 concentration (FIGURE 8–47).
- Thus, increased blood lactate may be influenced by elevated sympathetic drive during exercise, more so in hypoxia, rather than by a lower intracellular PO_2 per se.
- If it is systemic and not intracellular PO_2 that increases the catecholamine response in hypoxia, and therefore is responsible for higher lactate efflux, it would explain the observations by others of increased lactate efflux from nonexercising muscles in the upper extremity during lower extremity exercise.[312, 313]

FIGURE 8–45

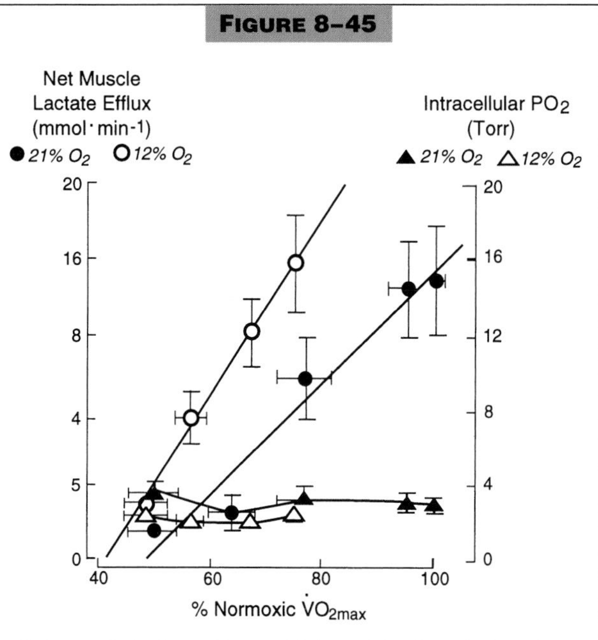

Net muscle lactate efflux and intracellular PO_2 displayed as a function of O_2 consumption ($\dot{V}O_2$) in normoxia and hypoxia in normal exercising subjects (for lactate efflux, r = 0.97 and 0.99 in normoxia and hypoxia, respectively). $\dot{V}O_2$ max = maximal O_2 consumption. (Modified after Richardson RS, Noyszewski EA, Leigh JS, et al: Lactate efflux from exercising human skeletal muscle: Role of intracellular PO_2. J Appl Physiol 85:627–634, 1998.)

FIGURE 8–46

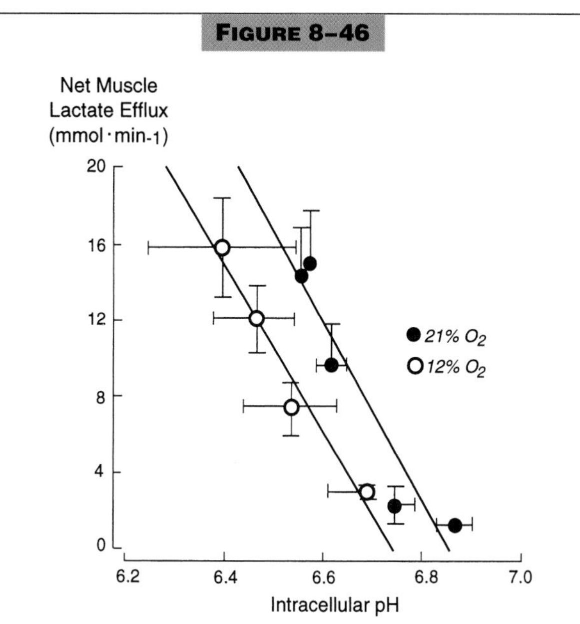

Relationship between net muscle lactate efflux and intracellular pH in hypoxia and normoxia in normal exercising subjects (r = 0.94 and 0.98 in normoxia and hypoxia, respectively). (Modified after Richardson RS, Noyszewski EA, Leigh JS, et al: Lactate efflux from exercising human skeletal muscle: Role of intracellular PO_2. J Appl Physiol 85:627–634, 1998.)

EXERCISE

CONTROVERSIAL ISSUES

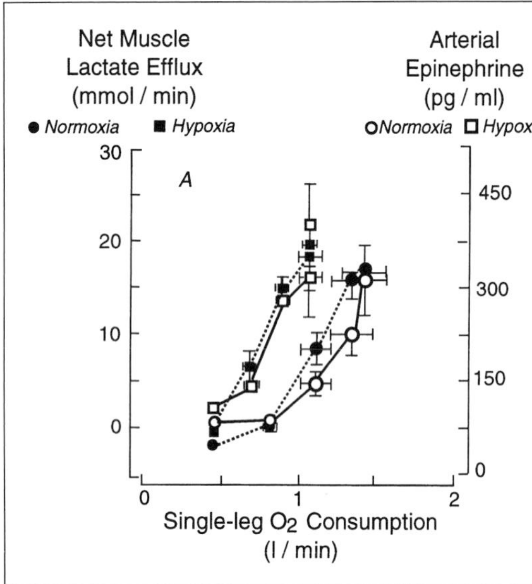

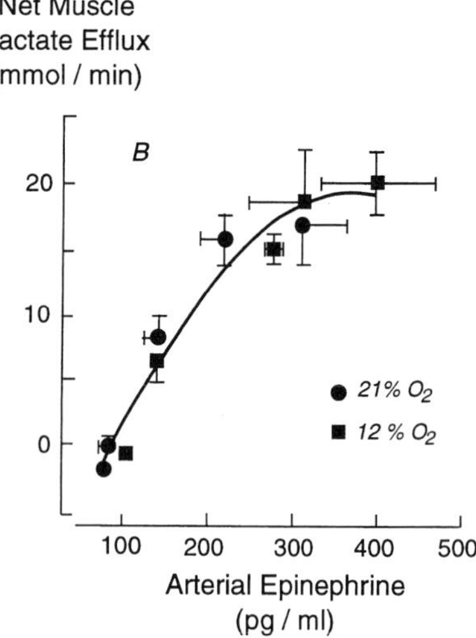

FIGURE 8-47

A, Relationships of net muscle lactate efflux and arterial epinephrine levels to $\dot{V}O_2$ in hypoxia and normoxia in exercising subjects. *B*, Relationship between net muscle lactate efflux and arterial epinephrine level is independent of inspired O_2 concentration. (Modified after Richardson RS, Noyszewski EA, Leigh JS, et al: Lactate efflux from exercising human skeletal muscle: Role of intracellular P_{O_2}. J Appl Physiol 85: 627–634, 1998.)

Disability Evaluation

- The ATS has suggested that in most cases, results of pulmonary function tests at rest are sufficient to predict the presence and degree of impairment during exercise.[317]
- The FEV_1/FVC criterion for severe impairment was set at less than or equal to 0.4, and categories were added for mild and moderate impairment using standard pulmonary function tests and $\dot{V}O_{2\ max}$.
- In most patients with mild to moderate abnormalities of resting function, the degree of exercise impairment cannot be predicted from pulmonary function tests performed at rest.
- In patients with pulmonary vascular obstruction, exercise impairment may not even be suspected on the basis of resting studies.[317a]
- Even in patients with clear-cut and severe chronic airway obstruction, it was not possible to predict exercise-induced hypoxemia.[318] If FEV_1/FVC exceeded 0.50 and DL_{CO} (SB) exceeded 20 mL/min/mm Hg, a fall in Pa_{O_2} during exercise could be excluded in all cases.
- In asymptomatic shipyard workers, as many as half had cardiovascular limitation unsuspected from clinical or laboratory studies performed at rest.[319]

CLINICAL APPLICATIONS

Heart Disease

- Patients with significant heart disease usually have limited exercise capacity:
- Thus, $\dot{V}O_{2\ max}$ is decreased, associated with increased heart rate relative to work rate and oxygen uptake at all levels of exercise, decreased O_2 pulse, but with normal ventilatory response.
- The slope of $\dot{V}O_2$ vs. work may be decreased, whereas slope of heart rate vs. oxygen uptake is increased.
- In patients with peripheral vascular disease, BP may increase dramatically, whereas in cardiomyopathy or coronary artery disease, BP may not increase normally and may even fall.
- If cardiac output is *very* limited, anaerobic threshold may be very low (less than 40% of predicted or observed $\dot{V}O_{2\ max}$).

EXERCISE

CLINICAL APPLICATIONS

Obstructive Ventilatory Defect

- These patients usually have increased VE_{O_2}, VE_{CO_2}, VD/VT, and (A − a)DO_2 and decreased breathing reserve.
- IC typically decreases (as end-expiratory volume, FRC, increases) and airflow limitation develops.
- With a moderate to severe defect, there is decreased $\dot{V}O_{2\,max}$, maximum heart rate, and breathing reserve.
- Respiratory rate is usually increased but below 40 breaths per minute with prolonged exhalation and concave expiratory flow pattern.
- Hypoxemia may be mild or severe.
- If the mechanical limitation is severe, alveolar ventilation may not increase sufficiently to meet the increased CO_2 production and arterial PCO_2 may rise.
- It is usually not possible to detect anaerobic threshold or ventilatory threshold by noninvasive methods, even though observed blood lactate accumulation and metabolic acidosis is demonstrable by arterial blood samples.
- Often, dyspnea limits exercise before lactate or ventilatory equivalents rise.

End-Expiratory Lung Volume

- In normal subjects during exercise, end-expiratory lung volume (EELV), which is really FRC, decreases.[320]
  - FRC decreases even during mild exercise and during heavy exercise FRC decreases 0.71 ± 0.7 L associated with increased abdominal pressure.
  - Reduced FRC during exercise aids inspiration by optimizing diaphragmatic length and permitting elastic recoil of the chest wall.
  - Similar results have been observed in older normal subjects: with exercise intensity at 50% to 70% $\dot{V}O_{2max}$, FRC decreased 0.38 L and flow limitation was present over 25% of VT.[321] As exercise increased, FRC increased to near resting levels permitting increased expiratory flow rates; during heavy exercise, FRC remained constant but end-inspiratory lung volume approached 90% of TLC, and more than 40% of VT was flow-limited.
- In patients with airflow obstruction, FRC increases during exercise:
  - Regnis and coworkers studied patients with cystic fibrosis to determine whether the severity of the disease correlated with the change in FRC during exercise.
  - The changes in FRC were highly correlated with resting lung function, indices of maximal expiratory flow, and maximal work.
  - Patients with severe airflow obstruction (mean FEV_1 29% ± 4% predicted) increased FRC during exercise, whereas patients with mild disease had near-normal ventilatory pattern during exercise.
  - Babb and colleagues showed that even mild airway obstruction is associated with an increase in FRC rather than the expected decrease observed in normal subjects.[322]
- Babb and Rodarte also showed that use of IC to estimate FRC during exercise with the assumption that TLC remained constant was supported by direct measurements of TLC and IC during exercise.[323]
- FRC increases during exercise in obese women, but not in lean women, suggesting that FRC increases during exercise may not be specific for obstructive ventilatory defect.[324]
- Thus, the diagnostic implication of the change in FRC during exercise requires further study.

EXERCISE

CLINICAL APPLICATIONS

Restrictive Ventilatory Defect (Interstitial Lung Disease)

- With mild restrictive defects, $\dot{V}O_{2\,max}$ may remain normal, but there is usually evidence of ventilation-perfusion mismatching and decreased breathing reserve associated with marked tachypnea (over 50 breaths per minute).
- This pattern may occur in patients with interstitial lung disease when lung function is normal at rest.
- Tachypnea usually reaches diagnostic levels (50 breaths/minute or more) without concurrent abnormalities in VT. In normal subjects:

$$\frac{V_T}{IC} < 0.7$$

$$\frac{V_T}{VC} < 0.55$$

With more severe restriction, PaO_2 usually falls, $(A - a)DO_2$ increases, and V_D/V_T remains elevated, even with mild disease.

- There is an abnormal drive to ventilation in addition to excessive wasted ventilation, so minute ventilation is excessive at all levels of exercise and ventilatory equivalents for CO_2 and O_2 are abnormally increased.

Pulmonary Vascular Obstruction

- There maybe marked effort dyspnea with pulmonary vascular obstruction despite normal physical findings and chest roentgenogram.
- Pulmonary function at rest may be completely normal except for decreased DL_{CO} and evidence of chronic alveolar hyperventilation.
- Characteristically, numerous regions of lung are poorly perfused in relation to their ventilation, so wasted ventilation is increased and VD/VT may also be abnormal.
- Patients usually have an abnormal drive to ventilation so minute ventilation is excessive at all work rates and ventilatory equivalents for CO_2 and O_2 are abnormally increased.
- The only abnormality in these patients may be the absolute value of physiologic dead space during exercise.
    - Thus it is vital to study patients suspected of pulmonary vascular obstruction with arterial blood gas samples.
    - If wasted ventilatory volume (VD, physiologic dead space) increases by more than twofold and exceeds 300 mL, be suspicious of pulmonary vascular obstruction; if VD exceeds 400 mL, cardiovascular and radiographic studies are mandatory.
- These patients usually have abnormal cardiovascular responses to exercise if the pulmonary vascular obstruction is severe; with a limited cardiac output response to exercise, $\dot{V}O_{2max}$ and O_2 pulse are often markedly reduced.

EXERCISE

CLINICAL APPLICATIONS

Obesity

- Excess deposition of fat in the abdomen and chest wall markedly increases the stress on the heart and lungs.
- At rest, cardiac output is increased to meet the increased oxygen uptake of the increased body mass relative to lean body weight; additional increased cardiac output during exercise is limited.
- O_2 uptake at rest is increased in proportion to the excess body mass, but increases normally during exercise.
- Ventilation-perfusion matching is usually abnormal at rest due to hypoventilation of dependent basal regions of the lungs.
- Ventilatory equivalents, VD/VT, and PaO_2 are usually abnormal at rest, but with increased tidal volume during exercise, hypoxemia, and evidence of $\dot{V}A/\dot{Q}c$ mismatching usually disappear.
- $\dot{V}O_{2max}$ and anaerobic threshold are decreased relative to observed body weight but normal when related to lean body weight.
- O_2 pulse is also normal or high when related to lean body weight. The O_2 pulse is often elevated (O_2 uptake increased relative to heart rate), so obese patients appear well conditioned.
- O_2 uptake is increased relative to external work by approximately 6 mL/minute/kg of excess body weight, but the increase in O_2 uptake with increased external work is normal.
- The response to exercise is limited because the metabolic rate and minute volume of ventilation is increased for a given work rate and O_2 consumption.[325]
- Metabolic cost of breathing is increased because of the increased chest wall mass and decreased distensibility and associated tachypnea.
- Work of breathing is abnormally increased and may be associated with pulmonary atelectasis.

Neuromuscular Disease

- Neuromuscular abnormalities may limit maximum ventilation during exercise far below levels expected from measurements of FEV_1 and FVC at rest.
- Therefore, we always measure maximal respiratory pressures and MVV directly in patients to be exercised, rather than predicting exercise ventilation on nomograms based on FEV_1 measured at rest.
- $PaCO_2$ may increase because of the inability to increase alveolar ventilation to meet metabolic needs despite decreased $\dot{V}O_{2\,max}$, maximum heart rate, and ventilatory capacity.

Poor Physical Condition

- $\dot{V}O_{2_{max}}$ is usually reduced, but the heart rate is excessive at all work levels.
- If motivated, these subjects may attain their maximal predicted heart rates and develop significant metabolic acidosis, but observed blood lactate accumulation (OBLA) is rarely less than 80% of predicted.
- Gas exchange, ECG, and BP responses are normal.

Anxiety

- Anxious persons often have marked tachypnea and irregular patterns of breathing, associated with acute alveolar hyperventilation.
- During exercise, these abnormalities usually disappear and the subject ventilates appropriately for the work rate in response to the neurohumoral stimuli of exercise.
- Unless these patients are studied with arterial blood samples, however, the pattern of response may resemble that of pulmonary vascular obstruction (patients with anxiety will have normal $PaCO_2$, VD, and VD/VT during exercise).

EXERCISE

CLINICAL APPLICATIONS

Poor Motivation

- Most subjects can be induced to perform well in the laboratory.
- Even patients involved in compensation cases can be made to understand that abnormalities in gas exchange, ventilation-perfusion relationships, and DL_{CO} may only become significantly abnormal at high work rates.
- With poor motivation, look for decreased values for $\dot{V}O_{2\,max}$, maximum heart rate, maximum minute ventilation, and normal gas exchange, and *no* evidence of metabolic acidosis.

Summary

- A basic system that measures only ventilation and heart rate provides enough information to meet many clinical needs; for laboratories unfamiliar with technical demands of more complex measurements, such a system has the advantage of increasing the likelihood that the measurements will be accurate.
- Using such a system allows technical and medical personnel to gain a better understanding of the advantages and limitations of exercise testing without the expense and confusion arising when sophisticated testing is attempted.
- If a laboratory elects to measure expired gas concentrations, and the derived values from these data as part of exercise testing, whether to assemble a system from components or purchase a complete commercial system is an important decision.
- Assembling a system from components enables one to use equipment a laboratory may already have, allows greater flexibility for changes in the future, and is often less expensive; the expertise and time required, however, are often considerable.
- Complete commercial exercise systems allow the obvious advantage of requiring minimal development time and are often engineered to maximize ease of operation and reduction of data. Many such systems are quite expensive, are not necessarily more accurate than the component systems, and usually offer less flexibility.
- As with other types of automated testing systems, data that confirm the accuracy of the measurements made by the system should be available prior to clinical use.
- Rigorous quality control procedures with automated systems are as important as with manual systems. Most desirable in microprocessors or computer systems are units that permit programming changes should they be needed in the future.

APPLICATIONS OF PULMONARY FUNCTION TESTS

SCREENING STUDIES

Goals

- Screening pulmonary function tests[326] should separate subjects who have normal lungs from those who have abnormal lungs in a few minutes of the patients' time, with little or no discomfort.
- The apparatus should be inexpensive and portable, and should require little or no technical training to operate.
- Tests should be free from error and should pinpoint the specific functional abnormality and its location in a quantitative manner.

APPLICATIONS OF PULMONARY FUNCTION TESTS

SCREENING STUDIES

Uses

Screening tests can be used for several purposes:

- Early detection of pulmonary or cardiopulmonary disease (e.g., emphysema, pulmonary fibrosis, pulmonary vascular disease)
- Differential diagnosis of patients with dyspnea
- Detection of the presence, location, and extent of regional disease
- Evaluation of patients prior to surgical procedures
- Determination of the risk of certain diagnostic procedures
- Early detection of respiratory failure and monitoring of treatment in critical care units
- Quantitative evaluation of specific treatment in patients with known pulmonary disease
- Periodic examination of pulmonary function in workers whose occupations are associated with known pulmonary hazards
- Epidemiologic studies of populations to provide clues regarding the pathogenesis of pulmonary disease
- Annual evaluation of any adult over the age of 40 years who smokes 20 or more cigarettes daily

Obstructive Ventilatory Defect

- In some laboratories, screening pulmonary function tests include
  - Static lung volumes by spirometry
  - Single-breath helium, neon, or methane dilution (as part of the measurement of single-breath CO diffusing capacity)
  - FVC and its subdivisions and flow-volume curves
  - Distribution of inspired gas using the single-breath N_2 washout method
- These tests permit diagnosis of obstructive ventilatory defects in asymptomatic patients on the basis of decreased $FEF_{25-75\%}$ from spirograms and decreased maximal flow at low lung volumes from flow-volume curves.
- In more advanced obstruction, FEV_1, FEV_1/FVC ratio, and maximal flows at all lung volumes may be abnormally decreased. The evidence of airway obstruction may be associated with uneven distribution of ventilation, as reflected by an abnormal single-breath N_2 washout test, and associated hyperinflation, as reflected by increased RV and FRC and decreased FVC.
- If the airway obstruction is severe (volume-corrected flow < 0.4 TLC/sec at 50% VC or FEV_1/FVC ratio < 0.4), the TLC measured by single-breath dilution may be underestimated significantly.[60, 61]

APPLICATIONS OF PULMONARY FUNCTION TESTS

SCREENING STUDIES

Obstructive Ventilatory Defect

Comparison with Restrictive Ventilatory Defects

- If airway function is normal, early development of a restrictive ventilatory defect may be suggested by the finding of increased FEV_1/FVC ratio associated with increased maximal expiratory airflow.
- With more advanced disease, TLC, VC, and associated lung volumes are decreased, with evidence of uneven distribution of ventilation.
- Interpretation of the spirogram in mixed ventilatory defects may be aided by examining FEV_1 as a percentage of predicted normal values rather than as a percentage of FVC.
- Mixed defects are more easily defined by measurement of TLC using a multiple-breath dilution technique or, preferably, body plethysmography.
- In patients with neither a restrictive nor obstructive ventilatory defect, the finding of an isolated decreased single-breath CO diffusing capacity may be the first clue to the presence of an interstitial process, emphysema, or pulmonary vascular obstruction.
- In general, the degree of severity of a particular pulmonary pattern is indicated by the decrease in percentage of predicted values, (TABLE 8-7).
- If the screening tests are normal, but the patient has symptoms, more complete pulmonary function studies are indicted (particularly if arterial blood gases show evidence of chronic hyperventilation).
- In patients with cough or a history of wheezing with respiratory tract infections, such studies should include bronchial provocation testing to determine whether the patient has abnormal airway reactivity. (See Chapter 4, Radiography and Imaging and Chapter 5, Nuclear Medicine and Applications.)

TABLE 8-7

Severity of Pulmonary Impairment

Impairment Assessment	VC*	FEV_1*	FEV_1/FVC†	$FEF_{25\%-75\%}$*	TLC*	DL_{CO}*
Normal	>80	>80	>70	>65	>80	>80
Mild	66–80	66–80	60–70	50–65	66–80	61–80
Moderate	50–65	50–65	45–59	35–49	50–65	40–60
Severe	<50	<50	<45	<35	<50	<40

* Percentage of predicted normal values.

† Absolute value.

VC = vital capacity; FEV_1 = forced expired volume in 1 second; FVC = forced vital capacity; $FEF_{25\%-75\%}$ = forced expired flow between 25% and 75% of FVC; TLC = total lung capacity; DL_{CO} = single breath carbon monoxide diffusing capacity.

APPLICATIONS OF PULMONARY FUNCTION TESTS

PATTERNS OF RESPONSE

Obstructive Ventilatory Defect

General Pattern

- The usual pattern of airway obstruction is summarized in TABLE 8–8.
- Supplementary data include RV and Raw, uneven distribution of ventilation, and significant reversibility of airway obstruction, with or without decreased diffusing capacity.
- Common causes of obstructive ventilatory defects, including those involving the upper airway, central and peripheral airways, as well as the lung parenchyma, are listed in TABLE 8–9.

TABLE 8–8

Obstructive Ventilatory Defect

Characteristics of Obstructive Ventilatory Defect	Supplemental Data Confirming Obstruction
Normal or decreased VC	• Increased RV
Decreased maximum expiratory airflow	• Increased airway resistance
Decreased MVV	• Abnormal distribution of inspired gas • Significant response to bronchodilator • Decreased DL_{CO} • Decreased lung elastic recoil

Source: Adapted from Welch MH: Ventilatory function of the lungs. *In* Guenter CA, Welch MH (eds): Pulmonary Medicine. Philadelphia, JB Lippincott, 1977, pp. 72–123.

TABLE 8–9

Common Causes of Obstructive Ventilatory Defects

Upper Airway
- Pharyngeal and laryngeal tumors, edema, infections
- Foreign bodies
- Tumors, collapse, and stenosis of trachea

Central and Peripheral Airway
- Bronchitis
- Bronchiectasis
- Bronchiolitis
- Bronchial asthma

Parenchymal Disease
- Emphysema

Source: Adapted from Welch MH: Ventilatory function of the lung. *In* Guenter CA, Welch MH (eds): Pulmonary Medicine. Philadelphia, JB Lippincott, 1977, pp. 72–123.

APPLICATIONS OF PULMONARY FUNCTION TESTS

PATTERNS OF RESPONSE

Obstructive Ventilatory Defect

Reversibility

- Assesment of reversibility of decreased expiratory airflow is included in the differential diagnosis of airflow obstruction.
- Reversibility may occur
  - Acutely in response to bronchodilator aerosols
  - Chronically in response to a variety of airway treatments
  - Spontaneously during remission of bronchial asthma
- Reversibility implies a better prognosis than for fixed obstruction and may have considerable significance when planning a treatment program.
- American Thoracic Society: VC (slow or forced) and FEV_1 are the primary spirometric indices to determine bronchodilator response.
  - Total expiratory time should be considered when using FVC to assess the bronchodilator response because FVC increases in obstructed patients when expiratory time increases.
  - A 12% increase above the prebronchodilator value *and* a 200-mL increase in either FVC or FEV_1 indicate a positive bronchodilator response in adults.
  - $FEF_{25-75\%}$ and instantaneous flow rates should only be considered secondarily in evaluating reversibility.
  - Flows must be volume-adjusted, or the effect of changing FVC must be considered in the interpretation (FIGURE 8–48).
  - Ratios such as FEV_1/VC should not be used to evaluate reversibility.[103, 327, 328, 329] (APPENDIX 5 lists recommended criteria for response to a bronchodilator in adults.)
- Conventional criteria for reversibility may still be misleading.[330]
  - These criteria are not useful to distinguish patients with asthma from those with other forms of chronic airway obstruction in a clinically defined population.
  - When applied to a patient population, these criteria selected the most obstructed patients (a contradiction of the definition of reversibility).
- Elisasson and Degraff suggested that the difference in FEV_1 before and after bronchodilator administration (expressed as an absolute value or as a percentage of predicted FEV_1) appeared more appropriate as an expression of reversibility.[330]
- Failure to demonstrate significant responses to acute bronchodilator therapy does not rule out reversible airway obstruction.
- Many reports demonstrate that asthmatic patients with completely reversible airway obstruction may initially fail to respond to inhaled bronchodilators.[66, 331]
- Corticosteroids enhance responsiveness to beta-adrenergic agonists.[332, 333]
  - In many laboratories, reversibility is evaluated by testing spirometry before and 10 to 20 minutes after inhalation of albuterol aerosol (inhaler, two puffs).
  - Because many patients with asthma or other forms of airway disease do not respond initially to beta-adrenergic agonists, particularly at low doses, it is worth considering evaluation of reversibility after ipratropium bromide aerosol (inhaler, two puffs).
  - It is advisable to remember, however, that the maximal effect of ipratropium bromide may take 30 to 45 minutes.
  - Furthermore, many patients with reversible airway obstruction will not respond to a standard clinical dose of either class of dilator, but will still reverse completely if treated with larger doses.
- Thus, in some patients with airway obstruction who have never been treated before and who do not respond to a standard clinical dose of inhaled dilator, a cumulative dose-response protocol may be useful: spirometry is measured before (baseline) and 15 minutes after a progressively increasing dose of albuterol or ipratropium bromide.
  - The aerosol is administered (inhaler, two puffs) every 15 minutes until maximal increase in FEV_1 or FVC is attained or limiting symptoms are reached.
  - At this time interval, both agents produce at least 80% of their maximal response and most patients respond maximally after receiving 8 to 10 puffs.

APPLICATIONS OF PULMONARY FUNCTION TESTS

PATTERNS OF RESPONSE

Obstructive Ventilatory Defect

Reversibility

FIGURE 8-48

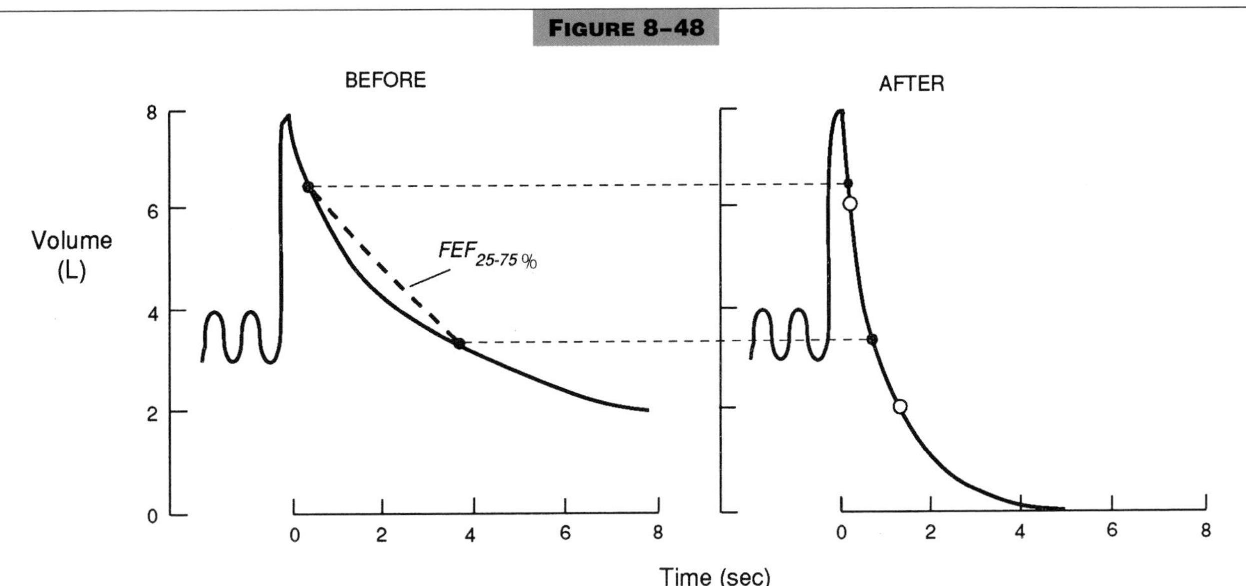

Schematic illustration of volume adjustment to calculate isovolume $FEF_{25-75\%}$. *Left,* Before administration of bronchodilator, the $FEF_{25-75\%}$ is calculated from a line connecting two points on the volume-time curve of the FVC. One solid circle indicates when 25% of the FVC is exhaled (6.5 L); the other solid circle indicates when 75% of the FVC is exhaled (3.5 L). This volume change (3.0 L) occurs in 3.4 seconds so $FEF_{25-75\%}$ is 0.88 L/sec. *Right,* After administration of bronchodilator, one open circle indicates when 25% of the FVC is exhaled (6.0 L) and the other open circle indicates when 75% of the FVC is exhaled (2.0 L). This volume change occurs in 1.3 seconds, so $FEF_{25-75\%}$ is 3.0 L/sec. The solid circles have been moved over from the "before" schematic based on the before volumes. The volume adjusted or isovolume $FEF_{25-75\%}$ is determined from a line connecting the solid circles on the "after" graph. In this case the volume change is the same as that observed in the "before" graph, or 3.0 L, but occurred in only 0.6 second so the isovolume $FEF_{25-75\%}$ is 5.0 L/sec, a marked improvement induced by the bronchodilator. This approach was developed because early reports indicated that some patients appeared to have significant improvement in FEV_1 but not $FEF_{25-75\%}$ when no volume adjustment was made in the calculation of $FEF_{25-75\%}$. When a volume adjustment was made in calculation of $FEF_{25-75\%}$, there was improvement in both FEV_1 and $FEF_{25-75\%}$, as illustrated here. (From Murray JF, Nadel JA (eds): Textbook of Respiratory Medicine. 3rd ed. Philadelphia, WB Saunders, 2000. p. 852).

Bronchial Provocation

- Provocation tests may be extremely useful in the diagnosis and management of patients with asthma, occupational asthma, and the differential diagnosis of patients with chronic cough, or wheezing, or intermittent dyspnea.
- Many laboratories use spirometry to evaluate the airway response, but the author relies on measurement of Raw in a body plethysmograph because Raw is
  - More sensitive
  - More specific for abnormalities in airway tone
  - Usually easier for the patient to perform than tests dependent on inspiration to TLC followed by a forced exhalation
- In limited numbers of patients, tests with specific allergens may be helpful in the evaluation of allergic asthma.
- In a small number of patients suspected of occupational asthma, specific challenge with agents found in the workplace may be useful in the diagnosis. Specific challenge tests are dangerous, tedious, and may not be useful if the patient is exposed to multiple agents in the workplace.

APPLICATIONS OF PULMONARY FUNCTION TESTS

PATTERNS OF RESPONSE

Obstructive Ventilatory Defect

Tests of Nonspecific Airway Responsiveness

- Abnormal airway responsiveness is viewed by many as a characteristic feature of asthma.
- Abnormal airway responsiveness also occurs in patients with chronic bronchitis and cystic fibrosis.
- Although a variety of stimuli have been used, including exercise and eucapneic ventilation, the most common stimuli are histamine and methacholine, which have good correlation and reproducibility.[334, 335]
- Methacholine is delivered in incremental concentrations until a desired effect on pulmonary function is achieved; usually, less than 0.1 mg/mL is the initial concentration to avoid inducing an inordinately severe reaction.
- The challenge begins with a saline control aerosol, and responses are reported relative to the saline value.
- Dose of agonist is expressed on the logarithmic abscissa as (1) cumulative inhalation breath units (the equivalent of one breath of a concentration containing 1 mg/mL); (2) cumulative amount of agonist in micromoles delivered from the nebulizer; and (3) the concentration inhaled (mg/mL).
- Endpoint: the dose causing a decrease in FEV_1 of 20%, a decrease in SGaw of 40%, or an increase of SRaw of 200%.
- Pulmonary function measurements should be made 3 to 5 minutes after delivery of the aerosol and repeated in 5 minutes.
- FEV_1 is the most common test used, although specific airway resistance may be more sensitive.
- Responses are influenced by medications, baseline airway function, respiratory infections, and exposure to specific allergens and chemical sensitizers.
- Bronchodilators, antihistamines, and calcium-channel blockers should probably be withheld before the test.

Test of Specific Airway Responsiveness

- Most commercial allergens are obtained as lyophilized extracts or as concentrated solutions.
- These retain potency indefinitely when stored at −20°C.
- Incremental allergen concentrations are given sequentially until the desired pulmonary function change occurs.
- The response to inhaled allergen depends on both allergic sensitivity as reflected by skin test as well as nonspecific airway responsiveness as reflected by histamine or methacholine responsiveness.
- Thus, the original guidelines of a starting concentration that produces a 2+ reaction (larger than 5-mm wheal) after intradermal injection is probably safe but may result in a very long test in some patients.
- With skin test 2+ at 0.0005 μg IgE/mL, use 0.025 μg AgE/mL; with 2+ reaction at 0.005 μg/mL, use 0.05 μg AgE/mL; and 0.05 μg AgE/mL when that dose causes a 2+ skin response.
- Aerosol delivery in North America is usually by (1) intermittent generation of aerosol during inspiration from a DeVilbiss 646 nebulizer connected to a dose-metering device that controls flow of compressed air at 20 psi for a fixed time, at a flow rate of 750 mL/minute or less,[299] or (2) Wright nebulizer with aerosol delivered to face mask with nebulizer output of 0.13 to 0.16 mL/minute.[334]
- Respiratory rate, tidal volume, and inspiratory flow rate are kept constant for a fixed time interval and volume of aerosol solution is 3 mL.
- Measurements of FEV_1 or airway resistance are most commonly used; usually the dose needed to decrease FEV_1 by 20% or more, or decrease specific airway conductance by 40% or more, are considered positive.

APPLICATIONS OF PULMONARY FUNCTION TESTS

PATTERNS OF RESPONSE

Obstructive Ventilatory Defect

Bullous Lung Disease

- In certain obstructive ventilatory defects, a variety of specific tests may prove useful.
- In a patient with a localized bulla who is being considered for surgical resection of the lesion, it is important to show that the bulla is responsible for the pulmonary function abnormalities and disability, and not intrinsic airway disease and/or emphysema.
- An exercise study will quantitate disability caused by the bulla, or associated disease.
- Physiologic studies relating Raw and $\dot{V}max$ to static transpulmonary pressure (Pstl) will differentiate the effects of loss of lung elastic recoil from those of intrinsic lung disease.
- Radioisotope perfusion lung scans, pulmonary angiograms, and thin-section CT scans will determine whether the vascular defects are localized (i.e., bullae) or diffuse (i.e., emphysema). (See Chapter 5, Nuclear Medicine Techniques and Applications.)
- These studies may also indicate whether the bulla is compressing normal lung tissue.
    - This possibility can be confirmed by a shunt study to determine whether compression of normal lung tissue by the bulla is having a "shunt-like effect" on arterial P_{O_2}.
- Radioisotope ventilation lung scans will also help determine whether the ventilatory defects are localized (i.e., bullae) or diffuse (i.e., emphysema).
- To evaluate further the possibility of concomitant emphysema, the single-breath DL_{CO} is useful.
- Measurement of "trapped gas" by comparison of TLC measured by single-breath gas dilution and body plethysmography should provide an estimate of the size of the bulla.
- Bronchograms or CT scans may be useful to determine the presence and extent of intrinsic airway disease.[74] (See Chapter 4, Radiography and Imaging.)

APPLICATIONS OF PULMONARY FUNCTION TESTS

PATTERNS OF RESPONSE

Obstructive Ventilatory Defect

Lung Volume Reduction Surgery

- Lung volume reduction surgery (LVRS) for emphysema is another example of a clinical problem in which a variety of specific physiologic tests combined with radiologic studies may prove useful. (See Chapter 4, Radiography and Imaging, and Chapter 5, Nuclear Medicine Techniques and Applications.)
- LVRS is based on the theory that reduction in lung volume in patients with diffuse emphysema will improve lung elastic recoil, increase radial traction on bronchi, and thus increase expiratory flow and relieve dyspnea.[336, 337]
- After initial disappointing results, this approach was revived as a therapy for COPD using the CO_2 laser in the early 1990s,[338] but it was not until Cooper reported his first 20 operations using the sternotomy approach in 1995 that enthusiasm for LVRS increased dramatically.[339]
- The published reports on LVRS, however, lack a uniform approach to selecting COPD patients and adequate and uniform assessments of Quality of Life.
  - Interpretation of this data is further complicated by variations in surgical technique and physiologic measurements.
  - Although some of the mechanisms for improvement with LVRS have been elucidated, much is still unknown regarding its effect on cardiopulmonary physiology and exercise tolerance.
  - Long-term results are not yet available; thus, the ability of LVRS to significantly alter the natural history of COPD remains unproved and awaits the results of a large controlled multicenter trial.[340, 341]
- The conventional explanations for the beneficial effects of LVRS are the increased elastic recoil[342] and increased ability of inspiratory muscles to generate force.[343]
- Increased inspiratory resistance is purported to predict poor outcomes.[344]
- An unusual explanation of the mechanism of LVRS has been proposed by Fessler and Permutt,[345] who have developed a mathematical analysis and graphic model of the mechanism affecting both vital capacity and expiratory airflow.
  - This analysis is based on their concept of the interaction between lung function and respiratory muscle function.
  - They extended their analysis from LVRS to previously published data on mechanical properties of the lungs in patients with $alpha_1$-antitrypsin deficiency, COPD, and asthma.
  - In each of these diseases, a major determinant of airflow limitation is the ratio of residual volume to total lung capacity (RV/TLC).
  - Furthermore, their analysis suggests that RV/TLC determines the improvement in pulmonary function following surgical treatment of emphysema.
  - Regardless of the underlying disease, impaired airflow appears to be due to the mismatch between the size of the lung and the size of the chest wall; surgery improves this mismatch.
  - They also suggest that their analysis can be used to guide patient selection for LVRS.

APPLICATIONS OF PULMONARY FUNCTION TESTS

PATTERNS OF RESPONSE

Restrictive Ventilatory Defects

• TABLE 8–10 summarizes the characteristics of the restrictive pattern. Supplementary data confirming restriction include decreased TLC, decreased single-breath diffusing capacity, uneven distribution of ventilation, chronic alveolar hyperventilation, and increased alveolar-arterial P_{O_2} pressure difference.
• Because static lung elastic recoil pressure depends on lung volume, the diagnosis of a restrictive ventilatory defect does not usually require measurement of pressure-volume curves of the lung.
• In patients with mixed disease or in whom poor cooperation is suspected, measurement of pressure-volume curves may be helpful.
• For common causes of restrictive ventilatory defects, see TABLE 8–11. (See Chapter 3, Pathology.)

TABLE 8–10

Restrictive Ventilatory Defect

Characteristics of Restrictive Ventilatory Defect	Supplemental Data Confirming Restrictive Pattern
Decreased VC	• Decreased TLC
Relatively normal expiratory flow rates	• Decreased lung compliance
Relatively normal MVV	• Chronic alveolar hyperventilation • Increased $(A - a)P_{O_2}$ • Abnormal distribution of inspired gas • Decreased $D_{L_{CO}}$

Source: Adapted from Welch MH: Ventilatory function of the lungs. *In* Guenter CA, Welch MH (eds): Pulmonary Medicine. Philadelphia, JB Lippincott, 1977, pp. 72–123.

TABLE 8–11

Common Causes of Restrictive Ventilatory Defects

Interstitial Lung Disease
- Interstitial pneumonitis
- Fibrosis
- Pneumoconiosis
- Granulomatosis
- Edema

Space-Occupying Lesions
- Tumor
- Cysts

Pleural Diseases
- Pneumothorax
- Hemothorax
- Pleural effusion, empyema
- Fibrothorax

Chest-Wall Diseases
- Injury
- Kyphoscoliosis
- Spondylitis
- Neuromuscular disease

Extrathoracic Conditions
- Obesity
- Peritonitis
- Ascites
- Pregnancy

Source: Adapted from Welch MH: Ventilatory function of the lungs. *In* Guenter CA, Welch MH (eds): Pulmonary Medicine. Philadelphia, JB Lippincott, 1977, pp. 72–123.

APPLICATIONS OF PULMONARY FUNCTION TESTS

PATTERNS OF RESPONSE

Pulmonary Vascular Obstruction

- Any patient who has dyspnea during exertion without evidence of obstructive or restrictive ventilatory defects deserves detailed pulmonary function studies of the pulmonary circulation.
- These studies should include exercise tests, especially when signs of pulmonary hypertension are absent and roentgenologic methods fail to demonstrate obstruction of large pulmonary arteries. (See Chapter 4, Radiography and Imaging, and Chapter 5, Nuclear Medicine Techniques and Applications.)
- Measurements of V_D/V_T may be normal at rest but increased during exercise, indicating ventilated but poorly perfused regions of lung.
- The diagnosis of pulmonary vascular obstruction may be made by V_D/V_T measurements during exercise, provided that no $\dot{V}_A/\dot{Q}_C$ abnormalities exist as a result of restrictive or obstructive ventilatory defects.
- Pulmonary vascular obstruction may cause abnormalities in V_D/V_T only during exercise for several reasons: poorly perfused regions may be poorly ventilated at rest, but ventilation may increase during exercise if deep breaths overcome smooth muscle constriction in peripheral airways.[346, 347]
    - At rest, bronchial blood flow may maintain normal carbon dioxide output from a poorly perfused region; during exercise, the collateral blood flow may not increase proportionately to ventilation.
    - If poorly ventilated regions are perfused by narrowed but not occluded arteries, these vessels may carry a smaller percentage of total flow during exercise than at rest.
    - Finally, inhalation of dead space gas containing CO_2 will increase P_{CO_2} in nonperfused alveoli; during exercise, increased V_T will dilute dead space gas more than at rest and the effect of the dead space gas will diminish during exercise.
- Acid-base status should be studied because patients with pulmonary vascular obstruction appear to have an abnormal drive to ventilation, resulting in rapid, shallow breathing and alveolar hyperventilation at rest and during exercise.
    - This results in decreased arterial P_{CO_2} and partially compensated respiratory alkalosis.
- Arterial P_{O_2} should be studied to determine whether O_2 transfer is impaired (TABLE 8–12); in many patients with pulmonary vascular obstruction, arterial P_{O_2} may be normal at rest but decreased during exercise (cases 3 and 9 in TABLE 8–12).
    - Breathing pure O_2 will demonstrate the presence of a right-to-left shunt, which is often dependent on posture (cases 3, 6, 9, 10) or exercise (cases 1, 9, 10, 11).
    - The shunt tends to increase under conditions that increase right-sided pressures relative to left-sided pressures, as occurs during increased venous return during exercise, or in the supine posture or at high vs. low lung volumes (cases 1, 3, 5, 6, 9, 10, 11 in TABLE 8–12).
- Confirmation of the results of these studies should be obtained by measuring pulmonary artery pressures and blood flow at rest and during exercise, and visualization of the vascular lesions by high-speed spiral CT, magnetic resonance imaging (MRI), or possibly angiography.
- In some cases, lung biopsy may be indicated to make a specific etiologic diagnosis and to choose the appropriate therapy.
- Because the response to exercise also depends on the patient's effort and cooperation, as well as possible underlying anatomic and functional disorders, the physician must assess the observed response in the context of the patient's subjective complaints, the severity of the exercise study, and evidence indicating that patient performed with maximal effort and cooperation.[29, 172, 348]

APPLICATIONS OF PULMONARY FUNCTION TESTS

PATTERNS OF RESPONSE

Pulmonary Vascular Obstruction

TABLE 8-12

Effects of Exercise, Respiratory Maneuvers, and Posture on Arterial Po_2(mm Hg) During Inhalation of Pure O_2

Case No.	Sitting				Supine	
	Rest	Slow Maximal Inspiration	Slow Maximal Expiration	Exercise	Rest	Slow Maximal Inspiration
1	410	370	512	122		
3	615 (105)	620	605	605 (83)	490	375
5	410	240		480	440	
7	389				487 (58)	384
9	572	395	463	96	520	
10	426 (72)			130	330 (62)	
11	350	120	390	180		

Notes: Case 1, patent foramen ovale; case 3, abnormal pleural-pulmonary vessels; cases 5 and 11, no shunt at cardiac catheterization; case 7, no abnormal pleural-pulmonary vessels; case 9, Po_2 is 73 mm Hg during exercise while supine, breathing pure oxygen; case 10, orthopnea relieved by breathing O_2 or sitting up. Numbers in parentheses indicate arterial Po_2 during inhalation of room air.

Poor Cooperation Pattern

- Pulmonary function tests in general depend heavily on the cooperation of the subject being tested.
- If a competent technician performs the procedures and recordings of the test tracings accompany the measurements, it is usually possible to determine the validity of the data in most cases.
- In some instances, particularly in compensation cases, the pulmonary function tests must be carried out only as part of a complete clinical evaluation, and the test results must be observed by the physician involved.
- Nevertheless, poor patient cooperation can usually be identified on the basis of the features listed in TABLE 8–13.
- The VC is decreased and does not show a smooth curve, reaching a maximum value asymptotically; it is often accompanied by relatively normal expiratory airflow, increased FEV_1/FVC ratio, and decreased MVV.
- Supplemental data confirming invalid test results include uneven, slurred, or notched curves on inspection; poor reproducibility on repeated testing; and decreased Pstl.
- A valid restrictive pattern differs from a test with poor effort in being reproducible and showing smooth expiratory curves on direct examination, increased lung elastic recoil (Pstl), and a normal or nearly normal MVV.

APPLICATIONS OF PULMONARY FUNCTION TESTS

PATTERNS OF RESPONSE

TABLE 8–13

Poor Cooperation

Characteristics of Poor Cooperation	Supplementary Results Confirming Pattern
Decreased VC	• Decreased TLC
Relatively normal expiratory airflows (increased FEV_1/FVC ratio)	• Decreased maximal Pstl
Decreased MVV	• Uneven, slurred, irregular recording of spirograms • Lack of reproducibility

Source: Adapted from Welch MH: Ventilatory function of the lungs. *In* Guenter CA, Welch MH (eds): Pulmonary Medicine. Philadelphia, JB Lippincott, 1977, pp. 72–123.

HIV-Related Pneumonia

- *Pneumocystis carinii* pneumonia (PCP) is a major pulmonary complication of HIV-related infections.
- Early diagnosis is important to successful treatment. (See Chapter 6, Bronchoscopy.)
- Chest roentgenograms, arterial blood gas measurements, gallium scans, exercise tests, and pulmonary function tests (including single-breath DL_{CO}) have all been used as screening tests. (See Chapter 5, Nuclear Medicine Techniques and Applications.)
- Chest roentgenograms, and arterial blood gas measurements are insensitive and nonspecific.
- Gallium scans are expensive, inconvenient, and nonspecific; involve a substantial delay in obtaining results; and involve radiation exposure.
- A value for DL_{CO} of less than 80% of predicted normal may be used as a screening test for PCP.
    - The use of DL_{CO} as a screening test is not without its disadvantages: It is expensive, requires special facilities, and requires specially trained individuals to perform and interpret the test. The test has a sensitivity of 98%,[349] but has a specificity as low as 26%.[350]
    - The poor specificity of the DL_{CO} has led to confusion about its significance.
- Ognibene and coworkers studied 24 asymptomatic HIV-seropositive patients and did not find any evidence of *Pneumocystis* infection by bronchoalveolar lavage or transbronchial biopsy, but 47% of the patients studied had diffuse interstitial pneumonitis.[351]
- This author studied 136 asymptomatic patients at UCSF prior to beginning inhaled pentamidine.
    - They were screened with a DL_{CO} test to detect occult pulmonary infections prior to instituting prophylactic PCP therapy: 46% of these patients had a decreased DL_{CO} and 13% of the patients with a decreased DL_{CO} had PCP; however, evidence of diffuse interstitial pneumonitis was not found.
    - The decreased DL_{CO} in the remaining patients may be due to an emphysema-like pulmonary disease that has been associated with HIV infection,[352] microembolization secondary to intravenous drug use, Kaposi's sarcoma, cytomegalovirus pneumonia, or other less common pathologies.
- The incidence of asymptomatic PCP, emphysema-like pulmonary disease, microembolization, and the other less common causes of a low DL_{CO} in an asymptomatic HIV-positive population have not been determined.
- A change in the alveolar-arterial oxygen pressure ($D(A - a)O_2$) or O_2 saturation during exercise has been suggested as a screening test for PCP, but neither has been standardized or studied in a prospective fashion.[353, 354]
- Several investigators have used pulse oximetry to detect O_2 desaturation during exercise to screen for PCP. These results suggest that the sensitivity and specificity of pulse oximetry during exercise may be increased above 80% if the work rate is increased sufficiently.[355, 356]

APPLICATIONS OF PULMONARY FUNCTION TESTS

PATTERNS OF RESPONSE

Obesity

General Pattern

Obesity may affect the results of studies. It

- Increases the risk from anesthesia and surgical procedures, especially involving the upper abdomen and thorax.
- Increases the work of breathing in pulmonary patients.
- Increases symptoms and adverse physiologic consequences of airway obstruction.
- Often is associated with sleep disorders and impaired regulation of ventilation.
- Limits exercise tolerance and makes physical conditioning more difficult to attain and maintain.

Physiologic Effects

- Increased mass of chest wall and abdominal wall and contents results in decreased outward recoil of the chest wall and increased pressure within the abdomen.
- Fatty infiltration of respiratory muscles may decrease maximum respiratory pressures, aggravate the abnormal lung volumes, and inhibit the capacity to respond to the increased work of breathing.
- ERV and FRC are decreased, especially when the obese subject is recumbent.[357, 358]
- The single-breath N_2 washout test is abnormally increased, and perfusion is increased to poorly ventilated, dependent lung zones at the bases.[359] This results in airway closure, often at lung volumes greater than FRC with associated arterial hypoxemia.[360]
- DL_{CO} is often increased and associated with increased red blood cell mass, cardiac output, and central blood volume.[361]
- Ventilatory response to CO_2 is often reduced; in some subjects, ventilatory response to both hypoxia and hypercapnia is reduced.[362]
- Obese patients with obstructive ventilatory defects usually have increased symptoms relative to the severity of the airway obstruction because they must breathe at low lung volumes at which airflow resistance is increased (TABLE 8–14). (See earlier section on Exercise for discussion of response to exercise in obesity.)

APPLICATIONS OF PULMONARY FUNCTION TESTS

PATTERNS OF RESPONSE

Obesity

Physiologic Effects

TABLE 8–14

Effects of Mild Obesity on Lung Function

	Grade 0	Grade I	Grade II
BMI*	20–24.9	25–29.9	30–40
Pack-years	29 (1–82)†	26 (1–123)†	27 (3–90)†
FRC (L)	3.45 ± 0.71‡	3.17 ± 0.69‡	2.66 ± 0.74‡
ERV (L)	1.10 ± 0.50	0.77 ± 0.37	0.59 ± 0.34
RV (L)	2.32 ± 0.48	2.36 ± 0.52	2.13 ± 0.54
TLC (L)	6.74 ± 0.97	6.58 ± 1.02	6.33 ± 0.91
FEV_1 (L)	3.15 ± 0.68	2.91 ± 0.56	3.14 ± 0.49
FVC (L)	4.12 ± 0.17	3.84 ± 0.71	3.94 ± 0.69
PEF (L/min)	456 ± 104	458 ± 98	470 ± 100

* Body mass index is the weight (in kilograms) divided by height (in meters) squared.

† Median ± range.

‡ Mean ± SD.

Source: Modified from Jenkins SC, Moxham J: The effects of mild obesity on lung function. Respir Med 85:309–311, 1991.

Aging Lung

Routine Test Results

- Older individuals tend to exhibit a decrease in maximal lung elastic recoil pressure and a displacement of the recoil curve up and to the left. There is also an increased index of curvature (K) in the exponential expression of lung elastic recoil (see earlier discussion of lung elastic recoil, reflecting increased alveolar size).[95, 363] Morphologic studies confirm increased alveolar dimensions with age.
- Effect of age on airflow rates depends on whether the data is based on cross-sectional studies or longitudinal studies. In longitudinal studies:
  - Progressive decline in FVC and FEV_1 did not begin until mid-30's and then FEV_1/FVC decreased linearly with age, independent of FVC, and was similar in men and women, and much less severe than that described in cross-sectional studies.[364]
  - Maximal flow decreased, but no change in lung elastic recoil pressure or airway resistance occurred with age, suggesting that age increased airway collapsibility.[365]
- RV and closing volume increase whereas VC decreases,[366, 367] suggesting that lung emptying is limited with increasing age because of airway closure (see earlier discussion of RV).
- MVV decreases about 30%, probably as a consequence of decreased maximal respiratory pressures, decreased distensibility of the total respiratory system, decreased lung elastic recoil, and impaired coordination of the respiratory system.
- Phase IV (closing volume) increases with age.

(continued)

APPLICATIONS OF PULMONARY FUNCTION TESTS

PATTERNS OF RESPONSE

The Aging Lung

Routine Test Results

- Arterial P_{CO_2} does not change with age, but arterial P_{O_2} declines[368] and the alveolar-arterial P_{O_2} differences widen[369] with age, probably reflecting increased closing volume relative to ERV.
- DL_{CO} decreases because DM decreases after 40 years of age; Vc is maintained until the seventh decade, and then decreases rapidly. This finding is consistent with morphologic studies of the aging lung, namely a decrease in alveolar surface area and capillary bed.[370]

Exercise

- Maximum O_2 uptake decreases after 40 years of age, by about 5 to 10% per decade.
- Because the anaerobic threshold is maintained with age, even elderly individuals are able to walk on the level, or even uphill, without developing metabolic acidosis; aerobic exercise training results in a significant improvement in maximal O_2 uptake.[371, 372]
- Limitations of maximal exercise capacity with age appear to result from a decrease in maximal cardiac output resulting from a decrease in maximal heart rate and decrease in stroke volume with age. The decline in stroke volume may be minimized by vigorous training, but the decline in maximal heart rate with age cannot.
- The difference between arterial and venous O_2 levels does not change with age, suggesting that the metabolic capacity of the skeletal muscles can be maintained by aerobic exercise.[373]
- Some elderly persons complain of limited exercise capacity because of dyspnea of unknown cause.
  - Dyspnea may be related to decreased maximal respiratory pressures with age[374] or to excessive ventilation relative to O_2 uptake.
  - The latter finding may be due to increased dead space[375] with age because the tracheal diameter increases,[376] and a marked increase in ventilation occurs when the anaerobic threshold is exceeded.
  - Nevertheless, aerobic exercise training increases maximal O_2 uptake by almost 30%, even in sedentary individuals.[377]

Abnormal Respiratory Muscle Function

General

- Abnormal function of respiratory muscle may be a cause of unexplained dyspnea or respiratory failure.
- Inspiratory muscles may become fatigued and fail to contract adequately despite effective neural stimulation.
- If the cause is not detected and treated adequately, respiratory failure may result.
- This problem may develop in patients with obstructive or restrictive ventilatory defects, neuromuscular disorders such as myasthenia gravis, cardiogenic shock, or sepsis.[27, 378–387]

Maximum Negative Airway Pressure

- Maximum negative airway pressure (PM_{max}) is generated by an inspiratory effort against an occluded airway.
- In this test, the subject inspires maximally from RV against an obstructed mouthpiece with a small leak (1 mm in diameter) to prevent closure of the glottis or development of pressure above the glottis by the muscles of the cheeks.
- A plateau pressure should be maintained for at least 1 second.
- Reproducible maximal values are difficult to obtain; the coefficient of variation is about 9% for duplicate tests for MIP and MEP.[374]

APPLICATIONS OF PULMONARY FUNCTION TESTS

PATTERNS OF RESPONSE

Abnormal Respiratory Muscle Function

Transdiaphragmatic Pressure

- Transdiaphragmatic pressure (Pdi_{max}) is determined by measuring the difference between intragastric and esophageal pressures during the same maneuver.
  - Pdi_{max} is measured at RV because PM_{max} is reduced at larger lung volumes.
  - Conversely, maximal expiratory pressures are greatest at TLC.
  - Because it is difficult to obtain cooperation from the patients to breathe to RV, PM_{max} and Pdi_{max} are often measured at FRC (which probably accounts in part for the reported variability).
- Healthy persons can sustain respiratory patterns requiring 40% of Pdi_{max} for long periods without fatigue.
- When a patient must increase Pdi/Pdi_{max} ratio to overcome a resistive load, endurance decreases in proportion to the resistive load (FIGURE 8–49).
- Normal subjects can inspire with varying degrees of diaphragm and rib cage contraction; thus, Pdi_{max} may be decreased because of marked recruitment of the rib cage during the test.
  - The range reported is accordingly large: 18 to 137 cm H_2O.
  - Training results in improved coordination and reproducible values with a coefficient of variation of 19%.[388]

FIGURE 8–49

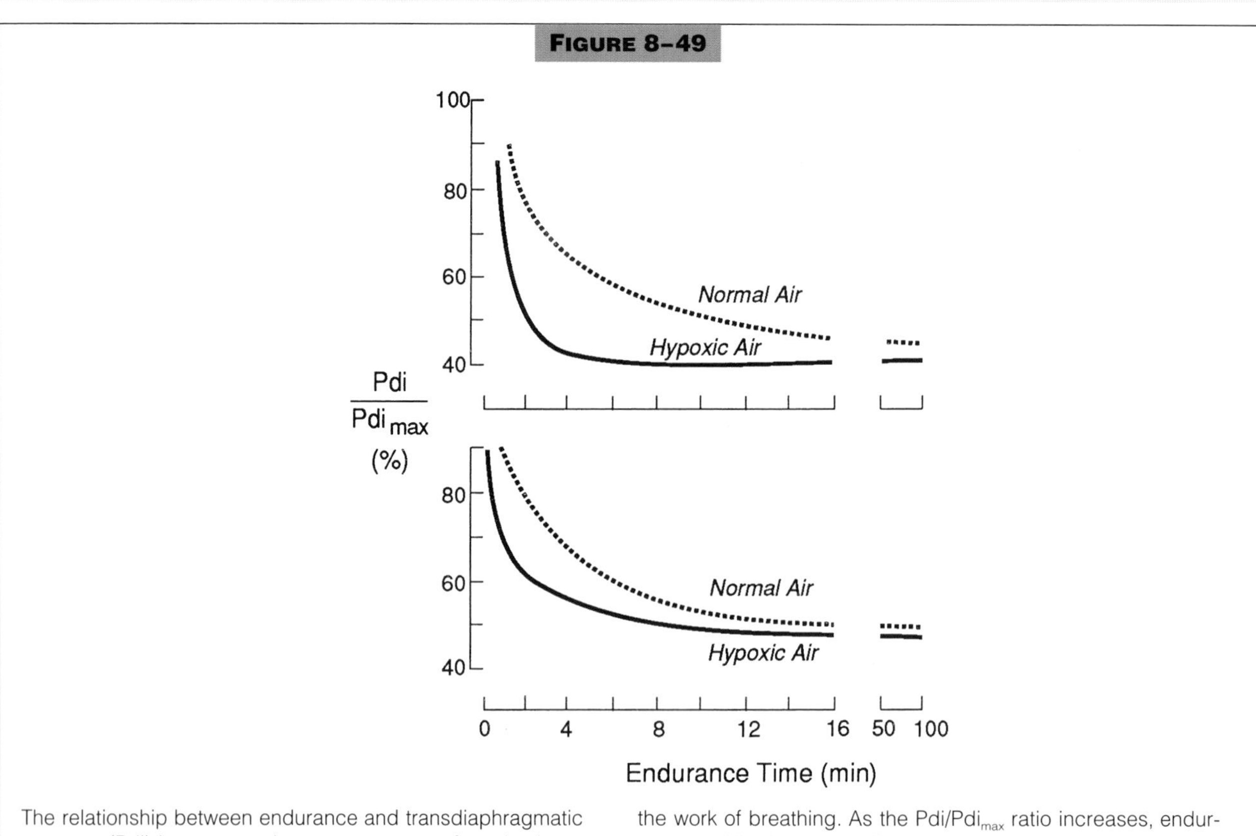

The relationship between endurance and transdiaphragmatic pressure (Pdi) is expressed as a percentage of maximal transdiaphragmatic pressure (Pdi_{max}). Data from two patients breathing normal and hypoxic air are shown. Added airway resistance leads to an increased Pdi/Pdi_{max} ratio and increases the work of breathing. As the Pdi/Pdi_{max} ratio increases, endurance rapidly decreases. This effect is more pronounced when the respiratory muscles are made hypoxic. (Modified after Roussos CS, Macklem PT: Diaphragmatic fatigue in man. J Appl Physiol 43:189–197, 1977.)

APPLICATIONS OF PULMONARY FUNCTION TESTS

PATTERNS OF RESPONSE

Abnormal Respiratory Muscle Function

Cervical Magnetic Stimulation

- Cervical magnetic stimulation (CMS) is a method of phrenic nerve stimulation.[389]
- Similowski and associates reported the results of comparisons of stimulated Pdi (Pdi_{stim}) with the maximal Pdi obtained during static combined expulsive Mueller maneuver (Pdi_{max}) and with the Pdi generated during a sniff test (Pdi_{sniff}). These values are comparable to those obtained in other studies with transcutaneous phrenic nerve stimulation.
- Subsequently, however, other studies showed that CMS stimulated many muscles of the upper thoracic cage as well as the diaphragm.[390, 391]
- Although initially promising, these studies have demonstrated difficulty in obtaining surface signals of acceptable quality.
- The variable shape and latency of the action potential induced by magnetic stimulation plus the shorter phrenic nerve conduction times with CMS compared with phrenic nerve stimulation indicate that diaphragm EMG after CMS is potentially unreliable, perhaps because chest wall electrodes also record electrical activity from other muscles.

Maximal Voluntary Ventilation

- Maximal voluntary ventilation (MVV) is used to assess muscle strength and endurance.
- Endurance decreases as $\dot{V}E$/MVV increases in a pattern similar to that observed with increasing Pdi/Pdi_{max} ratio.
- In the absence of an external resistance, the largest ventilation that can be sustained more than 15 minutes is about 60% of the MVV.

Diaphragmatic Electromyograph

- The diaphragmatic electromyograph is used to evaluate respiratory muscle strength and endurance.
- Changes in respiratory muscle electrical activity appear to reflect closely other aspects of muscle contraction.
  - Normally, the phrenic nerve stimulates the diaphragm at a mixture of frequencies between 20 and 400 Hz.
  - A graphic display of EMG signal strength against frequency is called the "power spectrum."
- When the power spectrum is analyzed over two limited frequency ranges (below 50 Hz and above 150 Hz), it shifts to the low-frequency range as the diaphragm fatigues. This change precedes failure of contraction, and therefore may be useful to predict decompensation of the respiratory muscle.
- Phrenic nerve conduction time may also be used to assess diaphragmatic paralysis or weakness. With recording electrodes placed over the rib cage above the diaphragm, the phrenic nerve is stimulated in the neck: normal conduction time is 7.7 ± 0.8 msec.

Fluoroscopy

- Fluoroscopy is used to evaluate diaphragmatic function.
- Decreased excursion should be evaluated with a lateral view using the "sniff test."
- Decreased excursion alone is nonspecific, but decreased excursion associated with paradoxical motion during the "sniff test" is very specific.
- False negative findings may occur during spontaneous breathing caused by contraction of abdominal muscles during exhalation, producing downward motion of the diaphragm when the abdominal muscles relax at the beginning of inspiration.
- False positive tests can be produced by paradoxical motion limited to the anterior portion of the diaphragm.

APPLICATIONS OF PULMONARY FUNCTION TESTS

PATTERNS OF RESPONSE

Abnormal Respiratory Muscle Function

Respiratory Muscle Failure

- *Increased work of breathing:* Higher airflow resistance or greater elastic recoil of lung or chest wall may increase the work of breathing and energy required of the respiratory muscles.
- *Decreased energy supply:*
  - Reduction in the supply of vital metabolic substrates may limit the efficiency of respiratory muscles under certain circumstances.
  - Reduction in cardiac output, arterial O_2 content, or extraction of O_2 from the blood may impair aerobic metabolism and compromise respiratory muscle function.
  - Decreased O_2 delivery may be critically important under conditions that increase respiratory work. O_2 consumption by respiratory muscles may rise 25-fold above baseline under conditions of high $\dot{V}_E$ and increased airway resistance, and may exceed supply.
  - Forceful muscle contraction alone impedes blood flow to respiratory muscles in animals breathing against increased respiratory workloads.
  - Other variables related to metabolism (e.g., hypercapnia, malnutrition, acidosis, electrolyte disorders) may also limit endurance.
- *Decreased muscular efficiency:*
  - The number and mix of fiber types determine inspiratory reserve.
  - Disease processes and training may alter the number and relative proportions of fibers in the diaphragm.
  - Under certain conditions, changes in the mix of fiber types or the loss of fibers may play an important role in the development or maintenance of respiratory failure.
  - For example, atrophy of all muscle fibers is a potentially important problem in patients undergoing long-term mechanical ventilation.[379]

Muscular Efficiency

- Muscular efficiency depends on mechanical factors as well as on structure.
  - The position and configuration of the diaphragm at the beginning of inspiration reflect resting muscle fiber length.
  - As FRC increases, the contour of the diaphragm flattens, and muscle fibers are not stretched to their optimal length.
  - Acute air-trapping (as in asthma) may cause a mechanical disadvantage of the diaphragm by fiber shortening, but when hyperinflation persists, the resting length of individual muscle fibers may return toward normal.
- Hyperinflation also causes mechanical disadvantage by flattening the diaphragm.
  - The Pdi_{max} is determined by the radius of curvature of the diaphragm at any value of muscle tension (Laplace's law).
  - Increasing the radius of curvature of the diaphragm greatly reduces its capacity to develop Pdi and change lung volume.
- Although abdominal muscles are usually regarded as expiratory, abdominal muscle tone may be needed to maintain the mechanical advantage of the diaphragm; thus, flaccidity of abdominal muscles contributes to the inefficient ventilation seen in paraplegic patients, especially when these patients are in upright positions.
- VC is a useful test of respiratory muscle weakness because normally a small fraction of the muscle strength is required to inflate the lung.
  - Furthermore, the curvilinear relationship between pressure and volume results in the fact that a greater loss of muscle strength (pressure) is required to produce a loss of volume.
  - Although MIP may be reduced markedly before a loss in lung volume, most patients with respiratory muscle weakness have decreased VC and decreased lung compliance.
- Decreased lung compliance is thought to result from atelectasis which may be detectable by chest roentgenograms.
- FRC, IC, ERV, and TLC may also be decreased associated with decreased lung elastic recoil; these changes are suggestive of decreased outward recoil of the chest wall.

APPLICATIONS OF PULMONARY FUNCTION TESTS

INFECTION CONTROL AND SAFETY

General

(See Chapter 7, Laboratory Diagnosis of Respiratory Tract Infections)

Patients with communicable infectious diseases present a potential risk to the technical and administrative staff of the pulmonary function laboratory, as well as to other patients who may be in the laboratory for studies at the same time.

Tuberculosis

- Pulmonary laboratory directors are familiar with the risk of spreading tuberculosis by aerosols produced by sputum-positive patients who cough and do not follow accepted precautions.
- There has also been the more theoretical possibility of transmitting tuberculosis from one patient to another via infected secretions, which may contaminate pulmonary function equipment.

Immunosuppressed Patients

Increasing numbers of immunosuppressed patients in cancer treatment and transplant programs have raised the possibility of increased risk of transmission of infection to such patients.

HIV Infection Protocol

- The administrative assistant responsible for the schedule makes certain the requisition is completed, which screens for possible HIV, tuberculosis, and other possible infectious diseases.
- When the patient arrives at the laboratory, the technicians check for possible communicable infectious diseases on the requisition, the medical record, and the questionnaire completed by the patient. If the screening protocol is negative, studies are performed.
- All patients are studied with the same equipment using a new sterile mouthpiece and filter that traps particles 0.2 μm in diameter and does not affect the results of physiologic tests.
- It is assumed that infectious particles, whether bacterial, fungal, parasite, or virus, will be carried in respiratory secretions of such a large size that all of them will be trapped by these filters.
- These assumptions are reinforced by this author's record of no infectious diseases transmitted from his equipment.
- The assumptions are also reinforced by the CDC that has not reported transmission of HIV or hepatitis virus via pulmonary function equipment.

Alternative HIV Protocol

- Careful screening of patients prior to testing is mandatory.
- Use disposable mouthpieces, discarded after single patient use, or use rubber mouthpieces that are changed between each patient and cleaned with high-level disinfection.
- Change external spirometer tubing between patients with high-level disinfection and drying of the tubing between each use.
- Change nose clips between each patient and discard or clean with high-level disinfection.
- Change water in water-sealed spirometers at least monthly.
- Technicians must wash hands thoroughly before and after pulmonary function testing and use gloves when blood samples are to be collected.

APPLICATIONS OF PULMONARY FUNCTION TESTS

SUMMARY

Respiratory Processes

- As mixed venous blood passes through the pulmonary circulation, a complex sequence of changes ensures that adequate amounts of O_2 are added and proper amounts of CO_2 are eliminated.
- Active movement of gas molecules proceeds from the atmosphere into the lungs and this fresh air is distributed to perfused airspaces (*ventilation*).
- Passive movement of O_2 and CO_2 molecules between the inspired gas and the mixed venous blood occurs at sites of gas exchange (*diffusion*).
- Venous blood moves into the lungs and is distributed to the sites of gas exchange (*blood flow*).
- Ventilation is regulated to meet the metabolic demands and voluntary needs of the individual (*regulation of ventilation*).

Physiologic Tests

- The accurate and precise measurement of these complex respiratory processes requires a large number of different physiologic tests.
- No single pulmonary function test provides all the information desired in any single subject.
- Nor are all these tests required in the management of each patient.
- Some tests are very simple and may be carried out in a small clinic or physician's office.
- Others require considerable technical experience, expensive apparatus, and usually are carried out in a hospital cardiopulmonary laboratory; still others are research procedures and are presently available only in a few major medical centers.
- Some tests (such as spirograms and flow-volume curves) should be performed on every patient with known or suspected cardiopulmonary disease just as measurement of blood pressure, urinalysis, and determination of hemoglobin are performed routinely on all patients.
- Pulmonary function tests are now an essential part of clinical practice as are tests of any other organ system.
- These tests have not supplanted other diagnostic procedures.
- They indicate only how disease has altered function.
- They cannot make a specific pathologic diagnosis.
- They reveal alterations only when the lesion disturbs function sufficiently so that presently available tests can detect with certainty the deviation from normal values.
- Pulmonary function tests will not even determine the existence of a lesion if it does not interfere with the function of the lung.
- Pulmonary function tests supplement but do not replace a good history and physical examination or radiologic, bacteriologic, bronchoscopic, and pathologic studies.
- This chapter reviews the physiologic concepts involved in each component of pulmonary function, the commonly used tests of each component, and examples of the clinical applications of the tests alone and in combination.

REFERENCES

1. Jones NL, Jones J, Edwards RHT: Exercise tolerance in chronic airway obstruction. Am Rev Respir Dis 103:477–491, 1971.

2. Pontoppidan H, Geffin B, Lowenstein E: Acute respiratory failure in the adult. N Engl J Med 287:690–698, 1972.

3. Gardner RM, Baker CD, Broennle AMJ, et al: ATS Statement—Snowbird workshop on standardization of spirometry. Am Rev Respir Dis 119:831–838, 1979.

4. Schoenberg JB, Beck GJ, Bouhuys A: Growth and decay of pulmonary function in healthy blacks and whites. Respir Physiol 33:367–393, 1978.

5. Knudson RJ, Slatin RC, Lebowitz MD, Burrows B: The maximal expiratory flow-volume curve: Normal standards, variability and effects of age. Am Rev Respir Dis 113:587–600, 1976.

6. Crapo RO, Morris AH, Gardner RM: Reference spirometric values using techniques and equipment that meet ATS recommendations. Am Rev Respir Dis 123:859–864, 1981.

REFERENCES

7. Morris JF, Koski A, Johnson LC: Spirometric standards for healthy nonsmoking adults. Am Rev Respir Dis 103:57–67, 1971.

8. DaCosta JL: Pulmonary function studies in healthy Chinese adults in Singapore. Am Rev Respir Dis 104:128–131, 1971.

9. Vestbo J, Knudsen K, Rasmussen F: Predictive value of the single-breath nitrogen test for hospitalization due to respiratory disease. Lung 168:93–101, 1990.

10. Marazzini L, Cavigioli G, Mastropasqua B, Pelucchi A: FEV_1 decline in asymptomatic young adults: Relationships with some tests of small airways function. Eur Respir J 2:817–821, 1989.

11. Pride N: Assessment of long-term changes in airway function. Agents Actions 30:21–34, 1990.

12. Jayr C, Matthay MA, Lampe G, et al: Preoperative hypoxemia is a reasonable predictor of severe post-operative pulmonary complications in patients undergoing major abdominal surgery. Am Rev Respir Dis 139:A151, 1989.

13. Burrows B, Huang N, Hughes R, et al: Terms and Symbols. A report of the ACCP-ATS Joint Committee on Pulmonary Nomenclature. Chest 67:583–598, 1975.

14. Kory RC: Clinical spirometry: Recommendation of the Section on Pulmonary Function Testing, Committee on Pulmonary Physiology, American College of Chest Physicians. Dis Chest 43:214–219, 1963.

15. Morris JF, Temple WP, Koski A: Normal values for the ratio of one-second forced expiratory volume to forced vital capacity. Am Rev Respir Dis 108:1000–1003, 1973.

16. McFadden ERJ, Linden DA: A reduction in maximum mid-expiratory flow rate. A spirographic manifestation of small airway disease. Am J Med 52:725–737, 1972.

17. Cosio M, Ghezzo H, Hogg JC, et al: The relations between structural changes in small airways and pulmonary-function tests. N Engl J Med 298:1277–1281, 1978.

18. Hyatt RE: Dynamic lung volumes. *In* Fenn WO, Rahn HS (eds): Handbook of Physiology: A Critical, Comprehensive Presentation of Physiological Knowledge and Concepts. Vol. 1. Washington, DC, American Physiological Society, 1955, pp. 1381–1397.

19. Mead J, Tumer JM, Macklem PT, Little JB: Significance of the relationship between lung recoil and maximum expiratory flow. J Appl Physiol 22:95–108, 1967.

20. Pride NB, Permutt S, Riley RL, Bromberger-Barnea B: Determinants of maximal expiratory flow from the lungs. J Appl Physiol 23:646–662, 1967.

21. McCarthy DS, Craig DB, Cherniak RM: Intraindividual variability in maximal expiratory flow-volume and closing volume in asymptomatic subjects. Am Rev Respir Dis 112:407–411, 1975.

22. Cochrane GM, Prieto F, Clark TJ: Intrasubject variability of maximal expiratory flow volume curve. Thorax 32: 171–176, 1977.

23. Wright BM, McKerrow CB: Maximum forced expiratory flow rate as a measure of ventilatory capacity: With a description of a new portable instrument for measuring it. Br J Med 5159:1041–1046, 1959.

24. Ferris BG: Epidemiology: Standardization project. Am Rev Respir Dis 118:1–120, 1978.

25. Gaensler EA, Wright GW: Evaluation of respiratory impairment. Arch Environ Health 12:146–189, 1966.

26. Rochester DF, Arora NS, Braun NMT, Goldberg SK: The respiratory muscles in chronic obstructive pulmonary disease (COPD). Bull Eur Physiopathol Respir 15:951–975, 1979.

27. Derenne J-PH, Macklem IT, Roussos CS: State of the art: The respiratory muscles: Mechanics, control, and pathophysiology. Part 1. Am Rev Respir Dis 118:119–133, 1978.

28. Comroe JHJ, Todd J, Gammon DD, et al: The effect of DFP upon patients with myasthenia gravis. Am J Med Sci 212:641–651, 1946.

29. Gelb AF, Gold WM, Wright RR, et al: Physiologic diagnosis of subclinical emphysema. Am Rev Respir Dis 107:50–63, 1973.

30. Berend N, Thurlbeck WM: Correlations of maximum expiratory flow with small airway dimensions and pathology. J Appl Physiol 52:346–351, 1982.

31. Berend N, Wright JL, Thurlbeck WM, et al: Small airways disease: Reproducibility of measurements and correlation with lung function. Chest 79:263–268, 1981.

32. Niewoehner DE, Knoke JD, Kleinerman J: Peripheral airways as a determinant of ventilatory function in the human lung. J Clin Invest 60:139–151, 1977.

33. Petty TL, Silvers GW, Stanford RE, et al: Small airway pathology is related to increased closing capacity and abnormal slope of phase III in excised human lungs. Am Rev Respir Dis 121:449–456, 1980.

34. Petty TL, Silvers GW, Stanford RE: Functional correlations with mild and moderate emphysema in excised lungs. Am Rev Respir Dis 124:700–704, 1981.

35. Knudson RJ, Burrows B, Lebowitz MD: The maximal expiratory flow-volume curve: Its use in the detection of ventilatory abnormalities in a population study. Am Rev Respir Dis 114:871–879, 1976.

36. Knudson RJ, Lebowitz MD, Holberg CJ, Burrows B: Changes in the normal maximal expiratory flow-volume curve with growth and aging. Am Rev Respir Dis 127:725–734, 1983.

REFERENCES

37. Miller RD, Hyatt RE: Evaluation of obstructing lesions of the trachea and larynx by flow-volume loops. Am Rev Respir Dis 108:475–481, 1973.

38. Despas PJ, Leroux M, Macklem PT: Site of airway obstruction in asthma as determined by measuring maximal expiratory flow breathing air and a helium-oxygen mixture. J Clin Invest 51:3235–3243, 1972.

39. Hutcheon M, Griffin P, Levison H, Zamel N: Volume of isoflow. A new test in detection of mild abnormalities of lung mechanics. Am Rev Respir Dis 110:458–465, 1974.

40. Lam S, Abboud RT, Chan-Yeung M, Tan F: Use of maximal expiratory flow-volume curves with air and helium-oxygen in the detection of ventilatory abnormalities in population surveys. Am Rev Respir Dis 123:234–237, 1981.

41. Li K-YR, Tan LT-K, Chong P, Dosman JA: Between-technician variation in the measurement of spirometry with air and helium. Am Rev Respir Dis 124:196–198, 1981.

42. Meadows JAI, Rodarte JR, Hyatt RE: Density dependence of maximal expiratory flow in chronic obstructive pulmonary disease. Am Rev Respir Dis 121:47–53, 1980.

43. Pappenheimer J, Comroe JHJ, Cournand A, et al: Standardization of definitions and symbols in respiratory physiology. Fed Proc 9:602–605, 1950.

44. Darling RC, Cournand A, Richards DWJ: Studies on the intrapulmonary mixture of gases: III. An open circuit method for measuring residual air. J Clin Invest 19:609–618, 1940.

45. Fleming GM, Chester EH, Sanlie J, Saidel GM: Ventilation in homogeneity using multibreath nitrogen washout: Comparison of moment ratios and other indexes. Am Rev Respir Dis 121:789–794, 1980.

46. Light RW, George RB, Meneely GR, et al: New method for analyzing multiple-breath nitrogen washout curves. J Appl Physiol 48:265–272, 1980.

47. Lewis SM, Evans JW, Japowayski AA: Continuous distributions of specific ventilation recovered from inert gas washout. J Appl Physiol 44:416–423, 1978.

48. Zelkowitz PS, Giammona ST: Cystic fibrosis. Pulmonary studies in children, adolescents, and young adults. Am J Dis Child 117:543–547, 1969.

49. Bouhuys A: Pulmonary nitrogen clearance in relation to age in healthy males. J Appl Physiol 18:297–300, 1963.

50. Turney ZS, Blumenfeld W: Heated Fleisch pneumotachometer: A calibration procedure. J Appl Physiol 34: 117–121, 1973.

51. von der Hardt H, Zywietz C: Reliability in pneumotachographic measurements. Respiration 33:416–424, 1976.

52. Schaanning CG, Gulsvik A: Accuracy and precision of helium dilution technique and body plethysmography in measuring lung volumes. Scand J Clin Lab Invest 32:271–277, 1973.

53. Meneely GR, Ball CO, Kory RC, et al: A simplified closed circuit helium dilution method for the determination of the residual volume of the lungs. Am J Med 28: 824–831, 1960.

54. Holmgren A: Determination of the functional residual volume by means of the helium dilution method. Scand J Clin Lab Invest 6:131–136, 1954.

55. Boren HG, Kory RC, Syner JC: The Veteran's Administratio–Army cooperative study of pulmonary function. II. The lung volume and its subdivisions in normal man. Am J Med 41:96–114, 1966.

56. Goldman H, Becklake M: Respiratory function tests. Normal values at median altitudes and the prediction of normal results. Am Rev Tuberc 79:457–467, 1959.

57. Briscoe WA, Becklake MR, Rose TF: The intrapulmonary mixing of helium in normal and emphysematous subjects. Clin Sci 10:37–51, 1951.

58. Grimby G, Soderholm B: Spirometric studies in normal subjects. III. Static lung volumes and maximum voluntary ventilation in adults with a note on physical fitness. Acta Med Scand 173:199–206, 1963.

59. Martin R, Macklem PT: Suggested Standardized Procedures for Closed Volume Determinations (Nitrogen Method). Bethesda, MD, Division of Lung Disease, National Heart and Lung Institute, NIH, 1973.

60. Mitchell MM, Renzettl AD Jr: Evaluation of a single-breath method of measuring total lung capacity. Am Rev Respir Dis 97:571–580, 1968.

61. Burns CB, Scheinhorn DJ: Evaluation of single-breath helium dilution total lung capacity in obstructive lung disease. Am Rev Respir Dis 97:580–583, 1984.

62. Harris TR, Pratt PC, Kilburn KH: Total lung capacity measured by roentgenograms. Am J Med 50:756–763, 1971.

62a. Lloyd HM, String TS, Dubois AB: Radiographic and plethysmographic determination of total lung capacity. Radiology 86:7–14, 1966.

63. Barnhard HB, Pierce JA, Joyce JW, Bates JH: Roentgenographic determination of total lung capacity. A new method evaluated in health, emphysema and congestive heart failure. Am J Med 28:51–60, 1960.

64. Clausen JL, Zarins L, Ries AL: Measurements of abnormal increases in pulmonary tissue in restrictive lung disease. Am Rev Respir Dis 117:322, 1978.

65. Clausen JL, Zarins LP: Estimation of lung volumes from chest radiographs. *In* Clausen JL (ed): Pulmonary Function Testing Guidelines and Controversies, Equipment Methods, and Normal Values. Orlando, FL, Grune & Stratton, 1984, pp. 155–163.

REFERENCES

66. Rebuck AS, Read J: Assessment and management of severe asthma. Am J Med 51:788–798, 1971.

67. Jacquemin CH, Varene P: The transfer function of the "man-in differential plethysmograph" system. *In* DuBois AB, van de Woestijne KP (eds): Body Plethysmography. Vol. 4. Basel, Switzerland, S. Karger, 1969, pp. 76–87.

68. Smidt U, Muysers K, Buchhein W: Electronic compensation of differences in temperature and water vapour between inspired and expired air and other signal handling in body plethysmography. Progr Respir Res 4:39–49, 1969.

69. Bryant GH, Hansen JE: An improvement in whole body plethysmography. Am Rev Respir Dis 112:464–465, 1975.

70. Stanescu DC, Rodenstein P, Cauberghs M, Van de Woestijne KP: Failure of body plethysmography in bronchial asthma. J Appl Physiol 52:939–948, 1982.

71. Rodenstein DO, Stanescu DC, Francis C: Demonstration of failure of body plethysmography in airway obstruction. J Appl Physiol 52:949–954, 1982.

72. Rodenstein DO, Stanescu DC: Reassessment of lung volume measurement by helium dilution and by body plethysmography in chronic air-flow obstruction. Am Rev Respir Dis 126:1040–1044, 1982.

73. DuBois AB: Resistance to breathing. *In* Fenn WO, Rahn H (eds): Handbook of Physiology: A Critical, Comprehensive Presentation of Physiological Knowledge and Concepts. Vol. 1. Washington, DC, American Physiological Society, 1964, pp. 451–462.

74. Gelb AF, Gold WM, Nadel JA: Mechanisms limiting airflow in bullous lung disease. Am Rev Respir Dis 107: 571–578, 1973.

75. Hahn HL, Graf PD, Nadel JA: Effect of vagal tone on airway diameters and on lung volume in anesthetized dogs. J Appl Physiol 41:581–589, 1976.

76. Butler J, Caro CG, Alcala R, DuBois AB: Physiological factors affecting airway resistance in normal subjects and in patients with obstructive airway disease. J Clin Invest 39:584–591, 1960.

77. Milic-Emili J, Mead J, Turner JM, Glausek EM: Improved technique for estimating pleural pressure from esophageal balloons. J Appl Physiol 19:207–211, 1964.

78. Leman R, Benson M, Jones JG: Absolute pressure measurements with hand-dipped and manufactured esophageal balloons. J Appl Physiol 37:600–603, 1974.

79. Begin R, Renzetti AD Jr, Bigler AH, Watanabe S: Flow and age dependence of airway closure and dynamic compliance. J Appl Physiol 38:199–207, 1975.

80. Woolcock AJJ, Vincent JN, Macklem PT: Frequency dependence of compliance as a test for obstruction in the small airways. J Clin Invest 48:1097–1105, 1969.

81. Dawson A: Elastic recoil and compliance. *In* Clausen JL (ed): Pulmonary Function Testing: Guidelines and Controversies. New York, Academic Press, 1982, pp. 193–204.

82. Knudson RJ, Clark DF, Kennedy TC, Knudson DE: Effect of aging alone on mechanical properties of the normal adult human lung. J Appl Physiol 43:1054–1062, 1977.

83. Turner JM, Mead J, Wohl ME: Elasticity of human lungs in relation to age. J Appl Physiol 25:664–671, 1968.

84. Bode FR, Dosman J, Martin RR, et al: Age and sex differences in lung elasticity, and in closing capacity in nonsmokers. J Appl Physiol 41:129–135, 1976.

85. Yernault JC, Baran D, Englert M: Effect of growth and aging on the static mechanical lung properties. Bull Eur Physiopathol Respir 13:777–778, 1977.

86. Zapletal A, Paul T, Samanek M: Pulmonary elasticity in children and adolescents. J Appl Physiol 40:953–961, 1976.

87. Gibson GJ, Pride NB: Lung distensibility. The static pressure-volume curve of the lungs and its use in clinical assessment. Br J Dis Chest 70:143–184, 1976.

88. Salazar E, Knowles JH: An analysis of pressure-volume characteristics of the lungs. J Appl Physiol 19:97–104, 1964.

89. Pengelly LD: Curve-fitting analysis of pressure-volume characteristics of the lungs. J Appl Physiol 42:111–116, 1977.

90. Colebatch HJH, Ng CKY, Nikov N: Use of an exponential function for elastic recoil. J Appl Physiol 46:387–393, 1979.

91. Gibson GJ, Pride NB, Davis T, Schroter RC: Exponential description of the static pressure-volume curve of normal and diseased lungs. Am Rev Respir Dis 120:799–811, 1979.

92. Colebatch HJH, Greaves IA, Ng CKY: Pulmonary mechanics in diagnosis. *In* de Kock MA, Nadel JA, Lewis CM (eds): Mechanisms of Airway Obstruction in Human Respiratory Disease: Proceedings of the International Symposium, Tygerberg, SA Cape Town, South Africa, AA Balkema, 1979, pp. 25–47.

93. Pare PD, Brooks LA, Bates J, et al; Exponential analysis of the lung pressure-volume curve as a predictor of pulmonary emphysema. Am Rev Respir Dis 126:54–61, 1982.

94. Thompson MJ, Colebatch HJ: Decreased pulmonary distensibility in fibrosing alveolitis and its relation to decreased lung volume. Thorax 44:725–731, 1989.

95. Colebatch HJH, Greaves IA, Ng CKY: Exponential analysis of elastic recoil and aging in healthy males and females. J Appl Physiol 47:683–691, 1979.

96. Greaves IA, Colebatch HJH: Elastic behavior and structure of normal and emphysematous lungs post mortem. Am Rev Respir Dis 121:127–136, 1980.

REFERENCES

97. Hetzel M: The pulmonary clock. Thorax 36:481–486, 1981.

98. Thurlbeck WM, Dunnill MS, Hartung W, et al: A comparison of three methods of measuring emphysema. Hum Pathol 1:215–226, 1970.

99. Gugger M, Gould G, Sudlow M, et al: Extent of pulmonary emphysema in man and its relation to the loss of elastic recoil. Clin Sci 80:353–358, 1991.

100. Morrison N, Abboud R, Ramadan F, et al: Comparison of single breath carbon monoxide diffusing capacity and pressure-volume curves in detecting emphysema. Am Rev Respir Dis 139:1179–1187, 1989.

101. West W, Nagai A, Hodkin J, Thurlbeck W: The National Institutes of Health Intermittent Positive Pressure Breathing Trail—Pathology studies. III. The diagnosis of emphysema. Am Rev Respir Dis 135:123–129, 1987.

102. Macklem P, Eidelman D: Reexamination of the elastic properties of emphysematous lungs. Respiration 57: 187–192, 1990.

103. American Thoracic Society: Lung function testing: Selection of reference values and interpretative strategies. Am Rev Respir Dis 144:1202–1216, 1991.

104. Townsend M: Spirometric forced expiratory volumes measured in the standing versus the sitting posture. Am Rev Respir Dis 130:123–124, 1984.

105. Liistro G, Stanescu D, Dooms G, et al: Head position modifies upper airway resistance in men. J Appl Physiol 64:1285–1288, 1988.

106. Melissinos C, Mead J: Maximum expiratory flow changes induced by longitudinal tension on trachea in normal subjects. J Appl Physiol 43:537–544, 1977.

107. Van de Woestijne K, Afschrift M: Airway dynamics during forced expiration in patients with chronic obstructive lung disease. *In* Orie N, Van der Lende R (eds): Bronchitis III. Assen, Royal Van Gorcium, 1970, pp. 195–206.

108. Krowka M, Enright P, Rodarte J, Hyatt RE: Effect of effort on measurement of forced expiratory volume in one second. Am Rev Respir Dis 136:829–833, 1987.

109. Gimeno F, Berg W, Sluiter H, Tammeling G: Spirometry-induced bronchial obstruction. Am Rev Respir Dis 105:68–74, 1972.

110. Clark T, Hetzel M: Diurnal variation of asthma. Br J Dis Chest 71:87–92, 1977.

111. McDermott M: Diurnal and weekly cyclical changes in lung airways resistance. J Physiol (London) 186:90, 1966.

112. De Millas H, Ulmer W: Circadian rhythms of airways resistance in healthy subjects and patients with obstructive airways disease. Pneumologie 144:237–252, 1971.

113. Kerr H: Diurnal variation of respiratory function independent of air quality. Arch Environ Health 26:144–152, 1973.

114. Halberg F: Chronobiology and the lung: Implications and applications. Bull Eur Physiopathol Respir 23: 529–531, 1987.

115. Minette A: Contribution to the chronobiology of lung function: Changes of baseline values of four lung function indices between 8h and 17h in patients with bronchitic complaints without asthmatic components. Bull Eur Physiopathol Respir 23:541–543, 1987.

116. Schwartz J, Katz S, Fegley R, Tockman M: Analysis of spirometric data from a national sample of healthy 6- to 24-year-olds (NHANES II). Am Rev Respir Dis 138:1405–1414, 1988.

117. Schwartz J, Katz S, Fegley R, Tockman M: Sex and race differences in the development of lung function. Am Rev Respir Dis 138:1415–1421, 1988.

118. Buist A, Vollmer W: The use of lung function tests in identifying factors that affect lung growth and aging. Stat Med 7:11–18, 1988.

119. Hibbert M, Lanigan A, Raven J, Phelan P: Relation of armspan to height and the prediction of lung function. Thorax 43:657–659, 1988.

120. Becklake M, Permutt S: Evaluation of tests of lung function for "screening" for early detection of chronic obstructive lung disease. *In* Macklem P, Permutt S (eds): The Lung in the Transition Between Health and Disease. New York, Marcel Dekker, 1979, pp. 345–388.

121. Cotes J: Lung Function: Assessment and Application in Medicine (4th ed.). Oxford, Blackwell Scientific Publishers, 1979.

122. Weisman I, Zeballos R: Lower single breath carbon monoxide diffusing capacity (DL_{CO}) in black subjects compared with Caucasians. Chest 92:142S, 1987.

123. Burrows B, Taussig L: As the twig is bent, the tree inclines (perhaps). Am Rev Respir Dis 122:813–816, 1980.

124. U.S. Department of Health and Human Services: The health consequences of smoking: Chronic obstructive lung disease, a report of the Surgeon General. Rockville, MD, Public Health Service Office on Smoking and Health, 1984.

125. Green M, Mead J, Turner JM: Variability of maximum expiratory flow-volume curves. J Appl Physiol 37:67–74, 1974.

126. Frisancho A: Functional adaptation to high altitude hypoxia. Science 187:313–319, 1975.

127. Heath D, Williams D: The lung at high altitude. Invest Cell Pathol 2:147–156, 1979.

128. Gautier H, Peslin R, Grassino A, et al: Mechanical properties of the lungs during acclimatization to altitude. J Appl Physiol 52:1407–1415, 1982.

REFERENCES

129. Holtzmann M, Cunningham J, Sheller J, et al: Effect of ozone on bronchial reactivity in atopic and nonatopic subjects. Am Rev Respir Dis 120:1059–1067, 1978.

130. Sheppard D, Epstein J, Bethel R, et al: Tolerance to sulfur dioxide–induced bronchoconstriction in subjects with asthma. Environ Res 30:412–419, 1983.

131. Bethel R, Epstein J, Sheppard D, et al: Sulfur dioxide–induced bronchoconstriction in freely breathing, exercising asthmatic subjects. Am Rev Respir Dis 128:987–990, 1983.

132. Lippman M: Health significance of pulmonary function responses to irritants. J Air Pollut Cont Assoc 38:881–887, 1988.

133. Linn W, Theodore G, Shamoo DA, et al: Respiratory effects of sulfur dioxide in heavily exercising asthmatics. Am Rev Respir Dis 127:278–283, 1983.

134. Nadel JA, Comroe JH Jr: Acute effects of inhalation of cigarette smoke on airway conductance. J Appl Physiol 16:713–716, 1961.

135. Susuki S, Sasaki H, Takashima T: Effects of smoking on dynamic compliance and respiratory resistance. Environ Health 38:133–137, 1983.

136. Fielding J, Phenow K: Health effects of involuntary smoking. N Engl J Med 319:1452–1460, 1988.

137. Lebowitz M: The relationship of socio-environmental factors to the prevalence of obstructive lung diseases and other chronic conditions. J Chronic Dis 30:599–611, 1977.

138. Gaensler EA: Clinical pulmonary physiology. N Engl J Med 252:177–184, 1955.

139. Engel LA, Grassino A, Anthonisen NR: Demonstration of airway closure in man. J Appl Physiol 38:1117–1125, 1975.

140. Daniels AU, Couvillon LA, Lebrizzi JM: Evaluation of nitrogen analyzers. Am Rev Respir Dis 112:571–575, 1975.

141. Craven N, Sidwall G, West P, et al: Computer analysis of the single-breath nitrogen washout curve. Am Rev Respir Dis 113:445–449, 1976.

142. Buist AS, Ross BB: Predicted values for closing volumes using a modified single breath nitrogen test. Am Rev Respir Dis 107:744–752, 1973.

143. Buist AS, Ghezzo H, Anthonisen NR, et al: Relationship between the single-breath N_2 test and age, sex, and smoking habit in three North American cities. Am Rev Respir Dis 120:305–318, 1979.

144. Buist AS, Ross BB: Quantitative analysis of the alveolar plateau in the diagnosis of early airway obstruction. Am Rev Respir Dis 108:1078–1087, 1973.

145. Knudson RJ, Lebowitz MD, Burton AP, Knudson DE: The closing volume test: Evaluation of nitrogen and bolus methods in a random population. Am Rev Respir Dis 115:423–434, 1977.

146. Becklake MR, Leclerc M, Strobach H, Swift J: The N_2 closing volume test in population studies: Sources of variation and reproducibility. Am Rev Respir Dis 111:141–147, 1975.

147. Hyatt RE, Rodarte JR: "Closing volume," one man's noise—other man's experiment. Mayo Clin Proc 50:17–27, 1975.

148. McFadden ER Jr, Holmes B, Kiker R: Variability of closing volume measurements in normal man. Am Rev Respir Dis 111:135–140, 1975.

149. Make B, Lapp NL: Factors influencing the measurement of closing volume. Am Rev Respir Dis 111:749–754, 1975.

150. Travis DM, Green M, Don H: Simultaneous comparison of helium and nitrogen expiratory "closing volume." J Appl Physiol 34:304–308, 1973.

151. Linn WS, Hackney JD: Nitrogen and helium "closing volumes": Simultaneous measurement and reproducibility. J Appl Physiol 34:396–399, 1973.

152. Fowler WS: Lung function studies: III. Uneven pulmonary ventilation in normal subjects and in patients with pulmonary disease. J Appl Physiol 2:283–299, 1949.

153. Comroe JH Jr, Fowler WS: Lung function studies: VI. Detection of uneven alveolar ventilation during a single breath of oxygen. Am J Med 10:408–413, 1951.

154. Cournand A, Baldwin EDF, Darling RC, Richards DW Jr: Studies on intrapulmonary mixture of gases: IV. The significance of the pulmonary emptying rate and a simplified open circuit measurement of residual air. J Clin Invest 20:681–689, 1941.

155. Darling RC, Cournand A, Richards DW Jr Studies on intrapulmonary mixture of gases: V. Forms of inadequate ventilation in normal and emphysematous lungs, analyzed by means of breathing pure oxygen. J Clin Invest 23:55–67, 1944.

156. Fowler WS, Cornish ER Jr, Kety SS: Lung function studies. VIII. Analysis of alveolar ventilation by pulmonary N_2 clearance curves. J Clin Invest 31:40–50, 1952.

157. Emmanuel G, Briscoe WA, Cournand A: Method for the determination of the volume of air in the lungs: Measurements in chronic pulmonary emphysema. J Clin Invest 40:329–337, 1961.

158. Meneely GR, Kaltreider NL: The volume of the lung determined by helium dilution: Description of the method and comparison with other procedures. J Clin Invest 28:129–139, 1949.

159. Hathirat S, Renzetti AD Jr, Mitchell M: Intrapulmonary gas distribution; a comparison of the helium mixing time and nitrogen single breath test in normal and diseased subjects. Am Rev Respir Dis 102:750–759, 1970.

REFERENCES

160. Hale FC, Cohen AA, Hemingway A: Reliability of the estimation of functional residual capacity in the emphysematous patient. Am Rev Respir Dis 87:820–829, 1963.

161. Robertson JS, Siri WE, Jones HB: Lung ventilation patterns determined by analysis of nitrogen elimination rates: Use of the mass spectrometer as a continuous gas analyzer. J Clin Invest 29:577–590, 1950.

162. Comroe JH Jr, Forster REI, DuBois AB, et al: Useful Data, Equations and Calculations. The Lung: Clinical Physiology and Pulmonary Function Tests (2nd ed.). Chicago, IL, Year Book Medical Publishers, 1962, pp. 323–364.

163. Ogilvie CM, Forster RE, Blakemore WS, Morton JW: A standardized breath holding technique for the clinical measurement of the diffusing capacity of the lung for carbon monoxide. J Clin Invest 36:1–17, 1957.

164. Krogh M: The diffusion of gases through the lungs of man. J Physiol (London) 49:271–296, 1915.

165. Jones FS, Mead F: A theoretical and experimental analysis of anomalies in the estimation of pulmonary diffusing capacity by the single breath method. Q J Exp Physiol 46:131–143, 1961.

166. Lilienthal JL Jr, Riley RL, Premmel DD, Franke RE: An experimental analysis in man of the O_2 pressure gradient from alveolar air to arterial blood during rest and exercise at sea level and at altitude. Am J Physiol 147:199–216, 1946.

167. Forster RE: Diffusion of gases. *In* Fenn WO, Rahn H (eds): Handbook of Physiology. Vol. 1. Washington, DC, American Physiological Society, 1964, pp. 839–872.

168. Berend NC, Woolcock AJ, Marlin GE: Correlation between the function and structure of the lung in smokers. Am Rev Respir Dis 119:695–705, 1979.

169. Bergin C, Muller N, Nichols D, et al: The diagnosis of emphysema. A computer tomography-pathologic correlation. Am Rev Respir Dis 133:541–546, 1986.

170. Morrison N, Abboud R, Muller N, et al: Pulmonary capillary blood volume in emphysema. Am Rev Respir Dis 141:53–61, 1990.

171. Matsuba K, Ikeda T. Nagai A, Thurlbeck W: The National Institutes of Health Intermittent Positive-Pressure Breathing Trial: Pathology Studies. IV. The Destructive Index. Am Rev Respir Dis 139:1439–1445, 1989.

172. Nadel JA, Gold WM, Burgess JH: Early diagnosis of chronic pulmonary vascular obstruction. Am J Med 44:16–25, 1968.

173. Cotes JE, Dabbs JM, Elwood PC, et al: Iron-deficiency anaemia: Its effect on transfer factor for the lung (diffusing capacity) and ventilation and cardiac frequency during sub-maximal exercise. Clin Sci 42:325–335, 1972.

174. Crapo RO, Morris AH: Standardized single breath normal values for carbon monoxide diffusing capacity. Am Rev Respir Dis 123:185–189, 1981.

175. Rankin J, McNeill RS, Forster RE: Influence of increased alveolar carbon dioxide tension on pulmonary diffusing capacity for CO in man. J Appl Physiol 15:543–549, 1960.

176. Karp RB, Graf PD, Nadel JA: Regulation of pulmonary capillary blood volume by pulmonary arterial and left atrial pressures. Circ Res 22:1–10, 1968.

177. Stokes D, Macintyre N, Nadel J: Nonlinear increases in diffusing capacity during exercise by seated and supine subjects. J Appl Physiol 51:858–863, 1981.

178. Carlin J, Hsia C, Cassidy S, et al: Recruitment of lung diffusing capacity with exercise before and after pneumonectomy in dogs. J Appl Physiol 51:858–863, 1981.

179. Ceretelli P, DiPrampero P: Gas exchange during exercise. Handbook of Physiology. The Respiratory System. Gas Exchange. Vol. IV. Bethesda, MD, American Physiological Society, 1987, pp. 297–339.

180. Kinker J, Haffor A-S, Stephan M, Clanton T: Kinetics of CO uptake on diffusing capacity in transition from rest to steady-state exercise. J Appl Physiol 72:1764–1772, 1992.

181. Okada O, Presson RJ, Kirk K, et al: Capillary perfusion patterns in single alveolar walls. J Appl Physiol 72: 1838–1844, 1992.

182. West J, Schneider A, Mitchell M: Recruitment in networks of pulmonary capillaries. J Appl Physiol 39:976–984, 1975.

183. Comroe JH Jr, Forster RE II, DuBois AB, et al: Diffusion: The Lung: Clinical Physiology and Pulmonary Function Tests (2nd ed.). Chicago, IL, Year Book Medical Publishers, 1962, pp. 111–139.

184. Forster RE II, Roughton FJW, Cander L, et al: Apparent pulmonary diffusing capacity for CO at varying alveolar O_2 tensions. J Appl Physiol 11:277–289, 1957.

185. Van Noord J, Clement J, Van de Woestijne K, Demedts M: Total respiratory resistance and reactance in patients with asthma, chronic bronchitis, and emphysema. Am Rev Respir Dis 143:922–927, 1991.

186. Stewart R: Carbon monoxide diffusing capacity in asthmatic patients with mild airflow limitation. Chest 94: 332–336, 1988.

187. Klein J, Gamsu G, Webb W, et al: High-resolution CT diagnosis of emphysema in symptomatic patients with normal chest radiographs and isolated low diffusing capacity. Radiology 182:817–821, 1992.

188. Gould G, Redpath A, Ryan M, et al: Lung CT density correlates with measurements of airflow limitation and the diffusing capacity. Eur Respir J 4:141–146, 1991.

189. Wall M, Moe E, Elsenberg J, et al: Pulmonary capillary blood volume in emphysema. Am Rev Respir Dis 141:

REFERENCES

53–161, 1990.

190. Gould G, MacNee W, McLean A, et al: CT measurements of lung density in life can quantitate distal airspace enlargement—an essential defining feature of human emphysema. Am Rev Respir Dis 137:380–392, 1988.

191. Thurlbeck W: Pathophysiology of chronic obstructive pulmonary disease. Clin Chest Med 11:389–403, 1990.

192. Eidelman D, Ghezzo H, Kim W, Cosio M: The destructive index and early lung destruction in smokers. Am Rev Respir Dis 144:156–159, 1991.

193. Neuth CJL, Cotton DJ, Nadel TA: Pulmonary diffusing capacity measurement at multiple intervals during a single exhalation in man. J Appl Physiol 43:617–625, 1970.

194. Gold WM, Youker J, Anderson S, Nadel JA: Pulmonary-function abnormalities after lymphangiography. N Engl J Med 273:519–524, 1965.

195. McNeill RS, Rankin J, Forster RE: The diffusing capacity of the pulmonary membrane and the pulmonary capillary blood volume in cardiopulmonary disease. Clin Sci 17:465–482, 1958.

196. Wessel HU, Kezdi P, Cugell DW: Respiratory and cardiovascular function in patients with severe pulmonary hypertension. Circulation 29:825–832, 1964.

197. West JB, Dollery CT, Naimaule A: Distribution of blood flow in isolated lung: Relation to vascular and alveolar pressures. J Appl Physiol 19:713–724, 1964.

198. Howell JBL, Permutt S, Proctor DF, Riley RL: Effects of inflation of the lung on different parts of pulmonary vascular bed. J Appl Physiol 16:71–76, 1961.

199. West JB, Dollery CT: Distribution of blood flow and the pressure-flow relations of the whole lung. J Appl Physiol 20:175–183, 1965.

200. Vanderstappen M, Momex J, Lahneche B, et al: Gallium-67 scanning in the staging of cryptogenetic fibrosing alveolitis and hypersensitivity pneumonitis. Eur Respir J 1: 517–522, 1988.

201. Rienmuller R, Behr J, Kalender W, et al: Standardized quantitative high resolution CT in lung diseases. J Comput Assist Tomog 15:742–749, 1991.

202. Schwartz D, Galvin J, Dayton C, et al: Determinants of restrictive lung function in asbestos-induced pleural fibrosis. J Appl Physiol 68:1932–1937, 1990.

203. Glanville A, Baldwin J, Hunt S, Theodore J: Long-term cardiopulmonary function after human heart-lung transplantation. Aust NZ J Med 20:208–214, 1990.

204. Otulana B, Higenbottam T, Scott J, et al: Lung function associated with histologically diagnosed acute lung rejection and pulmonary infection in heart-lung transplant patients. Am Rev Respir Dis 142:329–332, 1990.

204a. Clelland C, Higenbottam T, Otulana B, et al: Histologic prognostic indicators for the lung allografts of heart-lung transplants. J Heart Transplant 9:177–185, 1990.

205. de Hoyos A, Patterson G, Maurer J, et al: Pulmonary transplantation. Early and late results. The Toronto Lung Transplant Group. Thorac Cardiovasc Surg 103:295–306, 1992.

206. Novick R, Ahmad D, Menkis A, et al: The importance of acquired diffuse bronchomalacia in heart-lung transplant recipients with obliterative bronchiolitis. J Thorac Cardiovasc Surg 101:643–648, 1991.

207. Theodore J, Marshall S, Kramer M, et al: The "natural history" of the transplanted lung: Rates of pulmonary functional change in long-term survivors of heart-lung transplantation. Transplant Proc 23:1165–1166, 1991.

208. Theodore J, Stames V, Lewiston N: Obliterative bronchiolitis. Clin Chest Med 11:309–321, 1990.

209. Pasque M, Cooper J, Kaiser L, et al: Improved technique for bilateral lung transplantation: Rationale and initial clinical experience. Ann Thorac Surg 49:785–791, 1990.

210. Starnes V, Theodore J, Oyer P, et al: Evaluation of heart-lung transplant recipients with prospective, serial transbronchial biopsies and pulmonary function studies. J Thorac Cardiovasc Surg 98:683–690, 1989.

211. McGregor C, Dark J, Hilton C, et al: Early results of single lung transplantation in patients with end-stage pulmonary fibrosis. J Thorac Cardiovasc Surg 98:350–354, 1989.

212. Kindt G, Weiland J, Davis W, et al: Bronchitis in adults. A reversible cause of airway obstruction associated with airway neutrophils and neutrophil products. Am Rev Respir Dis 140:483–492, 1989.

213. Hutter J, Scott J, Deespins P, et al: Heart-lung transplantation at Papworth Hospital. Eur J Cardio-Thorac Surg 3:300–303, 1989.

214. Higenbottam T, Stewart S, Penketh A, Wallwork J: Transbronchial lung biopsy for the diagnosis of rejection in heart-lung transplant patients. Transplantation 46:532–539, 1988.

215. Severinghaus J, Ozanne G, Massuda Y: Measurement of the ventilatory response to hypoxia. Chest 70:121–124, 1976.

216. Lourenco RV: Clinical methods for the study of regulation of breathing. Chest 70:109–112, 1976.

217. Cherniack NS, Dempsey J, Fencl V, et al: Workshop on assessment of respiratory control in humans. I. Methods of measurement of ventilatory responses to hypoxia and hypercapnia: Conference Report. Am Rev Respir Dis 115:177–181, 1977.

218. Mithoefer JC: Breathholding. *In* Fenn WO, Rahn H (eds): Handbook of Physiology. Washington, DC, American Physiological Society, 1965, pp. 1011–1025.

REFERENCES

219. Davidson JT, Whipp BJ, Wesserman K, et al: Role of the carotid bodies in breath-holding. N Engl J Med 290: 819–822, 1974.

220. Read DJC: A clinical method for assessing the ventilatory response to carbon dioxide. Australas Ann Med 16: 20–32, 1967.

221. Irsigler GB: Carbon dioxide response lines in young adults: The limits of the normal response. Am Rev Respir Dis 114:529–536, 1976.

222. Patrick JM, Cotes JE: Hypoxic and hypercapnic ventilatory drives in man (correspondence). J Appl Physiol 40: 1012, 1976.

223. Rebuck AS, Campbell EJM: A clinical method for assessing the ventilatory response to hypoxia. Am Rev Respir Dis 109:345–350, 1974.

224. Rebuck AS, Woodley WE: Ventilatory effects of hypoxia and their dependence on P_{CO_2}. J Appl Physiol 38: 16–19, 1975.

225. Whitelaw WA, Derenne J, Milic-Emili J: Occlusion pressure as a measure of respiratory center output in conscious man. Respir Physiol 23:181–199, 1975.

226. Matthews AW, Howell JBL: The rate of isometric inspiratory pressure development as a measure of responsiveness to carbon dioxide in man. Clin Sci Mol Med 49: 57–68, 1975.

227. Kryger MH, Yacoub O, Dosman J, et al: Effect of meperidine on occlusion pressure responses to hypercapnia and hypoxia with and without external inspiratory resistance. Am Rev Respir Dis 114:333–340, 1976.

228. Gelb AF, Klein E, Schiffman P, et al: Ventilatory response and drive in acute and chronic obstructive pulmonary disease. Am Rev Respir Dis 116:9–16, 1977.

229. Wright BM: Discussion on measuring pulmonary ventilation. *In* Harbord RP, Woolmer R (eds): Symposium on Pulmonary Ventilation. Altrincham, England, John Sherratt and Son, 1959, p. 87.

230. Priban IP: An analysis of some short-term patterns of breathing in man at rest. J Physiol (London) 166:425–434, 1963.

231. Bendixen HH, Smith GM, Mead J: Pattern of ventilation in young adults. J Appl Physiol 19:195–198, 1964.

232. Allison RD, Holmes EL, Nyboer J: Volumetric dynamics of respiration as measured by electrical impedance plethysmography. J Appl Physiol 19:166–173, 1964.

233. Mead J, Peterson N, Grimby G, et al: Pulmonary ventilation measured from body surface movements. Science 156:1383–1384, 1967.

234. Mead J, Loring SH: Analysis of volume displacement and length changes of the diaphragm during breathing. J Appl Physiol 53:750–755, 1982.

235. Burwell CS, Robin ED, Whaley RD, Bickelmann AG: Extreme obesity associated with alveolar hypoventilation—A Pickwickian syndrome. Am J Med 21:811–818, 1956.

236. Fowler WS: Lung function studies. II. The respiratory dead space. Am J Physiol 154:405–416, 1948.

237. Fowler WS: Lung function studies. V. Respiratory dead space in old age and pulmonary emphysema. J Clin Invest 29:1439–1444, 1950.

238. Severinghaus JW, Stupfel M: Alveolar dead space as an index of distribution of blood flow in pulmonary capillaries. J Appl Physiol 10:335–348, 1957.

239. Bishop JM, Cole RB: The effects of inspired oxygen concentration, age and body position upon the alveolar-arterial oxygen tension difference (AaD) and physiological dead space. J Physiol (London) 162:60P, 1962.

240. Terman JW, Newton JL: Changes in alveolar and arterial gas tensions as related to altitude and age. J Appl Physio1 19:21–24, 1964.

241. Lenfant C: Measurement of ventilation/perfusion distribution with alveolar-arterial differences. J Appl Physiol 18:1090–1094, 1963.

242. Mellemgaard K: The alveolar-arterial oxygen difference: Size and components in normal man. Acta Physiol Scand 67:10–20, 1966.

243. West JB: Causes of carbon dioxide retention in lung disease. N Engl J Med 284:1232–1236, 1971.

244. Riley RL, Cournand A: Analysis of factors affecting partial pressures of oxygen and carbon dioxide in gas and blood of lungs: Theory. J Appl Physiol 4:77–101, 1951.

245. Andersen AM, Ladefoged J: Partition coefficient of ^{133}xenon between various tissues and blood in vivo. Scand J Clin Lab Invest 19:72–78, 1967.

246. Bryan AC, Bentivoglio LG, Beerel F, et al: Factors affecting regional distribution of ventilation and perfusion in the lung. J Appl Physiol 19:395–402, 1964.

247. Milic-Emili J, Henderson JA, Dolovich MB, et al: Regional distribution of inspired gas in the lung. J Appl Physiol 21:749–759, 1966.

248. Kaneko K, Milic-Emili J, Dolovich MB, et al: Regional distribution of ventilation and perfusion as a function of body position. J Appl Physiol 21:767–777, 1966.

249. Anthonisen NR, Milic-Emili J: Distribution of pulmonary perfusion in erect man. J Appl Physiol 21:760–766, 1966.

250. Dollfuss RE, Milic-Emili J, Bates DV: Regional ventilation of the lung studied with boluses of 133 xenon. Resp Physiol 2:234–246, 1967.

251. Wagner HN Jr, Sabiston DC Jr, Lio M, et al: Regional pulmonary blood flow in man by radioisotope scanning. J Am Med Assoc 187:601–603, 1964.

REFERENCES

252. Harding LK, Horsfield K, Singhal SS, Cumming G: The proportion of lung vessels blocked by albumin microspheres. J Nucl Med 14:579–581, 1973.

253. Gold WM, McCormack KR: Pulmonary-function response to radioisotope scanning of the lungs. J Am Med Assoc 197:146–148, 1966.

254. Wagner PD, Saltzman HA, West JB: Measurement of continuous distributions of ventilation-perfusion ratios: Theory. J Appl Physiol 36:588–599, 1974.

255. Wagner PD, Smith CM, Davies NJH, et al: Estimation of ventilation-perfusion inequality by inert gas elimination without arterial sampling. J Appl Physiol 59:376–383, 1985.

256. Mohler JG, Collier CR, Brandt W, et al: Blood gases. *In* Clausen JL (ed): Pulmonary Function Testing Guidelines and Controversies: Equipment, Methods, and Normal Values. Orlando, FL, Grune & Stratton, 1984, pp. 223–258.

257. Hansen JE, Clausen JL, Levy SE, et al: Proficiency testing materials for pH and blood gases; the California Thoracic Society experience. Chest 89:214–217, 1986.

258. Comroe JH Jr: Measurements on arterial blood. I. Collection and storage of blood. *In* Comroe JH Jr, Adams MH, Venning EH (eds): Methods in Medical Research. Vol 2. Chicago, Year Book, 1950, pp 138–180.

259. Kammer RE, Harris AH: Clinical Pulmonary Function Testing. Salt Lake City, UT, Intermountain Thoracic Society, 1975.

260. Clark LC Jr, Monitor and control of blood and tissue oxygen tensions. Trans Am Soc Artif Int Organs 2:41–48, 1956.

261. Hansen JE, Stone ME, Ong ST, Van Kessel AL: Evaluation of blood gas quality control and proficiency testing materials by tonometry. Am Rev Respir Dis 125: 480–483, 1982.

262. Noonan DC, Komjathy ZL: Long-term reproducibility of a new pH/blood-gas quality control system compared to two other procedures. Clin Chem 22:1817–1820, 1976.

263. Van Slyke DD, Neill JM: Determination of gases in blood and other solutions by vacuum extraction and manometric measurement. J Biol Chem 61:523, 1924.

264. Kusumi F, Butts WC, Ruff WL: Superior analytic performance by electrolytic cell analysis of oxygen content. J Appl Physiol 35:299–300, 1973.

265. van Kampen EJ, Zijlstra WG: Standardization of hemoglobinometry. II. The hemoglobincyanide method. Clin Chim Acta 6:538–544, 1961.

266. Levinsohn D, Gordon L, Sessler D: The Allen's test: Analysis of four methods. J Hand Surg 16A:279–282, 1991.

267. Cohen M, Rentrop K, Cohen B: Safety and efficacy of percutaneous entry of the brachial artery versus cutdown technique and arteriotomy for left-sided cardiac catheterization. Am J Cardiol 57:682–684, 1986.

268. Campagna A, Matthay M: Complications of invasive monitoring in the intensive care unit. Vol. 6. Northbrook IL, American College of Chest Physicians, 1991.

269. McQuitty JC, Lewiston NJ: Pulmonary function testing of children. *In* Clausen JL (ed): Pulmonary Function Testing Guidelines and Controversies: Equipment, Methods and Normal Values. Orlando, FL, Grune & Stratton, 1982, pp. 321–330.

270. Hess CE, Nichols AB, Hung WB, Suratt PM: Pseudohypoxemia secondary to leukemia and thrombocytosis. N Engl J Med 301:361–363, 1979.

271. Saunders NA, Powles ACP, Rebuck AS: Ear oximetry: Accuracy and practicability in the assessment of arterial oxygenation. Am Rev Respir Dis 113:745–749, 1976.

272. Dawson A: How should we report the oxygen saturation measured on the CO-oximeter? Cal Thorac Soc ABG Newsletter June:6–7, 1989.

273. Mendelson Y, Kent J, Shaharian A, et al: Evaluation of the Datascope Accusat pulse oximeter in healthy adults. J Clin Monit 4:59–63, 1988.

274. Mackenzie N: Comparison of a pulse oximeter with an ear oximeter and in-vitro oximeter. J Clin Monit 1:156–160, 1985.

275. Chapman KR, D'Urzo A, Rebuck AS: The accuracy and response characteristics of a simplified ear oximeter. Chest 83:860–864, 1983.

276. Eichorn J, Cooper J, Cullen D, et al: Standards for patient monitoring during anaesthesia at Harvard Medical School. JAMA 256:1017–1020, 1986.

277. Huch R, Huch A, Lumbers DW: Transcutaneous measurement of blood PO_2 ($tcPO_2$)—Method and application in perinatal medicine. J Perinat Med 1:183–191, 1973.

278. McDowell JW, Thiele WH: Usefulness of the transcutaneous PO_2 monitor during exercise testing in adults. Chest 78:853–855, 1980.

279. Vyas H, Helms P, Cheriyan G: Transcutaneous oxygen monitoring beyond the neonatal period. 16:844–847, 1988.

280. Prendiville A, Maxwell D, Rose A, Silverman M: Histamine-induced airway obstruction in infancy: Changes in oxygenation. Pediatr Pulmonol 4:164–168, 1988.

281. Martin R, Beoglos A, Miller M, et al: Increasing arterial carbon dioxide tension: Influence on transcutaneous carbon dioxide tension measurements. Pediatrics 81:684–687, 1988.

282. Kesten S, Chapman K, Rebuck A: Response characteristics of a dual transcutaneous oxygen/carbon dioxide monitoring system. Chest 99:1211–1215, 1991.

283. Naifeh K, Severinghaus J: Validation of a maskless CO_2-response test for sleep and infant studies. J Appl Physiol 64:391–396, 1988.

REFERENCES

284. Hess D: Capnometry and capnography: Technical aspects, physiologic aspects and clinical applications. Respir Care 35:537, 1990.

285. Morley T: Capnography in the intensive care unit. J Int Care Med 5:209, 1990.

286. Schwardt J, Gobran S, Neufeld G, et al: Sensitivity of CO_2 washout to changes in acinar structure in a single-path model of lung airways. Ann Biomed Eng 19:679–697, 1991.

287. Goldberg J, Rawle P, Zehnder J, Sladen R: Colorimetric end-tidal carbon dioxide monitoring for tracheal intubation. Anesth Analg 70:191–194, 1990.

288. Bhende M, Thompson A, Howland D: Validity of a disposable end-tidal carbon dioxide detector in verifying endotracheal tube position in piglets. Crit Care Med 19: 566–568, 1991.

289. Varon A, Morrina J, Civetta J: Clinical utility of a colorimetric end-tidal CO_2 detector in cardiopulmonary resuscitation and emergency intubation. J Clin Monitor 7: 289–293, 1991.

290. Thiele FA, van Kempen LH: A micro method for measuring the carbon dioxide release by small skin areas. Br J Dermatol 86:463–471, 1972.

291. McLellan PA, Goldstein RS, Ramcharan V, Rebuck AS: Transcutaneous carbon dioxide monitoring. Am Rev Respir Dis 124:199–201, 1981.

292. McGavin CR, Gupta SP, McHardy GJ: Twelve-minute walking test for assessing disability in chronic bronchitis. Br Med J 1:822–823, 1976.

293. Consolazio CF, Johnson RE, Pecora L: Physiological Measurements of Metabolic Functions in Man. New York, McGraw-Hill, 1963.

294. Jones NI, Campbell EJM: Clinical Exercise Testing (2nd ed.). Philadelphia, WB Saunders, 1982.

295. Sue DY, Hansen JE, Blais M, Wasserman K: Measurement and analysis of gas exchange during exercise using a programmable calculator. J Appl Physiol 49:456–461, 1980.

296. Wilmore JH, Costill DL: Semiautomated systems approach to the assessment of oxygen uptake during exercise. J Appl Physiol 36:618–620, 1974.

297. Cander L, Forster RE: Determination of pulmonary parenchymal tissue volume and pulmonary capillary blood flow in man. J Appl Physiol 14:541–551, 1959.

298. Whipp BJ, Davis JA, Torres F, Wasserman K: A test to determine the parameters of aerobic function during exercise. J Appl Physiol 50:217–221, 1981.

299. Chai H, Farr RS, Froehlich LA, et al: Standardization of bronchial inhalation challenge procedures. J Allergy Clin Immunol 56:323–327, 1975.

300. Townley RG: Guidelines for bronchial inhalation challenge with pharmacologic and antigenic agents. Am Thorac Soc News 6:11–19, 1980.

301. Wasserman K, Whipp BJ: Exercise physiology in health and disease. Am Rev Respir Dis 112:219–249, 1975.

302. Sorbini CA, Grassi V, Solinas E, Muiesan G: Arterial oxygen tension in relation to age in healthy subjects. Respiration 25:3–13, 1968.

303. Harris EA, Seelye ER, Whitlock RML: Revised standards for normal resting dead-space volume and venous admixture in men and women. Clin Sci Molec Med 55: 125–128, 1978.

304. Furuike AN, Sue DY, Hansen JE, Wasserman K: Comparison of physiologic dead space/tidal volume ratio and alveolar-arterial P_{O_2} difference during incremental and constant work exercise. Am Rev Respir Dis 126:579–583, 1982.

305. Borg GAV: Psychophysical bases of perceived exertion. Med Sci Sports Exerc 14:377–381, 1982.

306. Borg G, Noble B: Percieved exertion. *In* Wilmore JH (ed): Exercise and Sports Sciences Review. New York, Academic Press, 1974, pp. 131–153.

307. Simon P, Schwatzstein R, Weiss J, et al: Distinguishable sensations of breathlessness induced in normal volunteers. Am Rev Respir Dis 140:1021–1027, 1989.

308. Stark RD, Chatterjee SS: A new exercise test for clinical dyspnea. Practical Cardiol 9:86–95, 1983.

309. Stark RD, Gambles SA, Chatterjee SS: An exercise test to assess clinical dyspnea: Estimation of reproducibility and sensitivity. Br J Dis Chest 76:269–278, 1982.

310. Stark RD, Gambles SA: Effects of salbutamol, ipratropium bromide and disodium cromoglycate on breathlessness induced by exercise in normal subjects. Br J Clin Pharmacol 12:497–501, 1981.

311. Stark RD, Morton PB, Sharman R, et al: Effects of codeine on the respiratory response to exercise in healthy subjects. Br J Clin Pharm 15:355–359, 1983.

312. Donovan C, Brooks G: Endurance training affects lactate clearance, not lactate production. Am J Physiol 244 (Endocrinol Metab 7):E83–E92, 1983.

313. Donovan C, Pagliassotti M: Enhanced efficiency of lactate removal after endurance training. J Appl Physiol 68: 1053–1058, 1990.

314. Stanley W, Gertz E, Wisneski J, et al: Systemic lactate kinetics during graded exercise in man. Am J Physiol (Endocrin Metab 12) 249:E595–602, 1985.

315. Gladden L: Current "anaerobic threshold" controversies. The Physiologist 27:312–318, 1984.

316. Richardson R, Noyszewski E, Leigh J, Wagner P: Lactate efflux from exercising human skeletal muscle: Role of intracellular P_{O_2}. J Appl Physiol 85:627–634, 1998.

REFERENCES

317. American Thoracic Society: Evaluation of impairment/disability secondary to respiratory disorders. Am Rev Respir Dis 133:1205–1209, 1986.

317a. Wiedemann H: Evaluating pulmonary impairment: Appropriate use of pulmonary function and exercise tests. Cleve Clin J Med 58:148–152, 1991.

318. Ries A, Farrow J, Clausen J: Pulmonary function tests cannot predict exercise-induced hypoxemia in chronic obstructive pulmonary disease. Chest 93:454–459, 1988.

319. Oren A, Sue D, Hansen J, et al: The role of exercise testing in impairment evaluation. Am Rev Respir Dis 135: 230–235, 1987.

320. Henke K, Sharratt M, Pegelow D, Dempsey J: Regulation of end-expiratory lung volume during exercise. J Appl Physiol 64:135–146, 1988.

321. Johnson B, Redden W, Pegelow D, et al: Flow limitation and regulation of functional residual capacity during exercise in a physically active aging population. Am Rev Respir Dis 143:960–967, 1991.

322. Babb T, Viggiano R, Hurley B, et al: Effect of mild-to-moderate airflow limitation on exercise capacity. J Appl Physiol 70:223–230, 1991.

323. Babb T, Rodarte J: Lung volumes during low-intensity steady-state cycling. J Appl Physiol 70:934–937, 1991.

324. Babb T, Buskirk E, Hodgson J: Exercise end-expiratory lung volumes in lean and moderately obese women. Intl J Obesity 13:11–19, 1989.

325. Whipp B, Davis J: The ventilatory stress of exercise in obesity. Exercise testing in the dyspneic patient. Am Rev Respir Dis 129:S90–S92, 1984.

326. Comroe JH Jr, Nadel JA: Current concepts: Screening tests of pulmonary function. N Engl J Med 282:1249–1253, 1970.

327. Snider GL, Woolf CR, Kory RC, Ross J: Criteria for the assessment of reversibility in airways obstruction. Report of the Committee on Emphysema, American College of Chest Physicians. Chest 65:552–553, 1974.

328. Brand P, Quanje RP, Postma D, et al: A comparison of different ways to express bronchodilator response. Am Rev Respir Dis 141 (Part 2): A20, 1990.

329. Morris AH, Kanner RE, Crapo RO, Gardner RM: Spirometry. *In* Clinical Pulmonary Function Testing (2nd ed.). Salt Lake City, Intermountain Thoracic Society, 1984, pp 9–27.

330. Eliasson O, Degraff AC Jr: The use of criteria for reversibility and obstruction to define patient groups for bronchodilator trials. Influence of clinical diagnosis, spirometric, and anthropometric variables. Am Rev Respir Dis 132:858–864, 1985.

331. Shenfield GM, Hodson ME, Clarke SW, Paterson JW: Interaction of corticosteroids and catecholamines in the treatment of asthma. Thorax 30:430–435, 1975.

332. Kalsner S: Mechanism of hydrocortisone potentiation of responses to epinephrine and norepinephrine in rabbit aorta. Circ Res 24:383–395, 1969.

333. Davies AO, Lefkowitz RJ: Corticosteroid-induced differential regulation of beta-adrenergic receptors in circulating human polymorphonuclear leukocytes and mononuclear leukocytes. J Clin Endocrinol Metab 51:599–605, 1980.

334. Cockcroft D, Killian D, Melton J: Bronchial reactivity to inhaled histamine: A method and clinical survey. Clin Allergy 7:235–243, 1977.

335. Hargreave F, Ryan A, Thomson N: Bronchial responsiveness to histamine or methacholine in asthma: Measurement and clinical significance. J Allergy Clin Immunol 68:347–355, 1981.

336. Brantigan O: The surgical treatment of pulmonary emphysema. West Virg Med J 50:283–285, 1954.

337. Brantigan O, Mueller E, Kress M: A surgical approach to pulmonary emphysema. Am Rev Respir Dis 80: 194–202, 1959.

338. Wakabayashi A, Brenner M, Kayaleh R, et al: Thoracoscopic carbon dioxide laser treatment of bullous emphysema. Lancet 337:881–883, 1991.

339. Cooper J, Trulock E, Triantafillou G, et al: Bilateral pneumonectomy (volume reduction) for chronic obstructive pulmonary disease. J Thorac Cardiovasc Surg 109: 106–116, 1995.

340. Benditt J, Albert R: Lung reduction surgery. Great expectations and a cautionary note [editorial]. Chest 107: 297–298, 1995.

341. Make B, Fein A: Is volume reduction surgery appropriate in the treatment of emphysema? Am J Respir Crit Care Med 153:1205–1207, 1996.

342. Sciurba F, Rogers R, Keenan R, et al: Improvement in pulmonary function and elastic recoil after lung-reduction surgery for diffuse emphysema [see comments]. N Engl J Med 334:1095–1099, 1996.

343. Teschler H, Stamatis G, El-Raouf Farhat A, et al: Effect of surgical lung volume reduction on respiratory muscle function in pulmonary emphysema. Eur Respir J 9: 1779–1784, 1996.

344. Ingenito E, Evans R, Kaczka D, et al: Relation between preoperative inspiratory lung resistance and the outcome of lung-volume-reduction surgery for emphysema. N Engl J Med 338:1181–1185, 1998.

345. Fessler H, Permutt S: Lung volume reduction surgery and airflow limitation. Am J Respir Crit Care Med 157:715–722, 1998.

346. Severinghaus JW, Swenson EW, Finley TN, et al: Unilateral hypoventilation produced in dogs by occluding one pulmonary artery. J Appl Physiol 16:53–60, 1961.

347. Nadel JA, Colebatch HJH, Olsen CR: Location and mechanism of airway constriction after barium sulfate microembolism. J Appl Physiol 19:387–394, 1964.

REFERENCES

348. Coleman DL, Dodek PM, Golden JA, et al: Correlation between serial pulmonary function tests and fiberoptic bronchoscopy in patients with *Pneumocystis carinii* pneumonia and the acquired immune deficiency syndrome. Am Rev Respir Dis 129:491–493, 1984.

349. Hopewell P, Luce J: Pulmonary involvement in the acquired immunodeficiency syndrome. Chest 87:104–112, 1985.

350. Stover D, Meduri G: Pulmonary function tests. Clin Chest Med 9:473–479, 1988.

351. Ognibene F, Masur H, Rogers P, et al: Nonspecific interstitial pneumonitis without evidence of *Pneumocystis carinii* in asymptomatic patients infected with human immunodeficiency virus. Ann Intern Med 109:874–887, 1988.

352. Diaz P, Clanton T, Pacht E: Emphysema-like pulmonary disease associated with human immunodeficiency virus infection. Ann Intern Med 116:124–128, 1992.

353. Stover D, Greeno R, Gagliardi A: The use of a simple exercise test for the diagnosis of *Pneumocystis* pneumonia in patients with AIDS. Am Rev Respir Dis 139:1343–1346, 1989.

354. Tietjen P, Stover D: The use of exercise blood gas measurements and lactate dehydrogenase levels in the diagnosis of *Pneumocystis carinii* pneumonia. Am Rev Respir Dis 141:A27, 1990.

355. Smith D, McLuckie A, Wyatt J, Gazzard B: Severe exercise hypoxemia with normal or near normal X-rays: A feature of *Pneumocystis carinii* infection. Lancet 2:1049–1050, 1988.

356. Faetkenheuer G, Salzberger B, Allolio B, et al: Exercise oximetry for the early diagnosis of *Pneumocystis carinii* pneumonia. Lancet 1:222, 1989.

357. Rochester D, Enson Y: Current concepts in the pathogenesis of the obesity-hypoventilation syndrome. Am J Med 57:402–420, 1974.

358. Reichel G: Lung volumes, mechanical changes in arterial blood gases in obese patients and in Pickwickian syndrome. Bull Physiopathol Respir 18:1011–1020, 1972.

359. Partridge M, Ciofetta G, Hughes J: Topography of ventilation-perfusion ratios in obesity. Bull Eur Physiopathol Respir 14:765–773, 1979.

360. Sixt R, Bake B, Kral J: Closing volume and gas exchange before an intestinal bypass operation. Scand J Respir Dis 95:65–67, 1976.

361. Meyers D, Goldberg A, Bleecker M, et al: Relationship of obesity and physical fitness to cardiopulmonary and metabolic function in healthy older men. J Gerontol 46:M57–65, 1991.

362. Zwillich C, Sutton F, Peirson D, et al: Decreased hypoxic drive in the obesity-hypoventilation syndrome. Am J Med 59:343–348, 1975.

363. Knudson R, Kaltenborn W: Evaluation of lung elastic recoil by exponential curve analysis. Respir Physiol 46:29–42, 1981.

364. Burrows B, Lebowitz M, Camilli A, Knudson R: Longitudinal changes in forced expiratory volume in one second in adults. Am Rev Respir Dis 133:974–980, 1986.

365. Gelb A, Zamel N: Effect of aging on lung mechanics in healthy nonsmokers. Chest 68:538–541, 1975.

366. Crapo R, Morris A, Clayton P, Nixon C: Lung volumes in healthy nonsmoking adults. Bull Eur Physiopathol Respir 18:419–425, 1982.

367. Davis C, Cambell E, Openshaw P, et al: Importance of airway closure in limiting maximal expiration in normal man. J Appl Physiol Respir Environ Exercise Physiol 48: 695–701, 1980.

368. Amaducci S, Mandelli V, Morpugo M, Rampulla C: Aging, cigarette smoking, and respiratory function. Bull Eur Physiopathol Respir 13:523–532, 1977.

369. Hertle F, Georg E, Lange H-J: Die arteriellen Blutgsapartialdrucke und ihr Beziehungen zu alter und anthropometrischen Grössen. Respiration 28:1–130, 1971.

370. Georges R, Saumon GAL: The relationship of age to pulmonary membrane conductance and capillary blood volume. Am Rev Respir Dis 117:1069–1078, 1978.

371. Bottiger L: Regular decline in physical working capacity with age. Br Med J 3:270–271, 1978.

372. Hodgson JL, Buskirk, ER: Physical fitness and age, with emphasis on cardiovascular function in the elderly. J Am Geriatr Soc 25:285–292, 1977.

373. Fuchi T, Iwaoka K, Higuchi M, Hobayashi S: Cardiovascular changes associated with decreased aerobic capacity of aging in long-distance runners. Eur J Appl Physiol 58:884–889, 1989.

374. Black L, Hyatt R: Maximal respiratory pressures: Normal values and relationship to age and sex. Am Rev Respir Dis 99:696–702, 1969.

375. Malmberg P, Hedenstrom H, Fridriksson H: Reference values for gas exchange during exercise in healthy non-smoking and smoking men. Bull Eur Physiopathol Respir 23:131–138, 1987.

376. Gibellino F, Osmanliev D, Watson A, Pride N: Increase in tracheal size with age helps preserve peak expiratory flow rate in the face of loss of lung elastic recoil. Am Rev Respir Dis 132:784–787, 1985.

377. Grimby G: Physical activity and effects of muscle training in the elderly. Ann Clin Res 20:62–66, 1988.

378. Aubier M, Trippenbach T, Roussos C: Respiratory muscle fatigue during cardiogenic shock. J Appl Physiol 51:499–508, 1981.

REFERENCES

379. Wheeler AP, Marini JJ: Look to the physical examination for valuable diagnostic clues: Avoiding the consequences of respiratory muscle fatigue. J Respir Dis 6:107–125, 1985.

380. Cohen C, Zagelbaum G, Gross D, et al: Clinical manifestations of inspiratory muscle fatigue. Am J Med 73: 308–316, 1982.

381. Ford GT, Whitelew WA, Rosenal TW, et al: Diaphragm function after upper abdominal surgery in humans. Am Rev Respir Dis 127:431–436, 1983.

382. Gross D, Ladd HW, Riley EJ, et al: The effect of training on strength and endurance of the diaphragm in quadriplegia. Am J Med 68:27–35, 1980.

383. Leith DE, Bradley M: Ventilatory muscle strength and endurance training. J Appl Physiol 41:508–516, 1976.

384. Murciano D, Aubier M, Lecocguic Y, Pariente R: Effects of theophylline on diaphragmatic strength and fatigue in patients with chronic obstructive pulmonary disease. N Engl J Med 311:349–353, 1984.

385. Roussos C, Macklem PT: The respiratory muscles. N EngJ J Med 307:786–797, 1982.

386. Sharp JT, Drutz WS, Moisan T, et al: Postural relief of dyspnea in severe chronic obstructive pulmonary disease. Am Rev Respir Dis 122:201–211, 1980.

387. Hussain SNA, Simkus G, Roussos C: Respiratory muscle fatigue: A cause of ventilatory failure in septic shock. J Appl Physiol 58:2033–2040, 1985.

388. Davis J: Phrenic nerve conduction in man. J Neurol Neurosurg Psychol 30:420–426, 1967.

389. Similowski T, Fleury B, Launois S, et al: Cervical magnetic stimulation: A new painless method for bilateral phrenic nerve stimulation in conscious humans. J Appl Physiol 67:1311–1318, 1989.

390. Wragg S, Aquilina R, Morgan J, et al: Comparison of cervical magnetic stimulation and bilateral percutaneous electrical stimulation of the phrenic nerve in normal subjects. Eur Respir J 7:1788–1792, 1994.

391. Mador M, Rodis A, Magaland U, Ameen K: Comparison of cervical magnetic and transcutaneous phrenic nerve stimulation before and after threshold loading. Am J Respir Crit Care Med 154:448–453, 1996.

392. Cherniak R, Raber M: Normal standards for ventilatory function using an automated wedge spirometer. Am Rev Respir Dis 106:38–44, 1972.

393. Quanjer P (ed): Standardized lung function testing: Report of the working party. Bull Eur Physiopathol Respir 19:1–95, 1983.

394. Dockery D, Ware J, Ferris BJ, et al: Distribution of forced expiratory volume in one second and forced vital capacity in healthy, white, adult never-smokers in six U.S. cities. Am Rev Respir Dis 131:511–520, 1985.

395. Roca J, Sanchis J, Augusti-Vidal A, et al: Spirometric reference values from a Mediterranean population. Bull Eur Physiopathol Respir 22:217–224, 1986.

396. Paoletti P, Pistelli G, Fazzi P: Reference values for vital capcity and flow-volume curves from a general population study. Bull Eur Physiopathol Respir 22:451–459, 1986.

397. Miller A, Thornton J, Warshaw R, et al: Mean and instantaneous expiratory flows, FVC and FEV_1: Prediction equations from a probability sample of Michigan, a large industrial state. Bull Eur Physiopathol Respir 22:589–597, 1986.

398. Miller G, Ashcroft M, Swan A, Beadnell H: Ethnic variation in forced expiratory volume and forced vital capacity of African and Indian adults in Guyana. Am Rev Respir Dis 102:979–981, 1970.

399. Oscherwitz M, Edlavitch S, Baker T, et al: Differences in pulmonary functions in various racial groups. Am J Epidemiol 96:319–327, 1972.

400. Rossiter C, Weill H: Ethnic differences in lung function: Evidence for proportional differences. Int J Epidemiol 3:55–61, 1974.

401. Lap N, Amandus H, Hall R, Morgan W: Lung volumes and flow rates in black and white subjects. Thorax 29:185–188, 1974.

402. Cookson J, Blake G, Faranisi C: Normal values for ventilatory function in Rhodesian Africans. Br J Dis Chest 70:107–111, 1976.

403. Patrick J, Femi-Pearse D: Reference values for FEV_1 and FVC in Nigerian men and women: A graphical summary. Med J Nigeria 6:380–385, 1976.

404. Johannsen Z, Erasmus L: Clinical spirometry in normal Bantu. Am Rev Respir Dis 97:585–597, 1968.

405. Lindall A, Medina A, Grisner J: A re-evaluation of normal pulmonary function measurements in the adult female. Am Rev Respir Dis 95:1061–1064, 1967.

406. Kory R: The Veterans Administration–Army Cooperative Study of Pulmonary Function. I. Clinical spirometry in normal men. Am J Med 30:243–258, 1961.

407. Black L, Offord K, Hyatt R: Variability in the maximal expiratory volume curve in asymptomatic smokers and in nonsmokers. Am Rev Respir Dis 110:282–292, 1974.

408. Hall A, Heywood C, Cotes J: Lung function in healthy British women. Thorax 34:359–365, 1979.

409. American Thoracic Society: Single-breath carbon monoxide diffusing capacity (transfer factor). Recommendations for a standard technique. Am Rev Respir Dis 136: 1299–1307, 1987.

410. Billiet L, Baisier W, Naedts J: Effet de la taille, et du sexe de l'age sur la capacité de diffusion pulmonaire de l'adulte normal. J Physiol (Paris) 55:199–200, 1963.

REFERENCES

411. Cotes JE: Measurement of the Transfer Factor (Diffusing Capacity) for the Lung and its Subdivisions: Lung Function. Assessment and Application in Medicine (4th ed.). Oxford, Blackwell Scientific Publications, 1979, pp. 230–250.

412. Teculescu D, Stanescu D: Lung diffusing capacity. Normal values in male smokers and nonsmokers using the breath-holding technique. Scand J Respir Dis 51:137–149, 1970.

413. Van Ganse W, Ferris BJ, Cotes J: Cigarette smoking and pulmonary diffusing capacity (transfer factor). Am Rev Respir Dis 105:30–41, 1972.

414. Frans A, Stanescu D, Veriter C, et al: Smoking and pulmonary diffusing capacity. Scand J Respir Dis 56:165–183, 1975.

415. Marcq M, Minette A: Lung function changes in smokers with normal conventional spirometry. Am Rev Respir Dis 114:723–738, 1976.

416. Salorinne Y: Single-breath pulmonary diffusing capacity: Reference values and application in connective tissue diseases and in various lung diseases. Scand J Respir Dis 96(Suppl):1–86, 1976.

417. Miller A, Thornton J, Warshaw R, et al: Single breath diffusing capacity in a representative sample of the population of Michigan, a large industrial state. Am Rev Respir Dis 127:270–277, 1983.

418. Paoletti P, Viegi G, Pistelli G, et al: Reference equations for the single-breath diffusing capacity. A cross-sectional analysis and effect of body size and age. Am Rev Respir Dis 132:806–813, 1985.

419. Knudson R, Kaltenborn W, Knudson D, Burrows B: The single-breath carbon monoxide diffusing capacity. Reference equations derived from a healthy nonsmoking population and effects of hematocrit. Am Rev Respir Dis 135: 805–811, 1987.

420. Roca J, Rodriguez-Roisin R, Cobo E, et al: Single-breath carbon monoxide diffusing capacity prediction equations from a Mediterranean population. Am Rev Respir Dis 141:1026–1032, 1990.

421. Jones NL, Makrides L, Hitchcock C, et al: Normal standards for an incremental progressive cycle ergometer test. Am Rev Respir Dis 131:700–708, 1985.

APPENDICES

Reference Equations for Predicted Normal Values

APPENDIX 1

Predicted Values for FEV_1 and FVC Derived from Selected Studies of Nonsmoking Caucasian Men*

First Author, Year	Age Mean or Range	Number Studied	FEV_1† for Ht and Age	Regression Coefficients		RSD or SEE	FVC† for Ht and Age	Regression Coefficients		RSD or SEE
				Ht	Age			Ht	Age	
Morris, 1971[7]	20–84	517	3.63	3.62	−0.032	0.55	4.84	5.83	−0.025	0.74
Cherniack, 1972[392]	15–79	870	3.74	3.59	−0.023	NR	4.52	4.76	−0.014	NR
Quanjer, 1983[393]	21–64	189	3.59	4.05	−0.031	0.43	4.51	6.11	−0.032	0.64
Crapo, 1981[6]	15–91	125	3.96‡	4.14	−0.024	0.49	4.89‡	6.00	−0.021	0.64
Knudson, 1983[36]	25–84	86	3.81	6.65	−0.029	0.52	4.64	8.44	−0.030	0.56
Dockery, 1985[394]	25–74	624	3.78	Eq. nonlinear§		0.40	4.72	Eq. nonlinear§		0.47
Roca, 1986[395]	20–70	443	3.95	4.99	−0.021	0.44	5.15	6.78	−0.015	0.53
Paoletti, 1986[396]	29–64	59	3.83	4.94	−0.027	0.48	5.06	7.24	−0.027	0.58
Miller, 1986[397]	18–85	176	3.94	5.66	−0.023	0.41	4.84	7.74	−0.021	0.51

* To be included studies had to (1) include men and women; (2) adequately describe the methods used; (3) analyze spirometric values in terms of age and height. Instruments of measurement were water spirometer[6, 7, 394]; dry or wedge spirometer[392, 397]; pneumotachygraph.[393, 395]

† Predicted FEV_1 or FVC = predicted value for Ht 1.75 m, age 45 + Ht coefficient × (Ht − 1.75) + age coefficient × (age − 45).

‡ Studies carried out at an altitude of 1400 m.

§ $FEV_1 = Ht^2(1.54 - 4.06 \times 10^{-3}\ age - 6.14 \times 10^{-5}\ age^2)$; $FVC = Ht^2(1.75 - 1.35 \times 10^{-4}\ age - 1.01 \times 10^{-4}\ age^2)$.

Abbreviations: RSD = residual standard deviation; SEE = standard error of the estimate; NR = not reported.

Source: American Thoracic Society: Lung function testing: Selection of reference values and interpretive strategies. Am Rev Respir Dis 144:1202, 1991.

APPENDIX 2

Predicted Values for FEV_1 and FVC Derived from Selected Studies of Nonsmoking Caucasian Women*

First Author, Year	Age Mean or Range	Number Studied	FEV_1† for Ht and Age	Regression Coefficients		RSD or SEE	FVC† for Ht and Age	Regression Coefficients		RSD or SEE
				Ht	Age			Ht	Age	
Morris, 1971[7]	20–84	471	2.72	3.50	−0.025	0.47	3.54	4.53	−0.024	0.52
Cherniack, 1972[392]	15–79	452	2.87	2.37	−0.019	NR	3.36	3.08	−0.015	NR
Quanjer, 1983[393]	21–64	514	2.71	3.17	−0.031	0.35	3.39	4.64	−0.027	0.42
Crapo, 1981[6]	15–84	126	2.92‡	3.42	−0.026	0.33	3.54‡	4.91	−0.022	0.39
Knudson, 1983[36]	20–87	204	2.79	3.09	−0.020	0.39	3.36	4.27	−0.017	0.49
Dockery, 1985[394]	25–74	1830	2.79	Eq. nonlinear§		0.40	3.41	Eq. nonlinear§		0.47
Roca, 1986[395]	20–70	427	2.87	3.17	−0.025	0.31	3.72	4.54	−0.021	0.40
Paoletti, 1986[396]	21–64	313	2.84	2.43	−0.020	0.29	3.78	4.12	−0.015	0.39
Miller, 1986[397]	18–82	193	2.91	2.68	−0.025	0.33	3.59	4.14	−0.023	0.45

* To be included studies had to (1) include men and women; (2) adequately describe the methods used; (3) analyze spirometric values in terms of age and height. Instruments of measurement were water spirometer[6, 7, 394]; dry or wedge spirometer[392, 397]; pneumotachygraph.[393, 395]

† Predicted FEV_1 or FVC = predicted value for Ht 1.65 m, age 45 + Ht coefficient × (Ht − 1.65) + age coefficient × (age − 45).

‡ Studies carried out at an altitude of 1400 m.

§ $FEV_1 = Ht^2(1.332 - 4.06 \times 10^{-3}\ age - 6.14 \times 10^{-5}\ age^2)$; $FVC = Ht^2(1.463 - 1.35 \times 10^{-4}\ age - 1.01 \times 10^{-4}\ age^2)$.

Abbreviations: RSD = residual standard deviation; SEE = standard error of the estimate; NR = not reported.

Source: American Thoracic Society: Lung function testing: Selection of reference values and interpretive strategies. Am Rev Respir Dis 144:1202, 1991.

APPENDIX 3

Predicted Values for FEV_1 and FVC Derived from Selected Studies of Black Men and Women*

First Author, Year	Age Mean or Range	Number Studied	FEV_1 for Ht and Age†	Regression Coefficients		RSD or SEE	FVC for Ht and Age†	Regression Coefficients		RSD or SEE
				HT	AGE			HT	AGE	
MEN										
Johannsen, 1968[404]	20–50	120	2.96‡	2.87	−0.017	0.46	4.07	4.09	—	0.52
Miller, 1970[398]	35–54	96	3.05	3.40	−0.024	0.37	3.79	4.44	−0.024	0.46
Oscherwitz, 1972[399]	50.3 ± 6.6	110	2.94	2.99	−0.031	0.64	3.78	3.70	−0.027	0.68
Rossiter, 1974[400]	21–70	147	3.04	4.51	−0.027	0.52§	3.84	5.77	−0.019	0.59§
Lap, 1974[401]	34.9 ± 11.9	79	3.53	3.54	−0.025	0.23	4.11	3.94	−0.021	0.32
Cookson, 1976[402]	43.6 ± 15.1	141	3.12	2.20	−0.024	0.50	3.74	3.90	−0.017	0.65
Patrick, 1976[403]	18–65	213	3.11	4.23	−0.023	NR	3.72	3.51	−0.025	NR
WOMEN										
Johannsen, 1968[404]	20–50	100	2.25‡	2.18	−0.013	0.34	2.74‡	2.51	−0.015	0.35
Miller, 1970[398]	35–54	109	2.19	2.45	−0.018	0.31	2.74	3.15	−0.020	0.38
Cookson, 1976[402]	36.7 ± 11.6	102	2.35	2.40	−0.028	0.41	2.86	3.00	−0.019	0.42
Patrick, 1976[403]	18–65	117	2.10	1.49	−0.014	NR	2.64	3.17	−0.020	NR

* Instruments of measurement were: water spirometer,[400, 402, 404] dry or bellows spirometer,[398, 401] and various others.[399, 403] Predicted values for men and women are calculated as shown in footnotes to Appendices 1 and 2.

† Predicted value for a 45-year-old man 1.75 m tall and a 45-year-old woman 1.65 m tall.

‡ Corrected from ATPS to BTPS conditions, assuming spirometer temperature of 22°C.

§ Includes Caucasian subjects.

Abbreviations: RSD = residual standard deviation; SEE = standard error of the estimate; NR = not reported.

Source: American Thoracic Society: Lung function testing: Selection of reference values and interpretive strategies. Am Rev Respir Dis 144:1202, 1991.

APPENDIX 4

Predicted Values for FEV_1/FVC% Derived from Selected Studies of Caucasian and Black Men and Women*

First Author, Year	Age Mean or Range	n	FEV_1/FVC%† for Ht 1.75 m and Age 45 Yr	Regression Coefficients: Ht	Regression Coefficients: Age	RSD or SEE	n	FEV_1/FVC%† for Ht 1.65 m and Age 45 Yr	Regression Coefficients: Ht	Regression Coefficients: Age	RSD or SEE
		CAUCASIAN MEN					**CAUCASIAN WOMEN**				
Quanjer, 1983[393]	21–64	189	78.4	—	−0.16	5.3	514	80.2	—	−0.24	6.4
Crapo, 1981[6]	15–91	125	80.9‡	−13.0	−0.15	4.8	126	81.9‡	−20.2	−0.25	5.3
Knudson, 1983[36]	25–85	86	82.0	—	−0.11	6.3	204	82.6	−18.5	−0.19	7.6
Paoletti, 1986[396]	8–64	263	75.9	−5.3	−0.23	6.1	538	70.5	−4.3‖	−0.31	5.8
Miller 1986[397]	18–85	176	80.5	−13.1	−0.15	5.6	193	82.3	−21.5	−0.15	6.8
		BLACK MEN					**BLACK WOMEN**				
Johannsen, 1968[404]	20–50	120	75.0	—	−0.29	8.6	—	—	—	—	—
Oscherwitz, 1972[399]	50.3 ± 6.6	110	77.7	4.2	−0.32	10.2	—	—	—	—	—
Rossiter, 1974[400]	21–70	147	77.2	0.62	−0.34	7.2§	—	—	—	—	—
Cookson, 1976[402]	43.6 ± 15.1	141	81.4	—	−0.25	10.7	102	82.3	—	−0.38	11.7

* Table comprises studies cited in Appendices 1 and 2, which also reported values for FEV_1/FVC% analyzed in relation to height and age. For the instruments of measurement used, see footnotes to Appendices 1 and 2. Note: studies of Caucasian subjects were confined to nonsmokers; studies of black subjects included all smoking categories. Predicted values for FEV_1/FVC are calculated as shown in footnotes to Appendices 1 and 2. Only one study gives equations for black women.

† Predicted value for a 45-year-old man 1.75 m tall and a 45-year-old woman 1.65 m tall.

‡ Studies carried out at an altitude of 1400 m.

§ Includes Caucasian subjects.

‖ Coefficient not significant.

Source: American Thoracic Society: Lung function testing: Selection of reference values and interpretive strategies. Am Rev Respir Dis 144:1202, 1991.

APPENDIX 5

Recommended Criteria for Response to a Bronchodilator in Adults

Organization	FVC (%)	FEV_1 (%)	$FEF_{25\%-75\%}$	Comments
Am Coll Chest Phys[327]	15–25	15–25	15–25	% of baseline in at least two of three tests
Intermountain Thoracic Soc[329]	15	12	45	% of baseline
ATS[103]	12	12	—	% of baseline and an absolute change of 200 mL

Source: American Thoracic Society: Lung function testing: Selection of reference values and interpretive strategies. Am Rev Respir Dis 144:1202, 1991.

Appendix 6

Reference Equations for Minute Volume of Ventilation (MVV) (L/min)

Sex	Height Factor (cm)	Age Factor (yr)	Constant	95% Confidence Interval	Reference
Women	0.807 H	−0.57 A	−5.50	±21.0	405
Men	1.34 H	−1.26 A	−21.4	±56.8	406

Appendix 7

Predicted Values for Total Lung Capacity (TLC) and Residual Volume (RV) Derived from Selected Studies of Men and Women*

First Author, Year	Age Mean or Range	Number Studied	TLC† for Ht and Age	Regression Coefficients		RSD or SEE	RV† for Ht and Age	Regression Coefficients		RSD or SEE
				Ht	Age			Ht	Age	
Men										
Goldman, 1959[56]	44 ± 17	44	6.61	9.40	−0.015	0.65	2.04	2.70	0.017	0.39
Cotes, 1979[121]	19–72	127	6.68	8.67	—	0.91	NR	NR	NR	NR
Boren, 1966[55]	20–62	422	6.35	7.80	—	0.87	1.62	1.90	0.012	0.53
Black, 1974[407]	16–59	83	6.84	7.80	—	0.68	2.15	3.80	0.034	0.57
Crapo, 1982[366]	15–91	123	6.72	7.95	0.003	0.79	1.87	2.16	0.021	0.37
Women										
Goldman, 1959[56]	38 ± 16	50	5.18	7.90	−0.008	0.53	1.78	3.20	0.009	0.37
Grimby, 1963[58]	18–72	58	5.05	7.31	−0.016	0.52	1.44	2.92	0.008	0.35
Black, 1974[407]	16–59	110	5.20	6.40	—	0.62	1.76	2.30	0.021	0.46
Hall, 1979[408]	27–74	113	5.30	7.46	−0.013	0.51	1.80	2.80	0.016	0.31
Crapo, 1982[366]	17–84	122	5.20	5.90	—	0.54	1.73	1.97	0.020	0.38

* Only one[366] of these studies conforms strictly to the ATS recommendations for spirometry[409]; references 55, 121, 407, and 408 included all smoking categories, and in two[56, 58] smoking status was not defined. Residual volume was measured as follows: helium rebreathing,[56, 58, 121, 408] whole-body plethysmograph,[407] single-breath helium dilution,[366] and helium rebreathing or open-circuit N_2 washout in one study.[55] Predicted values for TLC and RV are calculated as shown in footnotes to Appendices 1 and 2.

† Predicted value for a 45-year-old man 1.75 m tall and a 45-year-old woman 1.65 m tall.

Abbreviations: RSD = residual standard deviation; SEE = standard error of the estimate; NR = not reported.

Source: American Thoracic Society: Lung function testing: Selection of reference values and interpretive strategies. Am Rev Respir Dis 144:1202, 1991.

APPENDIX 8

Comparison of Inspiratory and Expiratory Pressure-Volume Curves in Five Normal Subjects

Normal Subject (No.)	Exp. K cm H_2O^{-1}	Insp. K cm H_2O^{-1}	Exp. Vmax (L)	Insp. Vmax (L)	Exp. R^2	Insp. R^2	Exp. Runs Test	Insp. Runs Test
1	0.072	0.055	7.26	7.27	0.983	0.993	P	P
2	0.164	0.078	6.57	7.36	0.991	0.964	P	P
3	0.111	0.105	8.19	8.13	0.990	0.988	P	P
4	0.099	0.088	7.11	7.01	0.991	0.993	P	P
5	0.087	0.041	6.78	7.58	0.990	0.985	P	P

Abbreviations: Exp. = expiratory; K = constant; Vmax = volume (V) extrapolated to infinite pressure (P) from the equation $V = Vmax - Ae^{-KP}$; Insp. = inspiratory; R^2 = proportion of total variance accounted for by the regression equation; P = passed; K = a constant $\times$ (6.64×10^{-4}) $\times$ age (years) + 0.082; Vo/Vmax% = 0.601 $\times$ age (years) − 8.49.

Source: Gibson GJ, Pride NB, Davis T, Schroter RC: Exponential description of the static pressure-volume curve of normal and diseased lungs. Am Rev Respir Dis 120:799, 1979.

APPENDIX 9

Regressions of Flow-Volume Parameters on the Height and Age in Normal Subjects by Age Group

Flow Rates	n	Mean	SD	r	Constant	Coefficients			$S_{y,x}$
						HEIGHT (CM)	AGE (YR)	AGE² (YR)	
MALES	**AGE: ≥6 < 12 YR**			**HEIGHT 111.8–154.9 CM**					
$\dot{V}max_{50}$	105	2.416	0.793	0.571	−2.5454	—	—	—	0.6538
$\dot{V}max_{75}$	105	1.234	0.542	0.379	−1.0149	0.0171	—	—	0.5037
MALES	**AGE: ≥12 < 25 YR**			**HEIGHT 139.7–193.0 CM**					
$\dot{V}max_{50}$	131	4.800	1.504	0.674	−6.3851	0.0543	0.1150	—	1.1196
$\dot{V}max_{75}$	131	2.388	0.890	0.539	−4.2421	0.0397	−0.0057*	—	0.7551
MALES	**AGE: >25 YR**			**HEIGHT 157.5–195.6 CM**					
$\dot{V}max_{50}$	86	4.808	0.618	−5.5409	0.0684	−0.0366	—	—	1.2915
$\dot{V}max_{75}$	86	1.917	0.884	0.634	−2.4827	0.0310	−0.0230	—	0.6917
FEMALES	**AGE: ≥6 < 11 YR**			**HEIGHT 106.7–143.3 CM**					
$\dot{V}max_{50}$	75	2.256	0.717	0.377	0.7362	—	0.1846	—	0.6689
$\dot{V}max_{75}$	75	1.225	0.508	0.211	−0.1657	0.0109	—	—	0.4999
FEMALES	**AGE: ≥11 < 20 YR**			**HEIGHT 132.1–182.9 CM**					
$\dot{V}max_{50}$	96	3.943	1.074	0.469	−2.3040	0.0288	0.1111	—	0.9585
$\dot{V}max_{75}$	96	2.126	0.763	0.421	−4.4009	0.0243	0.2923	−0.0075	0.7202
FEMALES	**AGE: ≥20 YR**			**Height 147.3–180.3 cm**					
$\dot{V}max_{50}$	204	3.573	1.178	0.572	0.6088	0.0268	−0.0289	—	0.9709
$\dot{V}max_{75}$	204	1.436	0.848	0.647	1.1177	0.0096	−0.0259	—	0.6499
FEMALES	**AGE: ≥20 < 70 YR**			**HEIGHT 147.3–180.3 CM**					
$\dot{V}max_{50}$	176	3.761	1.105	0.475	−0.4371	0.0321	−0.0240	—	0.9778
$\dot{V}max_{75}$	176	1.558	—	0.601	−0.1822	0.0174	−0.0254	—	0.6612
FEMALES	**AGE: ≥70 YR**			**HEIGHT 147.3–167.6 CM**					
$\dot{V}max_{50}$	27	2.307	0.817	0.456	6.2402	0.0118	−0.0755	—	0.7569
$\dot{V}max_{75}$	27	0.570	0.249	0.312	1.8894	—	−0.0172	—	0.2409

Abbreviations: n = number of subjects; SD = standard deviation; r = multiple correlation coefficient; $S_{y,x}$ = standard deviation around regression line; $\dot{V}max_{50}$ and $\dot{V}max_{75}$ = maximal flow after exhalation of 50% and 75% of forced vital capacity.[36]

Predicted value = constant + [height coefficient × height (cm)] + [age coefficient × age² (years)] + [age² coefficient × age² (years)].

* This age coefficient is not significant. The value of the coefficient itself is not different from 0, and the amount of variance accounted for by age is also not significant.

Source: American Thoracic Society: Lung function testing and selection of reference values and interpretive strategies. Am Rev Respir Dis 144:1202–1216, 1991.

APPENDIX 10

Single-Breath Nitrogen Test: Normal Values for Nonsmokers

Reference	Population Studied		No.	Regression Equation
	SEX	AGE IN YEARS		
Buist and Ross[142]	M and F	—	284	CV/%VC = 0.318 A + 1.919 ± 4.61 SEE
				CC/%TLC = 0.525 A + 14.348 ± 4.34 SEE
Buist et al.[143]	Normal M	—	95	CV/%VC = 0.40 A − 1.89 ± 4.56 SD
				CC/%TLC = 0.53 A + 13.25 ± 4.00 SD
				$\Delta\%N_2/L$ = 0.001 A + 0.81 ± 0.59 SD
	Normal F	—	145	CV/%VC = 0.40 A − 2.90 ± 4.56 SD
				CC/%TLC = 0.53 A + 15.70 ± 4.00 SD
				$\Delta\%N_2/L$ = 0.001 A + 1.07 ± 0.59 SD
Buist and Ross[144]	M	—	137	$\Delta\%N_2/L$ = 0.01 A + 0.710 ± 0.43 SEE
	F	<60	203	$\Delta\%N_2/L$ = 0.009 A + 1.036 ± 0.57 SEE
	F	>60	203	$\Delta\%N_2/L$ = 0.0058 A + 1.777 ± 1.30 SEE
Knudson et al.[145]	—	25–54	147	CV/%VC = 0.269 A − 0.882
	—	25–54	148	CC/%TLC = 0.471 A + 11.942
	—	8–19	189	$\Delta\%N_2/L$ = 1.771 − 0.018 H
	—	20–54	239	$\Delta\%N_2/L$ = 1.717 − 0.0002 A − 0.018 H
	—	55+	164	$\Delta\%N_2/L$ = 1.599 − 0.026 A − 0.036 H

Abbreviations: A = age in years; H = height in inches; SD = standard deviation; SEE = standard error of the estimate; CC = closing capacity; CV = dosing volume; TLC = total lung capacity; VC = vital capacity; $\Delta\%N_2/L$ = slope of phase III.

APPENDIX 11

Predicted Values for Diffusing Capacity (DL_{CO}) and KCO (DL_{CO}/VA) Derived from Selected Studies of Men and Women*

First Author, Year	Age Mean or Range	n	DL_{co}† for Ht and Age	Regression Coefficients		RSD or SEE#	DL_{co}/VA† for Ht and Age	Regression Coefficients		RSD or SEE
				HT	AGE			HT	AGE	
MEN										
Billiet, 1963[410]	20–75	57	35.3	57.6	−0.24	4.2	4.96	—	−0.04	0.92
Cotes, 1979[411]	19–72	127	30.3	32.5	−0.20	5.1	4.83	—	−0.04	0.81
Teculescu, 1970[412]	19–67	47	32.6	33.3	−0.30	4.2	5.17†	—	−0.04	0.73
Van Ganse, 1972[413]	25–79	70	29.3	16.4	−0.20	3.8	5.60	−0.90	−0.03	1.07
Frans, 1975[414]	39 ± 12	64	33.3	28.5	−0.14	4.2	NR	—	—	—
Marcq, 1976[415]	17–79	64	29.9	10.4	−0.20	3.9	4.59	—	−0.03	0.65
Salorinne, 1976[416]	20–69	69	30.7	14.2	−0.23	3.6	5.02	−3.53	−0.03	0.63
Crapo, 1981[174]	15–91	123	36.6§	41.6	−0.22	4.8	5.45§	—	−0.03	0.84
Miller, 1983[417]	43 ± 16	74	31.4	16.4	−0.23	4.8	4.77	−2.24	−0.03	0.73
Paoletti, 1985[418]	16–64	80	37.1‖	44.1	−0.19	5.8	4.81‖	−0.12††	−0.02	0.71
Knudson, 1987[419]	25–84	71	38.4‖	35.5	−0.27	4.6	5.61‖	−2.35††	−0.04	0.80
Roca, 1990[420]	20–70	194	33.6	36.7	−0.20	4.4	Eq. nonstandard¶		—	—
WOMEN										
Billiet, 1963[410]	20–68	41	25.2	21.9	−0.16	3.6	5.55	—	−0.03	0.85
Van Ganse, 1972[413]	24–76	72	20.3	16.8	−0.16	3.6	5.61	−0.17	−0.01	0.99
Salorinne, 1976[416]	20–69	101	25.0	21.9	−0.12	2.8	5.27	−3.96	−0.01	0.74
Hall, 1979[408]	27–74	113	30.1**	28.3	−0.19	4.1	5.66**	—	−0.02	0.74
Crapo, 1982[174]	17–84	122	27.4§	25.6	−0.14	3.6	5.46§	—	−0.03	0.78
Miller, 1983[417]	43 ± 15	130	23.7	16.0	−0.11	4.0	4.62	−1.81	−0.02	0.80
Paoletti, 1985[418]	18–64	291	27.9‖	15.7	−0.07	4.3	4.85‖	−2.51	−0.02	0.85
Knudson, 1987[419]	20–86	99	28.2‖	18.7	−0.15	4.5	5.37‖	−2.78††	−0.03	0.85

* Appendix refers to DL_{co} and includes predicted values from published reports in which the number of subjects studied and their ages were given and in which equations for DL_{co} were described in terms of height and age according to ATS recommendations.[409] All but one study[411] refer to nonsmokers. Residual volume or FRC was measured as follows: single-breath helium dilution,[174, 412, 414–420] multiple-breath helium dilution,[408, 410] open-circuit N_2.[413] Predicted values for DL_{co} and DL_{co}/VA are calculated as shown in footnotes to Appendices 1 and 2.

† Predicted value for 45-year-old man 1.75 m tall and a 45-year-old woman 1.65 m tall.

‡ Results adjusted to BTPS.

§ Measurements made at an altitude of 1400 m.

‖ Correction for breath-holding time as in the Epidemiology Standardization Project.[418, 419] Note that calculated DL is sensitive to the methods used to calculate breath-hold time.

¶ Form of equation not recommended by the ATS.

** Results calculated for all smoking categories and adjusted for smoking effect.

†† Coefficient not significant.

Abbreviations: RSD = residual standard deviation; SEE = standard error of the estimate.

Source: American Thoracic Society: Lung function testing and selection of reference values and interpretive strategies. Am Rev Respir Dis 144:1202, 1991.

Appendix 12

Normal Response to Hypercapnia

Reference	No. Subjects	$\Delta\dot{V}E$*		
		MEAN	SD	RANGE
Read, 1967[220]	21	2.65	1.21	1.16–6.18
Irsigler, 1976[221]	126	2.6	1.2	0.47–6.22

* ΔL/min BTPS^{-1}/end-tidal CO_2 mm Hg.

Appendix 13

Normal Response to Hypoxia

Reference	No. Subjects	$\Delta\dot{V}E$*			End-tidal P_{CO_2} (mm Hg)	
		MEAN	SD	RANGE	MEAN	SD
Rebuck and Campbell, 1974[223]	9	1.65	1.20	0.26–4.12	51.2	3.7
Rebuck and Woodley, 1975[224]	11	0.56	0.42	0.16–1.76	39†	1.4
		2.20	1.07	1.21–4.90	51.7‡	2.1

* ΔL/min BTPS/1% desaturation.

† The increase in $\dot{V}E$ observed at a normal end-tidal P_{CO_2}.

‡ The increase in $\dot{V}E$ observed at an increased end-tidal P_{CO_2}, equivalent to mixed venous P_{CO_2}, in the same 11 subjects.

APPENDIX 14

Predictive Equations for Variables at Maximal Power Output*

Variable	Sex	Height (cm)	Age (yr)	Weight (kg)	Constant	SEE	r
Power output (kpm/min)	M	25.3	−9.06	—	−2759	245	0.721
	F	9.5	−9.21	6.1	−756	177	0.668
	−288	20.4	−8.7	—	−1902	216	0.858
	−249	16.2	−9.5	5.6	−1569	213	0.863
Oxygen intake (L/min)	M	0.034	−0.028	0.022	−3.76	0.483	0.799
	F	0.025	−0.018	0.010	−2.26	0.388	0.655
	−0.624	0.046	−0.021	—	−4.31	0.458	0.869
	−0.492	0.032	−0.024	0.019	−3.17	0.441	0.881
Heart rate (beats/min)	M	—	−0.80	—	206	11.6	0.723
	F	—	−0.63	—	198	8.9	0.730
		—	−0.72	—	202	10.3	0.721
Oxygen pulse (mL/beat)	M	0.342	—	—	−44.0	3.3	0.593
	F	0.190	—	—	−21.4	2.3	0.414
	−3.3	0.284	—	—	−26.9	2.8	0.865

* For equations applicable to both sexes, male is coded 0, female is coded 1. Blank spaces indicate an insignificant effect for the variable in question.

Abbreviations: SEE = standard error of the estimate; r = correction coefficient.

Source: Jones NL, Makrides L, Hitchcock C, et al: Normal standards for an incremental progressive cycle ergometer test. Am Rev Respir Dis 131:700, 1985.

APPENDIX 15

Measurements at 300 kpm/min in Age Categories (Males)

Age (yr)	$\dot{V}O_2$ (L/min)	$\dot{V}CO_2$(L/min)	R	$\dot{V}E$ (L/min)	VT (L)	HR (beats/min)	SBP (mm Hg)
15–24	1.00	0.82	0.81	22.9	1.60	104	130
SD	0.190	0.166	0.065	4.08	0.859	11.7	13.3
25–34	0.95	0.79	0.83	24.5	1.91	95	127
SD	0.153	0.199	0.128	10.5	0.719	10.1	*
35–44	0.91	0.73	0.81	24.3	1.78	92	125
SD	0.109	0.100	0.077	5.62	0.525	15.5	*
45–54	0.87	0.71	0.82	22.8	1.34	93	125
SD	0.125	0.121	0.074	5.85	0.264	9.7	*
55+	0.88	0.73	0.83	23.5	1.44	95	167
SD	0.105	0.086	0.073	2.78	0.314	10.9	*
Total	0.92	0.76	0.82	23.6	1.63	96	133
SD	0.146	0.143	0.083	6.37	0.604	12.1	*

*Too few observations to calculate SD.

Abbreviations: $\dot{V}O_2$ = O_2 intake; $\dot{V}CO_2$ = CO_2 output; R = respiratory exchange ratio; $\dot{V}E$ = minute ventilation; VT = tidal volume; HR = heart rate; SBP = systolic blood pressure; SD = standard deviation.

Source: Jones NL, Makrides L, Hitchcock C, et al: Normal standards for an incremental progressive cycle ergometer test. Am Rev Respir Dis 131:700, 1985.

APPENDIX 16

Measurements at 300 kpm/min in Age Categories (Females)

Age (yr)	$\dot{V}O_2$ (L/min)	$\dot{V}CO_2$ (L/min)	R	$\dot{V}E$ (L/min)	VT (L)	HR (beats/min)	SBP (mm Hg)
15–24	0.82	0.67	0.82	20.7	1.10	123	138
SD	0.061	0.062	0.063	2.61	0.104	16.2	*
25–34	0.87	0.72	0.84	21.7	1.23	124	142
SD	0.162	0.114	0.157	2.74	0.305	20.6	*
35–44	0.82	0.71	0.87	23.0	1.26	111	146
SD	0.084	0.053	0.067	2.20	0.231	13.4	*
45–54	0.85	0.70	0.82	22.0	1.31	117	151
SD	0.111	0.093	0.065	4.42	0.213	15.6	*
55–65	0.79	0.69	0.87	22.5	1.08	121	155
SD	0.138	0.132	0.056	5.02	0.269	13.6	*
Total	0.83	0.70	0.85	21.9	1.19	119	133
SD	0.116	0.094	0.089	3.7	0.243	15.9	15.0

* Too few observations to calculate SD.

Abbreviations: $\dot{V}O_2$ = O_2 intake; $\dot{V}CO_2$ = CO_2 output; R = respiratory exchange ratio; $\dot{V}E$ = minute ventilation; VT = tidal volume; HR = heart rate; SBP = systolic blood pressure; SD = standard deviation.

Source: Jones NL, Makrides L, Hitchcock C, et al: Normal standards for an incremental progressive cycle ergometer test. Am Rev Respir Dis 131:700, 1985.

APPENDIX 17

Measurements at 300 kpm/min in Height Categories*

Height (cm)	$\dot{V}O_2$ (L/min)	$\dot{V}CO_2$ (L/min)	R	$\dot{V}E$ (L/min)	VT (L)	HR (beats/min)		SBP (mm Hg)	RPE
						M	F		
<160	0.83	0.74	0.90	22.5	1.14	—	128	143	3.3
SD	0.152	0.139	0.098	3.89	0.229	—	11.4	31.8	†
160–165	0.80	0.68	0.85	21.4	1.16	—	118	143	2.0
SD	0.096	0.090	0.065	4.16	0.232	—	15.3	28.1	†
165–170	0.82	0.66	0.81	20.9	1.23	97	115	131	1.8
SD	0.112	0.066	0.075	3.47	0.256	15.4	16.3	25.2	†
170–175	0.88	0.72	0.82	22.9	1.48	96	114	130	2.0
SD	0.135	0.121	0.068	4.79	0.330	12.5	21.1	†	†
175–180	0.91	0.71	0.79	22.4	1.60	94	—	125	2.0
SD	0.066	0.068	0.068	4.46	0.634	17.0	—	†	†
180–185	0.95	0.80	0.84	25.3	1.51	98	—	135	1.7
SD	0.081	0.101	0.084	3.71	0.311	11.0	—	†	†
>185	1.09	0.93	0.86	28.3	2.27	94	—	120	1.0
SD	0.178	0.167	0.129	10.1	0.920	11.0	—	†	†
Total	0.87	0.73	0.83	22.7	1.40	96	119	132	†
SD	0.139	0.124	0.087	5.08	0.502	12.4	15.7	23.2	†

*There were no significant differences between males and females except for heart rate.

†Too few observations to calculate SD.

Abbreviations: RPE = rating of perceived exertion; $\dot{V}O_2$ = O_2 intake; $\dot{V}CO_2$ = CO_2 output; R = respiratory exchange ratio; $\dot{V}E$ = minute ventilation; VT = tidal volume; HR = heart rate; SBP = systolic blood pressure; SD = standard deviation.

Source: Jones NL, Makrides L, Hitchcock C, et al: Normal standards for an incremental progressive cycle ergometer test. Am Rev Respir Dis 131:700, 1985.

APPENDIX 18

Measurements at 600 kpm/min in Height Categories*

Height (cm)	$\dot{V}O_2$ (L/min)	$\dot{V}CO_2$ (L/min)	R	$\dot{V}_E$ (L/min)	V_T (L)	HR (beats/min) M	HR (beats/min) F	SBP (mm Hg)	RPE
<160	1.30	1.54	1.19	43.2	1.65	—	163	159	6.0
SD	0.117	0.199	0.144	6.46	0.196	—	9.6	13.9	†
160–165	1.30	1.44	1.11	41.7	1.72	—	153	151	4.7
SD	0.119	0.189	0.138	7.43	0.258	—	10.8	16.1	†
165–170	1.33	1.29	0.97	36.4	1.78	124	147	144	4.1
SD	0.128	0.178	0.123	6.56	0.391	18.4	12.3	12.3	†
170–175	1.42	1.38	0.98	38.9	1.89	115	144	158	3.9
SD	0.153	0.156	0.148	7.63	0.369	10.8	21.5	31.6	†
175–180	1.51	1.31	0.87	36.8	2.24	114	—	150	3.0
SD	0.145	0.079	0.077	5.43	0.679	21.7	—	17.0	†
180–185	1.44	0.32	0.92	37.0	2.01	111	—	153	3.1
SD	0.086	0.099	0.063	2.41	0.353	11.3	—	13.0	†
>185	1.55	1.36	0.88	36.3	2.86	109	—	149	2.4
SD	0.105	0.113	0.042	4.7	1.109	17.3	—	18.0	†
Total	1.39	1.36	0.99	38.4	1.96	116	151	151	†
SD	0.148	0.167	0.147	6.49	0.582	15.0	13.0	18.2	†

*There were no significant differences between males and females except for heart rate.

† Too few observations to calculate SD.

Abbreviations: RPE = rating of perceived exertion; $\dot{V}O_2$ = O_2 intake; $\dot{V}CO_2$ = CO_2 output; R = respiratory exchange ratio; $\dot{V}_E$ = minute ventilation; V_T = tidal volume; HR = heart rate; SBP = systolic blood pressure; SD = standard deviation..

Source: Jones NL, Makrides L, Hitchcock C, et al: Normal standards for an incremental progressive cycle ergometer test. Am Rev Respir Dis 131:700, 1985.

APPENDIX 19

Measurements at 600 kpm/min in Age Categories (Males)

Age (yr)	$\dot{V}O_2$ (L/min)	$\dot{V}CO_2$ (L/min)	R	$\dot{V}E$ (L/min)	VT (L)	HR (beats/min)	SBP (mm Hg)
15–24	1.53	1.39	0.92	25.9	2.31	122	152
SD	0.115	0.088	0.073	2.62	1.06	14.6	11.8
25–34	1.48	1.28	0.86	34.0	2.31	112	143
SD	0.093	0.123	0.083	6.00	0.656	12.6	25.9
35–44	1.50	1.32	0.88	37.8	2.35	111	148
SD	0.144	0.075	0.074	5.21	0.656	20.1	10.3
45–54	1.42	1.28	0.90	36.5	1.92	112	157
SD	0.092	0.102	0.065	2.73	0.360	11.6	12.5
55–65	1.35	1.35	1.00	38.7	2.07	123	178
SD	0.140	0.149	0.100	4.32	0.262	13.0	24.9
Total	1.46	1.35	0.91	36.5	2.19	116	154
SD	0.128	0.115	0.089	4.33	0.68	15.0	19.7

Abbreviations: $\dot{V}O_2$ = O_2 intake; $\dot{V}CO_2$ = CO_2 output; R = respiratory exchange ratio; $\dot{V}E$ = minute ventilation; VT = tidal volume; HR = heart rate; SBP = systolic blood pressure; SD = standard deviation.

Source: Jones NL, Makrides L, Hitchcock C, et al: Normal standards for an incremental progressive cycle ergometer test. Am Rev Respir Dis 131:700, 1985.

APPENDIX 20

Measurements at 600 kpm/min in Age Categories (Females)

Age (yr)	$\dot{V}O_2$ (L/min)	$\dot{V}CO_2$ (L/min)	R	$\dot{V}E$ (L/min)	VT (L)	HR (beats/min)	SBP (mm Hg)
15–24	1.30	1.30	0.99	36.1	1.40	156	140
SD	0.129	0.241	0.122	8.65	0.193	15.0	12.4
25–34	1.38	1.27	0.93	36.3	1.70	150	144
SD	0.190	0.149	0.168	7.87	0.280	17.7	16.2
35–44	1.31	1.44	1.10	41.2	1.81	154	152
SD	0.106	0.123	0.123	3.78	0.312	13.8	10.3
45–54	1.35	1.48	1.10	42.3	1.85	151	157
SD	0.120	0.180	0.129	5.38	0.260	12.1	11.3
55–65	1.27	1.53	1.21	46.8	1.76	155	162
SD	0.136	0.199	0.118	8.00	0.271	12.2	20.5
Total	1.32	1.40	1.07	40.4	1.70	153	149
SD	0.137	0.203	0.132	6.95	0.266	14.2	13.8

Abbreviations: $\dot{V}O_2$ = O_2 intake; $\dot{V}CO_2$ = CO_2 output; R = respiratory exchange ratio; $\dot{V}E$ = minute ventilation; VT = tidal volume; HR = heart rate; SBP = systolic blood pressure; SD = standard deviation.

Source: Jones NL, Makrides L, Hitchcock C, et al: Normal standards for an incremental progressive cycle ergometer test. Am Rev Respir Dis 131:700, 1985.

INDEX

Note: Page numbers followed by the letter f refer to figures; those followed by the letter t refer to tables.

E

F

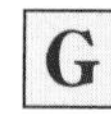

J

K

L

N

O

Q

R

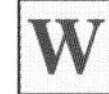

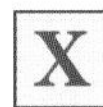

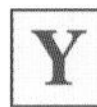

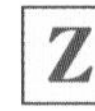